Glioblastoma and New Therapeutic Drugs and Approaches

Athanasios Alexiou
https://orcid.org/0000-0002-2206-7236
Novel Global Community Education Foundation, Australia

Md. Habibur Rahman
Novel Global Community Educational Foundation, Australia

Muhasina K.M.
https://orcid.org/0000-0001-6421-8859
Prime College of Pharmacy, Palakkad, India

Chenmala Karthika
https://orcid.org/0000-0001-7874-6521
JSS College of Pharmacy, India

Priti Tagde
Amity Institute Pharmacy, India

IGI Global
Scientific Publishing
Publishing Tomorrow's Research Today

Vice President of Editorial Melissa Wagner
Director of Acquisitions Mikaela Felty
Director of Book Development Jocelynn Hessler
Production Manager Mike Brehm
Cover Design Jose Rosado

Published in the United States of America by
IGI Global Scientific Publishing
701 East Chocolate Avenue
Hershey, PA, 17033, USA
Tel: 717-533-8845 | Fax: 717-533-7115
Website: https://www.igi-global.com E-mail: cust@igi-global.com

Library of Congress Cataloging-in-Publication Data

LCCN: 2025026281 (CIP Data Pending)
ISBN13: 9798337326955
Isbn13Softcover: 9798337326962
EISBN13: 9798337326979

British Cataloguing in Publication Data
A Cataloguing in Publication record for this book is available from the British Library.

Table of Contents

Detailed Table of Contents

Glioblastoma multiforme (GBM) is an aggressive primary brain tumor marked by rapid progression, diffuse infiltration, and poor prognosis. Conventional treatments—surgical resection, radiotherapy, and temozolomide chemotherapy—offer limited success due to intratumoral heterogeneity, the blood-brain barrier (BBB), glioma stem-like cells. Novel immunotherapeutic strategies, including immune checkpoint inhibitors, CAR T and CAR-NK cells, dendritic cell vaccines, and oncolytic virotherapy, are under investigation to improve immune-mediated tumor eradication. Tumor-treating fields (TTFs) and targeted molecular therapies show additional promise. This chapter explores the molecular and metabolic landscape of GBM, reviews current and emerging therapies, and underscores the urgent need for integrated, personalized treatment strategies to improve patient outcomes.

Glioblastoma is the most common and malignant primary brain tumor, having a high fatality rate. It is distinguished by fast development, medication resistance, a poor prognosis, and few therapeutic choices. These obstacles are caused by variables such as molecular heterogeneity, complicated genetic composition, and the blood-brain barrier, which prevents efficient medication administration. Nonetheless, recent improvements provide optimism. Personalized medicine and molecular-targeted treatments tailor treatment to a tumor's unique genetic makeup. Nanotechnology, CRISPR-Cas9 gene editing, and innovative drug delivery technologies have improved bioavailability and therapeutic accuracy. Furthermore, sophisticated imaging methods and liquid biopsies aid in early detection, real-time monitoring, and therapy optimization. This chapter provides a detailed overview of current glioblastoma management difficulties and focuses on developing treatments that have the potential to alter therapy results.

Glioblastoma (GBM) is a model of resistance to therapy. Despite the formation of lethal DNA lesions by alkylating agents, including temozolomide, GBM cells utilize error-prone double-strand break (DSB) repair pathways to escape death. New findings demonstrate that hypoxia, which is a key feature of the GBM microenvironment, reshuffles the response to DNA damage response networks by increasing the expression of POLQ. This change induces chromosomal rearrangements and radiation resistance but generates targetable vulnerabilities. Several lines of evidence have shown that POLQ silencing sensitized hypoxic GBM cells to poly(ADP–ribose) polymerase inhibitors through disabling backup repair pathways. This chapter reviews ongoing efforts to elucidate DSB repair plasticity in the context of treatment failure and describes opportunities to leverage that plasticity for therapeutic gain.

This chapter focuses on current drugs that are using in clinical trial on glioblastoma. According to the ClinicalTrials.gov, 2077 clinical trials are going on glioblastoma until May 2025. Different small molecules and alkylating agents that are already approved for marketing like Temozolomide, Carmustine, Lomustine, Tinostamustine, Cyclophosphamide are still using. Enzyme inhibitors are the mostly used therapies and different enzyme inhibitors like protease inhibitor, tyrosine kinase inhibitor, ATM kinase inhibitor, BET inhibitor, mTOR inhibitor, ornithine decarboxylase inhibitor, histone deacetylase inhibitor are common treatment strategies. In addition, many receptor inhibitors like inhibitors of fibroblast growth factor receptor and epidermal growth factor receptor are also used in many clinical trials. In different clinical trials, other approaches like using human monocolonized antibodies, vaccines, toxins and anti-fungal drugs are used as a potential treatment strategy.

Glioblastoma (GBM) is the most aggressive form of primary brain tumor in adults, marked by rapid growth, widespread infiltration, and resistance to standard therapies. A key challenge in treating GBM is the blood-brain barrier (BBB), which restricts the delivery of therapeutic agents to the central nervous system (CNS). Drug repurposing—finding new therapeutic uses for existing drugs—offers a promising, cost-effective strategy to overcome this hurdle. This chapter explores the structural and functional complexities of the BBB, emphasizing its transport mechanisms and recent advances in drug delivery strategies, such as nanocarriers, focused

Preface

INTRODUCTION

Glioblastoma (GBM) continues to stand as one of the most formidable challenges in contemporary oncology. Its aggressive growth, invasive behavior, and remarkable resistance to conventional therapies have made it a focus of intense scientific and clinical inquiry. Despite decades of research, the standard multimodal treatment—surgical resection followed by radiation and chemotherapy—remains limited in its ability to eliminate infiltrative tumor cells. Recurrence is not only common but often results in an even more resilient form of the disease, underscoring an urgent need for more effective therapeutic strategies.

In preparing this edited volume, *Glioblastoma and New Therapeutic Drugs and Approaches*, we sought to bring together leading advances that reflect both the complexity of GBM biology and the promise of emerging therapeutic innovations. Among these innovations, drug repurposing has gained exceptional traction. The ability to identify new anticancer potential in medications already approved for other clinical indications offers a powerful, time-efficient, and cost-effective avenue for accelerating treatment discovery. Increasingly, such agents have been shown to modulate GBM-associated signaling pathways, inhibit tumor progression, and in some cases disrupt the survival mechanisms of glioblastoma stem cells (GSCs)—a subpopulation now widely recognized as a major contributor to tumor recurrence following surgery.

As the chapters in this book illustrate, many repurposed drugs are advancing through preclinical studies, while others have reached clinical evaluation. Yet, formidable obstacles remain. Chief among them is the blood–brain barrier (BBB), which restricts therapeutic agents from achieving effective intratumoral concentrations. As a result, the field continues to push forward with multidimensional strategies, integrating molecular targeting, novel delivery systems, nanotechnology, and computational approaches to better understand and ultimately overcome the therapeutic barriers inherent to GBM.

Our goal with this reference work is to provide readers with a comprehensive overview of emerging research directions, methodological advancements, and translational efforts that define the current landscape of GBM investigation. We hope the insights contained herein will inspire new hypotheses, promote collaborative endeavors, and support the development of interventions that may one day shift the prognosis of this devastating disease.

This book is designed for a diverse and multidisciplinary readership, including:

- Professors, lecturers, and educators in Neuroscience, Medicine, Biochemistry, Biophysics, Biomedical Informatics, Bioinformatics, Neuroinformatics, Nanotechnology, and related fields
- Senior undergraduate, Master's, and PhD students pursuing advanced training in biomedical and life sciences
- Researchers, postdoctoral fellows, and senior investigators engaged in cancer biology, neuro-oncology, translational medicine, and therapeutic development
- Clinicians, rehabilitation specialists, caregivers, and professionals in geriatric and occupational therapy
- Industry professionals working in biomedical, pharmaceutical, and biotechnological sectors focused on neuro-oncology and neurodegenerative disorders

As editors, we express our deep appreciation to the contributors who have dedicated their expertise to this volume, and to the scientific community whose continuous efforts move the field forward. We present this book with the hope that it will serve as a valuable resource and a catalyst for future breakthroughs in the fight against glioblastoma.

ORGANIZATION OF THE BOOK

Chapter 1: Current Treatment Modalities and Their Merits and Demerits

Chapter 1 surveys the full spectrum of current therapeutic strategies used in glioblastoma care, beginning with traditional approaches such as surgery, radiotherapy, and temozolomide chemotherapy. It highlights the biological barriers—intratumoral heterogeneity, treatment-resistant stem-like cells, and the restrictive blood–brain barrier—that limit the success of these methods. The chapter also introduces promising innovations, including immune checkpoint inhibitors, CAR T and CAR-NK cell therapies, dendritic cell vaccines, oncolytic viruses, and tumor-treating fields. By integrating molecular and metabolic insights, this chapter underscores the need for personalized and combination-based therapeutic strategies.

Chapter 2: Current Challenges and Significant Innovations for Glioblastoma

Chapter 2 delves deeper into the biological and translational challenges that define glioblastoma research, including genomic instability, molecular diversity, and inadequate drug penetration. It highlights emerging innovations aimed at overcoming these obstacles, such as molecular-targeted therapies, nanotechnology-enabled delivery systems, and CRISPR-based gene editing. Advances in imaging and liquid biopsy technologies are also discussed, demonstrating their potential to enhance early detection and treatment monitoring. Together, these developments present a landscape of cautious optimism for future therapeutic breakthroughs.

Chapter 3: DNA Lesions and Double-Strand Breaks in Glioblastoma

This chapter explores one of the central mechanisms underlying glioblastoma's resilience: its remarkable capacity to evade DNA damage–induced cell death. The authors focus on double-strand break repair pathways, emphasizing the role of hypoxia-induced POLQ expression in promoting genomic instability and treatment failure. They also highlight compelling evidence that inhibiting POLQ can sensitize GBM cells to PARP inhibitors, especially under hypoxic conditions. By examining the plasticity of DNA repair systems, this chapter identifies promising molecular vulnerabilities for therapeutic intervention.

Chapter 4: Drug Regimens Used for Glioblastoma—Chemical Structures and Mechanisms of Action

In Chapter 4, the authors provide a comprehensive overview of chemotherapeutic agents commonly used in GBM—including temozolomide, carmustine, lomustine, and bevacizumab—along with their molecular mechanisms and structural features. They assess the limitations of standard regimens and explore emerging targeted agents, immunotherapies, and gene- and virus-based therapies. This chapter serves as a foundation for understanding both current clinical practice and evolving therapeutic landscapes.

Chapter 5: Resistance Mechanisms and the Nanotheranostic Approach

Chapter 5 examines the shortcomings of traditional therapies—ranging from toxicity to poor drug accumulation at the tumor site—and explains how nanotheranostics can address these limitations. By integrating diagnostic and therapeutic functions into a single platform, nanostructures such as nanoparticles, dendrimers, and exosomes offer improved targeting, controlled drug release, and enhanced imaging capabilities. This chapter demonstrates how these dual-function systems can potentially increase treatment efficacy while reducing collateral damage to healthy tissue.

Chapter 6: In-Vitro and In-Vivo Models for Glioblastoma

Preclinical modeling is essential for understanding GBM biology and testing new therapies, and Chapter 6 provides a rigorous evaluation of current in vitro and in vivo systems. The authors compare traditional cell lines with next-generation approaches such as organoids, bioprinted constructs, genetically engineered models, and tumor-on-chip technologies. Despite progress, limitations in clinical translation persist, prompting a call for hybrid, ethically aligned, and physiologically relevant models that can better predict therapeutic outcomes.

Chapter 7: Drugs Under Clinical and Pre-Clinical Research for Glioblastoma

This chapter provides an up-to-date overview of the extensive pipeline of therapeutics undergoing clinical evaluation for glioblastoma. Drawing on thousands of active trials, it covers small molecules, alkylating agents, a wide array of enzyme inhibitors, receptor-targeted therapies, monoclonal antibodies, vaccines, toxins, and antifungal agents repurposed for anticancer activity. The chapter emphasizes how diverse mechanistic approaches—from kinase inhibition to immune modulation—reflect the urgent need to broaden the therapeutic arsenal against GBM.

Chapter 8: Drug Repurposing and Overcoming the Blood–Brain Barrier

Chapter 8 focuses on the promise of drug repurposing as a rapid and cost-effective approach to GBM therapy. It reviews the structural and functional complexities of the blood–brain barrier and discusses cutting-edge delivery strategies such as nanocarriers, focused ultrasound, and receptor-mediated transcytosis. The authors highlight several repurposed agents with demonstrated BBB penetration and anti-tumor activity, and propose integrated frameworks to enhance CNS drug delivery and therapeutic success.

Chapter 9: Novel Drug Delivery and Dosage Forms for Glioblastoma

Expanding on earlier discussions of delivery challenges, Chapter 9 explores innovative dosage forms designed to bypass biological barriers and overcome tumor heterogeneity. These include nanoparticle-based carriers, exosome-mediated delivery, stem-cell–based vehicles, biodegradable implants such as Gliadel® wafers, and hydrogels for localized therapy. Additional emphasis is placed on intranasal delivery and focused ultrasound as minimally invasive methods to transiently bypass the BBB. The chapter concludes with reflections on the translational challenges that must be addressed for these technologies to reach clinical practice.

Chapter 10: Nanomaterial-Based Strategies for Overcoming the Blood–Brain Barrier

The concluding chapter explores advanced nanomaterial systems aimed specifically at navigating or bypassing the blood–brain barrier. The authors review the pathological drivers of GBM that complicate drug delivery—including hypoxia, glioma-initiating cells, and tumor heterogeneity—and evaluate nanotechnology-based approaches such as liposomes, micelles, dendrimers, solid lipid nanoparticles, and biomimetic carriers. While early clinical trials have shown only modest benefits, this chapter underscores the growing promise of nanomedicine and the critical need for personalized, delivery-optimized strategies in future GBM therapy.

CONCLUSION

As we conclude this volume, we reflect on the remarkable breadth and depth of the work presented across its chapters—each contributing essential insights into the intricate biological, clinical, and technological challenges that define glioblastoma research and treatment today. From foundational epidemiology to the molecular mechanics of DNA repair, from the exploration of drug resistance to the evolving landscape of nanotechnology, this book underscores both the complexity of GBM and the unwavering commitment of the scientific community to confront it.

The recurring themes woven throughout these chapters—tumor heterogeneity, therapeutic resistance, the formidable blood–brain barrier, and the persistent threat of recurrence—highlight the multifaceted nature of this disease. Yet, the avenues for innovation are equally compelling. Advances in immunotherapy, repurposed drugs, precision delivery systems, stem cell–based therapeutics, and nanomedicine collectively signal a shifting paradigm in GBM research. These innovations, coupled with increasingly sophisticated preclinical models and integrative diagnostic approaches, provide a foundation for more effective, personalized interventions.

As editors, we recognize that much work lies ahead. Glioblastoma remains a relentless adversary, demanding continued collaboration across disciplines—neuroscience, oncology, molecular biology, pharmacology, biomedical engineering, computational sciences, and clinical medicine. The progress reflected in these chapters represents not only scientific achievement but also hope: hope for extended survival, improved quality of life, and ultimately, transformative therapies that will change the trajectory of this devastating disease.

We extend our sincere gratitude to the authors whose expertise has shaped this volume, and to the broader research and medical communities whose dedication drives the field forward. It is our aspiration that this book serves as both a resource and a catalyst—empowering researchers, clinicians, students, and innovators to explore new directions and accelerate meaningful breakthroughs in glioblastoma care.

Chapter 1

Current Treatment Modalities Associated With Glioblastoma and Its Merits and Demerits

Rizwan Ahamad
https://orcid.org/0009-0005-9649-3376
Jamia Hamdard, New Delhi, India

Nazreen Tabassum
Jamia Hamdard, New Delhi, India

Arshi Aquil
Jamia Hamdard, New Delhi, India

Prerna Saxena
https://orcid.org/0009-0006-9130-7703
Jamia Hamdard, New Delhi, India

Rabnoor Alam
https://orcid.org/0000-0002-8901-5414
Jamia Hamdard, New Delhi, India

Suruchi Khanna
Jamia Hamdard, New Delhi, India

Mohd Akhtar
Jamia Hamdard, New Delhi, India

Mohd Aqil
Jamia Hamdard, New Delhi, India

Mohd Mujeeb
Jamia Hamdard, New Delhi, India

ABSTRACT

Glioblastoma multiforme (GBM) is an aggressive primary brain tumor marked by rapid progression, diffuse infiltration, and poor prognosis. Conventional treatments—surgical resection, radiotherapy, and temozolomide chemotherapy—offer limited success due to intratumoral heterogeneity, the blood-brain barrier (BBB), glioma stem-like cells. Novel immunotherapeutic strategies, including immune checkpoint inhibitors, CAR T and CAR-NK cells, dendritic cell vaccines, and oncolytic virother-

DOI: 10.4018/979-8-3373-2695-5.ch001

apy, are under investigation to improve immune-mediated tumor eradication. Tumor-treating fields (TTFs) and targeted molecular therapies show additional promise. This chapter explores the molecular and metabolic landscape of GBM, reviews current and emerging therapies, and underscores the urgent need for integrated, personalized treatment strategies to improve patient outcomes.

INTRODUCTION

Gliomas constitute a significant category of primary brain neoplasms, comprising roughly 30% of all brain tumor diagnoses and nearly 80% of malignant tumors confined to CNS. These tumors originate from glial cells and are known for their heterogeneity in terms of morphology, genetic alterations, and clinical behavior, necessitating a nuanced approach to diagnosis and treatment (Wang et al., 2022). The global incidence of gliomas ranges from 3 to 4 cases per 100,000 individuals annually in the United States. IDH-wild-type GBM is the most prevalent and aggressive subtype of glioma, constituting approximately 45–50% of all adult-type diffuse gliomas. The likelihood of developing gliomas rises with age, with diagnoses typically happening in people older than 50. Notably, GBM exhibits a higher prevalence in males compared to females, with an approximate gender ratio of 1.5:1 (Grochans et al., 2022).GBM encompass inherited syndromes such as Li-Fraumeni Syndrome, Turcot syndrome, and Neurofibromatosis type 1. Additionally, specific oncogenic mutations are critical in GBM pathogenesis, including alterations in TP53, PTEN, and EGFR, as well as NF1 mutations. Moreover, relevant chromosomal abnormalities, including trisomy of chromosome 7 and monosomy of chromosome 10, further contribute to the tumorigenic landscape of GBM. (Sloan et al., 2020). The outlook for people diagnosed with GBM is poor, with a projected median survival time of 14 months (Mohammed et al., 2022). Conventional treatment modalities for GBM encompass surgical excision, radiation, and chemotherapy, frequently utilizing temozolomide. These therapies, while frequently used, face significant challenges, particularly because of the tumor's extensive invasion into surrounding brain tissue and the presence of the blood-brain barrier (BBB), which restricts the efficacy of the medications. Moreover, the heterogeneity and elevated recurrence rate of GBM provide further challenges in therapy. The adverse effects of radiotherapy are often classified into three categories: acute, early-delayed, and late-delayed, depending on the timing of symptom development after treatment delivery. Acute effects occur soon after treatment, early-delayed effects appear within weeks to months, and late-delayed effects may emerge months to year's later (Chatzikonstantinou et al., 2019). Recent advancements in molecular biology, technological innovations, and the development of immunotherapeutic strategies are driving the exploration of novel therapeutic approaches for GBM. The rise of targeted therapies and personalized medicine techniques is capturing significant attention within the oncology community, paving the way for more effective treatment paradigms. This encompasses pharmacological approaches targeting specific molecular alterations in GBM cells, including aberrations in the EGFR, PDGFRA, and MGMT genes. Recent advancements in immunotherapy are being explored, particularly with PD-1/PD-L1 inhibitors, therapeutic vaccines, and adoptive cell transfer techniques such as CAR-T cell therapy. Furthermore, innovative therapeutic approaches such as tumor-treating fields (TTFs) are currently undergoing evaluation to assess their clinical efficacy and safety profiles in the treatment of GBM (Laba &Ziółkowski, 2021).

Histopathology of GBM

GBM is the most aggressive form of astrocytic tumor, arising from glial progenitor cells and typically involving the cerebral white matter. Histologically, GBM shows marked cellular pleomorphism, nuclear atypia, high mitotic activity, and areas of necrosis with surrounding microvascular proliferation. The tumor's infiltrative growth pattern, following deep white matter tracts, contributes to its poor surgical resectability. Despite its variable microscopic appearance, these features remain consistent hallmarks for diagnosis.

Detailed Histopathology of GBM

Gliomas likely arise from glial progenitor cells, which are categorized into subgroups based on malignancy grade and accessed via histological and genetic techniques (Wang et al., 2023). GBM often presents with signs of elevated intracranial pressure due to mass effect, typically infiltrating the white matter of the cerebral hemispheres, mostly intraparenchymally. Grossly, neurosurgical specimens show ill-defined margins, heterogeneous cut surface pigmentation, and gray tumor tissue with yellow necrotic foci (Lipková et al., 2022). Formalin fixation reveals tumor fragmentation and a softer consistency with grey–pink edges adjacent to neural tissue (Linkous & Yazlovitskaya, 2011). Some tumors contain macroscopic cysts with turbid fluid, reflecting liquefied necrosis. Microscopically, GBM exhibits significant morphological heterogeneity — the basis for its historical name "glioblastoma multiforme" (Urbanska et al., 2014). Tumor cells may be spindle-shaped, gemistocytic, lipidized, epithelioid, giant, small, or undifferentiated (Shan et al., 2022). Invasion occurs along deep white matter tracts (Riemenschneider et al., 2010). Hallmark features include prominent nuclear atypia, high cellularity, abundant mitotic figures, and nuclear pleomorphism, with regional heterogeneity that may complicate diagnosis, particularly in small stereotactic biopsy samples (Shan et al., 2022).

Classification of Glioblastoma

In 2021, the WHO adopted a new categorization for glioma tumors. This classification defines three categories of adult-type diffuse gliomas: astrocytoma (isocitrate dehydrogenase-IDH-mutant, grades 2–4), oligodendroglioma (IDH-mutant, 1p/19q-codeleted, grades 2–3), and glioblastoma (IDH wild-type, grade 4). The diagnosis of IDH-wild-type glioblastoma is contingent upon the identification of specific histological and genetic criteria. The main characteristics consist of microvascular growth, tissue death, mutations in the TERT promoter, amplification of the EGFR gene, and chromosomal changes, including +7 and -10 alterations (Louis et al., 2021). The presence of wild-type IDH1/2, TERT promoter mutations, chromosome 7 gain, loss of chromosome 10, and EGFR amplification are recognized as definitive molecular hallmarks of glioblastoma. These molecular characteristics can arise independently of the typical histopathological features associated with lower-grade diffuse gliomas.de diffuse gliomas (Stichel et al., 2018).

The most common mutations in GBM occur in TP53 (31–39%), PTEN (24–37%), IDH1 (12–20%), EGFR (14–15%), and NF1 (15–17%). However, TP53 and PTEN mutations are not GBM-specific, as they are frequent in various cancers. A hallmark GBM alteration is EGFRvIII, characterized by an in-frame deletion of exons 2–7, removing 267 amino acids from the extracellular domain. Other commonly altered genes include PIK3CA and PIK3R1 (Bleeker et al., 2012).

Integrated genomic analysis has identified four GBM subtypes: mesenchymal, proneural, neural, and classical. The neural subtype, mostly non-malignant cells, was excluded by Wang et al., while the classical subtype features EGFR amplification and TP53 alterations (Verhaak et al., 2010). The mesenchymal GBM tumors were observed to include mutations in NFI, PTEN, and RB1 have been shown in Figure 1. Histological examination demonstrated that the classic subtype displayed astrocytic characteristics, while the proneural subtype showed features akin to oligodendrocytes. In contrast, the mesenchymal subtype exhibited morphological traits reminiscent of both astroglial and microglial cells (Becker et al., 2021).

Figure 1. Mutation in GBM

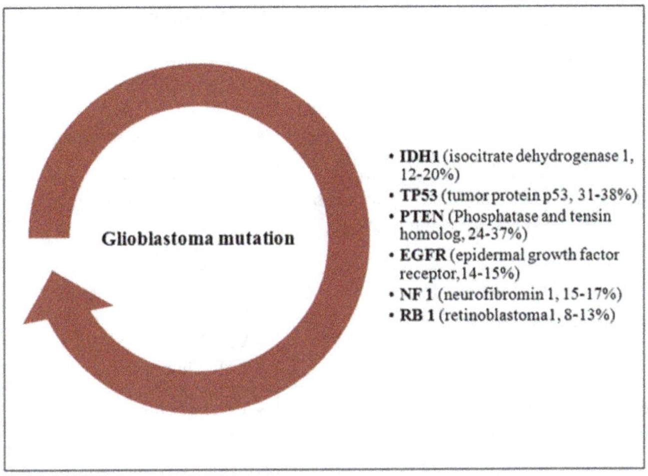

Current Therapeutic Approaches for GBM

Current therapeutic modalities for brain tumors include surgical intervention, systemic chemotherapy, and localized radiation therapy. These approaches are often employed in a multimodal framework to optimize outcomes and address the complex nature of these neoplasms mentioned in Table 1. Recent advancements in therapeutic interventions for patients with brain tumors have resulted in enhanced clinical outcomes for this population.

Table 1. An overview of various treatment approaches for glioblastoma multiforme

S. No.	Therapeutic Approach	Mechanism of action	Treatment type
1.	Radiation therapy	DNA double-strand breaks and ROS	• 2Dconventional • 3Dconformal • Intensity-modulated • Stereotactic radiosurgery Brachytherapy • Particle RT (Proton therapy)
2.	Chemotherapy	Alkylation in DNA base	• Temozolomide • Carmustine • Lomustine • Fotemustine
3.	Surgery based on image	Tumor resection	• Intraoperative ultrasonography • Intraoperative MRI • Intraoperative fluorescence imaging

continued on following page

Table 1. Continued

S. No.	Therapeutic Approach	Mechanism of action	Treatment type
4.	Nanoformulation	• 2B3–101PEGylatedliposomes • SGT-53Cationicliposomes • Liposomal irinotecan	• Target GSH/GSH transporters • Target Scfv/TfR • Convection enhanced delivery
5.	Immunotherapy	• Cemiplimab, Nivolumab • CAR-T cell therapy	• CheckpointinhibitorthatbindstoPD-1 • Engineered T cells express receptors against tumor markers.
6.	Inhibitor-based therapy	• Imatinib, Sunitinib • Erlotinib, Gefitinib • Bevacizumab • Niraparib	• Tyrosine kinase inhibitor • EGFR inhibitor • VEGF-A inhibition • PARP Inhibition
7.	Other approaches	• Laser interstitial thermal therapy • Tumor Treating Fields	• Thermal ablation of tumor tissue • Disrupts mitotic cell division

(Becker et al., 2021)

SURGICAL INTERVENTIONS IN GBM

Surgical removal has traditionally been seen as a vital part of treating brain tumors. Surgery serves as the first step in the treatment of GBM, fulfilling two objectives at the same time. The main goals of surgical resection are to reduce tumor size and improve overall survival rates (Karschnia et al., 2021). During neurosurgical procedures, neurosurgeons obtain tumor specimens essential for diagnosing neoplasms, utilizing the most recent WHO classification (Louis et al., 2021). Optimization of tumor resection in surgical techniques has been advanced, particularly through the use of intraoperative neuronavigation. (Rainer Wirtz et al., 2000) and fluorescence-guided resection (Leroy, 2015). The integration of intraoperative magnetic resonance (MR) imaging has further enhanced resection success rates, ultimately improving overall survival (OS) outcomes (Pichierri et al., 2019). Maximizing tumor resection is ideal, but tumors near eloquent brain areas require careful, patient-specific surgical planning. As shown in Figure 2, surgical options range from supramaximal resection to biopsy, depending on tumor extent and location.

Figure 2. Neurosurgical strategies for GBM resection

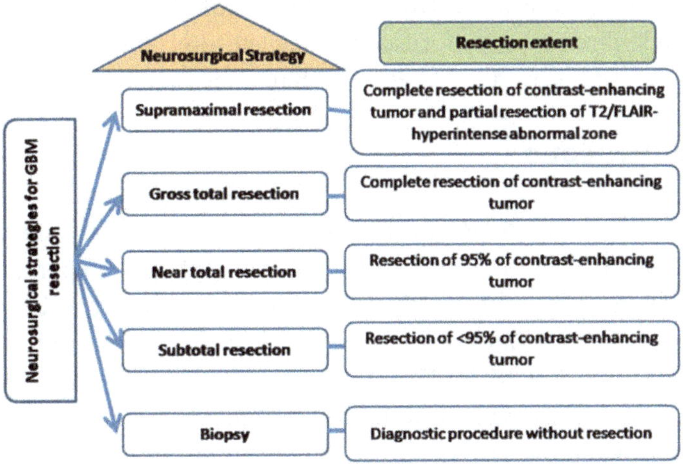

Supramaximal Resection

The SMR method is founded on the principle that GBM cells may infiltrate areas undetected through standard imaging techniques such as MRI and PET scans (Kickingereder et al., 2019). Research from multiple studies suggests that patients who have a GBM resection, achieving around 50% removal of the T2/FLAIR hyperintense abnormal area, demonstrate improved results (Pessina et al., 2017). While the exact resection level in SMR is not clearly established, class III data indicate that this surgical approach may enhance overall and progression-free survival (Dimou et al., 2020). It is critical to recognize that SMR may be particularly advantageous in cases where tumors are near vital brain structures. To comprehensively clarify the advantages of Surgical Management of Resectable GBM, it is essential to adopt a robust approach. There is a pressing need for rigorously designed clinical trials with well-defined technical, radiological, and outcome parameters.

Gross Total Resection

Gross Total Resection (GTR) is a key surgical approach for GBM, now more precisely defined as the complete removal of the contrast-enhancing tumor (Karschnia et al., 2021). While similar to SMR, the optimal minimum tumor resection percentage required to classify an intervention as GTR remains poorly defined. Some literature posits that a minimum of 90% resection of the contrast-enhancing tumor volume must be classified as GTR (Pessina et al., 2017). However, the predominant consensus among studies defines GTR as the total excision of these enhancing tumor components (Suchorska et al., 2016). The definition of GTR varies, highlighting the need for a standardized criterion focused on complete resection of contrast-enhancing tumors. Such clarity is essential to enhance future research on surgical outcomes.

Near Total Resection

Near-Total Resection (NTR) involves removing at least 80% of the tumor without exceeding the contrast-enhancing region. Sanai et al., 2011 reported significant outcome differences even within the 95–100% resection range. Karschnia et al. proposed that only the removal of at least 95% of the contrast-enhancing tumor should be categorized as NTR. The divergence in definitions of NTR, similar to the challenges associated with GTR, limits the ability to compare outcomes across different surgical approaches effectively. Nonetheless, pertinent studies regarding NTR indicate that optimal results are achieved in patients whose postoperative imaging reveals less than 1 cm^3 of residual tumor, or who acted as per Karschina et al.

Subtotal Resection

Sub-Total Resection (STR) involves partial tumor removal, leaving significant residual volume. While debated, current guidelines suggest that removing at least 80% of the contrast-enhancing tumor offers clinical benefit (Molinaro et al., 2020). STR is proposed when postoperative imaging indicates a residual volume of less than 5 cm^3 of contrast-enhancing tumor (Incekara, F. et al., 2020). Resections not meeting these criteria are classified as partial tumor reductions or biopsies.

Biopsy

Biopsy, though not therapeutic, is essential for diagnosis and treatment planning. It is typically used in elderly or low-KPS patients who cannot tolerate more invasive surgery (Chaichanaet al., 2011). Moreover, biopsy is often used to obtain a tissue sample in inoperable GBM cases.

Improvements in Surgical Treatment of GBM

The use of neuronavigation technology in neurosurgery has become a common practice globally, increasing the degree of tumor removal and simultaneously boosting the overall survival rates for GBM patients (Kubben et al., 2014). Additionally, Fluorescence-guided surgery with 5-aminolevulinic acid (5-ALA) has improved

GBM management by increasing resection extent and enhancing progression-free survival, as shown in randomized trials (Eljamel et al., 2008).

While several molecular targeting therapies are currently under development and show promising results, these treatments have not yet been incorporated into routine clinical practice (Senders et al., 2017). Furthermore, Intraoperative mass spectrometry is a promising innovation to improve GBM resection. Combined with awake craniotomy, motor mapping, image guidance, and augmented reality, it enhances glioma removal in the motor cortex (Turcotte et al., 2023).

RADIOTHERAPY

Whole-brain radiation therapy (WBRT) is increasingly used when SRS or surgery isn't feasible and improves survival in brain metastases patients. However, it is also associated with long-term cognitive decline. Over the past decade, cancer treatment has shifted from WBRT to targeted radiation, offering a cost-effective alternative to SRS. Like surgery, systemic medication is often combined with SRS to control CNS tumors and limit metastasis.

Recent studies support SRS for lesions ≤3 cm with minimal edema or in surgically challenging areas. A phase 3 trial compared cognitive and survival outcomes between SRS and WBRT. Nguyen et al. (2019) endorsed single-fraction partitioned SRS using Gamma Knife Icon (GKI-SPARE) for 10–30 metastases, showing dosimetric benefits over HA-WBRT.

SRS is the preferred adjuvant therapy, while WBRT is used for patients ineligible for SRS or with leptomeningeal disease. Surgical resection and SRS offer similar local control alone, but combining both yields the best outcomes, improving local control and reducing corticosteroid use (Patil et al., 2017). In addition, the radiation therapy possesses immunomodulatory properties that can alter the tumor and potentially rejuvenate immune responses (Hamilton et al., 2018). Current research focuses on how immunomodulatory effects influence immunotherapy efficacy and the outcomes of combining surgery with radiation. Overall, efforts aim to optimize treatment while minimizing radiation-related cognitive effects.

Radiation Therapy and Its Complications

Radiation therapy for brain metastases can cause side effects classified as acute, early-delayed, or late-delayed. Acute encephalopathy may develop within hours to weeks, worsening neurological symptoms and causing nausea, vomiting, and headaches (West & Barnett, 2011). Although immediate adverse effects can lead to herniation and death in individuals with sizable tumors, these issues are often controllable. Receiving a high radiation dose per fraction (more than 20 Gy) is the leading risk factor for developing acute encephalopathy. Early-delayed side effects typically appear one to six months after radiotherapy (Helson, 2018). During this period, patients may experience fatigue, increased sleep needs, and short-term cognitive or neurological issues, warranting imaging to rule out tumor growth. Late, often permanent, complications can arise six months post-radiotherapy (Wilke et al., 2018)

CHEMOTHERAPY IN GBM MANAGEMENT

Chemotherapy for glioblastoma can cause "chemobrain," involving lasting cognitive deficits due to hippocampal inflammation and neural damage. In rodent models, transplanting human neural stem cells into the hippocampus improved cognition by reducing inflammation and promoting regeneration (Acharya et al., 2015). For safety purposes, a clinical trial analyzing these approaches is feasible. The selection of the chemotherapy strategy for secondary brain cancers is influenced by the type of tumor and the presence of systemic disease. Table 2 provides an overview of some randomized controlled studies evaluating combinations of drugs for the treatment of glioblastoma.

Table 2. An overview of some randomized controlled studies evaluating combinations of drugs for the treatment of glioblastoma (Acharya et al., 2015)

S.No.	Clinical trial ID	Drug combination	Class	Mechanism of action	Phase/ status
1.	NCT00329719	Sorafenib; Temsirolimus	Recurrent GBM	Tyrosine kinase inhibitor; mTOR inhibitor	Phase I/II, Completed
2.	NCT00615927	Recurrent/ progressive grade II low-grade Glioma	Imatinib; Hydroxyurea	Tyrosine kinase inhibitor; ribonucleoside diphosphate reductase inhibitor	Phase II/ Completed
3.	NCT00921167	Bevacizumab; Irinotecan	Recurrent Gliomas	Anti-VEGF antibody; Topoisomerase I inhibitor	Phase II/ Completed
4.	NCT00621686	Bevacizumab; Sorafenib	Recurrent GBM	Anti-VEGF antibody; Tyrosine protein kinases	Phase II/ Completed
5.	NCT02340156	Temozolomide; SGT-53	Recurrent GBM	Alkylating agent; Liposome-p53 DNA	Phase II/ Completed
6.	NCT00800917	Bevacizumab; Temsirolimus	Recurrent GBM	Anti-VEGF antibody; mTOR inhibitor	Phase II/ Completed

continued on following page

Table 2. Continued

S.No.	Clinical trial ID	Drug combination	Class	Mechanism of action	Phase/ status
7.	NCT00671970	Bevacizumab; Erlotinib	Recurrent GBM	Anti-VEGF antibody; Tyrosine kinase inhibitor;	Phase II/ Completed
8.	NCT00672243	Erlotinib; Sirolimus	Recurrent GBM	Tyrosine kinase inhibitor; mTOR inhibitor	Phase II/ Completed
9.	NCT00613093	O6-Benzylguanine; Temozolomide	Temozolomide resistant malignant glioma	O6-alkylguanine-DNA alky ltransferase inhibitor; Alkylating agent	Phase II/ Completed
10.	NCT00777153	Cediranib; Lomustine	Recurrent GBM	Tyrosine kinase; Alkylating agent	Phase III/ Completed

BIOMARKER-GUIDED THERAPY FOR GBM

Biomarker- guided treatment of patients with glioblastoma is currently relies on the detection of specific markers linked to prognosis or anticipated therapeutic benefit. Nonetheless, as therapy alternatives proliferate, a growing complexity is becoming evident (Yan et al., 2019). Biomarker profiling is increasingly used in glioblastoma, though actionable targets remain limited. MGMT promoter methylation predicts better response to temozolomide, especially in older patients. Targeted therapies exist for rare mutations like BRAF V600E and NTRK fusions, while IDH1/2 mutations define a distinct subgroup but lack standard targeted options. EGFR-targeted treatments, such as rindopepimut, have not improved survival. Comprehensive molecular testing at diagnosis is recommended, though most patients still rely on standard multimodal therapy (Wick et al., 2014).

TARGETED THERAPIES INCLUDING IMMUNOTHERAPY, GENE THERAPY, CELL THERAPY AND VACCINE THERAPY

The CNS operates in an immune-restricted environment due to the blood-brain barrier, lack of lymphatics, low MHC II expression, scarce APCs, and immunosuppressive cytokines like TGF-β. These factors limit effective T cell-mediated immune responses (Jackson et al., 2014). Louveau et al. in 2015 introduced a functional lymphatic system within the CNS. This newly identified system facilitates the transport of immune cells and fluid derived from cerebrospinal fluid, altering our perception of immune surveillance in this region (Louveau et al., 2015).

In parallel, immunotherapy has gained traction as a cornerstone in cancer treatment strategies, particularly following breakthroughs in immune checkpoint blockade and the development of CAR-modified T cell therapies (Queirolo et al., 2014;Blanding & Gibney, 2023).These innovations have yielded improved clinical outcomes for many cancer patients, resulting in a notable uptick in FDA approvals for immunotherapeutic agents targeting immune checkpoints such as cytotoxic T-lymphocyte-associated protein 4 (CTLA-4), programmed cell death protein 1 (PD-1), and programmed cell death ligand 1 (PD-L1). CAR T cell therapies fall within this expanding arsenal.

Despite these advances, the landscape for GBM remains challenging, with a notable absence of FDA-approved immunotherapies tailored for this aggressive tumor type (McGranahan et al., 2019, Topalian et al., 2015). Immune checkpoint inhibitors have improved survival in some melanoma patients with brain metastases, highlighting immunotherapy's potential in CNS cancers. However, GBM's immune suppression and molecular heterogeneity hinder treatment response, making it crucial to address these challenges to advance effective immunotherapies (Jackson et al., 2019). An overview of various immunotherapies currently under investigation is summarized in Table 3.

Immunotherapy faces limitations, with immune checkpoint inhibitors showing low and variable response rates across solid tumors. As of 2018, only 12.46% of eligible cancer patients responded, despite 43.6% being considered suitable candidates (Magee et al., 2020).

Table 3. Highlights the ongoing clinical trials and associated therapies

S. No.	Clinical Trials ID	Name	Drug	Combination	status
1.	NCT03018288	Vaccines	PD-1 (pembrolizumab)	HSPPC-96	Phase I
	NCT02529072		PD-1 (nivolumab)	pp65DC	
	NCT03014804			DCVAX-L	
2.	NCT02798406	Virus	PD-1 (pembrolizumab)	DNX-2401	
3.	NCT02311920	Dual Check Point Blocker	CTLA-4 (ipilimumab)	PD-1 (nivolumab) therapy	
	NCT02658981			Anti-LAG-3 (BMS986016)/ antiCD137(urelumab)	
	NCT02335918		PD-1 (nivolumab)	anti-CD-27 (varlilumab)	Phase I/II
	NCT03058289			IntratumoralIDO1 inhibitor(INT230-6)	
	NCT02327078			IDO1inhibitor (epacadostat)	
	NCT02794883		PD-L1 (durvalumab)	CTLA-4 (tremelimumab)	PhaseII
4.	NCT02829723	CSF-1Rinibitor	PD-1(PDR001)	CSF-1rinhibitor (FPA008)	PhaseI
	NCT02526017		Nivo	CSF-1rinhibitor (BLZ945)	Phase I/II
5.	NCT02311582	Laser Treatment	MK-3475	MRI-guided laser ablation	
6.	NCT02866747	Radiation Therapy	PD-L1 (durvalumab)	Hypo fractionated stereotactic irradiation	
	NCT02313272		Pembro		Phase I
	NCT02648633		Nivo	SRS+Valproic acid	
7.	NCT04277221	Autologous Dendritic Cell/ Tumor Antigen (ADCTA)	ADCTA vaccine with Bevacizumab as a standard therapy vs. standard therapy alone	Recruiting (Status)	Phase III

(Naser et al., 2022)

GENE THERAPY

As of August 2018, no gene therapies have been approved for GBM in the United States or Europe. Gene therapy for glioblastoma (GBM) has seen progress, with 77 clinical trials registered in the U.S. It can complement surgery, replace traditional therapies, or treat recurrent and chemo-resistant tumors. Advances in imaging and delivery methods enable minimally invasive treatment of early-stage tumors. The first HSV-TK/ganciclovir trial began 25 years ago (Shah et al., 2025). The advancements in gene therapy methods have since emerged, with over 100 preclinical studies currently underway worldwide to find effective glioblastoma treatments (Jain, 2018). Figure 3 summarizes various gene therapy strategies for GMB.

Figure 3. Gene therapy strategies for GBM

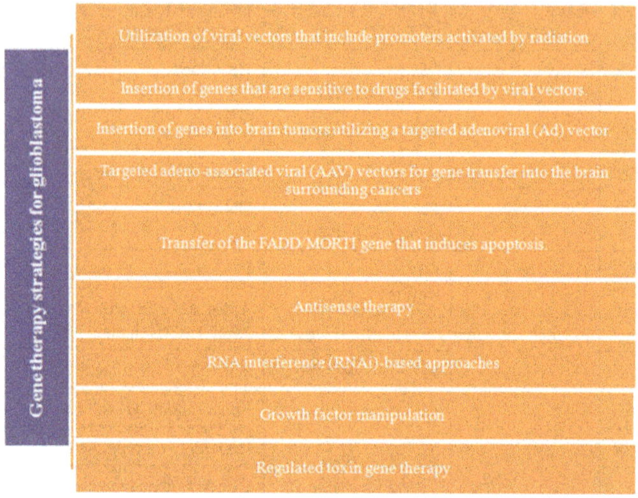

High-dose chemotherapy is limited by myelosuppression and neurotoxicity. Gene therapy using P140K-modified hematopoietic stem cells protects the blood system, allowing safer treatment in glioblastoma patients with poor prognosis, improving survival without significant side effects (Adair et al., 2012). GBMs frequently become tolerant to temozolomide, a challenge that can be partially addressed with the co-administration of O6-benzylguanine (O6BG). However, this combination therapy is associated with significant myelosuppression. A clinical trial suggested that gene therapy utilising P140K-modified hematopoietic stem cells can confer resistance to O6BG, improve chemotherapy tolerance, and enhance clinical outcomes for patients afflicted with this malignancy (Adair et al., 2014).

CELL THERAPY

Neural stem cells (NSCs) migrate toward GBM tumors, making them promising delivery vehicles for gene and personalized therapies. While their attraction mechanisms are unclear, tumor-secreted chemoattractants and microenvironmental changes are suspected, warranting further study to improve NSC-based treatments (Bagó et al., 2015). Intratumoral delivery of IL-12-secreting NSCs in rodent glioma models significantly extends survival by inducing strong antitumor immunity. Engineered NSCs selectively target glioblastoma, inhibit tumor growth, and activate cytochrome P450 2B6 to metabolize cyclophosphamide locally (Namba et al., 2015).The importance of NSCs in brain tumors is rooted in its ability to leverage the tumor-targeting properties of these cells to administer efficient, tumor-specific treatment for brain cancer (Tang et al., 2021).

VACCINE THERAPY

Cancer vaccines are carefully designed to specifically focus on tumor-associated antigens, thereby eliciting a robust immune response aimed at combating malignant tumors (Saxena et al., 2021). The limited number of glioblastoma-specific antigens typically indicates that the primary source for glioblastoma antigens is usually tumor-associated antigens, which restricts patient participation. EGFRvIII is a thoroughly studied antigen that is specific to tumors; it is a mutated variant of EGFR that remains functional and occurs in approximately 25–30% of GBM cases (Hu et al., 2018).The utilization of genetic engineering to modify T cells for the expression of CARs targeting specific tumor cell antigens has emerged as a state-of-the-art technique in oncology. Table 4 offers a comprehensive summary of various vaccination strategies. The selection of the appropriate antigen and vaccination approach is critical to success. Current clinical trials for GBM vaccines are yielding suboptimal outcomes; however, ongoing advancements in this field hold the potential to refine these therapies into a transformative treatment modality. It is crucial to increase financial investment in the research and development of GBM vaccines to harness their full potential (Sadelain et al., 2017). The target selection and immunization strategy require improvement. Glioblastoma microenvironment has many immunosuppressive mechanisms that can hinder the efficacy of current vaccinations. A study is being undertaken on adjuvant compounds that may enhance immunotherapy responses. Immunotherapy might provide more enduring results in glioblastoma patients if an appropriate target and vaccination technique are integrated with an immunomodulator that can reduce or enhance the body's immune response to the tumor, various vaccine based approaches for GBM are summarized in Table 4 (Zhao et al., 2022). While table 5 illustrates the combination of Innovative with conventional therapies.

Table 4. Vaccine therapy in GBM (Zhao et al., 2022)

S.No.	Clinical trial ID	Name	Class	Status
1.	NCT01967758	ADU-623	rAA, rGBM	Phase I
2.	NCT01480479	Rindopepimut	Newly diagnosed GBM (nGBM)	Phase III
	NCT00458601			Phase II
	NCT01498328		rGBM	
3.	NCT00905060	HSPPC-96	nGBM	
	NCT01814813		rGBM	
	NCT03018288		nGBM	
4.	NCT02455557	SurVax M		
5.	NCT01567202	DCs vaccine (autogenic gliomastem-like cells (A2B5+) loaded)		
6.	NCT01204684	DCs vaccine (tumor lysate loaded)	nAA, rAA, nAO, rAO, nGBM, rGBM	
7.	NCT02754362	Bevacizumab and TAA, Poly-ICLC,KLH	rGBM	

Table 5. Combination of Innovative with conventional therapies

S.No.	Innovative approaches	Applications	References/Sources
1.	Combination of gene therapy with chemotherapy	The study, grant #NCT02414165, titled "Toca 511 & Toca FC vs. Standard of Care in Patients With Recurrent High Grade Glioma," explores the integration of gene therapy and chemotherapy. This randomized, open-label Phase II/III trial investigates the retroviral vector Voc imageneamiretrorepvec (Toca 511), which targets rapidly proliferating tumor cells to enable the introduction of the cytosine deaminase gene with 5-fluorocytosine.	(Cloughesy et al., 2018)
2.	Combination of gene therapy and CAR-T	Immunosuppressive Tregs, TAMs, and MDSCs inhibit cytotoxic T cell anticancer activity and immunotherapy efficacy in the glioblastoma microenvironment.	(Kamran et al., 2017)
3.	Chip for individualized pharmacological screening of brain cancers	Selecting the best GBM treatment is difficult. Conventional 2D cell cultures inadequately represent tumors and their three-dimensional microenvironments. A photo-polymerizable poly(ethylene) glycol diacrylate (PEGDA) hydrogel 3D brain cancer chip employs proliferating glioblastoma cells to generate cancerous tissues, serving as a prospective drug screening approach.	(Fan et al., 2016)
4.	Personalized/precision approaches	Customizes treatment to the patient's genetic and surroundings.	(Sarhangi et al., 2024)

continued on following page

Table 5. Continued

S.No.	Innovative approaches	Applications	References/Sources
5.	Animal models	A s.c.Xenograft of a human glioblastoma cell line in an immunodeficient rodent model. A constraining factor of intracranial xenografts is their short survival period. The ideal mouse model is transgenic, as genetic modification enables the precise incorporation of mutations associated with human glioblastomas.	(Miyai et al., 2017)
6.	Countering drug resistance	Considering the prevalent activation of mammalian target of rapamycin (mTOR) signaling in GBM, tumors demonstrate resistance to mTOR-targeted treatment.	(Iwanami et al., 2013)
7.	Induced neural stem cells	Genetically modified iNSCs containing tumoricidal gene products maintain their differentiation ability while inducing an apoptotic response in co-cultured human GBMcells.	(Bagó et al., 2016)
8.	Genomic analysis	When merging with mutation analysis, gene expression profiling is crucial for advancing rational personalized therapy for GBM.	(Lee et al., 2017)

CURRENT NANOCARRIERS AND NANOCARRIER-RELATED APPROACHES FOR THE MANAGEMENT OF GLIOBLASTOMA

Nanoformulations facilitate effective and targeted delivery of anticancer agents to tumors over the BBB at lower dosages than standard formulations, hence diminishing chemotherapy toxicity. The nanocarrier-based combination treatment for GBMs offers several benefits, including the ease of administering drugs sequentially, synergism, and improved targeting of anticancer medications directly at the tumor location (M. Zhao et al., 2020).

Nanoparticles are the most prevalent agents employed in the treatment of GBMs and summarize the clinical trials in table 6 and different nanocarriers are showed in figure 4. They are categorized according to the colloidal drug carrier type from which they are obtained, including liposomes, solid lipid nanoparticles, polymeric micelles, polymeric nanoparticles, silica, and dendrimers.

Figure 4. Nanocarrier for the treatment of GBM

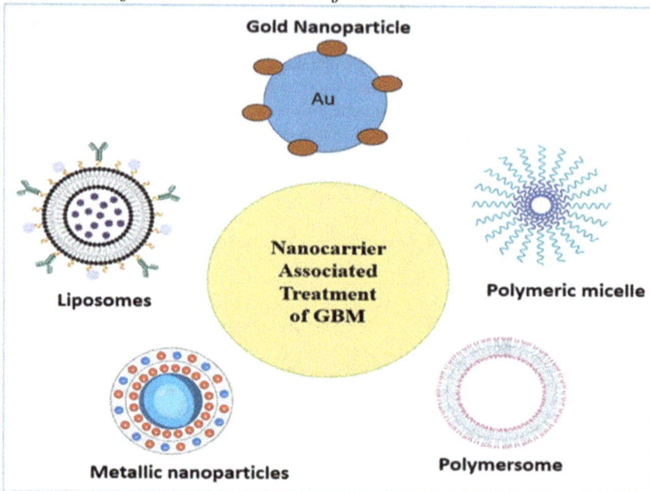

Liposomes

Liposomes exhibit a structural architecture akin to cellular membranes, featuring a hydrophilic core encapsulated by a phospholipid bilayer. This unique configuration significantly augments lipophilicity, facilitating the translocation of lipophilic macromolecules across the BBB. These nanoparticles provide numerous benefits, such as simple synthesis, high encapsulation efficiency for various anticancer drugs, excellent biocompatibility, lack of immunogenicity, enhanced solubility for therapeutic substances, and proven commercial potential (Glaser et al., 2017).Numerous unique receptors and antigens overexpressed on glioblastoma cells present promising targets for therapeutic intervention. Research involving liposomal doxorubicin targeted at IL-4 and IL-13 receptors in rodent models has demonstrated considerable decreases in tumor size compared to treatments that use unconjugated liposomes (Yang et al., 2015).

Polymeric Micelles

Polymeric micelles are formed with a lipophilic core composed of polymers and an outer hydrophilic shell. This structure results from the self-assembly of block copolymers, and the design can affect both the effectiveness of drug loading and the pace of sustained release for chemotherapy agents (Karim et al., 2016).The distinctive core-shell structure and the size range of 10 to 100 nm shield the drug-loaded core from engaging with the system and being targeted by macrophages through phagocytic processes. This design significantly improves the circulation time of the nanoparticles, yielding a half-life that exceeds 10 hours (Nishiyama et al., 2016). Micelles for brain tumors can serve as carriers for anticancer agents like temozolomide to improve delivery to glioblastoma.

Dendrimers

Dendrimers are nanoscale macromolecules, typically under 12 nm in size, recognized for their highly branched and compact scaffold architecture. This structural design enhances the delivery and stability of siRNA by facilitating its transport and protecting it from enzymatic degradation during circulation (Stenström et al., 2018). When methotrexate is encapsulated within dendrimers, it exhibits improved therapeutic potency and an increased ability to cross the BBB. However, the dendrimers are subject to rapid clearance by the reticuloendothelial system, which can limit their bioavailability. Additionally, their interactions with cellular membranes can induce cytotoxic effects in healthy tissues. Furthermore, the controlled release profiles of dendrimers can be less optimal compared to other drug delivery systems (Qiu et al., 2018).

Metal Particles

Metal polymeric micelles feature a hydrophobic core of polymers surrounded by a hydrophilic outer covering, which can notably enhance radiosensitization in GBM cells. Preclinical studies using animal models have demonstrated that treatment with metal particles before radiation therapy results in extensive DNA damage within the tumor cells (Bobyk et al., 2013).These metal nanoparticles exhibit high X-ray attenuation, unique electrical properties, and notable synthetic versatility, positioning them as promising candidates for use as radiosensitizers. Specifically, iron oxide nanoparticles, including superparamagnetic iron oxide nanoparticles (SPIONs), leverage their super paramagnetism to enhance magnetic resonance imaging (MRI) precision in localizing brain tumors and facilitate the delivery of chemotherapeutic agents directly to the neoplastic tissue nanoparticles (SPION), which have superparamagnetic characteristics and have been beneficial in MRI for accurately locating brain cancers and delivering chemotherapy agents directly to the tumors (Her et al., 2017).

Silica

Silica nanoparticles (SiNPs) offer numerous advantages due to their excellent biocompatibility, extensive outer surface for drug loading, and inherent durability.

However, concerns regarding their cytotoxicity, potential for DNA damage, and the production of reactive oxygen species have raised significant challenges. These issues may hinder the effective utilization of SiNPs in areas such as biomarker development, cancer therapy, and drug delivery systems (Krętowski et al., 2017).

Nanoparticle-Induced Hyperthermia

Hyperthermia, along with radiation and chemotherapeutic agents, has been explored as a treatment strategy. The mechanisms by which hyperthermia enhances radiosensitization and chemosensitization involve several key processes: the impairment of DNA repair mechanisms, heat-mediated suppression of the AKT signaling pathway, augmented apoptotic signaling, and alterations to the blood-brain barrier. Experimental studies indicate that localized temperatures exceeding 45°C can induce apoptosis in GBM cells within murine models (Mahmoudi et al., 2018).

Table 6. Summary of nanotechnology used in glioblastoma clinical trials (Naser et al., 2022).

S. No.	Therapeutic agent	Therapeutic strategy	Recruitment status	Status
1.	Polysiloxane Gd-Chelates based nanoparticles (AGuIX)	AGuIX Nanoparticles with Radiotherapy Plus Concomitant Temozolomide	Recruiting	Phase I and II (randomized) NCT04881032
2.	NU-0129 based on Spherical Nucleic Acid (SNA) platform	NU-0129 IV plus standard of care tumor resection within 8-48 h.	Completed	Early Phase I NCT03020017
3.	ABI-009 (nab-Rapamycin)	ABI-009 (alone) ABI-009 + bevacizumab ABI-009 + temozolomide ABI-009 + lomustine ABI-009 + temozolomide + radiotherapy ABI-009 + marizomib	Active, not recruiting	Phase II NCT03463265
4.	Nanoliposomal CPT-11 (NL CPT-11)	NL CPT-11 in patients with recurrent high-grade gliomas: glioblastoma multiforme (GBM), gliosarcoma (GS), anaplastic astrocytoma (AA), anaplastic oligodendroglioma (AO), anaplastic mixed oligoastrocytoma (AMO), or malignant astrocytoma NOS (not otherwise specified	Completed	Phase I NCT00734682

FUTURE DIRECTIONS

The prognosis for individuals with brain tumors continues to be disheartening, despite substantial efforts to decipher the intricate mechanisms governing their pathogenesis and biological behavior. Addressing these challenges requires implementing a personalized precision medicine approach that considers the unique traits and molecular profile of each patient's tumor. This approach aims to tailor therapeutic interventions to the unique biological context, enhancing treatment efficacy and improving patient outcomes. It is essential to use a systems biology approach to accomplish this goal, which includes a thorough comprehension of several steps of the organization related to the onset and course of sickness. Tumor reduction alone is insufficient because the patient will eventually die from recurrences and the tumor's rapid advancement. Improvements in targeted therapy delivery are crucial for the tumor to be destroyed effectively and safely. Finding receptors specific to glioblastoma is a future problem, and selective delivery to the treatment of glioblastoma may necessitate a multi-receptor approach due to the tumor's complex biology. Progress in nanobiotechnology has enabled the creation of innovative diagnostic and treatment methods that improve the effectiveness of drug delivery through different biological obstacles. Given that even minimal residual tumor cells can lead to catastrophic recurrences, the objective remains total tumor eradication.

Immunotherapy is a hope for treating GBMs, particularly when combined with adjuvants. Clinical trials have explored a range of vaccination therapies utilizing autologous tumor antigens or specific peptide antigens in GBM patients.A pivotal study will evaluate immunotherapy checkpoint inhibition alongside vaccination as part of a unified therapeutic approach. In light of glioblastoma's resilience, immunotherapy is increasingly integrated into multimodal treatment regimens that also encompass chemotherapy and radiation, aiming to leverage the synergistic effects of these modalities. Recognizing that no single therapeutic intervention suffices for glioblastoma, adopting multimodal therapy is essential. Until the advent of a non-invasive or minimally invasive alternative, surgical intervention will remain a cornerstone of the comprehensive treatment strategy for this aggressive malignancy.

CONCLUSION

Glioblastoma multiforme presents significant therapeutic challenges owing to its aggressive behavior, high propensity for recurrence, and resistance to established treatments. The conventional treatment paradigm, which encompasses surgical resection, radiotherapy, and chemotherapy (primarily with temozolomide), yields limited survival benefits and fails to achieve curative outcomes. Surgical intervention aims to reduce tumor burden and alleviate neurological symptoms; however, complete resection remains infrequently attainable due to the infiltrative characteristics of GBM. Radiotherapy contributes to local control but is often undermined by intrinsic and acquired resistance mechanisms and collateral damage to surrounding normal tissue. Chemotherapy faces additional hurdles, primarily due to the less permeable BBB and inherent resistance pathways.

In recent times, new therapeutic approaches have attracted interest for their possibilities in the treatment of GBM. Tumor-treating fields, targeted therapies, and various immunotherapeutic approaches—including immune checkpoint inhibitors, CAR-T and CAR-NK cell therapies, dendritic cell vaccines, and oncolytic virotherapyhave shown promise in early-stage studies. Nevertheless, these innovative strategies encounter several challenges, such as limited tumor microenvironment penetration, the immunosuppressive milieu associated with GBM, and the risk of adverse effects.

In conclusion, despite substantial progress in elucidating GBM pathobiology and developing novel treatment strategies, clinical outcomes remain inadequate. There is an urgent imperative to pursue multimodal and personalized treatment approaches that synergistically integrate conventional and emerging therapies. The ongoing advancement of translational research, coupled with the execution of comprehensive and well-structured clinical trials, is critical in fostering improved prognostic outcomes and enhancing the overall standard of living for GBM patients. By integrating novel therapeutic approaches, innovative treatment modalities, and personalized medicine strategies, the medical community can better address the complex challenges associated with GBM, ultimately leading to more effective interventions and support systems for affected individuals.

REFERENCES

Acharya, M. M., Martirosian, V., Chmielewski, N. N., Hanna, N., Tran, K. K., Liao, A. C., Christie, L. A., Parihar, V. K., & Limoli, C. L. (2015). Stem cell transplantation reverses chemotherapy-induced cognitive dysfunction. *Cancer Research, 75*(4), 676–686. DOI: 10.1158/0008-5472.CAN-14-2237 PMID: 25687405

Adair, J. E., Beard, B. C., Trobridge, G. D., Neff, T., Rockhill, J. K., Silbergeld, D. L., Mrugala, M. M., & Kiem, H. P. (2012). Extended survival of glioblastoma patients after chemoprotective HSC gene therapy. *Science Translational Medicine, 4*(133). Advance online publication. DOI: 10.1126/scitranslmed.3003425 PMID: 22572881

Adair, J. E., Johnston, S. K., Mrugala, M. M., Beard, B. C., Guyman, L. A., Baldock, A. L., Bridge, C. A., Hawkins-Daarud, A., Gori, J. L., Born, D. E., Gonzalez-Cuyar, L. F., Silbergeld, D. L., Rockne, R. C., Storer, B. E., Rockhill, J. K., Swanson, K. R., & Kiem, H. P. (2014). Gene therapy enhances chemotherapy tolerance and efficacy in glioblastoma patients. *The Journal of Clinical Investigation, 124*(9), 4082–4092. DOI: 10.1172/JCI76739 PMID: 25105369

Bagó, J. R., Alfonso-Pecchio, A., Okolie, O., Dumitru, R., Rinkenbaugh, A., Baldwin, A. S., Miller, C. R., Magness, S. T., & Hingtgen, S. D. (2016). Therapeutically engineered induced neural stem cells are tumour-homing and inhibit progression of glioblastoma. *Nature Communications, 7*(1), 10593. Advance online publication. DOI: 10.1038/ncomms10593 PMID: 26830441

Bagó, J. R., Sheets, K. T., & Hingtgen, S. D. (2015). Neural stem cell therapy for cancer. *Methods (San Diego, Calif.), 99*, 37–43. DOI: 10.1016/j.ymeth.2015.08.013 PMID: 26314280

Becker, A. P., Sells, B. E., Jaharul Haque, S., & Chakravarti, A. (2021). Tumor Heterogeneity in Glioblastomas: From Light Microscopy to Molecular Pathology. *Cancers (Basel), 13*(4), 1–25. DOI: 10.3390/cancers13040761 PMID: 33673104

Blanding, W. M., & Gibney, B. C. (2023). Commentary: Neoadjuvant immunotherapy: A brave new world. *The Journal of Thoracic and Cardiovascular Surgery, 166*(2), 356. DOI: 10.1016/j.jtcvs.2022.12.019 PMID: 36774207

Bleeker, F. E., Molenaar, R. J., & Leenstra, S. (2012). Recent advances in the molecular understanding of glioblastoma. *Journal of Neuro-Oncology, 108*(1), 11–27. DOI: 10.1007/s11060-011-0793-0 PMID: 22270850

Bobyk, L., Edouard, M., Deman, P., Vautrin, M., Pernet-Gallay, K., Delaroche, J., Adam, J. F., Estève, F., Ravanat, J. L., & Elleaume, H. (2013). Photoactivation of gold nanoparticles for glioma treatment. *Nanomedicine; Nanotechnology, Biology, and Medicine*, *9*(7), 1089–1097. DOI: 10.1016/j.nano.2013.04.007 PMID: 23643529

Chaichana, K. L., Garzon-Muvdi, T., Parker, S., Weingart, J. D., Olivi, A., Bennett, R., Brem, H., & Quinones-Hinojosa, A. (2011). Supratentorial glioblastoma multiforme: The role of surgical resection versus biopsy among older patients. *Annals of Surgical Oncology*, *18*(1), 239–245. DOI: 10.1245/s10434-010-1242-6 PMID: 20697823

Chatzikonstantinou, G., Ulrich, P., Archavlis, E., Zamboglou, N., Strouthos, I., Zoga, E., Baltas, D., & Tselis, N. (2019). Interstitial high-dose-rate brachytherapy in the primary treatment of inoperable glioblastoma multiforme. *Journal of Contemporary Brachytherapy*, *11*(3), 215–220. DOI: 10.5114/jcb.2019.85722 PMID: 31435428

Cloughesy, T. F., Landolfi, J., Vogelbaum, M. A., Ostertag, D., Elder, J. B., Bloomfield, S., Carter, B., Chen, C. C., Kalkanis, S. N., Kesari, S., Lai, A., Lee, I. Y., Liau, L. M., Mikkelsen, T., Nghiemphu, P., Piccioni, D., Accomando, W., Diago, O. R., Hogan, D. J., & Walbert, T. (2018). Durable complete responses in some recurrent high-grade glioma patients treated with Toca 511 + Toca FC. *Neuro-Oncology*, *20*(10), 1383–1392. DOI: 10.1093/neuonc/noy075 PMID: 29762717

Dimou, J., Beland, B., & Kelly, J. (2020). Supramaximal resection: A systematic review of its safety, efficacy and feasibility in glioblastoma. *Journal of Clinical Neuroscience*, *72*, 328–334. DOI: 10.1016/j.jocn.2019.12.021 PMID: 31864830

Eljamel, M. S., Goodman, C., & Moseley, H. (2008). ALA and Photofrin® Fluorescence-guided resection and repetitive PDT in glioblastoma multiforme: A single centre Phase III randomised controlled trial. *Lasers in Medical Science*, *23*(4), 361–367. DOI: 10.1007/s10103-007-0494-2 PMID: 17926079

Fan, Y., Nguyen, D. T., Akay, Y., Xu, F., & Akay, M. (2016). Engineering a Brain Cancer Chip for High-throughput Drug Screening. *Scientific Reports*, *6*(1), 25062. Advance online publication. DOI: 10.1038/srep25062 PMID: 27151082

Glaser, T., Han, I., Wu, L., & Zeng, X. (2017). Targeted nanotechnology in glioblastoma multiforme. *Frontiers in Pharmacology*, *8*(MAR), 238646. DOI: 10.3389/FPHAR.2017.00166/PD PMID: 28408882

Grochans, S., Cybulska, A. M., Simińska, D., Korbecki, J., Kojder, K., Chlubek, D., & Baranowska-Bosiacka, I. (2022). Epidemiology of Glioblastoma Multiforme-Literature Review. *Cancers (Basel)*, *14*(10), 2412. Advance online publication. DOI: 10.3390/cancers14102412 PMID: 35626018

Hamilton, A. J., Seid, J., Verdecchia, K., & Chuba, P. (2018). Abscopal Effect after Radiosurgery for Solitary Brain Metastasis from Non-small Cell Lung Cancer. *Cureus, 10*(12). Advance online publication. DOI: 10.7759/cureus.3777 PMID: 30854265

Helson, L. (2018). Radiation-induced Demyelination and Remyelination in the Central Nervous System: A Literature Review. *Anticancer Research, 38*(9), 4999–5002. DOI: 10.21873/anticanres.12818 PMID: 30194143

Her, S., Jaffray, D. A., & Allen, C. (2017). Gold nanoparticles for applications in cancer radiotherapy: Mechanisms and recent advancements. *Advanced Drug Delivery Reviews, 109*, 84–101. DOI: 10.1016/j.addr.2015.12.012 PMID: 26712711

Hu, Z., Ott, P. A., & Wu, C. J. (2018). Towards personalized, tumour-specific, therapeutic vaccines for cancer. *Nature Reviews. Immunology, 18*(3), 168–182. DOI: 10.1038/nri.2017.131 PMID: 29226910

Incekara, F., Smits, M., Van der Voort, S. R., Dubbink, H. J., Atmodimedjo, P. N., Kros, J. M., Vincent, A. J. P. E., & van den Bent, M. (2020). The association between the extent of glioblastoma resection and survival in light of MGMT promoter methylation in 326 patients with newly diagnosed IDH-wildtype glioblastoma. *Frontiers in Oncology, 10*, 1087. DOI: 10.3389/fonc.2020.01087 PMID: 32766140

Iwanami, A., Gini, B., Zanca, C., Matsutani, T., Assuncao, A., Nael, A., Dang, J., Yang, H., Zhu, S., Kohyama, J., Kitabayashi, I., Cavenee, W. K., Cloughesy, T. F., Furnari, F. B., Nakamura, M., Toyam, Y., Okano, H., & Mischel, P. S. (2013). PML mediates glioblastoma resistance to mammalian target of rapamycin (mTOR)-targeted therapies. *Proceedings of the National Academy of Sciences of the United States of America, 110*(11), 4339–4344. DOI: 10.1073/pnas.1217602110 PMID: 23440206

Jackson, C. M., Choi, J., & Lim, M. (2019). Mechanisms of immunotherapy resistance: Lessons from glioblastoma. *Nature Immunology, 20*(9), 1100–1109. DOI: 10.1038/s41590-019-0433-y PMID: 31358997

Jackson, C. M., Lim, M., & Drake, C. G. (2014). Immunotherapy for brain cancer: Recent progress and future promise. *Clinical Cancer Research, 20*(14), 3651–3659. DOI: 10.1158/1078-0432.CCR-13-2057 PMID: 24771646

Jain, K. K. (2018). A critical overview of targeted therapies for glioblastoma. *Frontiers in Oncology, 8*(OCT), 418128. DOI: 10.3389/fonc.2018.00419 PMID: 30374421

Kamran, N., Kadiyala, P., Saxena, M., Candolfi, M., Li, Y., Moreno-Ayala, M. A., Raja, N., Shah, D., Lowenstein, P. R., & Castro, M. G. (2017). Immunosuppressive Myeloid Cells' Blockade in the Glioma Microenvironment Enhances the Efficacy of Immune-Stimulatory Gene Therapy. *Molecular Therapy : the Journal of the American Society of Gene Therapy, 25*(1), 232–248. DOI: 10.1016/j.ymthe.2016.10.003 PMID: 28129117

Karim, R., Palazzo, C., Evrard, B., & Piel, G. (2016). Nanocarriers for the treatment of glioblastoma multiforme: Current state-of-the-art. *Journal of Controlled Release, 227*, 23–37. DOI: 10.1016/j.jconrel.2016.02.026 PMID: 26892752

Karschnia, P., Vogelbaum, M. A., van den Bent, M., Cahill, D. P., Bello, L., Narita, Y., Berger, M. S., Weller, M., & Tonn, J. C. (2021). Evidence-based recommendations on categories for extent of resection in diffuse glioma. *European Journal of Cancer, 149*, 23–33. DOI: 10.1016/j.ejca.2021.03.002 PMID: 33819718

Kickingereder, P., Isensee, F., Tursunova, I., Petersen, J., Neuberger, U., Bonekamp, D., Brugnara, G., Schell, M., Kessler, T., Foltyn, M., Harting, I., Sahm, F., Prager, M., Nowosielski, M., Wick, A., Nolden, M., Radbruch, A., Debus, J., Schlemmer, H.-P., & Maier-Hein, K. H. (2019). Automated quantitative tumour response assessment of MRI in neuro-oncology with artificial neural networks: A multicentre, retrospective study. *The Lancet. Oncology, 20*(5), 728–740. DOI: 10.1016/S1470-2045(19)30098-1 PMID: 30952559

Krętowski, R., Kusaczuk, M., Naumowicz, M., Kotyńska, J., Szynaka, B., &Cechowska-Pasko, M. (2017). The Effects of Silica Nanoparticles on Apoptosis and Autophagy of Glioblastoma Cell Lines. *Nanomaterials 2017, Vol. 7, Page 230, 7*(8), 230. .DOI: 10.3390/nano7080230

Kubben, P. L., Scholtes, F., Schijns, O. E., ter Laak-Poort, M. P., Teernstra, O. P., Kessels, A. G., van Overbeeke, J. J., Martin, D. H., & Van Santbrink, H. (2014). Intraoperative magnetic resonance imaging versus standard neuronavigation for the neurosurgical treatment of glioblastoma: A randomized controlled trial. *Surgical Neurology International, 5*(1), 70. DOI: 10.4103/2152-7806.132572 PMID: 24991473

Laba, A. E., & Ziółkowski, P. (2021). Trends in glioblastoma treatment research: An analysis of clinical trials and literature. *Neurologia i Neurochirurgia Polska, 55*(3), 269–280. DOI: 10.5603/PJNNS.a2021.0024 PMID: 33710606

Lee, J. K., Wang, J., Sa, J. K., Ladewig, E., Lee, H. O., Lee, I. H., Kang, H. J., Rosenbloom, D. S., Camara, P. G., Liu, Z., Van Nieuwenhuizen, P., Jung, S. W., Choi, S. W., Kim, J., Chen, A., Kim, K. T., Shin, S., Seo, Y. J., Oh, J. M., & Nam, D. H. (2017). Spatiotemporal genomic architecture informs precision oncology in glioblastoma. *Nature Genetics*, *49*(4), 594–599. DOI: 10.1038/ng.3806 PMID: 28263318

Leroy, H. A., Vermandel, M., Lejeune, J. P., Mordon, S., & Reyns, N. (2015). Fluorescence guided resection and glioblastoma in 2015: A review. *Lasers in Surgery and Medicine*, *47*(5), 441–451. DOI: 10.1002/lsm.22359 PMID: 25946082

Linkous, , A., & Yazlovitskaya, E. (2011). Angiogenesis in glioblastoma multiforme: Navigating the maze. *Anti-cancer Agents in Medicinal Chemistry*, *11*(8), 712–718. DOI: 10.2174/187152011797378643 PMID: 21707499

Lipková, J., Menze, B., Wiestler, B., Koumoutsakos, P., & Lowengrub, J. S. (2022). Modelling glioma progression, mass effect and intracranial pressure in patient anatomy. *Journal of the Royal Society, Interface*, *19*(188), 20210922. Advance online publication. DOI: 10.1098/rsif.2021.0922 PMID: 35317645

Louis, D. N., Perry, A., Wesseling, P., Brat, D. J., Cree, I. A., Figarella-Branger, D., Hawkins, C., Ng, H. K., Pfister, S. M., Reifenberger, G., Soffietti, R., Von Deimling, A., & Ellison, D. W. (2021). The 2021 WHO Classification of Tumors of the Central Nervous System: A summary. *Neuro-Oncology*, *23*(8), 1231–1251. DOI: 10.1093/neuonc/noab106 PMID: 34185076

Louveau, A., Smirnov, I., Keyes, T. J., Eccles, J. D., Rouhani, S. J., Peske, J. D., Derecki, N. C., Castle, D., Mandell, J. W., Lee, K. S., Harris, T. H., & Kipnis, J. (2015). Structural and functional features of central nervous system lymphatic vessels. *Nature*, *523*(7560), 337–341. DOI: 10.1038/nature14432 PMID: 26030524

Magee, D. E., Hird, A. E., Klaassen, Z., Sridhar, S. S., Nam, R. K., Wallis, C. J. D., & Kulkarni, G. S. (2020). Adverse event profile for immunotherapy agents compared with chemotherapy in solid organ tumors: A systematic review and meta-analysis of randomized clinical trials. *Annals of Oncology : Official Journal of the European Society for Medical Oncology*, *31*(1), 50–60. DOI: 10.1016/j.annonc.2019.10.008 PMID: 31912796

Mahmoudi, K., Bouras, A., Bozec, D., Ivkov, R., & Hadjipanayis, C. (2018). Magnetic hyperthermia therapy for the treatment of glioblastoma: a review of the therapy's history, efficacy and application in humans. *International Journal of Hyperthermia : The Official Journal of European Society for Hyperthermic Oncology. International Journal of Hyperthermia, 34*(8), 1316–1328. DOI: 10.1080/02656736.2018.1430867 PMID: 29353516

McGranahan, T., Therkelsen, K. E., Ahmad, S., & Nagpal, S. (2019). Current State of Immunotherapy for Treatment of Glioblastoma. *Current Treatment Options in Oncology, 20*(3), 24. Advance online publication. DOI: 10.1007/s11864-019-0619-4 PMID: 30790064

Miyai, M., Tomita, H., Soeda, A., Yano, H., Iwama, T., & Hara, A. (2017). Current trends in mouse models of glioblastoma. *Journal of Neuro-Oncology, 135*(3), 423–432. DOI: 10.1007/s11060-017-2626-2 PMID: 29052807

Mohammed, S., Dinesan, M., & Ajayakumar, T. (2022). Survival and quality of life analysis in glioblastoma multiforme with adjuvant chemoradiotherapy: A retrospective study. *Reports of Practical Oncology and Radiotherapy : Journal of Greatpoland Cancer Center in Poznan and Polish Society of Radiation Oncology, 27*(6), 1026–1036. DOI: 10.5603/RPOR.a2022.0113 PMID: 36632307

Molinaro, A. M., Hervey-Jumper, S., Morshed, R. A., Young, J., Han, S. J., Chunduru, P., Zhang, Y., Phillips, J. J., Shai, A., Lafontaine, M., Crane, J., Chandra, A., Flanigan, P., Jahangiri, A., Cioffi, G., Ostrom, Q., Anderson, J. E., Badve, C., Barnholtz-Sloan, J., & Berger, M. S. (2020). Association of maximal extent of resection of contrast-enhanced and non–contrast-enhanced tumor with survival within molecular subgroups of patients with newly diagnosed glioblastoma. *JAMA Oncology, 6*(4), 495–503. DOI: 10.1001/jamaoncol.2019.6143 PMID: 32027343

Namba, H., Kawaji, H., & Yamasaki, T. (2015). Use of genetically engineered stem cells for glioma therapy. *Oncology Letters, 11*(1), 9–15. DOI: 10.3892/ol.2015.3860 PMID: 26870161

Nguyen, T. K., Sahgal, A., Detsky, J., Soliman, H., Myrehaug, S., Tseng, C. L., Husain, Z. A., Carty, A., Das, S., Yang, V., Lee, Y., Sarfehnia, A., Chugh, B. P., Yeboah, C., & Ruschin, M. (2019). Single-Fraction Stereotactic Radiosurgery Versus Hippocampal Avoidance Whole Brain Radiation Therapy for Patients With 10 to 30 Brain Metastases: A Dosimetric Analysis. *International Journal of Radiation Oncology, Biology, Physics, 105*(2), 394–399. DOI: 10.1016/j.ijrobp.2019.06.2543 PMID: 31283978

Nishiyama, N., Matsumura, Y., & Kataoka, K. (2016). Development of polymeric micelles for targeting intractable cancers. *Cancer Science, 107*(7), 867–874. DOI: 10.1111/cas.12960 PMID: 27116635

Patil, C. G., Pricola, K., Sarmiento, J. M., Garg, S. K., Bryant, A., & Black, K. L. (2017). Whole brain radiation therapy (WBRT) alone versus WBRT and radiosurgery for the treatment of brain metastases. *Cochrane Database of Systematic Reviews, 9*(9). Advance online publication. DOI: 10.1002/14651858.CD006121.pub4 PMID: 28945270

Pessina, F., Navarria, P., Cozzi, L., Ascolese, A. M., Simonelli, M., Santoro, A., Clerici, E., Rossi, M., Scorsetti, M., & Bello, L. (2017). Maximize surgical resection beyond contrast-enhancing boundaries in newly diagnosed glioblastoma multiforme: Is it useful and safe? A single institution retrospective experience. *Journal of Neuro-Oncology, 135*(1), 129–139. DOI: 10.1007/s11060-017-2559-9 PMID: 28689368

Pichierri, A., Bradley, M., & Iyer, V. (2019). Intraoperative magnetic resonance imaging–guided glioma resections in awake or asleep settings and feasibility in the context of a public health system. *World Neurosurgery: X, 3*, 100022. DOI: 10.1016/j.wnsx.2019.100022 PMID: 31225516

Qiu, J., Kong, L., Cao, X., Li, A., Wei, P., Wang, L., Mignani, S., Caminade, A. M., Majoral, J. P., & Shi, X. (2018). Enhanced Delivery of Therapeutic siRNA into Glioblastoma Cells Using Dendrimer-Entrapped Gold Nanoparticles Conjugated with β-Cyclodextrin. *Nanomaterials (Basel, Switzerland), 8*(3), 131. Advance online publication. DOI: 10.3390/nano8030131 PMID: 29495429

Queirolo, P., Spagnolo, F., Ascierto, P. A., Simeone, E., Marchetti, P., Scoppola, A., Del Vecchio, M., Di Guardo, L., Maio, M., Di Giacomo, A. M., Antonuzzo, A., Cognetti, F., Ferraresi, V., Ridolfi, L., Guidoboni, M., Guida, M., Pigozzo, J., & Chiarion Sileni, V. (2014). Efficacy and safety of ipilimumab in patients with advanced melanoma and brain metastases. *Journal of Neuro-Oncology, 118*(1), 109–116. DOI: 10.1007/s11060-014-1400-y PMID: 24532241

Rainer Wirtz, W. S., Albert, F. K., Schwaderer, M., Heuer, C., Staubert, A., Tronnier, V. M., Knauth, M., & Kunze, S. (2000). The benefit of neuronavigation for neurosurgery analyzed by its impact on glioblastoma surgery. *Neurological Research, 22*(4), 354–360. DOI: 10.1080/01616412.2000.11740684 PMID: 10874684

Riemenschneider, M. J., Jeuken, J. W. M., Wesseling, P., & Reifenberger, G. (2010). Molecular diagnostics of gliomas: State of the art. *Acta Neuropathologica, 120*(5), 567–584. DOI: 10.1007/s00401-010-0736-4 PMID: 20714900

Sadelain, M., Rivière, I., & Riddell, S. (2017). Therapeutic T cell engineering. *Nature, 545*(7655), 423–431. DOI: 10.1038/nature22395 PMID: 28541315

Sanai, N., Polley, M. Y., McDermott, M. W., Parsa, A. T., & Berger, M. S. (2011). An extent of resection threshold for newly diagnosed glioblastomas. *Journal of Neurosurgery, 115*(1), 3–8. DOI: 10.3171/2011.2.JNS10998 PMID: 21417701

. Sarhangi, N., Patrinos, G. P., Aghaei Meybodi, H. R., Nikfar, S., Sarrami, B., Kiani, P., Larijani, B., Khodayari, N., &Hasanzad, M. (2024). Personalized Medicine and Therapeutics. *A Glimpse at Medicine in the Future*, 111–127. .DOI: 10.1007/978-981-97-4974-4_7

Saxena, M., van der Burg, S. H., Melief, C. J. M., & Bhardwaj, N. (2021, June). (202*1). Therapeutic cancer* vaccines. *Nature Reviews. Cancer, 21*(6), 360–378. DOI: 10.1038/s41568-021-00346-0 PMID: 33907315

Senders, J. T., Muskens, I. S., Schnoor, R., Karhade, A. V., Cote, D. J., Smith, T. R., & Broekman, M. L. (2017). Agents for fluorescence-guided glioma surgery: A systematic review of preclinical and clinical results. *Acta Neurochirurgica, 159*(1), 151–167. DOI: 10.1007/s00701-016-3028-5 PMID: 27878374

Shah, S., Green, J., Graff, S. A., Li, Q., & Heiss, J. D. (2025). Gene Therapy for Glioblastoma Multiforme. *Viruses, 17*(1), 118. Advance online publication. DOI: 10.3390/v17010118 PMID: 39861907

Shan, F. Y., Zhao, D., Tirado, C. A., Fonkem, E., Zhang, Y., Feng, D., Huang, J. H., Shan, F. Y., Zhao, D., Tirado, C. A., Fonkem, E., Zhang, Y., Feng, D., & Huang, J. H. (2022). *Glioblastomas: Molecular Diagnosis and Pathology*. Glioblastoma - Current Evidence., DOI: 10.5772/intechopen.105472

Sloan, E. A., Hilz, S., Gupta, R., Cadwell, C., Ramani, B., Hofmann, J., Kline, C. N., Banerjee, A., Reddy, A., Oberheim Bush, N. A., Chang, S., Braunstein, S., Chang, E. F., Raffel, C., Gupta, N., Sun, P. P., Kim, J. Y. H., Moes, G., Alva, E., & Solomon, D. A. (2020). Gliomas arising in the setting of Li-Fraumeni syndrome stratify into two molecular subgroups with diver*gent clinicopathologi*c *fea*tures. *Acta Neuropathologica, 139*(5), 953–957. DOI: 10.1007/s00401-020-02144-8 PMID: 32157385

. Stenström, P., Manzanarcs, D., Zhang, Y., Ceña, V., &Malkoch, M. (2018). Evaluation of Amino-Functional Polyester Dendrimers Based on Bis-MPA as Nonviral Vectors for siRNA Delivery. *Molecules 2018, Vol. 23, Page 2028, 23*(8), 2028. .DOI: 10.3390/molecules23082028

Stichel, D., Ebrahimi, A., Reuss, D., Schrimpf, D., Ono, T., Shirahata, M., Reifenberger, G., Weller, M., Hänggi, D., Wick, W., Herold-Mende, C., Westphal, M., Brandner, S., Pfister, S. M., Capper, D., Sahm, F., & von Deimling, A. (2018). Distribution of EGFR amplification, combined chromosome 7 gain and chromosome 10 loss, and TERT promoter mutation in brain tumors and their potential for the reclassification of IDHwt astrocytoma to glioblastoma. *Acta Neuropathologica, 136*(5), 793–803. DOI: 10.1007/s00401-018-1905-0 PMID: 30187121

Suchorska, B., Weller, M., Tabatabai, G., Senft, C., Hau, P., Sabel, M. C., Herrlinger, U., Ketter, R., Schlegel, U., Marosi, C., Reifenberger, G., Wick, W., Tonn, J. C., & Wirsching, H. G. (2016). Complete resection of contrast-enhancing tumor volume is associated with improved survival in recurrent glioblastoma—Results from the DIRECTOR trial. *Neuro-Oncology, 18*(4), 549–556. DOI: 10.1093/neuonc/nov326 PMID: 26823503

Tang, X., Zuo, C., Fang, P., Liu, G., Qiu, Y., Huang, Y., & Tang, R. (2021). Targeting Glioblastoma Stem Cells: A Review on Biomarkers, Signal Pathways and Targeted Therapy. *Frontiers in Oncology, 11*, 701291. DOI: 10.3389/fonc.2021.701291 PMID: 34307170

Topalian, S. L., Drake, C. G., & Pardoll, D. M. (2015). Immune checkpoint blockade: A common denominator approach to cancer therapy. *Cancer Cell, 27*(4), 450–461. DOI: 10.1016/j.ccell.2015.03.001 PMID: 25858804

Turcotte, E. L., Jones, B. A., Chhabra, N., Porter, A. B., Donev, K., Hu, L. S., & Bendok, B. R. (2023). Awake microsurgical resection of a motor cortex glioma with cortical and subcortical motor mapping, image guidance, and augmented reality: 2-dimensional operative video. *Operative Neurosurgery (Hagerstown, Md.), 24*(2), e122. DOI: 10.1227/ons.0000000000000525 PMID: 36637320

Urbanska, K., Sokolowska, J., Szmidt, M., & Sysa, P. (2014). Glioblastoma multiforme - an overview. *Contemporary Oncology = Współczesna Onkologia, 18*(5), 307–312. DOI: 10.5114/wo.2014.40559 PMID: 25477751

Verhaak, R. G. W., Hoadley, K. A., Purdom, E., Wang, V., Qi, Y., Wilkerson, M. D., Miller, C. R., Ding, L., Golub, T., Mesirov, J. P., Alexe, G., Lawrence, M., O'Kelly, M., Tamayo, P., Weir, B. A., Gabriel, S., Winckler, W., Gupta, S., Jakkula, L., & Hayes, D. N. (2010). Integrated genomic analysis identifies clinically relevant subtypes of glioblastoma characterized by abnormalities in PDGFRA, IDH1, EGFR, and NF1. *Cancer Cell, 17*(1), 98–110. DOI: 10.1016/j.ccr.2009.12.020 PMID: 20129251

Wang, Y., Luo, R., Zhang, X., Xiang, H., Yang, B., Feng, J., Deng, M., Ran, P., Sujie, A., Zhang, F., Zhu, J., Tan, S., Xie, T., Chen, P., Yu, Z., Li, Y., Jiang, D., Zhang, X., Zhao, J. Y., & Ding, C. (2023). Proteogenomics of diffuse gliomas reveal molecular subtypes associated with specific therapeutic targets and immune-evasion mechanisms. *Nature Communications*, *14*(1), 505. Advance online publication. DOI: 10.1038/s41467-023-36005-1 PMID: 36720864

Wang, Y., Wang, Z., Hua, C., Xu, Y., Li, Y., & Zhao, G. (2022). Primary Malignant Brain Tumors following Systemic Malignancies: A Population-Based Analysis. *Neuroepidemiology*, *56*(6), 452–459. DOI: 10.1159/000527437 PMID: 36244332

West, C. M., & Barnett, G. C. (2011). Genetics and genomics of radiotherapy toxicity: Towards prediction. *Genome Medicine*, *3*(8), 52. Advance online publication. DOI: 10.1186/gm268 PMID: 21861849

Wick, W., Weller, M., Van Den Bent, M., Sanson, M., Weiler, M., Von Deimling, A., Plass, C., Hegi, M., Platten, M., & Reifenberger, G. (2014). MGMT testing—The challenges for biomarker-based glioma treatment. *Nature Reviews. Neurology*, *10*(7), 372–385. DOI: 10.1038/nrneurol.2014.100 PMID: 24912512

Wilke, C., Grosshans, D., Duman, J., Brown, P., & Li, J. (2018). Radiation-induced cognitive toxicity: Pathophysiology and interventions to reduce toxicity in adults. *Neuro-Oncology*, *20*(5), 597–607. DOI: 10.1093/neuonc/nox195 PMID: 29045710

Yan, C., Wang, J., Yang, Y., Ma, W., & Chen, X. (2019). Molecular biomarker-guided anti-angiogenic targeted therapy for malignant glioma. *Journal of Cellular and Molecular Medicine*, *23*(8), 4876–4882. DOI: 10.1111/jcmm.14417 PMID: 31210419

Yang, C. Y., Liu, H. W., Tsai, Y. C., Tseng, J. Y., Liang, S. C., Chen, C. Y., Lian, W. N., Wei, M. C., Lu, M., Lu, R. H., Lin, C. H., & Jiang, J. K. (2015). Interleukin-4 receptor-targeted liposomal doxorubicin as a model for enhancing cellular uptake and antitumor efficacy in murine colorectal cancer. *Cancer Biology & Therapy*, *16*(11), 1641–1650. DOI: 10.1080/15384047.2015.1095397 PMID: 26436767

Zhao, M., van Straten, D., Broekman, M. L. D., Préat, V., & Schiffelers, R. M. (2020). Nanocarrier-based drug combination therapy for glioblastoma. *Theranostics*, *10*(3), 1355–1372. DOI: 10.7150/thno.38147 PMID: 31938069

Zhao, T., Li, C., Ge, H., Lin, Y., & Kang, D. (2022). Glioblastoma vaccine tumor therapy research progress. *Chinese Neurosurgical Journal*, *8*(1), 2. Advance online publication. DOI: 10.1186/s41016-021-00269-7 PMID: 35045874

Chapter 2
Current Challenges and Significant Innovations for Glioblastoma

Amritha Chakkittukandiyil
https://orcid.org/0000-0002-2683-8341
Department of Pharmacology, National College of Pharmacy, Kerala University of Health Sciences, Manassery, India

Deepak Vasudevan Sajini
https://orcid.org/0000-0003-2200-8401
Department of Pharmacology, National College of Pharmacy, Kerala University of Health Sciences, Manassery, India

S. Venkatesh
Department of Pharmacology, College of Pharmacy, Kannur Medical College, Anjarakandy, India

Sujith Varma K.
https://orcid.org/0000-0002-0866-5571
Department of Pharmaceutics, National College of Pharmacy, Kerala University of Health Sciences, Manassery, India

ABSTRACT

Glioblastoma is the most common and malignant primary brain tumor, having a high fatality rate. It is distinguished by fast development, medication resistance, a poor prognosis, and few therapeutic choices. These obstacles are caused by variables such as molecular heterogeneity, complicated genetic composition, and the blood-brain barrier, which prevents efficient medication administration. Nonetheless, recent improvements provide optimism. Personalized medicine and

DOI: 10.4018/979-8-3373-2695-5.ch002

molecular-targeted treatments tailor treatment to a tumor's unique genetic makeup. Nanotechnology, CRISPR-Cas9 gene editing, and innovative drug delivery technologies have improved bioavailability and therapeutic accuracy. Furthermore, sophisticated imaging methods and liquid biopsies aid in early detection, real-time monitoring, and therapy optimization. This chapter provides a detailed overview of current glioblastoma management difficulties and focuses on developing treatments that have the potential to alter therapy results.

1. INTRODUCTION

Glioblastoma multiforme (GBM) is the most common and aggressive malignant brain tumor found in adults. GBMs occur primarily in the brain but can also affect the brainstem, cerebellum, and spinal cord. Astrocytic tumor cells with poor differentiation, nuclear atypia, microvascular proliferation, and necrosis are among the histological characteristics of GBM. About sixty-one percent of all primary gliomas occur in the four lobes of the brain: frontal (25%), temporal (20%), parietal (13%), and occipital (3%) (Davis, 2016). The WHO Classification of CNS Tumors states that GB is the most aggressive and deadly of all primary brain tumors and the highest and worst prognostic-grade, or "grade IV," glioma (Brat et al., 2008). The GBM grade IV is recognized by its increased cellular density, microvascular proliferation, nuclear abnormalities, necrosis, and invasiveness. The GBM is a fast-growing and aggressive brain tumor that is more commonly detected in older persons (Ohgaki et al., 2004). According to data gathered in the Central Brain Tumor Registry of the United States (CBTRUS) from 2014 to 2018, GB accounted for 14.5% of all CNS tumors and 48.6% of the malignant ones, despite being regarded as an uncommon tumor with an incidence rate of around 3 per 100,000 persons (Ostrom et al., 2020).

It was thought that GBM originates when cells in the brain or spinal cord undergo DNA alterations caused by mutations or variances. GBM can be broadly classified into primary, or de novo arising without a known precursor, and secondary, where a low-grade tumor transforms over time into GBM. The etiology of GBM is still unknown. Ionizing radiation is considered as a common risk factor associated with GBM (Ellor et al., 2014). The radiation-induced GBMs are seen after years of therapeutic radiation prescribed for another tumor or conditions (Johnson et al., 2015). Other environmental factors contributing to GBM are exposure to vinyl chloride, smoking, pesticides, petroleum refining, and the manufacture of synthetic rubber. Studies have shown that the use of electromagnetic fields, formaldehyde, mobile phones, and non-ionizing radiation will trigger the incidence of GBM (Alifieris & Trafalis, 2015). Age is also considered as a factor for the development of GBM (Liguori, 2024). Specific genetic diseases like neurofibromatosis 1 and 2, Li

Fraumeni syndrome, tuberous sclerosis, and retinoblastoma can increase the risk of glioma development. Common symptoms linked with GBM include headaches that intensify, muscular weakness in the face, arms, or legs, difficulties with balance and coordination, altered sense of touch, nausea and vomiting, blurred or double vision, difficulty speaking, seizures, and memory loss. The symptoms might vary widely depending on the size and location of the tumor, as well as the anatomical components of the affected brain region (Young et al., 2015). It was previously considered that GBM develops when cells in the brain or spinal cord suffer DNA changes caused by mutations or variations (Perry et al., 2006; Schiff et al., 2015). The first-line treatment for glioblastoma is surgery, which can aid with diagnosis and cytoreduction, followed by stereotactic radiation and chemotherapy. There are currently just a few FDA-approved medications for GB, including temozolomide (TMZ), Bevacizumab, CCNU, and BiCNU (Bae et al., 2024). The most safe surgical resection, radiation treatment (RT), and chemotherapy with TMZ have been the standard of care (Ng et al., 2024). TMZ's anti-tumor activity is restricted by its poor capacity to penetrate the BBB (only reaching 20% of blood concentration) and cellular processes that impart therapeutic resistance. New therapeutic alternatives are urgently needed (Grochans et al., 2022). With a median progression-free survival (mPFS) of 6.7 months and a median overall survival (mOS) of 20.9 months, the prognosis is still dismal. In recurrent illness, where there is no standard of treatment and the mOS from the initial recurrence is around 6.5 months, the therapeutic results are considerably worse (Bae et al., 2024; van Linde et al., 2017).

GBM has become the enemy of contemporary medicine, with current therapy techniques failing to dramatically improve patient outcomes after decades of study. This brain tumor has a median overall survival time of less than two years and a nearly 100% death rate under current treatment methods. The primary cause of treatment failure in the case of GBM is the inadequate passage of medicament to the targeted area through the blood-brain barrier (BBB). Recent investigations have uncovered numerous major hurdles to GBM biology, including its amazing heterogeneity, capacity to elude immune responses, and the protective BBB, which restricts treatment delivery. The discovery of innovative and more effective therapy techniques will help to extend the lives of GBM patients. One such strategy is nanoparticle-based therapy, which interacts with specialized transport mechanisms that can traverse the BBB to boost therapeutic efficacy while minimizing systemic toxicity and drug degradation. The polymeric nanoparticles are designed to deliver drugs to the brain with minimal systemic adverse effects (Chiariello et al., 2023).

2. KEY CHALLENGES IN GLIOBLASTOMA TREATMENT

GBM has a poor prognosis and progresses quickly. Treating GBM is still extremely difficult despite advancements in medical science because of a number of internal and external causes (Sadowski et al., 2024).

2.1. Tumor Molecular Heterogeneity and Infiltration

One of the main characteristics of GBM is the high intra- and intertumoral heterogeneity. Heterogeneity indicates that the cells found within the same tumor and between individuals have distinct genetic, molecular, and phenotypic profiles (Becker et al., 2021; Friedmann-Morvinski, 2014). This further leads to resistance towards the targeted therapies and promotes recurrence. This variety presents a considerable obstacle for targeted medication administration. Heterogeneity can have an impact on tumor diagnosis and characterization since it is difficult to obtain a complete description of the entire genetic signature in such a heterogeneous tumor using surgical specimens. Multiple biopsies should be conducted and repeated during the course of GB to have a greater probability of correct diagnosis. This approach is not realistic nor sustainable for the patient (Del Bene et al., 2022). Furthermore, the variability of GBs makes it exceedingly difficult to target all tumor cells within the same patient and to treat different patients with the same therapy (Reardon & Wen, 2015). Genetic diversity in GBM involves changes in crucial signalling pathways, including the PI3K/AKT/mTOR, p53, and RAS/MAPK pathways, resulting in varied treatment responses among patients. Even in one tumor, various areas can show unique genetic characteristics, leading to different drug responses and the emergence of resistant subclones (Degl'Innocenti et al., 2020; Parker et al., 2016). This unpredictability is made much more difficult by the tumor's highly infiltrative nature, which makes total surgical excision impossible since cancer cells invade healthy brain tissue beyond the visible tumor boundaries by spreading along blood arteries and white-matter pathways. As a result, remaining infiltrative cells, which often have stem-like and treatment-resistant traits, evade standard treatments like radiation, chemotherapy, and surgery, which eventually causes tumor recurrence and adverse patient outcomes (Seker-Polat et al., 2022; Malhotra & Rahman, 2024).

2.2. Impact of BBB on Drug Delivery

The blood-brain barrier (BBB) serves as the brain's own security system, carefully monitoring what enters and exits to maintain the central nervous system's equilibrium. It protects the brain from hazardous chemicals in the circulation, such as viruses and other infections, while still letting important nutrients to flow through.

This protective barrier is made up of closely linked, non-fenestrated endothelial cells that line the brain's small blood arteries, strengthened by specific junctions, and surrounded by glial cells' supporting end feet (Liguori, 2024). Although the BBB protects the brain, it also makes it more difficult for many treatments to reach the brain, thereby limiting the therapeutic use of the drug. About 95% of systemic medications cannot reach tumors due to the BBB, and the hypoxic areas of GBM further diminish the effectiveness of medications (Oliver et al., 2021). The BBB uses a variety of mechanisms to restrict drug delivery, including efflux transporters like P-glycoprotein (P-gp) and Multidrug Resistance-associated Proteins (MRPs), which aggressively pump out medicines that manage to enter endothelial cells. Furthermore, the BBB's high production of metabolic enzymes destroys therapeutic medicines before they reach their target within the brain (Rajendran & Vadakkepushpakath, 2024). Overcoming the BBB is one of the primary objectives of GBM research. Methods including medication delivery by nanoparticles, targeted ultrasound-assisted BBB rupture, and the production of BBB-penetrating peptides are also being researched (Barzegar-Fallah et al., 2022). Furthermore, because the barrier functions in both ways, the passage of chemicals from the brain to the circulation is similarly reduced, decreasing the diagnostic value of liquid biopsies based on blood samples for brain illnesses (Del Bene et al., 2022).

2.3. Immunosuppressive Microenvironment

The immunosuppressive nature of the tumor microenvironment (TME) is one of the important aspects of the tumor to escape from the immune response. The major characteristic features of TME that make the treatment more difficult are hypoxia, immune suppression, and a rich extracellular matrix (ECM). GBM exhibits hypoxia or low oxygen levels inside the tumor, thereby making the tumor more resistant to radiation and therapy (Feldman, 2024). ECM is made of collagen and hyaluronic acid which serves as a excellent barrier to medication penetration physically. Myeloid-derived suppressor cells (MDSCs) and tumor-associated macrophages in the TME aid in tumor growth and immune evasion. Effective immunotherapy is further hampered by the presence of regulatory T cells and the production of immunosuppressive cytokines. Through interactions with cellular receptors that trigger survival pathways, this extracellular matrix can trap therapeutic drugs, preventing them from accessing the tumor cells, and contribute to treatment resistance (Zhang et al., 2022; Lin et al., 2024).

2.4. Resistance to Existing Therapies

Therapeutic resistance is one of the leading reasons of poor prognosis in GB patients. This characteristic worsens over time, undermining existing treatment options for recurrent GB. In most situations, resection is no longer viable, and chemotherapy and radiation fail to prevent tumor development (Yekula et al., 2021). The typical chemotherapeutic drug given to patients with GBM is temozolomide, approved by the FDA in 2005. GBM-temozolomide resistance is a significant barrier to successful therapy and is caused by several interconnected pathways. Therapeutic resistance increases with time due to the molecular alterations that occur throughout GB development. The main cause for this resistance is the overexpression of O6-methylguanine-DNA methyltransferase (MGMT), a DNA repair enzyme that directly reverses the cytotoxic DNA lesions caused by temozolomide and prevents tumor cell death. Patients whose tumors have a methylated (silenced) MGMT promoter typically respond better to temozolomide, whereas patients with high MGMT expression show resistance. The mismatch repair (MMR) system, which typically detects and handles temozolomide-induced DNA mismatches, might have flaws that allow tumor cells to withstand DNA damage without dying. These flaws are one of the additional resistance mechanisms (Woo et al., 2019). Overexpression of Histone deacetylase 6 (HDAC6) in GBM has also been shown to provide resistance to temozolomide-mediated cell growth suppression and apoptosis induction (Wang et al., 2016).

2.5. Recurrence and Lack of Curative Options

GBM has a poor prognosis with a median survival period of 14 months. Even after intensive initial treatment with surgery, radiation, and chemotherapy, GBM has a nearly universal recurrence rate (Vaz-Salgado et al., 2023). Every patient with GBM has the potential to relapse. Almost all GB tumors reappear after surgery, radiation, and chemotherapy, and have a reduced response rate to standard treatments, leaving relatively little therapeutic alternatives available. Following first-line therapy, further treatment options become limited, making the treatment for the disease recurrence more challenging. The main cause of recurrence is the tumor's heterogeneous and infiltrative character, which makes total eradication challenging. The majority of recurrences happen around the original tumor location, indicating microscopic illness that persists after the first therapy. Recurrent GBM is often treated with systemic chemotherapy, targeted medicines, re-irradiation, repeat surgery, and, more recently, novel treatments such as immunotherapy and oncolytic virus therapy. Controversy surrounds the most effective treatment method for recurring illness, and there is no therapeutic standard for this condition (Birzu et al., 2021). Despite the lack of evidence suggesting that a second surgery for GBM significantly improves survival, clinicians usually give surgical intervention when it is thought to be practical. This ongoing lack of treatment alternatives is a result of a number of particular difficulties, including the tumor's resistance to cell death, its capacity to adjust to treatments, the BBB's protective environment, and, in the majority of instances, the lack of obvious molecular targets. For recurrence, systemic therapy is frequently advised, with nitrosoureas (such as lomustine) being the most prevalent kind. Nevertheless, nitrosourea-based treatment has little efficacy (Wick et al., 2010). Since no recurrence treatment is better than any other, the course of treatment is determined by the preferences of the particular center and the unique features of each patient, including age, performance status, tumor location, time to recurrence, and usage of corticosteroids (Carson et al., 2007; Mineo et al., 2007). Thus, GBM recurrence continues to be the main barrier to recovery, and novel treatment approaches are desperately needed to help afflicted people.

2.6. Limitations of Current Imaging and Diagnostic Tools

The standard therapeutic strategy, which includes radiation, chemotherapy, and surgical excision, has significant drawbacks, especially when it comes to dealing with the invasive nature of gliomas. When describing the features of a tumor, typical diagnostic techniques such as computed tomography (CT), magnetic resonance imaging (MRI), and positron emission tomography (PET) are essential. Nevertheless, they have drawbacks, including low biological specificity and difficulties in identifying areas of active tumors. In the fight against this difficult brain tumor, the continuous advancement of diagnostic instruments and treatment strategies offers a complex and exciting new battlefield (Thenuwara et al., 2203). In certain therapeutic settings, access to advanced imaging modalities may be restricted due to their high cost and limited availability (Pulumati et al., 2023).

3. INNOVATIVE TREATMENT STRATEGIES FOR GBM

The currently available standard of care for GBM consists of surgically removing the tumor, followed by radiation therapy that is concurrent with chemotherapy and temozolomide (Stupp et al., 2005). In recent decades, there have been notable advancements and innovations in treating GBM. Nevertheless, recurrence is frequently unavoidable, and patient survival is still dismal despite the advancements. Tumor complexity, the presence of the BBB, and the presence of GBM cancer stem cells are some of the factors that make it difficult to find an effective therapeutic option. As a result, it is necessary to improve current treatment approaches and look into new treatment alternatives to improve GBM treatment strategies (Aldoghachi et al., 2022).

3.1. Immunotherapy in GBM

This seeks to use the patient's immune system to combat the tumor. The strategies include vaccinations, oncolytic viruses, immune checkpoint inhibitors, and adoptive cell transfer (such as CAR-T treatment). Among these, immune checkpoint inhibitors have demonstrated great results in a patient population with melanomas and other malignancies. Therapeutic vaccinations are also emerging as promising cancer therapies, with now three therapeutic cancer vaccines licensed by the FDA (Bausart et al., 2022).

The main goal of immunotherapies is to overcome the immunosuppressive environment by activating both innate and adaptive immune responses (Majc et al., 2021). However, the majority of patients still do not react to immunotherapy, despite the fact that it has been proven to improve survival for a certain percentage of patients with solid tumors. Immune checkpoint inhibitors now have a response rate of less than 15% for cancer patients (Haslam & Prasad, 2019). The GBM microenvironment's immunosuppressive characteristics, along with the brain's unique immunological privilege, provide substantial challenges to successful immunotherapy adoption (Zhang et al., 2022).

An important development is the DCVax-L vaccine, which in a Phase III study showed a statistically significant improvement in median survival when compared to standard-of-care (19.3 months versus 16.5 months). Although the inclusion of an external control group reduces the quality of the data, this is one of the first Phase III immunotherapy trials in GBM to be effective (Ng et al., 2024).

One of the primary targets for GBM monotherapy is glioma-associated macrophages (GAMs), which play an important role in tumor formation, immune suppression, and treatment resistance. GAMs promote the proliferation of tumor cells by directly interacting with the glioma cells (Ng et al., 2024). This includes several strategies like reprogramming GAMs from an immunosuppressive M2 phenotype to a pro-inflammatory M1 phenotype to improve the anti-tumor response (Chen et al., 2022). Depleting GAMs with CSF-1R inhibitors is an additional tactic that lowers the quantity of macrophages that support tumors. Additionally, treatments that target pro-tumor signalling pathways like PI3K and CCL2/CCR2 try to stop tumor growth that is driven by macrophages. To specifically alter GAM function and enhance treatment efficacy, cutting-edge techniques such as delivery via nanoparticles are being investigated (Eckert et al., 2025).

Making artificial lymph node structures to boost anti-tumor immune responses is one really creative strategy. To stop glioma recurrence, researchers have created an in situ sprayed exosome-cross-linked gel that acts as a synthetic lymph node by directly stimulating T cells that have infiltrated tumors. A bio-orthogonal interaction between alkyne-modified alginate polymers and azide-modified chimeric exosomes produces this gel. The gel structure delays the immune system's rapid clearance of the chimeric exosomes, which are made from dendritic cell-tumor hybrid cells, extending the duration of antitumor immunity while enabling strong T-cell activation (Bao et al., 2024).

An additional novel immunotherapeutic approach for GBM involves the use of bispecific antibodies (biAbs). These altered proteins enable targeted immune responses by their capability to simultaneously attach to two different antigens, typically one on immune cells and another on tumor cells. B7-H3 (CD276), part of the B7 superfamily associated with low survival rates in GBM patients, has recently been investigated as a possible target for biAb therapy. Scientists have developed recombinant anti-B7-H3×CD3 biAbs to forge a direct link between T cells and GBM cells that express B7-H3. The development of nanoparticles activated by matrix metalloproteinase-2 (MMP-2) that include these B7-H3 bispecific antibodies is a significant progress in this area. The engineered S-biAb/dEGCG@NPs demonstrated enhanced intracranial accumulation, with levels that were 4.1-, 9.5-, and 12.3-fold greater than those of biAb/dEGCG@NPs, biAb/dEGCG complexes, and free biAbs, respectively (Fan et al., 2023).

3.2. Molecular and genetically targeted therapies

One of the most often studied targets in GBM, especially in the classical subtype, is the epidermal growth factor receptor (EGFR). Despite a large number of clinical trials, EGFR-targeted therapies have not yet resulted in significant clinical benefits for GBM patients. The development of more specialized agents and an understanding of the mechanisms underlying resistance to these therapies are still priorities. These resistance mechanisms include tumor heterogeneity, EGFR's kinase-independent pro-survival functions, poor BBB penetration, mutations, and compensatory signalling pathways (Begagić et al., 2023; Rodriguez et al., 2023).

Additional commonly targeted pathways consist of the mammalian target of rapamycin (mTOR), vascular endothelial growth factor (VEGF), and mitogen-activated protein kinase (MEK). These pathways play a role in cell development, blood vessel formation, and survival. Inhibitors aimed at these have been assessed in both preclinical and clinical environments, showing differing levels of effectiveness. Research is underway on combination therapies that simultaneously target various pathways to address resistance and enhance outcomes (Begagić et al., 2023).

Another strategy being explored is targeting regulators of the cell cycle and the tumor microenvironment. These strategies seek to hinder the spread of GBM cells and alter the supportive surroundings that foster tumor development (Zhao et al., 2024). An improved prognosis is linked to isocitrate dehydrogenase (IDH) mutations, which are frequently seen in secondary GBMs. Novel strategies include IDH inhibitors and medications that target the epigenetic changes brought on by these mutations, such as DNA methylation. The potential of DNA methyltransferase and histone deacetylase inhibitors to control tumor development is being investigated (Han et al., 2020).

3.3. Gene Therapy and Oncolytic Viruses

With subgroups (mesenchymal, classical, and proneural) exhibiting distinct genetic profiles and treatment responses, GBM is incredibly diverse. To match treatments to the biological traits of each GBM subtype, precision medicine techniques, including gene editing and customized gene delivery, are being developed; however, practical translation is still difficult because of patient heterogeneity and trial design constraints (Koes et al., 2025). In gene therapy, therapeutic approaches include blocking oncogenic miRNAs using antagomiRs or re-establishing tumor-suppressive miRNAs with synthetic mimics. Viral vectors, lipid nanoparticles, or exosome-based systems that can penetrate the BBB and reach tumor cells are used to deliver these compounds. Furthermore, miRNAs are useful indicators for diagnosis and prognosis that aid in the creation of tailored treatments for GBM (Rajput, 2025).

Gene therapy typically depends on vectors to transport therapeutic genes into GBM cells. Viral vectors (such as adenovirus, lentivirus, and adeno-associated virus) are effective for gene delivery but can trigger immune reactions. Non-viral vectors (such as lipid nanoparticles and polymers) provide reduced immunogenicity and can be designed for tumor selectivity. These systems are employed to deliver genes that trigger apoptosis, block oncogenic signalling, or alter the tumor microenvironment (Rajput, 2025)

Oncolytic virotherapy, which employs viruses designed to target and lyse tumor cells while promoting anti-tumor immunity specifically, has become a viable treatment approach for GBM (Hamad et al., 2023). Oncolytic viruses (OVs) have two main effects: direct destruction of tumors and stimulation of the immune system. In GBM patients, Ovs alter the tumor microenvironment (TME), prompting a shift in tumor-associated macrophages/microglia (TAMs) phenotypes, decreasing immunosuppressive M2-like TAMs while boosting pro-inflammatory M1-like populations (Blitz et al., 2022; van den Bossche et al., 2018). Clinical trials have evaluated more than 20 oncolytic viruses for the treatment of GB. These include poliovirus, Ad, Reovirus, MVs, NDVs, and HSV-1. The convection-enhanced delivery (CED) of the recombinant non-pathogenic polio-rhinovirus chimera (PVSRIPO) is an example of how novel OV delivery approaches have been refined to circumvent the BBB constraint. CED is a cutting-edge novel method that transfers medicinal chemicals in the CNS's interstitial spaces via a pressure gradient in a catheter. For virotherapy to be effective, oncolytic viruses must be delivered safely and effectively (Hamad et al., 2023).

3.4. Tumor-Treating Fields (TTF)

TTF therapy involves administering alternating electrical fields produced by a portable battery-operated device, transmitted to the tumor through 4 (2 pairs) transducer arrays positioned on the patient's skin around the tumor site (Khagi et al., 2024). The portability of the device enables its use at home and while performing daily tasks, thereby integrating it into patients' everyday lives. TTF works through a variety of methods, including disrupting cancer cell mitosis, inhibiting DNA replication and damage response, interfering with cell motility, and enhancing systemic antitumor immunity (Khagi et al., 2024). According to new research, TTF can alter the tumor microenvironment to enhance anticancer immune responses (Park et al., 2019). Increased leukocyte recruitment, improved dendritic cell phagocytosis of cancer cells, and activation of dendritic cell maturation are all components of the antitumor immune response brought on by TTF (Voloshin et al., 2020). The delivery of TTF is being optimized through the development of sophisticated computer modeling and individualized treatment planning techniques, with a focus on enhancing field intensity at the tumor site while avoiding negative effects on nearby healthy tissue (Mikic et al., 2024).

3.5. Nanotechnology-Based Therapies

Nanoparticles are becoming more frequently utilized to enhance drug delivery to the brain by bypassing the BBB, aiming at tumor cells, and minimizing systemic toxicity. Lipid-based nanoparticles, dendrimers, and polymeric nanoparticles can enclose chemotherapeutic agents, siRNA, or CRISPR elements. For example, nanoparticles loaded with temozolomide or doxorubicin have demonstrated improved penetration and effectiveness in preclinical GBM models (Liu et al., 2023). Nanocarriers can be designed to encapsulate a range of therapeutic agents, such as chemotherapy medications, small molecule inhibitors, nucleic acids for gene treatment, and even mixtures of several agents for enhanced effects. Their dimensions generally vary from 10 to 200 nm, where smaller dimensions (10–50 nm) enable improved tumor infiltration, cellular absorption, and TME dispersion, whereas larger dimensions (100–200 nm) encourage extended circulation, increased retention at the tumor location, and diminished clearance via renal filtration (Yusuf et al., 2023). Only a small number of liposomal techniques have advanced to clinical trials in GB, despite all the advancements in this sector. Several phase I/II clinical studies were conducted on CaelyxTM, a pegylated liposomal formulation of doxorubicin (DOX), either alone or in combination treatment (with temozolomide, tamoxifen, RT, or a combination of these) as one of the primary candidates under investigation (Horta et al., 2025). To evaluate the effectiveness of liposomal curcumin in conjunction with radiation and temozolomide, a new phase I clinical trial at Johns Hopkins University (NCT05768919) is presently accepting participants. The restricted effectiveness noted so far in these clinical trials indicates that although nanoparticle-based systems can enhance drug delivery, additional optimization in formulation and the creation of new targeting strategies are needed to improve their clinical effectiveness in treating GB (Horta et al., 2025).

3.6. In situ delivery system

In situ delivery includes injecting medicines directly into the tumor cavity or surrounding brain tissue following surgical excision. Currently, in situ delivery is accomplished using convection-enhanced delivery (CED) (Clinical Trial: NCT03043391), which involves gently pushing medications into the tumor (Sperring et al., 2023). New formulations for in situ administration seek to optimize the effects of first-generation anti-glioblastoma drugs like carmustine and temozolomide, either alone or together. To optimize therapeutic results, consider combining TMZ with the O6 alkylguanine DNA alkyltransferase inhibitor dialdehyde O6 benzylguanine (DABG), which has been studied in xenografts and may be given intracranially to minimize peripheral toxicity (Chen et al., 2022; Chu et al., 2022). In situ administration can target the tumor microenvironment and stimulate the immune system that suppresses tumors. Hyaluronic acid (HA) was recently exploited as an injectable delivery platform for combinatory therapies (Catania et al., 2023). Innovative biomaterials including smart materials, polymeric matrices, and hydrogels provide for more adaptive materials that can cling to surgical resection margins.

3.7. Drug repurposing

Drug repurposing is a successful method of using previously authorized medications for new indications other than their original application, acting as an alternative to de novo drug development (Chakkittukandiyil et al., 2024). Compared to new drug creation, repurposing medications provides a number of benefits. Because many medications have previously been thoroughly examined for safety profiles and pharmacokinetic characteristics, drug repurposing can be substantially less expensive and time-consuming than new drug research (Alomari et al., 2021). Numerous medications that have previously received approval for clinical usage in the treatment of other conditions have been repurposed to treat GBM once it was discovered that they target the signaling pathways linked to GBM. Some of these medications are at the clinical trial stage, while many are still undergoing pre-clinical testing. A few of the drugs in clinical trials for GBM are Memantine, Levetiracetam, Valproic Acid, Dimethyl Fumarate, Sertraline, Sulfasalazine, Nelfinavir, Captopril, Mefloquine etc (Alomari et al., 2021). Auranofin (AF), an inhibitor of TrxR1, and flubendazole, an inhibitor of microtubule development that triggers autophagy and STAT3-dependent apoptosis, can be taken either by themselves or in conjunction with the prooxidant menadione for GBM (74). Anticancer medications that have shown promise in vitro but have not produced therapeutic results in vivo, or that have unacceptably high off-target effects when given systematically, might be given a second chance of life through local distribution. For instance, systemic treatment of Placlitaxel in conjunction with albumin to promote osmotic opening of the BBB (NCT04528680) or intranasal delivery of Temozolomide (TMZ) (Clinical Trial: NCT04091503) are being studied (Chiariello et al., 2023).

4. TECHNOLOGICAL BREAKTHROUGHS IN GLIOBLASTOMA MANAGEMENT

GBM is the most aggressive and deadly kind of primary brain tumor, distinguished by its fast proliferation, diffuse infiltration, and resistance to conventional therapy. With a median lifespan of about 12 to 15 months, the prognosis remains dire despite years of clinical research and proven treatments, including radiation therapy, chemotherapy, and surgical excision. There is an urgent need for innovative technologies that can revolutionize GBM diagnosis, monitoring, and therapy due to the limitations of traditional approaches. Significant technical developments in recent years have changed how glioblastoma is treated.

4.1. Role of Nanotechnology in Enhancing Treatment

The recent development in cancer nanotechnology has opened new avenues for treating GB. The nanoparticle measuring less than 100 nm in hydrodynamic size is used in the treatment of various cancers (Hayashi et al., 1997). The use of biocompatible nanomaterials loaded with chemotherapeutic agents has shown a sustained release effect, which can lower systemic toxicity and increase antitumor effects. Nanoparticles that can cross the blood-brain barrier after systemic administration, which were developed for distribution in the brain to target GB cells shown promising results. The nanoparticle, when compared with conventional nanoparticles, can be targeted with precise drug delivery to the target site. These nanoparticles, when triggered by specific stimuli or modified by corresponding factors, can lead to aggregation at the target level and release the payloads to have a smart treatment mode (Sun et al., 2023). The specific materials and components of smart nanoparticles could respond to external and internal stimuli, like pH, temperature, enzymes, optical & magnetic regulation. The rapid development of nanotechnology has provided new options to develop nano-imaging technology for the diagnosis and treatment of GB (Lee Bredlau et al., 2017). A variety of imaging techniques with high sensitivity, high resolution, high specificity, and deep tissue penetration and contrast agents utilizing small particle sizes are being developed (Tang et al., 2019; Manek & Petroianu, 2021). The unique paramagnetic properties of magnetic nanoparticles, which enable their detection by MRI, are also been developed. The superparamagnetic iron oxide (SPIOs) smaller than 50 nm is most commonly used as an MRI contrast agent (Ndoum et al., 2012). These nanoparticles can provide a longer contrast period and are eliminated through the kidneys (Aime & Caravan, 2009). The SPIOs can be taken up by tumor cells and by reactive phagocytic cells to provide a safe alternative for patients at risk for nephrogenic systemic fibrosis and have no adverse renal effects (Neuwelt et al., 2007). Liposomes are small spherical vesicles with single or multiple lipid bilayers of either natural or synthetic origin and are compatible with the lipid layer of the BBB (Wei et al., 2023). Liposomes can be used as a carrier of chemotherapeutic drugs for glioblastoma and allow target delivery to glioma tissue. The incorporation of daunorubicin and doxorubicin in liposomal vesicles has been developed and shown to be transported to glioma tissue (Zhao et al., 2016).

The study with lactoferrin (LF), an iron-binding protein, can bind to transferrin receptors, like TFR and CD71, and is used for overexpression in tumor cells. The drug carriers modified with LF can cross the BBB via receptor-mediated endocytosis. These LF modified nanocarriers are incorporated with daunorubicin via an active drug loading method and found to inhibit angiogenesis mimicking channels (VM) and block the nutrient source that fuels tumor cells (Liu et al., 2017; Gruden & Poklar Ulrih, 2021). The polymeric micelles are vesicles of nanometer diameter that can infiltrate into the tumor via junctions of damaged endothelial cells and get internalized. This process is considered a potential force for the precision treatment of glioblastoma (Wei et al., 2023; Clay et al., 2017; Mohan et al., 2018; Ghosh & Biswas, 2021). The hyperbranched macromolecules called dendrimers can bind covalently to a large number of drugs to nanoparticles. The most common dendrimer, polyamide amine (PAMAM), has high solubility and low toxicity. The PAMAM-based dendrimer carriers is a promising drug targeting for cancer treatment due to their rich peripheral amino groups and internal cavity structures, which can be modified by various ligands and encapsulate chemotherapeutic agents (Dias et al., 2020; Filipczak et al., 2021). The nanomaterials can be co-labelled with radioisotopes to target the molecules to reach the glioblastoma site for increasing the amount of contrast agents (Liu et al., 2012). Injection of nanomaterials labelled with radioisotopes into the glioblastoma site allows for visualization of the image for treating glioblastoma. The most commonly used contrast agent is iodine, which has a short imaging time and causes side effects. The gold nanoparticles have been shown to provide clear and durable images with better stability and long residence time in vivo. A study with polyethyleneimine as template and sequentially modified with PEG and glioma-specific peptide embedded in gold nanoparticles has shown to be a useful nanoprobe for imaging and radionuclide therapy of glioma cells in a subcutaneous tumor model (Zhao et al., 2019). The photothermal therapy uses photothermal converters accumulated in the tumor to absorb light energy to generate heat and ablate tumor cells. Photothermal nanoprobes can be used for thermal imaging with high detection depth, high spatial resolution, and high imaging contrast. The Au NPs, pyrazino [2,3-g] quinoxaline-based NPs with strong absorption in the near-infrared region, can produce a sharp contrast of the biological tissue image in the infrared light region. These NPs have a high photothermal conversion rate, which can be used for photothermal treatment of tumors and allow the integration of tumor diagnosis and treatment (Shang et al., 2017; Zhang et al., 2021).

4.2. Latest Innovative Drug Delivery Mechanism

The largest area of research in GB is the incorporation of nanocarriers into drug delivery to the localized regions with glioma tumors. The complex and endless combinations of nanocarrier characteristics create huge possibilities for improving target specificity with improved safety and efficacy of therapeutic agents to treat glioma. The availability of datasets and the use of computational algorithms have opened new methods in the drug discovery process. Machine learning and deep learning have helped in drug designing by creating molecules that are more selective to the target protein, which optimizes the binding activity. The microfluidic devices and microrobots in conjunction with nanocarriers are the upcoming development that pose advantages in drug delivery of therapeutic agents to treat glioma (Damiati et al., 2018; Hu et al., 2020; D'Amico et al., 2021). The microfluidic devices are microscopic devices containing different channels. The change of liquid pressure and movement of liquid through these channels can be utilized in areas like drug encapsulation, nanoparticle preparation, drug delivery, and targeting of drugs (Niculescu et al., 2021). The advantages of microfluidic devices for use in drug delivery include allowing the creation of uniform particles and can deliver multiple drugs in the same particle or droplet. This will be advantageous in GB, as combinatory treatments are necessary to effectively treat patient tumors that are heterogeneous in composition. The device allows precise dosage, with sustained or controlled release of drugs with few side effects (Mancera-Andrade et al., 2018). The promising innovation in drug delivery is the use of microrobots capable of delivering drugs to the target site. These microrobots can be driven electrically, chemically, magnetically, or by light to overcome the Brownian motion to pass the BBB and deliver the therapeutic moiety to the target site (Hu et al., 2020). Magnetic nanorobots were developed and can pass through the BBB both in vitro and in vivo. These robots use bacterial motion to enter the target tumor area to release glioma drugs (Zhang et al., 2021).

4.3. Applications of CRISPR-Cas9 and Gene Editing Techniques

The CRISPR and Cas9 technology has gained recognition since it was incorporated into genome editing technology and used in gene therapy and other applications (Gostimskaya, 2022). CRISPR/Cas9 is the most powerful tool to identify oncogenes, a gene with transformative capabilities that results in a tumor cell. The CRISPR/Cas9 technology is powerful in the world for personalized medicine, offering tailored interventions based on an individual's unique genetic profile. The technology helps to remove disease-causing genes, but also has therapeutic effects by inserting 'protective' genes (Jhu et al., 2023). A study has revealed that CRISPR/Cas9-mediated ATG5 could knock out the gene that promotes the transformation of 'bad' or malignant cells to 'good' cells (Wang et al., 2022; Hazafa et al., 2020). In gene therapy, the CRISPR/Cas9 technology has emerged as a powerful tool for precise and targeted modifications to the DNA sequences of cells (Gupta et al., 2021). This capability will help to correct genetic defects, opening new avenues for therapeutic interventions. Gene therapy holds great promise for treating various genetic disorders, as the CRISPR/Cas9 system allows for the direct correction of harmful mutations within the genome. This approach offers a potential cure for diseases with a known genetic basis, addressing the root cause rather than merely managing symptoms. Initially, viral vector delivery of therapeutic transgenes, mainly for cancer treatment or monogenic diseases, marked the early stages of gene therapy (Zhang, 2021). The CRISPR/Cas system, particularly CRISPR/Cas9, has gained prominence due to its low cost, ease of use, and efficient and precise performance (Yu & Wu, 2019). The study with CRISPR/Cas9-mediated endogenous T cell receptor (TRAC),β-2microglobulin (B2M), and PD-1(PDCD1) multi-gene disrupted (CAR-T Cells has shown intensive anti-tumor activity in preclinical models of glioma, but needs further studies to ensure the safety and efficacy of these cell products in humans (Choi et al., 2019).

5. ADVANCES IN DIAGNOSIS AND MONITORING OF GLIOBLASTOMA

Timely and precise diagnosis is vital for enhancing patient outcomes, while efficient monitoring is crucial for assessing treatment response and identifying recurrence. Conventional diagnostic techniques, including magnetic resonance imaging (MRI) and histopathological examination, exhibit limitations in sensitivity, specificity, and speed. In recent years, improvements in imaging tech, molecular diagnostics, liquid biopsies, and artificial intelligence (AI) have greatly improved the capability to diagnose and track GBM with increased accuracy.

5.1. Liquid Biopsy

Liquid biopsies present a hopeful, non-invasive method for diagnosing and monitoring GBM by identifying tumor-related biomarkers in body fluids like blood or cerebrospinal fluid (CSF). These biopsies can detect circulating tumor DNA (ctDNA), microRNAs (miRNAs), and extracellular vesicles such as exosomes that contain tumor-specific genetic and proteomic data. Although ctDNA identification in blood is constrained by the blood-brain barrier's restrictive characteristics, CSF-based liquid biopsies exhibit enhanced sensitivity for obtaining the molecular profile of GBM. Liquid biopsies facilitate real-time tracking of tumor development, treatment effectiveness, and new resistance mechanisms, which could help tailor individualized therapy. In addition, they offer potential for the early identification of recurrence and may supplement or lessen the necessity for additional surgical or imaging procedures (De Lima et al., 2025).

5.2. Neuroimaging Techniques

Advanced neuroimaging methods have dramatically improved the diagnosis and surgical treatment of GBM. Advanced imaging techniques, including diffusion-weighted MRI, perfusion-weighted MRI, magnetic resonance spectroscopy (MRS), and positron emission tomography (PET) imaging, have been widely used to address diagnostic problems in the context of initial diagnosis, treatment planning, and follow-up. Diffusion-weighted MRI assesses the cellularity, perfusion-weighted imaging (PWI) evaluates vascularity, and MRS analyzes metabolic profiles. Functional MRI (fMRI) and tractography help safeguard essential brain functions during surgical procedures. PET, especially when utilizing radiolabelled amino acids, aids in distinguishing genuine tumor advancement from treatment-induced alterations like pseudo progression. Moreover, intraoperative imaging techniques such as intraoperative MRI and fluorescence-guided surgery utilizing 5-ALA enhance the scope of tumor removal while reducing harm to healthy brain tissue (Henssen et al., 2023).

5.3. Radiomics

Radiomics entails obtaining numerous quantitative characteristics from medical images through algorithms that characterize data. When combined with clinical and genomic information, radiomics can assist in forecasting tumor type, grade, molecular subtype, and treatment response (McCague et al., 2023).

Radiomics derives intricate imaging characteristics from MRI scans of glioblastomas that exceed human perception abilities. By examining a wide range of quantitative data, radiomics can differentiate GBM from other brain tumors and recognize unique molecular subtypes with varying prognoses. This sophisticated method improves diagnostic precision and speed, thereby enabling earlier and more tailored treatment strategies that boost patient outcomes (Kwiatkowska-Miernik et al., 2023).

5.4. AI and machine learning

AI and machine learning are revolutionizing the diagnosis and monitoring of GBM by improving MRI analysis with unmatched accuracy. AI-powered models facilitate automated tumor segmentation and classification, as shown by the BraTS Challenge and sophisticated networks such as SKIPNet, which effectively outline tumor subregions and distinguish GBM from lower-grade gliomas (The 2024 Brain Tumor Segmentation (BraTS) Challenge: Glioma segmentation on post-treatment MRI, n.d.; Mendiratta et al., 2024). Deep learning additionally forecasts essential molecular biomarkers like IDH mutations and 1p/19q codeletions directly from images, reducing the necessity for invasive examinations (Farahani et al., 2024). Multimodal systems combine tumor grading, segmentation, and radio genomic classification, providing a holistic diagnostic method (Liu et al., 2025). Predictive models mimic tumor development and treatment reactions, aiding personalized therapies, whereas topological data analysis monitors changes after treatment (Rucco et al., 2020). Moreover, advanced technologies such as image-guided radionuclide therapy and treatment-informed predictive MRI improve real-time observation. Transfer learning enhances accessibility by modifying advanced AI models for low-resource environments, thereby improving GBM diagnosis globally (Zhao et al., 2024).

5.5. New and Emerging Technologies

Cutting-edge technologies like biosensors, Raman spectroscopy, and optical coherence tomography (OCT) are under investigation for real-time tumor boundary identification and early diagnosis in glioblastoma during surgery (Thenuwara et al., 2023; Burström et al., 2024). These imaging methods provide high-resolution, non-invasive information that can improve surgical accuracy. Simultaneously, the advancement of intelligent biopsies and robotic-assisted technologies driven by real-time imaging and molecular responses is enhancing the precision of tissue sampling, reducing procedural risks, and allowing focused examination of particular tumor areas (Lanza et al., 2023). Collectively, these developments offer the potential for improved diagnostics and individualized treatment strategies.

6. CHALLENGES IN ADAPTING NEW IDEAS TO CLINICAL PRACTICE

Despite promising developments in research and innovation, integrating these discoveries into effective clinical practice remains difficult. The intricacy of GBM biology, the specific environment of the brain, and systemic challenges in research and healthcare delivery are all important barriers. Though strategies like targeted ultrasound, implanted drug delivery devices, nanoparticles, and optically modulated BBB permeability are being investigated, there are still issues with repeatability, toxicity, and immunogenicity when transferring these techniques from animal models to humans (Dong, 2018). Intra-tumor variety and resistance mechanisms are major reasons why several targeted medicines and clinical studies have not shown significant survival gains. To address this, innovations like logic-gated chimeric antigen receptors and combination treatments are being explored; nevertheless, biomarker identification and accurate patient selection are still challenging (Li et al., 2022). Modular CAR designs, immune checkpoint co-inhibition, and tailored microenvironments are being investigated by researchers; however, bringing these intricate approaches to the clinic will require overcoming immune-related side effects and inconsistent effectiveness (Zhang et al., 2025). The intricacy of human GBM is not adequately represented by many preclinical models, especially when it comes to its invasive nature and interactions with the immune system. Furthermore, therapeutic techniques are sometimes not immediately transferable due to size disparities between people and animal models (Klein et al., 2020). Advanced diagnostic techniques, including metabolomic signatures, extracellular vesicle detection, and ctDNA profiling, need more testing before they can be incorporated into standard clinical practice (Bae et al., 2024). Because GBM is somewhat uncommon, it can be difficult to find enough patients for reliable clinical studies, particularly for tailored or targeted treatments (Yalamarty et al., 2023).

7. CONCLUSION

GBM is a formidable challenge in neuro oncology due to its invasive nature, heterogeneity, infiltration and strong BBB, which interferes with the effective drug administration. Adding to this, the immunosuppressive microenvironment and resistance to conventional treatments make the outcome more complicated. Novel approaches like immunotherapy, gene therapy, targeted medicines, and the use of oncolytic viruses were developed. Technologies like TTF and CRISPR-Cas9 gene editing are creating new avenues for individualised and specific treatments. Meanwhile, advancements in monitoring and diagnostic methods are making it possible for more precise prognosis, real-time monitoring, and early detection of the disease.

Even though GBM still presents numerous clinical difficulties, the combination of interdisciplinary advances has enormous potential to change the way that GBM is treated in the future. To eventually convert these developments into significant clinical advantages for patients, more research and the incorporation of these innovative approaches are necessary.

REFERENCES

Aime, S., & Caravan, P. (2009). Biodistribution of gadolinium-based contrast agents, including gadolinium deposition. *Journal of Magnetic Resonance Imaging, 30*(6), 1259–1267. DOI: 10.1002/jmri.21969 PMID: 19938038

Aldoghachi, A. F., Aldoghachi, A. F., Breyne, K., Ling, K. H., & Cheah, P. S. (2022). Recent advances in the therapeutic strategies of glioblastoma multiforme. *Neuroscience, 491*, 240–270. DOI: 10.1016/j.neuroscience.2022.03.030 PMID: 35395355

Alifieris, C., & Trafalis, D. T. (2015). Glioblastoma multiforme: Pathogenesis and treatment. *Pharmacology & Therapeutics, 152*, 63–82. DOI: 10.1016/j.pharmthera.2015.05.005 PMID: 25944528

Alomari, S., Zhang, I., Hernandez, A., Kraft, C. Y., Raj, D., Kedda, J., & Chitneni, S. K. (2021). Drug repurposing for glioblastoma and current advances in drug delivery—A comprehensive review of the literature. *Biomolecules, 11*(12), 1870. Advance online publication. DOI: 10.3390/biom11121870 PMID: 34944514

Bae, W. H., Maraka, S., & Daher, A. (2024). Challenges and advances in glioblastoma targeted therapy: The promise of drug repurposing and biomarker exploration. *Frontiers in Oncology, 14*, 1441460. Advance online publication. DOI: 10.3389/fonc.2024.1441460 PMID: 39439947

Bae, W. H., Maraka, S., & Daher, A. (2024). Challenges and advances in glioblastoma targeted therapy: The promise of drug repurposing and biomarker exploration. *Frontiers in Oncology, 14*, 1441460. Advance online publication. DOI: 10.3389/fonc.2024.1441460 PMID: 39439947

Bao, P., Gu, H. Y., Jiang, Y. C., Wang, J. W., Wu, M., Yu, A., Wang, X., & Zhang, X. (2024). In situ sprayed exosome-cross-linked gel as artificial lymph nodes for postoperative glioblastoma immunotherapy. *ACS Nano, 18*(20), 13266–13276. DOI: 10.1021/acsnano.4c02425 PMID: 38709874

Barzegar-Fallah, A., Gandhi, K., Rizwan, S. B., Slatter, T. L., & Reynolds, J. N. (2022). Harnessing ultrasound for targeting drug delivery to the brain and breaching the blood–brain tumour barrier. *Pharmaceutics, 14*(10), 2231. Advance online publication. DOI: 10.3390/pharmaceutics14102231 PMID: 36297666

Bausart, M., Préat, V., & Malfanti, A. (2022). Immunotherapy for glioblastoma: The promise of combination strategies. *Journal of Experimental & Clinical Cancer Research : CR, 41*(1), 35. Advance online publication. DOI: 10.1186/s13046-022-02251-2 PMID: 35078492

Becker, A. P., Sells, B. E., Haque, S. J., & Chakravarti, A. (2021). Tumor heterogeneity in glioblastomas: From light microscopy to molecular pathology. *Cancers (Basel), 13*(4), 761. Advance online publication. DOI: 10.3390/cancers13040761 PMID: 33673104

Begagić, E., Pugonja, R., Bečulić, H., Čeliković, A., Tandir Lihić, L., Kadić Vukas, S., & Dorić, M. (2023). Molecular targeted therapies in glioblastoma multiforme: A systematic overview of global trends and findings. *Brain Sciences, 13*(11), 1602. Advance online publication. DOI: 10.3390/brainsci13111602 PMID: 38002561

Birzu, C., French, P., Caccese, M., Cerretti, G., Idbaih, A., Zagonel, V., & Lombardi, G. (2021). Recurrent glioblastoma: From molecular landscape to new treatment perspectives. *Cancers (Basel), 13*(1), 47. Advance online publication. DOI: 10.3390/cancers13010047 PMID: 33375286

Blitz, S. E., Kappel, A. D., Gessler, F. A., Klinger, N. V., Arnaout, O., Lu, Y., Peruzzi, P. P., Smith, T. R., Chiocca, E. A., Friedman, G. K., & Bernstock, J. D. (2022). Tumor-associated macrophages/microglia in glioblastoma oncolytic virotherapy: A double-edged sword. *International Journal of Molecular Sciences, 23*(3), 1808. Advance online publication. DOI: 10.3390/ijms23031808 PMID: 35163730

Brat, D. J., Prayson, R. A., Ryken, T. C., & Olson, J. J. (2008). Diagnosis of malignant glioma: Role of neuropathology. *Journal of Neuro-Oncology, 89*(3), 287–311. DOI: 10.1007/s11060-008-9618-1 PMID: 18712282

Burström, G., Amini, M., El-Hajj, V. G., Arfan, A., Gharios, M., Buwaider, A., & Edström, E. (2024). Optical methods for brain tumor detection: A systematic review. *Journal of Clinical Medicine, 13*(9), 2676. Advance online publication. DOI: 10.3390/jcm13092676 PMID: 38731204

Carson, K. A., Grossman, S. A., Fisher, J. D., & Shaw, E. G. (2007). Prognostic factors for survival in adult patients with recurrent glioma enrolled on New Approaches to Brain Tumor Therapy "NABTT" CNS Consortium Phase I and II clinical trials. *Journal of Clinical Oncology, 25*(18), 2601–2606. DOI: 10.1200/JCO.2006.08.1661 PMID: 17577040

Catania, G., Rodella, G., Vanvarenberg, K., Préat, V., & Malfanti, A. (2023). Combination of hyaluronic acid conjugates with immunogenic cell death inducer and CpG for glioblastoma local chemo-immunotherapy elicits an immune response and induces long-term survival. *Biomaterials, 294*, 122006. Advance online publication. DOI: 10.1016/j.biomaterials.2023.122006 PMID: 36701998

Chakkittukandiyil, A., Chakraborty, S., Kothandan, R., Rymbai, E., Muthu, S. K., Vasu, S., & Sajeev, A. (2024). Side effects based network construction and drug repositioning of ropinirole as a potential molecule for Alzheimer's disease: An in-silico, in-vitro, and in-vivo study. *Journal of Biomolecular Structure & Dynamics*, *42*(20), 10785–10799. DOI: 10.1080/07391102.2023.2258968 PMID: 37723871

Chen, S., Qiu, Q., Wang, D., She, D., Yin, B., Gu, G., & Chen, J. (2022). Dual-sensitive drug-loaded hydrogel system for local inhibition of post-surgical glioma recurrence. *Journal of Controlled Release*, *349*, 565–579. DOI: 10.1016/j.jconrel.2022.07.011 PMID: 35835399

Chen, X., Ma, X., Liu, X., Li, X., Jiang, S., & Zhang, Q. (2022). Origin, activation, and targeted therapy of glioma-associated macrophages. *Frontiers in Immunology*, *13*, 974702. Advance online publication. DOI: 10.3389/fimmu.2022.974702 PMID: 36275720

Chiariello, M., Inzalaco, G., Barone, V., & Gherardini, L. (2023). Overcoming challenges in glioblastoma treatment: Targeting infiltrating cancer cells and harnessing the tumor microenvironment. *Frontiers in Cellular Neuroscience*, *17*, 1327621. Advance online publication. DOI: 10.3389/fncel.2023.1327621 PMID: 38188666

Choi, B. D., Yu, X., Castano, A. P., Darr, H., Henderson, D. B., Bouffard, A. A., & Maus, M. V. (2019). CRISPR-Cas9 disruption of PD-1 enhances activity of universal EGFRvIII CAR T cells in a preclinical model of human glioblastoma. *Journal for Immunotherapy of Cancer*, *7*(1), 304. Advance online publication. DOI: 10.1186/s40425-019-0806-7 PMID: 31727131

Chu, C., Jablonska, A., Gao, Y., Lan, X., Lesniak, W. G., Liang, Y., & Zhang, Y. (2022). Hyperosmolar blood-brain barrier opening using intra-arterial injection of hyperosmotic mannitol in mice under real-time MRI guidance. *Nature Protocols*, *17*(1), 76–94. DOI: 10.1038/s41596-021-00634-x PMID: 34903870

Clay, N. E., Whittenberg, J. J., Leong, J., Kumar, V., Chen, J., Choi, I., & Lee, K.-B. (2017). Chemical and mechanical modulation of polymeric micelle assembly. *Nanoscale*, *9*(16), 5194–5204. DOI: 10.1039/C6NR08414A PMID: 28397883

D'Amico, R. S., Aghi, M. K., Vogelbaum, M. A., & Bruce, J. N. (2021). Convection-enhanced drug delivery for glioblastoma: A review. *Journal of Neuro-Oncology*, *151*(3), 415–427. DOI: 10.1007/s11060-020-03408-9 PMID: 33611708

Damiati, S., Kompella, U. B., Damiati, S. A., & Kodzius, R. (2018). Microfluidic devices for drug delivery systems and drug screening. *Genes*, *9*(2), 103. Advance online publication. DOI: 10.3390/genes9020103 PMID: 29462948

Davis, M. E. (2016). Glioblastoma: Overview of disease and treatment. *Clinical Journal of Oncology Nursing*, *20*(5, Suppl.), S2–S8. DOI: 10.1188/16.CJON.S1.2-8 PMID: 27668386

De Lima, B. P., Ferraz, L. S., Devalle, S., & Borges, H. L. (2025). Liquid biopsy-derived tumor biomarkers for clinical applications in glioblastoma. *Biomolecules*, *15*(5), 658. Advance online publication. DOI: 10.3390/biom15050658 PMID: 40427551

Degl'Innocenti, A., Di Leo, N., & Ciofani, G. (2020). Genetic hallmarks and heterogeneity of glioblastoma in the single-cell omics era. *Advanced Therapeutics*, *3*(1), 1900152. Advance online publication. DOI: 10.1002/adtp.201900152 PMID: 31942443

Del Bene, M., Osti, D., Faletti, S., Beznoussenko, G. V., DiMeco, F., & Pelicci, G. (2022). Extracellular vesicles: The key for precision medicine in glioblastoma. *Neuro-Oncology*, *24*(2), 184–196. DOI: 10.1093/neuonc/noab229 PMID: 34581817

Dias, A. P., da Silva Santos, S., da Silva, J. V., Parise-Filho, R., Ferreira, E. I., El Seoud, O., & Giarolla, J. (2020). Dendrimers in the context of nanomedicine. *International Journal of Pharmaceutics*, *573*, 118814. Advance online publication. DOI: 10.1016/j.ijpharm.2019.118814 PMID: 31759101

Dong, X. (2018). Current strategies for brain drug delivery. *Theranostics*, *8*(6), 1481–1493. DOI: 10.7150/thno.21254 PMID: 29556336

Eckert, T., Walton, C., Bell, M., Small, C., Rowland, N. C., Rivers, C., & Mehta, A. (2025). The basis for targeting the tumor macrophage compartment in glioblastoma immunotherapy. *Cancers (Basel)*, *17*(10), 1631. Advance online publication. DOI: 10.3390/cancers17101631 PMID: 40427130

Ellor, S. V., Pagano-Young, T. A., & Avgeropoulos, N. G. (2014). Glioblastoma: Background, standard treatment paradigms, and supportive care considerations. *The Journal of Law, Medicine & Ethics*, *42*(2), 171–182. DOI: 10.1111/jlme.12133 PMID: 25040381

Fan, R., Chen, C., Mu, M., Chuan, D., Liu, H., Hou, H., Zhang, X., & Wang, J. (2023). Engineering MMP-2 activated nanoparticles carrying B7-H3 bispecific antibodies for ferroptosis-enhanced glioblastoma immunotherapy. *ACS Nano*, *17*(10), 9126–9139. DOI: 10.1021/acsnano.2c12217 PMID: 37097811

Farahani, S., Hejazi, M., Tabassum, M., Ieva, A. D., Mahdavifar, N., & Liu, S. (2024). Diagnostic performance of deep learning for predicting gliomas' IDH and 1p/19q status in MRI: A systematic review and meta-analysis. arXiv. Retrieved May 17, 2025, from https://arxiv.org/abs/2411.02426

Feldman, L. (2024). Hypoxia within the glioblastoma tumor microenvironment: A master saboteur of novel treatments. *Frontiers in Immunology*, *15*, 1384249. Advance online publication. DOI: 10.3389/fimmu.2024.1384249 PMID: 38994360

Filipczak, N., Yalamarty, S. S. K., Li, X., Parveen, F., & Torchilin, V. (2021). Developments in treatment methodologies using dendrimers for infectious diseases. *Molecules (Basel, Switzerland)*, *26*(11), 3304. Advance online publication. DOI: 10.3390/molecules26113304 PMID: 34072765

Friedmann-Morvinski, D. (2014). Glioblastoma heterogeneity and cancer cell plasticity. *Critical Reviews in Oncogenesis*, *19*(5), 327–336. DOI: 10.1615/CritRevOncog.2014011777 PMID: 25404148

Ghosh, B., & Biswas, S. (2021). Polymeric micelles in cancer therapy: State of the art. *Journal of Controlled Release*, *332*, 127–147. DOI: 10.1016/j.jconrel.2021.02.016 PMID: 33609621

Gostimskaya, I. (2022). CRISPR–Cas9: A history of its discovery and ethical considerations of its use in genome editing. *Biochemistry (Moscow)*, *87*(8), 777–788. DOI: 10.1134/S0006297922080090 PMID: 36171658

Grochans, S., Cybulska, A. M., Simińska, D., Korbecki, J., Kojder, K., Chlubek, D., & Baranowska-Bosiacka, I. (2022). Epidemiology of glioblastoma multiforme–Literature review. *Cancers (Basel)*, *14*(10), 2412. Advance online publication. DOI: 10.3390/cancers14102412 PMID: 35626018

Gruden, Š., & Poklar Ulrih, N. (2021). Diverse mechanisms of antimicrobial activities of lactoferrins, lactoferricins, and other lactoferrin-derived peptides. *International Journal of Molecular Sciences*, *22*(20), 11264. Advance online publication. DOI: 10.3390/ijms222011264 PMID: 34681923

Gupta, S., Kumar, A., Patel, R., & Kumar, V. (2021). Genetically modified crop regulations: Scope and opportunity using the CRISPR-Cas9 genome editing approach. *Molecular Biology Reports*, *48*(5), 4851–4863. DOI: 10.1007/s11033-021-06477-9 PMID: 34114124

Hamad, A., Yusubalieva, G. M., Baklaushev, V. P., Chumakov, P. M., & Lipatova, A. V. (2023). Recent developments in glioblastoma therapy: Oncolytic viruses and emerging future strategies. *Viruses*, *15*(2), 547. Advance online publication. DOI: 10.3390/v15020547 PMID: 36851761

Han, S., Liu, Y., Cai, S. J., Qian, M., Ding, J., Larion, M., Gilbert, M. R., & Yang, C. (2020). IDH mutation in glioma: Molecular mechanisms and potential therapeutic targets. *British Journal of Cancer*, *122*(11), 1580–1589. DOI: 10.1038/s41416-020-0814-x PMID: 32291392

Haslam, A., & Prasad, V. (2019). Estimation of the percentage of US patients with cancer who are eligible for and respond to checkpoint inhibitor immunotherapy drugs. *JAMA Network Open*, *2*(5), e192535. Advance online publication. DOI: 10.1001/jamanetworkopen.2019.2535 PMID: 31050774

Hayashi, C., Ueda, R., & Tasaki, A. (1997). *Ultra-fine particles: Exploratory science and technology*. Noyes Publications.

Hazafa, A., Mumtaz, M., Farooq, M. F., Bilal, S., Chaudhry, S. N., Firdous, M., Naeem, M., Ullah, M. O., Yameen, M., Mukhtiar, M. S., & Zafar, F. (2020). CRISPR/Cas9: A powerful genome editing technique for the treatment of cancer cells with present challenges and future directions. *Life Sciences*, *263*, 118525. Advance online publication. DOI: 10.1016/j.lfs.2020.118525 PMID: 33031826

Henssen, D., Meijer, F., Verburg, F. A., & Smits, M. (2023). Challenges and opportunities for advanced neuroimaging of glioblastoma. *The British Journal of Radiology*, *96*(1141), 20211232. Advance online publication. DOI: 10.1259/bjr.20211232 PMID: 36062962

Horta, M., Soares, P., Leite Pereira, C., & Lima, R. T. (2025). Emerging approaches in glioblastoma treatment: Modulating the extracellular matrix through nanotechnology. *Pharmaceutics*, *17*(2), 142. Advance online publication. DOI: 10.3390/pharmaceutics17020142 PMID: 40006509

Hu, M., Ge, X., Chen, X., Mao, W., Qian, X., & Yuan, W. E. (2020). Micro/nanorobot: A promising targeted drug delivery system. *Pharmaceutics*, *12*(7), 665. Advance online publication. DOI: 10.3390/pharmaceutics12070665 PMID: 32679772

Jhu, M. Y., Ellison, E. E., & Sinha, N. R. (2023). CRISPR gene editing to improve crop resistance to parasitic plants. *Frontiers in Genome Editing*, *5*, 1289416. Advance online publication. DOI: 10.3389/fgeed.2023.1289416 PMID: 37965302

Johnson, D. R., Fogh, S. E., Giannini, C., Kaufmann, T. J., Raghunathan, A., Theodosopoulos, P. V., & Jenkins, R. B. (2015). Case-based review: Newly diagnosed glioblastoma. *Neuro-Oncology Practice*, *2*(3), 106–121. DOI: 10.1093/nop/npv020 PMID: 31386093

Khagi, S., Kotecha, R., Gatson, N. T. N., Jeyapalan, S., Abdullah, H. I., Avgeropoulos, N. G., & Mehta, M. P. (2024). Recent advances in Tumor Treating Fields (TTFields) therapy for glioblastoma. *The Oncologist*, *30*(2), oyae227. Advance online publication. DOI: 10.1093/oncolo/oyae227 PMID: 39401002

Klein, E., Hau, A.-C., Oudin, A., Golebiewska, A., & Niclou, S. P. (2020). Glioblastoma organoids: Pre-clinical applications and challenges in the context of immunotherapy. *Frontiers in Oncology*, *10*, 604121. Advance online publication. DOI: 10.3389/fonc.2020.604121 PMID: 33364198

Koes, N., Taisto, M., Tschida, B. R., Carlson, D. F., Aftabizadeh, M., Thirimanne, H. N., & Largaespada, D. A. (2025). Abstract 6511: Immunocompetent large animal model of mesenchymal glioblastoma achieved through somatic gene editing technology. *Cancer Research*, *85*(8, Supplement_1), 6511. DOI: 10.1158/1538-7445.AM2025-6511

Kwiatkowska-Miernik, A., Mruk, B., Sklinda, K., Zaczyński, A., & Walecki, J. (2023). Radiomics in the diagnosis of glioblastoma. *Polish Journal of Radiology / Polish Medical Society of Radiology*, *88*, e461–e466. DOI: 10.5114/pjr.2023.132168 PMID: 38020501

Lanza, C., Carriero, S., Buijs, E. F. M., Mortellaro, S., Pizzi, C., Sciacqua, L. V., & Venturini, M. (2023). Robotics in interventional radiology: Review of current and future applications. *Technology in Cancer Research & Treatment*, *22*, 15330338231152084. DOI: 10.1177/15330338231152084 PMID: 37113061

Lee Bredlau, A., Dixit, S., Chen, C., & Broome, A.-M. (2017). Nanotechnology applications for diffuse intrinsic pontine glioma. *Current Neuropharmacology*, *15*(1), 104–115. DOI: 10.2174/1570159X14666160223121002 PMID: 26903150

Li, X., Li, M., Huang, M., Lin, Q., Fang, Q., Liu, J., Chen, X., Liu, L., Zhan, X., Shan, H., Lu, D., Li, Q., Li, Z., & Zhu, X. (2022). The multi-molecular mechanisms of tumor-targeted drug resistance in precision medicine. *Biomedicine and Pharmacotherapy*, *150*, 113064. Advance online publication. DOI: 10.1016/j.biopha.2022.113064 PMID: 35658234

Liguori, G. L. (2024). Challenges and promise for glioblastoma treatment through extracellular vesicle inquiry. *Cells*, *13*(4), 336. Advance online publication. DOI: 10.3390/cells13040336 PMID: 38391949

Lin, H., Liu, C., Hu, A., Zhang, D., Yang, H., & Mao, Y. (2024). Understanding the immunosuppressive microenvironment of glioma: Mechanistic insights and clinical perspectives. *Journal of Hematology & Oncology*, *17*(1), 31. Advance online publication. DOI: 10.1186/s13045-024-01544-7 PMID: 38720342

. Liu, D., Dai, X., Ye, L., Wang, H., Qian, H., Cheng, H., & Zhang, J. (2023). Nanotechnology meets glioblastoma multiforme: Emerging therapeutic strategies. Wiley Interdisciplinary Reviews: Nanomedicine and Nanobiotechnology, 15(1), Article e1838. DOI: 10.1002/wnan.1838

Liu, S., Zhang, S. M., Ju, R. J., Xiao, Y., Wang, X., Song, X. L., Liu, Y., & Li, X. T. (2017). Antitumor efficacy of Lf modified daunorubicin plus honokiol liposomes in treatment of brain glioma. *European Journal of Pharmaceutical Sciences*, *106*, 185–197. DOI: 10.1016/j.ejps.2017.06.002 PMID: 28583810

Liu, Y., Cui, Z., Li, L., You, J., Feng, X., Wang, J., & Zhang, Y. (2025). Glioma multimodal MRI analysis system for tumor layered diagnosis via multi-task semi-supervised learning. arXiv. Retrieved May 17, 2025, from https://arxiv.org/abs/2501.17758

Majc, B., Novak, M., Kopitar-Jerala, N., Jewett, A., & Breznik, B. (2021). Immunotherapy of glioblastoma: Current strategies and challenges in tumor model development. *Cells*, *10*(2), 265. Advance online publication. DOI: 10.3390/cells10020265 PMID: 33572835

Malhotra, P., & Rahman, R. (2024). Tumour heterogeneity and disease infiltration as paradigms of glioblastoma treatment resistance. *Onco*, *4*(4), 349–358. DOI: 10.3390/onco4040024

Mancera-Andrade, E. I., Parsaeimehr, A., Arevalo-Gallegos, A., Ascencio-Favela, G., & Parra-Saldivar, R. (2018). Microfluidics technology for drug delivery: A review. *Frontiers in Bioscience (Elite Edition)*, *10*(1), 74–91. DOI: 10.2741/e809 PMID: 28930605

Manek, E., & Petroianu, G. A. (2021). Brain delivery of antidotes by polymeric nanoparticles. *Journal of Applied Toxicology*, *41*(1), 20–32. DOI: 10.1002/jat.4029 PMID: 32666582

McCague, C., Ramlee, S., Reinius, M., Selby, I., Hulse, D., Piyatissa, P., & Davies, R. (2023). Introduction to radiomics for a clinical audience. *Clinical Radiology*, *78*(2), 83–98. DOI: 10.1016/j.crad.2022.08.149 PMID: 36639175

Mendiratta, K., Singh, S., & Chattopadhyay, P. (2024). SKIPNet: Spatial attention skip connections for enhanced brain tumor classification. arXiv. Retrieved May 17, 2025, from https://arxiv.org/abs/2412.07736v1

Mikic, N., Gentilal, N., Cao, F., Lok, E., Wong, E. T., Ballo, M., & Kesari, S. (2024). Tumor-treating fields dosimetry in glioblastoma: Insights into treatment planning, optimization, and dose–response relationships. *Neuro-Oncology Advances*, *6*(1), vdae032. Advance online publication. DOI: 10.1093/noajnl/vdae032 PMID: 38560348

Mineo, J. F., Bordron, A., Baroncini, M., Ramirez, C., Maurage, C. A., Blond, S., & Dam-Hieu, P. (2007). Prognosis factors of survival time in patients with glioblastoma multiforme: A multivariate analysis of 340 patients. *Acta Neurochirurgica*, *149*(3), 245–253. DOI: 10.1007/s00701-006-1092-y PMID: 17273889

Mohan, A., Nair, S. V., & Lakshmanan, V.-K. (2018). Polymeric nanomicelles for cancer theragnostics. *International Journal of Polymeric Materials*, *67*(2), 119–130. DOI: 10.1080/00914037.2017.1309540

Neuwelt, E. A., Várallyay, C. G., Manninger, S., Solymosi, D., Haluska, M., Hunt, M. A., Nesbit, G., Stevens, A., Jerosch-Herold, M., Jacobs, J. M., & Hoffman, J. M. (2007). The potential of ferumoxytol nanoparticle magnetic resonance imaging, perfusion, and angiography in central nervous system malignancy: A pilot study. *Neurosurgery*, *60*(4), 601–612. DOI: 10.1227/01.NEU.0000255350.71700.37 PMID: 17415196

Ng, A. T., Steve, T., Jamouss, K. T., Arham, A., Kawtharani, S., & Assi, H. I. (2024). The challenges and clinical landscape of glioblastoma immunotherapy. *CNS Oncology*, *13*(1), 2415878. Advance online publication. DOI: 10.1080/20450907.2024.2415878 PMID: 39469854

Niculescu, A.-G., Chircov, C., Bîrcă, A. C., & Grumezescu, A. M. (2021). Fabrication and applications of microfluidic devices: A review. *International Journal of Molecular Sciences*, *22*(4), 2011. Advance online publication. DOI: 10.3390/ijms22042011 PMID: 33670545

Ohgaki, H., Dessen, P., Jourde, B., Horstmann, S., Nishikawa, T., Di Patre, P.-L., Burkhard, C., Schüler, D., Probst-Hensch, N. M., Maiorka, P. C., Baeza, N., Pisani, P., Yonekawa, Y., Yasargil, M. G., Lütolf, U. M., & Kleihues, P. (2004). Genetic pathways to glioblastoma: A population-based study. *Cancer Research*, *64*(19), 6892–6899. DOI: 10.1158/0008-5472.CAN-04-1337 PMID: 15466178

Ostrom, Q. T., Patil, N., Cioffi, G., Waite, K., Kruchko, C., & Barnholtz-Sloan, J. S. (2020). CBTRUS statistical report: Primary brain and other central nervous system tumors diagnosed in the United States in 2013–2017. *Neuro-Oncology*, *22*(Suppl. 1), iv1–iv96. DOI: 10.1093/neuonc/noaa200 PMID: 33123732

Park, J. I., Song, K. H., Jung, S. Y., Ahn, J., Hwang, S. G., Kim, J., Kim, E. H., & Kim, J. S. (2019). Tumor-treating fields induce RAW264.7 macrophage activation via NK-κB/MAPK signaling pathways. *Technology in Cancer Research & Treatment*, *18*, 1533033819868225. DOI: 10.1177/1533033819868225 PMID: 31401938

Parker, N. R., Hudson, A. L., Khong, P., Parkinson, J. F., Dwight, T., Ikin, R. J., Zhu, Y., Chen, J., Wheeler, H. R., & Howell, V. M. (2016). Intratumoral heterogeneity identified at the epigenetic, genetic and transcriptional level in glioblastoma. *Scientific Reports*, *6*(1), 22477. Advance online publication. DOI: 10.1038/srep22477 PMID: 26940435

Perry, J., Zinman, L., Chambers, A., Spithoff, K., Lloyd, N., & Laperriere, N. (2006). The use of prophylactic anticonvulsants in patients with brain tumours—A systematic review. *Current Oncology (Toronto, Ont.)*, *13*(6), 222–229. DOI: 10.3747/co.v13i6.107 PMID: 22792022

. Pulumati, A., Pulumati, A., Dwarakanath, B. S., Verma, A., & Papineni, R. V. L. (2023). Technological advancements in cancer diagnostics: Improvements and limitations. Cancer Reports, 6(2), Article e1764. DOI: 10.1002/cnr2.1764

Rajendran, A. T., & Vadakkepushpakath, A. N. (2024). Targeting glioblastoma: Advances in precision drug delivery. *Journal of Young Pharmacists : JYP*, *16*(4), 697–705. DOI: 10.5530/jyp.2024.16.89

Rajput, T. A. (2025). The role of microRNAs in glioblastoma: Gene therapy and diagnostic potentials. *Medical Science and Discovery*, *12*(5), 154–162. DOI: 10.36472/msd.v12i5.1276

Reardon, D. A., & Wen, P. Y. (2015). Glioma in 2014: Unravelling tumour heterogeneity—Implications for therapy. *Nature Reviews. Clinical Oncology*, *12*(2), 69–70. DOI: 10.1038/nrclinonc.2014.223 PMID: 25560529

Rodriguez, S. M. B., Kamel, A., Ciubotaru, G. V., Onose, G., Sevastre, A.-S., Sfredel, V., & Mirea, A. (2023). An overview of EGFR mechanisms and their implications in targeted therapies for glioblastoma. *International Journal of Molecular Sciences*, *24*(13), 11110. Advance online publication. DOI: 10.3390/ijms241311110 PMID: 37446288

Rucco, M., Falsetti, L., & Viticchi, G. (2020). Towards personalized diagnosis of glioblastoma in fluid-attenuated inversion recovery (FLAIR) by topological interpretable machine learning. arXiv. Retrieved May 17, 2025, from https://arxiv.org/abs/1912.08167

Sadowski, K., Jażdżewska, A., Kozłowski, J., Zacny, A., Lorenc, T., & Olejarz, W. (2024). Revolutionizing glioblastoma treatment: A comprehensive overview of modern therapeutic approaches. *International Journal of Molecular Sciences*, *25*(11), 5774. Advance online publication. DOI: 10.3390/ijms25115774 PMID: 38891962

Schiff, D., Lee, E. Q., Nayak, L., Norden, A. D., Reardon, D. A., & Wen, P. Y. (2015). Medical management of brain tumors and the sequelae of treatment. *Neuro-Oncology*, *17*(4), 488–504. DOI: 10.1093/neuonc/nou304 PMID: 25358508

Seker-Polat, F., Pinarbasi Degirmenci, N., Solaroglu, I., & Bagci-Onder, T. (2022). Tumor cell infiltration into the brain in glioblastoma: From mechanisms to clinical perspectives. *Cancers (Basel)*, *14*(2), 443. Advance online publication. DOI: 10.3390/cancers14020443 PMID: 35053605

Shang, W., Zeng, C., Du, Y., Hui, H., Liang, X., Chi, C., Wang, K., Wang, Z., & Tian, J. (2017). Core–shell gold nanorod@metal–organic framework nanoprobes for multimodality diagnosis of glioma. *Advanced Materials*, *29*(3), 1604381. Advance online publication. DOI: 10.1002/adma.201604381 PMID: 27859713

Sperring, C. P., Argenziano, M. G., Savage, W. M., Teasley, D. E., Upadhyayula, P. S., Winans, N. J., Canoll, P., & Bruce, J. N. (2023). Convection-enhanced delivery of immunomodulatory therapy for high-grade glioma. *Neuro-Oncology Advances*, *5*(1), vdad044. Advance online publication. DOI: 10.1093/noajnl/vdad044 PMID: 37215957

Stupp, R., Mason, W. P., van den Bent, M. J., Weller, M., Fisher, B., Taphoorn, M. J. B., Belanger, K., Brandes, A. A., Marosi, C., Bogdahn, U., Curschmann, J., Janzer, R. C., Ludwin, S. K., Gorlia, T., Allgeier, A., Lacombe, D., Cairncross, J. G., Eisenhauer, E., & Mirimanoff, R. O. (2005). Radiotherapy plus concomitant and adjuvant temozolomide for glioblastoma. *The New England Journal of Medicine*, *352*(10), 987–996. DOI: 10.1056/NEJMoa043330 PMID: 15758009

Sun, L., Liu, H., Ye, Y., Lei, Y., Islam, R., Tan, S., & Fu, Y. (2023). Smart nanoparticles for cancer therapy. *Signal Transduction and Targeted Therapy*, *8*(1), 418. Advance online publication. DOI: 10.1038/s41392-023-01642-x PMID: 37919282

Tang, W., Fan, W., Lau, J., Deng, L., Shen, Z., & Chen, X. (2019). Emerging blood–brain-barrier-crossing nanotechnology for brain cancer theranostics. *Chemical Society Reviews*, *48*(11), 2967–3014. DOI: 10.1039/C8CS00805A PMID: 31089607

The 2024 Brain Tumor Segmentation (BraTS) Challenge: Glioma segmentation on post-treatment MRI. (n.d.). arXiv. Retrieved May 17, 2025, from https://arxiv.org/html/2405.18368

Thenuwara, G., Curtin, J., & Tian, F. (2023). Advances in diagnostic tools and therapeutic approaches for gliomas: A comprehensive review. *Sensors (Basel)*, *23*(24), 9842. Advance online publication. DOI: 10.3390/s23249842 PMID: 38139688

van den Bossche, W. B. L., Kleijn, A., Teunissen, C. E., Voerman, J. S. A., Teodosio, C., Noske, D. P., van den Bent, M. J., van den Bent, M. J., & van den Bent, M. J. (2018). Oncolytic virotherapy in glioblastoma patients induces a tumor macrophage phenotypic shift leading to an altered glioblastoma microenvironment. *Neuro-Oncology*, *20*(11), 1494–1504. DOI: 10.1093/neuonc/noy082 PMID: 29796615

van Linde, M. E., Brahm, C. G., de Witt Hamer, P. C., Reijneveld, J. C., Bruynzeel, A. M. E., Vandertop, W. P., van de Ven, P. M., Wagemakers, M., van der Hoeven, A. M., Enting, R. H., & Verheul, H. M. W. (2017). Treatment outcome of patients with recurrent glioblastoma multiforme: A retrospective multicenter analysis. *Journal of Neuro-Oncology*, *135*(1), 183–192. DOI: 10.1007/s11060-017-2564-z PMID: 28730289

Vaz-Salgado, M. A., Villamayor, M., Albarrán, V., Alía, V., Sotoca, P., Chamorro, J., & García-Barbero, J. (2023). Recurrent glioblastoma: A review of the treatment options. *Cancers (Basel)*, *15*(17), 4279. Advance online publication. DOI: 10.3390/cancers15174279 PMID: 37686553

Voloshin, T., Kaynan, N., Davidi, S., Porat, Y., Shteingauz, A., Schneiderman, R. S., Zeevi, E., Munster, M., Blumberg, G., & Giladi, M. (2020). Tumor-treating fields (TTFields) induce immunogenic cell death resulting in enhanced antitumor efficacy when combined with anti-PD-1 therapy. *Cancer Immunology, Immunotherapy : CII*, *69*(7), 1191–1204. DOI: 10.1007/s00262-020-02534-7 PMID: 32144446

Wang, S. W., Gao, C., Zheng, Y. M., Yi, L., Lu, J. C., Huang, X. Y., & Li, B. (2022). Current applications and future perspective of CRISPR/Cas9 gene editing in cancer. *Molecular Cancer*, *21*(1), 57. Advance online publication. DOI: 10.1186/s12943-022-01518-8 PMID: 35189910

Wang, Z., Hu, P., Tang, F., Lian, H., Chen, X., Zhang, Y., He, X., Liu, Y., Wu, J., & Wang, Z. (2016). HDAC6 promotes cell proliferation and confers resistance to temozolomide in glioblastoma. *Cancer Letters*, *379*(1), 134–142. DOI: 10.1016/j.canlet.2016.06.001 PMID: 27267806

Wei, D., Zhang, N., Qu, S., Wang, H., & Li, J. (2023). Advances in nanotechnology for the treatment of GBM. *Frontiers in Neuroscience*, *17*, 1180943. Advance online publication. DOI: 10.3389/fnins.2023.1180943 PMID: 37214394

Wick, W., Puduvalli, V. K., Chamberlain, M. C., van den Bent, M. J., Carpentier, A. F., Cher, L. M., Mason, W., Weller, M., Hong, S., Musib, L., & Hedley, D. W. (2010). Phase III study of enzastaurin compared with lomustine in the treatment of recurrent intracranial glioblastoma. *Journal of Clinical Oncology*, *28*(7), 1168–1174. DOI: 10.1200/JCO.2009.23.2595 PMID: 20124186

Woo, P. Y. M., Li, Y., Chan, A. H. Y., Ng, S. C. P., Loong, H. H. F., Chan, D. T. M., Wong, G. K. C., & Poon, W. S. (2019). A multifaceted review of temozolomide resistance mechanisms in glioblastoma beyond O-6-methylguanine-DNA methyltransferase. *Glioma (Mumbai, India)*, *2*(2), 68–82. DOI: 10.4103/glioma.glioma_3_19

Yalamarty, S. S. K., Filipczak, N., Li, X., Subhan, M. A., Parveen, F., Ataide, J. A., & Torchilin, V. P. (2023). Mechanisms of resistance and current treatment options for glioblastoma multiforme (GBM). *Cancers (Basel)*, *15*(7), 2116. Advance online publication. DOI: 10.3390/cancers15072116 PMID: 37046777

Yekula, A., Taylor, A., Beecroft, A., Kang, K. M., Small, J. L., Muralidharan, K., & Carter, B. S. (2021). The role of extracellular vesicles in acquisition of resistance to therapy in glioblastomas. *Cancer Drug Resistance (Alhambra, Calif.)*, *4*(1), 1–16. DOI: 10.20517/cdr.2020.94 PMID: 35582008

Young, R. M., Jamshidi, A., Davis, G., & Sherman, J. H. (2015). Current trends in the surgical management and treatment of adult glioblastoma. *Annals of Translational Medicine*, *3*(9), 121. Advance online publication. DOI: 10.3978/j.issn.2305-5839.2015.05.10 PMID: 26207249

Yu, W., & Wu, Z. (2019). Use of AAV vectors for CRISPR-mediated in vivo genome editing in the retina. In Castle, M. J. (Ed.), *Adeno-associated virus vectors* (pp. 123–139). Springer., DOI: 10.1007/978-1-4939-9139-6_7

Yusuf, A., Almotairy, A. R. Z., Henidi, H., Alshehri, O. Y., & Aldughaim, M. S. (2023). Nanoparticles as drug delivery systems: A review of the implication of nanoparticles' physicochemical properties on responses in biological systems. *Polymers*, *15*(7), 1596. Advance online publication. DOI: 10.3390/polym15071596 PMID: 37050210

Zhang, B. (2021). CRISPR/Cas gene therapy. *Journal of Cellular Physiology*, *236*(4), 2459–2481. DOI: 10.1002/jcp.30064 PMID: 32959897

Zhang, H., Li, Z., Gao, C., Fan, X., Pang, Y., Li, T., & Zhang, Z. (2021). Dual-responsive biohybrid neutrobots for active target delivery. *Science Robotics*, *6*(52), eaaz9519. Advance online publication. DOI: 10.1126/scirobotics.aaz9519 PMID: 34043546

. Zhang, L., Zhang, Z., He, J., Zhang, Z., Zhou, H., Jiang, Y., & Wang, Y. (2025). Dual challenges and innovative strategies in chimeric antigen receptor T-cell therapy for glioblastoma. Oncology Advances, 0(000), 0–0. https://doi.org/ (advance online publication)DOI: 10.1002/onav.10000

Zhang, L. P., Kang, L., Li, X., Liu, S., Liu, T., & Zhao, Y. (2021). Pyrazino[2,3-g] quinoxaline-based nanoparticles as near-infrared phototheranostic agents for efficient photoacoustic-im imaging-guided photothermal therapy. *ACS Applied Nano Materials*, *4*(2), 2019–2029. DOI: 10.1021/acsanm.0c03346

Zhang, X., Zhao, L., Zhang, H., Zhang, Y., Ju, H., Wang, X., Ren, X., & Li, W. (2022). The immunosuppressive microenvironment and immunotherapy in human glioblastoma. *Frontiers in Immunology*, *13*, 1003651. Advance online publication. DOI: 10.3389/fimmu.2022.1003651 PMID: 36466873

Zhao, J., Ma, X., Gao, P., Han, X., Zhao, P., Xie, F., & Liu, Z. (2024). Advancing glioblastoma treatment by targeting metabolism. *Neoplasia : an International Journal for Oncology Research*, *51*, 100985. Advance online publication. DOI: 10.1016/j.neo.2024.100985 PMID: 38479191

Zhao, L., Li, Y., Zhu, J., Sun, N., Song, N., Xing, Y., Huang, H., Zhao, J., & Sun, J. (2019). Chlorotoxin peptide-functionalized polyethylenimine-entrapped gold nanoparticles for glioma SPECT/CT imaging and radionuclide therapy. *Journal of Nanobiotechnology*, *17*(1), 30. Advance online publication. DOI: 10.1186/s12951-019-0462-6 PMID: 30782154

Zhao, W. Y., Zhang, C. X., Liu, L., Mu, L. M., Zeng, F., Ju, R. J., Xie, H.-J., Yan, Y., Zhao, Y., & Lu, W.-L. (2016). Construction of functional targeting daunorubicin liposomes used for eliminating brain glioma and glioma stem cells. *Journal of Biomedical Nanotechnology*, *12*(7), 1404–1420. DOI: 10.1166/jbn.2016.2266 PMID: 29336535

Zhao, Y., Bai, L., Zhang, Z., Wu, Y., Islam, M., & Ren, H. (2024). Transferring knowledge from high-quality to low-quality MRI for adult glioma diagnosis. arXiv. Retrieved May 17, 2025, from https://arxiv.org/abs/2410.18698

Chapter 3
DNA Lesions and Double-Strand Breaks for Glioblastoma

Vidyasrilekha Sanapalli
School of Pharmacy and Technology Management, SVKM's Narsee Monjee Institute of Management Studies (NMIMS), Jadcherla, India

Anitha Kuttiappan
School of Pharmacy and Technology Management, SVKM's Narsee Monjee Institute of Management Studies (NMIMS), Shirpur, India

Krishna Swaroop Akey
Department of Pharmaceutical Chemistry, Shri Vile Parle Kelavani Mandal's College of Pharmacy, Shirpur, India

Pavan Kumar Chintamaneni
GITAM School of Pharmacy, GITAM University-Hyderabad Campus, Rudraram, India

Ashwini Deshpande
School of Pharmacy and Technology Management, SVKM's Narsee Monjee Institute of Management Studies (NMIMS), Jadcherla, India

Bharat Kumar Reddy Sanapalli
https://orcid.org/0000-0002-9162-5553
School of Pharmacy and Technology Management, SVKM's Narsee Monjee Institute of Management Studies (NMIMS), Jadcherla, India

ABSTRACT

Glioblastoma (GBM) is a model of resistance to therapy. Despite the formation of lethal DNA lesions by alkylating agents, including temozolomide, GBM cells utilize error-prone double-strand break (DSB) repair pathways to escape death. New findings demonstrate that hypoxia, which is a key feature of the GBM microenvironment, reshuffles the response to DNA damage response networks by increasing the expression of POLQ. This change induces chromosomal rearrangements and radiation resistance but generates targetable vulnerabilities. Several lines of evidence have

DOI: 10.4018/979-8-3373-2695-5.ch003

shown that POLQ silencing sensitized hypoxic GBM cells to poly(ADP–ribose) polymerase inhibitors through disabling backup repair pathways. This chapter reviews ongoing efforts to elucidate DSB repair plasticity in the context of treatment failure and describes opportunities to leverage that plasticity for therapeutic gain.

INTRODUCTION

Glioblastoma (GBM), a Grade IV astrocytoma, affects over 13,000 people annually in the U.S. alone. Despite maximal therapy, including surgical resection, Temozolomide (TMZ), and radiation, the median survival remains dismal at 15 months (Angom, Nakka, & Bhattacharya, 2023). Resistance genes are ultimately derived from the genomic chaos of GBM, characterized by hypermutated genomes, epidermal growth factor receptor (EGFR) amplification, and the O6-methylguanine-DNA methyltransferase (MGMT) promoter methylation state, which drive therapeutic responses (Woo et al., 2019). Nevertheless, it is becoming increasingly clear that an imbalance in double-strand break (DSB) repair is a key determinant of treatment resistance. GBM relies on genomic instability, but it cannot tolerate the lethal burdens of mutations. Unlike other cancers with preserved DNA damage response (DDR) pathways, GBM presents a state of regulated chaos, inactivating specific repair nodes, such as MSH6 mutations in TMZ-resistant recurrences, while overregulating others, such as the DNA-dependent protein kinase catalytic subunit (DNA-PKcs) in radioresistant niches (Vilar, Christmann, & Tomicic, 2022). This homeostasis also allows tumor adaptation without inducing apoptosis (Mazzoleni et al., 2024). For instance, Zhang et al. (2025) conducted single-cell sequencing and reported that subclonal BRCA2 deletions were associated with GBM, with the acquisition of homologous recombination (HR) deficiency in treatment-exposed regions and retention of HR proficiency in quiescent cells (Zhang & Wang, 2025). DSBs in GBM are not merely passive lesions but rather active modulators of oncogenic signaling. Radiation-induced breaks that activate NF-κB via ATM drive pro-survival cytokine secretion (Hasegawa, Saga, & Hosokawa, 2023). Similarly, TMZ-generated O_6-methylguanine (O_6MeG) mispairs form DSBs during replication, but GBM cells highjack alternative end-joining (Alt-EJ) to fuse distant chromosomal regions, thus generating double-minute chromosomes carrying oncogenic myelocytomatosis (MYC) (Agnihotri et al., 2012; Bora, Pal, Mandi, & Dutta, 2024). DSB repair must be temporally and spatially coordinated. Although poly(ADP–ribose) polymerase inhibitors (PARPis) appear to hold great potential in the treatment of MGMT-unmethylated GBM, the results from some phase I trials (e.g., NCT03581292) have been less favorable, especially because patients were not selected for such therapies (Bonm & Kesari, 2021; Sim, Galanis, & Khasraw, 2022). This underscores the importance of the utility of real-time biomarkers to monitor adaptive repair pathway switching, for example, ctDNA profiles for TP53 and RAD51 mutations (Reina, Šabanović, Lazzari, Gregorc, & Heeschen, 2024).

SPECTRUM OF DNA LESIONS IN GLIOBLASTOMA

The resistance of GBM to therapy is based on its capacity to handle and adapt to various types of DNA damage. Although DSBs are frequently cited as key lesions, genomic instability is the consequence of the interplay of oxidative lesions, alkylation damage, and replication stress (Annovazzi, Mellai, & Schiffer, 2017). To counteract these consequences, different challenges are emerging for the DNA repair machinery, ultimately enabling GBM cells to progress and develop resistance to treatment.

TMZ therapy induces alkylation damage, the signature lesion, which is frequently caused by a struggle between O_6MeG adducts and the MGMT repair protein (Strobel et al., 2019). Nevertheless, TMZ produces a wider range of lesions, including N_7-methylguanine (N_7MeG) and N_3-methyladenine (N_3MeA), which together constitute more than 85% of the total DNA adducts (Yang et al., 2019). The O_6MeG lesions, however, disrupt replication forks by inducing conformational changes in DNA. More recently, we reported that replication forks formed from N_3MeA adducts are not just obstacles but also smart killers of mitotic cells (Groth et al., 2010). For example, human GBM cells lacking functional Fanconi anemia (FA) pathway proteins, such as Fanconi anemia complementation group D2 (FANCD2), fail to reinforce these forks, and this inability is associated with massive generation of mitotic DSBs (Drzewiecka et al., 2023). This sensitivity to alkylation damage is intriguing since FA pathway mutations are rare in primary GBM, whereas the recurrent tumor arising in the presence of TMZ reveals epigenetic silencing of FA genes, providing evidence for the presence of positive selection each time the cells are exposed to alkylation damage to favor cells that no longer require tolerance to fork collapse (Lozinski, Bowden, Graves, Fay, & Tooney, 2021). This evolutionary struggle highlights the Janus-faced nature of alkylating agents — they wipe out sensitive populations, yet paradoxically, they favor the survival of clones able to compromise replication stress responses.

Oxidative DNA damage, which is mediated by the hypoxic microenvironment of the GBM, adds another dimension to its complexity. 8-Oxoguanine and other oxidized bases can be generated due to mitochondrial dysfunction and reactive oxygen species (ROS) formation during hypoxia (Attique et al., 2025; Krawczynski, Godlewski, & Bronisz, 2020). Nuclear DNA repair systems, including base excision repair (BER), have traditionally been described as part of the 'housekeeping' machinery that sustains the integrity of the nuclear genome against oxidative stress (Whitaker, Schaich, Smith, Flynn, & Freudenthal, 2017). However, recent discoveries have demonstrated that a mtDNA DDR that operates independently of the nuclear machinery (Lyakhovich, Graifer, Stefanovie, & Krejci, 2016). In GBM, mitochondrial ROS signal through the kinases ataxia-telangiectasia mutated (ATM) and Parkin RBR E3 ubiquitin protein ligase (PARK2) to mark defective mitochondria for elimination by mitophagy (Liu et al., 2020; Xie et al., 2021). While this mechanism may be beneficial in the short term, it inhibits therapeutic use (W. Li & Xu, 2023). Blocking ATM in hypoxic GBM cells perturbs mitochondrial quality control, which is followed by the generation of ROS that exceed the antioxidant capacity. Preclinical models have shown that the combination of ATM inhibitors and radiation induces ferroptosis—a form of iron-dependent cell death—in treatment-resistant GBM stem cells (Dalma, 2020). This finding changes the paradigm: rather than considering therapies that target the nuclear DDR only, those that increase mitochondrial oxidative stress may overcome crude resistance mechanisms.

Oncogene activation and misregulation of the cell cycle result in replication stress, which introduces a unique class of DNA lesions. Amplification of EGFR, which occurs in more than 50% of GBMs, promotes ectopic activation of replication origins via ataxia telangiectasia and Rad3-related (ATR) (Gousias, Theocharous, & Simon, 2022). The encounter of replication with the transcription machinery generates both RNA–DNA hybrids (R loops) and single-stranded DNA gaps. These lesions are of particular concern because they escape recognition by classical DDR sensors such as ATR-interacting protein (ATRIP) (Paull, 2019). Rather, GBM cells depend on dedicated enzymes such as RAD51 and FANCD2 to reinitiate a stalled fork, which can come at the cost of increased mutagenesis (Drzewiecka et al., 2023). For example, replication stress in EGFRVIII-mutant GBM increases the reliance on error-prone DNA polymerases, such as DNA polymerase eta (POLH), for low-fidelity lesion bypass (Jung, 2022). This "translesion synthesis" allows tumor cells to complete replication but introduces mutations that fuel heterogeneity. Recent single-molecule sequencing studies have mapped replication stress hotspots in GBM genomes, revealing preferential localization near oncogenes such as MYC and platelet-derived growth factor receptor alpha (PDGFRA) (Sun, Wang, Cheng, Su, & Ou, 2019). These regions, termed "replication catastrophe zones," are enriched for chromosomal rearrangements and may serve as biomarkers for tumors susceptible to ATR inhibitors (Anand et al., 2023; Azam, 2021).

The interplay between these lesions creates a vicious cycle of genomic instability. Alkylation damage-induced fork collapse generates DSBs, which are repaired via error-prone mechanisms under oxidative stress (Fahrer & Christmann, 2023). On the other hand, replication stress augments mutagenesis by promoting cell endurance through irresolute or erroneous DNA synthesis (Bostian & Eoff, 2016). This interdependence is not arbitrary but spatially organized within the complex architecture of GBM. For example, perinecrotic areas with strong hypoxia promote Alt-EJ of DSBs because of low levels of BRCA1, whereas in vascularized parts of a tumor, HR remains functional (Majumder, Nataraj, Maitreyi, & Datta, 2024) (**Figure 1**). This heterogeneity of tissues presents a challenge for therapy, since a drug is not only differentially effective in one niche versus another. Emerging techniques such as spatial transcriptomics are beginning to map DDR pathway activity throughout the GBM microenvironment, which offers hope for such spatially informed combination therapeutics (Chen, Larsson, Swarbrick, & Lundeberg, 2024; J. Liu et al., 2024; Robinson et al., 2025).

Figure 1. Hypoxia-driven repair pathway switching in glioblastoma

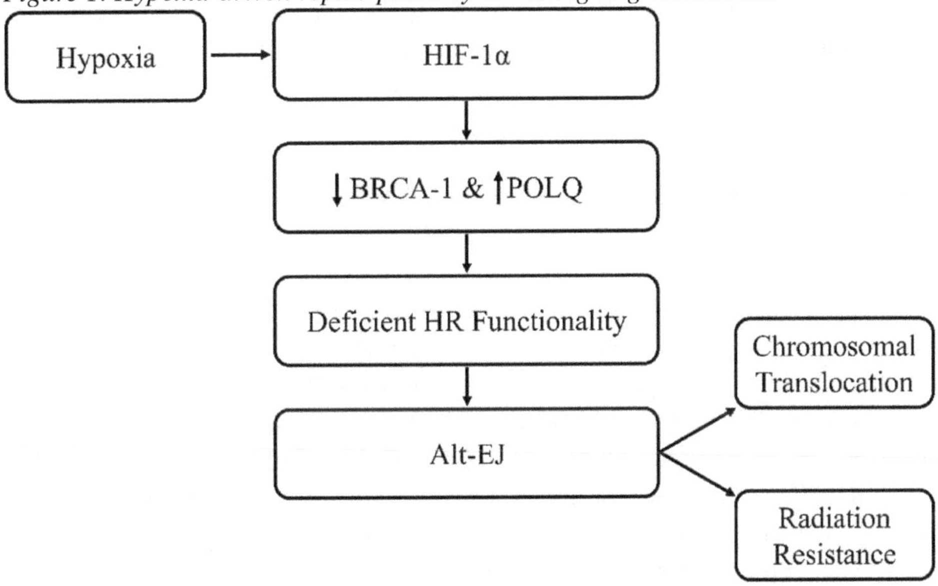

Hypoxia reprograms DNA double-strand break (DSB) repair in glioblastoma. In hypoxic niches, HIF-1α suppresses BRCA1 and upregulates POLQ, shifting repair to error-prone alternative end joining (Alt-EJ). This promotes chromosomal translocations (e.g., EGFR–MGMT fusions) and radiation resistance.

Crucially, the cocktail of DNA damage present in GBM is not only a biological oddity but also a therapeutic soft spot. Alkylation and oxidative lesions also decrease nucleotide levels through the induction of repair enzymes such as PARP-1, the latter of which can be reversed by salvage pathways such as the mitochondrial thymidine kinase (TK2) pathway (Wang, Luo, & Wang, 2019). Pharmacological inhibition of TK2 in TMZ-exposed GBM cells elicits increased replication stress, which is leveraged for synthetic lethality (Nafe & Hattingen, 2023). Consistently, replication stress itself might sensitize cells to immune recognition via increased neoantigen load as a result of polymerase errors (Amodio, Vitiello, Bardelli, & Germano, 2024). To exploit this synergy, combinations of DDR inhibitors, such as ATRs and PARPis, with agents targeting immune checkpoint inhibitors are under investigation in early-phase clinical trials (Shi et al., 2022). However, these strategies require more accurate patient selection because tumors with hypermutated genomes might behave differently from those with copy number-driven instability.

In conclusion, the DNA lesion landscape of GBM is a dynamic network influenced by therapy-induced damage, microenvironmental stress, and intrinsic replication errors. This ecosystem should be addressed via a complex approach that takes into consideration lesion type and, in a broader sense, spatial context and evolutionary selection. The next part of this review explores how the GBM has harnessed DSB repair pathways for survival amidst the genomic upheaval, thereby transforming a basic cellular process into a resistance mechanism.

THE MACHINERY OF DOUBLE-STRAND BREAK REPAIR IN GLIOBLASTOMA

The survival of glioblastoma relies on its capacity to repair DNA DSBs, the most deleterious form of DNA damage. Unlike normal cells, which tire burning at both ends in normal repair and genomic stability, GBM cells hijack DSB repair pathways to create orderly chaos-allowing errors for the purpose of driving evolution but avoid deadly genomic meltdown (Erasimus, Gobin, Niclou, & Van Dyck, 2016; Maksoud, 2022). This level of homeostasis is maintained through a combination of dysregulated repair, microenvironmental forces, and oncogene-driven adaptations, all of which represent targetable vulnerabilities.

A hallmark repair pathway behind the treatment resistance of GBM is the use of nonhomologous end joining (NHEJ), a nontemplated, mutagenic repair mechanism that links DNA ends without a homologous template (Ly et al., 2019). This ability to work independently of the cell cycle makes NHEJ the most prevalent pathway in most cancers, but NHEJ is upregulated to pathological levels in GBM (Esemen et al., 2022). The NHEJ kinase DNA-PKcs is upregulated by hyperactivation of the PI3K-AKT pathway in >50% of GBMs with EGFR amplification (Nahar Metu et al., 2023). This results in fast but imprecise repair of radiation-induced lesions, which enables the tumor cells to survive ionizing radiation but accrue heterogeneity, promoting mutations. Some recent studies have revealed that NHEJ is neither a static phenomenon in glioblastoma nor a universally derepressed process but is instead dynamically regulated by niches within tumors (Onciul et al., 2024). For example, in oxygenated and nutritionally abundant perivascular regions, classical-NHEJ (c-NHEJ), which depends on DNA-PKcs and XRCC4-like factor or Cernunnos (XLF), is preferred, whereas in hypoxic regions, the dominance of c-NHEJ is altered in favor of Alt-EJ, where microhomology and DNA polymerase theta (PolQ) facilitate the end-bridging process (Bhargava et al., 2018). This spatial segregation explains the paradoxical treatment response whereby radiation may be effective at controlling the vascularized portions of a tumor but is largely ineffective at controlling the hypoxic cores where Alt-EJ promotes resistance.

High-fidelity HR is also believed to be compromised radically through hypoxia and the common loss of tumor suppressors such as phosphatase and TENsin homolog deleted on chromosome 10 (PTEN) in GBM (Ahuja, Gupta, Ajay, & Ghorai, 2025; Tang, Bolderson, O'Byrne, & Richard, 2021). However, HR is not disappearing altogether—instead, it is smothered. In necrotic tumor regions, hypoxia-inducible factor 1-alpha (HIF-1α) is highly expressed and is capable of transcriptional repression of BRCA1 and RAD51, members of the SR family of partners (Singh, Tomar, & Rath, 2015). This repression force leads cells to rely on error-prone pathways yet reveal cryptic vulnerabilities. For example, when reoxygenated after anti-angiogenic treatment (by bevacizumab), HR proficiency can be temporarily restored, which inadvertently reduces the potency of the killing effect of PARPis on tumor cells (Ledermann & Luvero, 2015). This highlights the factor of timing in the HR status-based targeted therapy of cancer cells, as very likely, there are only temporary repair landscapes due to microenvironment instabilities within cells (**Figure 2**).

Figure 2. Spatial heterogeneity of DNA repair in glioblastoma

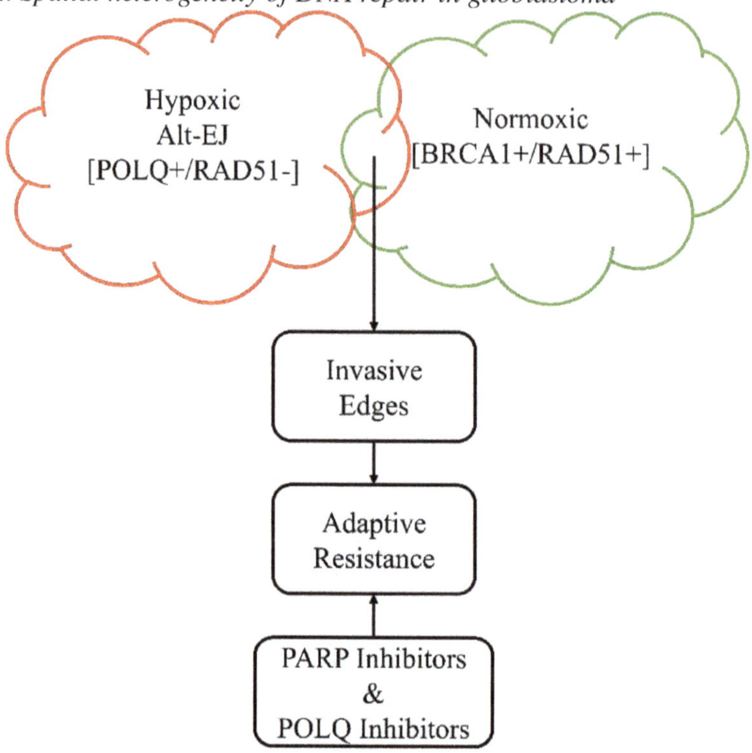

Spatial transcriptomics map of DSB repair activity across glioblastoma niches. The pronecrotic regions (hypoxic) show Alt-EJ dominance (POLQ+/RAD51−), whereas the perivascular zones (normoxic) retain HR activity (BRCA1+/RAD51+). Invasive margins exhibit mixed repair signatures, reflecting adaptive resistance. Therapeutic strategies must account for this heterogeneity, e.g., POLQ inhibitors for hypoxic cores and PARP inhibitors for HR-deficient margins.

Contrary to previous assumptions, the findings reveal that what was traditionally considered a secondary or backup response is, in fact, a functionally equivalent pathway for repair. This Alt-EJ was beginning to look increasingly like a node in GBM adaptive resistance. The Alt-EJ mode, as determined by microhomology sequence usage and POLQ-dependent activity, is heavily involved in some types of oxidative stress and is predominantly confined to telomeric regions for replication. Similarly, in glioblastoma stem cells (GSCs), POLQ acts as a surface intermediate for regulating the formation of branched DNA-repair ligase complexes and diagnosing so-called resistant sterically blocked breaks made by TMZ into more manageable forms that can be removed. By pressing large sections of the genome up against each other, which may be miles apart in space, Alt-EJ not only employs patches for repair but also creates cancer-driving swaps, such as EGFR-VIII deletions (Chung et al., 2025). Single-cell sequencing has revealed that therapy-resistant clones bearing the signature of Alt-EJ in recurrent GBM could represent a target to prevent aggressive subpopulations from burgeoning.

Repair pathway choice is also modulated by chromatin structure. Posttranslational modifications of histones, such as histone H3 lysine 9 (H3K9) trimethylation, form condensed chromatin and inhibit HR machinery access (Millán-Zambrano, Burton, Bannister, & Schneider, 2022). GBM takes advantage of this, overexpressing histone methyltransferases, such as Suppressor of Variegation 3-9 Homolog 1 (SUV39H1), which promote a chromatin state that is more conducive to NHEJ (Ciechomska, Jayaprakash, Maleszewska, & Kaminska, 2020; B. Li, Zheng, & Yang, 2019; Ozair et al., 2023). Alternatively, histone deacetylase (HDAC) inhibitors decompact the chromatin structure in a manner that unexpectedly promotes HR in certain contexts (Bose, Dai, & Grant, 2014). This dichotomy complicates the development of epigenetic-based strategies but provides opportunities for combination strategies. For example, HDAC inhibitors sensitize HR-competent tumor subpopulations to PARPis but render Alt-EJ-dependent niches sensitive to POLQ inhibition (Paul, Sinha, & Kundu, 2022).

The pharmacological exploitation of DSB repair is further hampered by the rewiring of metabolism by GBM (Meng, Palmer, Siedow, Haque, & Chakravarti, 2022). The high glucose uptake of the tumor and the production of lactate make the milieu acidic, which restricts important repair enzymes. Lactate, for example, interferes with the formation of the BRCA1-Partner and Localizer of BRCA2 (BRCA1-PALB2) complex, leading to even greater inhibition of HR (Simhadri et al., 2014). This metabolic underminement can be leveraged therapeutically: agents that further induce acidosis, including monocarboxylate transporter inhibitors, act in combination with radiation to exceed repair capacity. In contrast, the glucose-limiting ketogenic diet is under investigation in clinical trials as a means to sensitize patients to DDR-targeted therapies.

However, challenges exist in the development of therapeutic interventions. Intratumoral heterogeneity guarantees that one size does not fit all, and identification of alternative pathways is needed to overcome resistance. BBB penetration is a challenge for several DDR inhibitors, but nanoparticle formulations and focused ultrasound are promising in preclinical models (Brar, Jose, Wu, & Sharma, 2022; Duan et al., 2024). Furthermore, DSB repair-targeted therapies need to be designed so as not to attack normal neural stem cells (NSCs), which have some repair requirements in common with those of GSCs, with catastrophic toxicity. In the following section, we discuss how these mechanistic insights translate into clinical strategies, ranging from synthetic lethality to immune modulation, and the biomarkers for patient selection.

EXPLOITING DNA REPAIR VULNERABILITIES FOR THERAPEUTIC BENEFIT IN GLIOBLASTOMA

The dependence of glioblastoma on defective DNA repair offers a double-edged sword—genetically determined susceptibility to survival under genotoxic stress also imposes an unshielded vulnerability (Tian et al., 2015). Promising advances in cancer treatment are seeking to shift the balance from controlled genomic chaos to catastrophic cell death by leveraging synthetic lethal interactions, metabolic vulnerabilities and immune priming. We review these strategies below with an eye toward recent breakthroughs and unanswered questions.

Synthetic Lethality and the PARP Inhibition

PARPis, such as olaparib and niraparib, have transformed the treatment of BRCA-mutant cancers. In GBM, context-dependent HR deficiencies (such as PTEN loss and hypoxia-induced BRCA1 suppression) can be exploited via the use of PARPis in combination with TMZ to promote synthetic lethality (Veneris, Matulonis, Liu, & Konstantinopoulos, 2020) (**Figure 3**). In a 2023 phase II trial (NCT04564027), the MGMT-unmethylated disease, which is not typically TMZ sensitive, was associated with increased PFS in patients who were treated with TMZ plus veliparib (Aggarwal et al., 2024). This effect stems from PARP trapping at alkylation-induced single-strand breaks, which collapse replication forks into double-strand breaks (DSBs). However, resistance emerges via *RAD51* upregulation in hypoxic niches, highlighting the need for spatial targeting. Novel brain-penetrating PARP inhibitors, such as AZD9574, are now in clinical trials, with preclinical data showing enhanced efficacy in GSCs with PTEN mutations (Durant et al., 2018).

Figure 3. Synthetic lethality of PARP inhibitors in MGMT-unmethylated glioblastoma

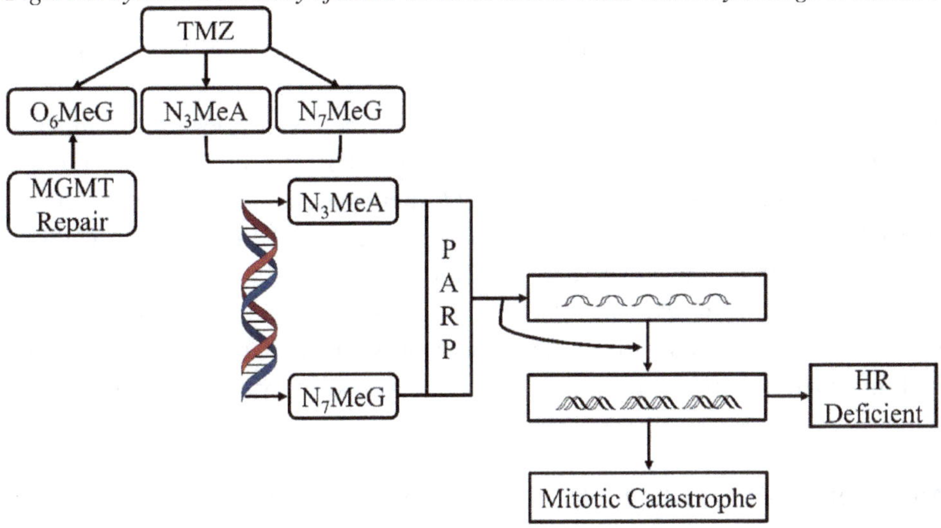

Mechanism of the synergistic effects of a PARP inhibitor (PARPi) with Temozolomide (TMZ) on MGMT-unmethylated glioblastoma. TMZ-induced N3-methyladenine and N7-methylguanine lesions stall replication forks. PARP trapping at these sites prevents repair, converting single-strand breaks (SSBs) into lethal double-strand breaks (DSBs) during replication. In HR-deficient tumors (e.g., those with PTEN loss), unrepaired DSBs trigger mitotic catastrophe.

POLQ and Alt-EJ: Targeting Error-Prone Repair

The Alt-EJ and POLQ have emerged as linchpins in the adaptive resistance of GBM. POLQ facilitates microhomology-mediated repair of TMZ-induced DSBs, enabling GSCs to evade death while accumulating oncogenic fusion proteins (e.g., EGFR-MGMT). A groundbreaking 2023 study by Gonzalo et al. demonstrated that the POLQ inhibitor ART558, combined with radiation, reduced tumor volume by 70% in orthotopic GBM models (Rodriguez-Berriguete et al., 2023). POLQ inhibition forces cells into a repair crisis, as unresolved DSBs activate cyclic GMP-AMP synthase-stimulator of interferon genes (cGAS-STING) signaling, triggering immunogenic cell death (Oh et al., 2023). This dual mechanism—direct cytotoxicity and immune activation—positions POLQ as a high-priority target, with two clinical trials (NCT05664243 and NCT05838768) recruiting GBM patients (Drew, Zenke, & Curtin, 2025; Fukuta, Shaha, da Silva-Candal, Zhao, & Mitragotri, 2025).

Combining DDR Inhibitors With Immunotherapy

DNA damage not only destabilizes genomes but also enhances tumor immunogenicity by increasing neoantigen load. However, the immunosuppressive microenvironment of GBM often nullifies this effect. Recent strategies have combined DDR inhibitors with immune checkpoint blockers (ICBs) to convert "cold" tumors into "hot" tumors (Ngoi, Peng, & Yap, 2022). For example, Hardaker et al. (2024) showed that ATR inhibition (ceralasertib) upregulates PD-L1 expression in GSCs, sensitizing them to anti-PD-1 therapy (Hardaker et al., 2024). Similarly, PARP inhibitors increase the amount of cytosolic DNA, activating STING-dependent interferon signaling. Olaparib was tested with durvalumab in recurrent GBM, with preliminary data showing prolonged stabilization in a subset of hypermutated tumors (Drew et al., 2024).

Metabolic Interventions to Exacerbate DNA Damage

The Warburg metabolism of GBM—marked by high glycolysis and lactate production—directly impairs DNA repair (Zhou & Wahl, 2019). Lactate acidosis inhibits the BRCA1–PALB2 interaction, crippling HR, whereas glucose deprivation depletes the nucleotides required for repair (**Figure 4**). Capitalizing on this, Martuscello et al. (2016) demonstrated that a ketogenic diet (90% fat, 10% carbohydrates) synergizes with TMZ in murine models, reducing tumor growth by 50% compared with TMZ alone (Martuscello et al., 2016). Clinical trials (NCT04631445) are evaluating this combination, with positron emission tomography (PET) imaging confirming enhanced DNA damage in diet-responsive patients (Mercier et al., 2022; Qin, Zhang, & Gao, 2024).

Figure 4. Metabolic regulation of DNA repair in glioblastoma

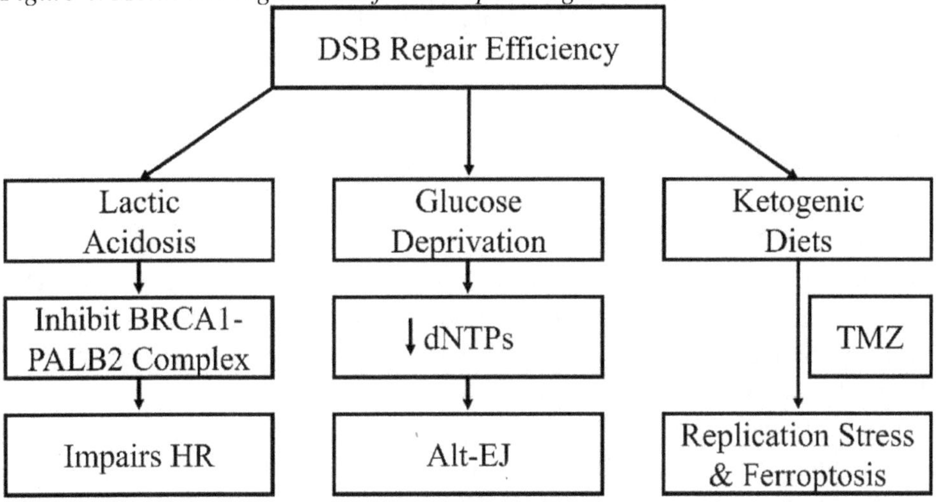

Metabolic adaptations influence DSB repair efficiency. Lactate acidosis inhibits BRCA1–PALB2 complex formation, impairing HR. Glucose deprivation depletes nucleotides (dNTPs), forcing reliance on error-prone repair. Ketogenic diets exacerbate these effects, synergizing with TMZ to induce replication stress and ferroptosis.

Blood–Brain Barrier Penetration and Toxicity Mitigation

A persistent challenge is delivering DDR inhibitors to the invasive margins of GBM. Nanoparticle formulations, such as poly(lactic-co-glycolic acid) (PLGA) carriers loaded with DNA-PKcs inhibitors, have shown promise in preclinical studies, achieving 10-fold higher intratumoral concentrations than free drugs. Focused ultrasound with microbubbles (FUS/MBs), which transiently disrupts the BBB, was tested in a first-in-human trial (NCT05370508) with the PARP inhibitor talazoparib. Early results indicate a 40% increase in drug delivery efficiency, although the risk of neuroinflammation remains ; .

THERAPEUTIC EXPLOITATION OF DNA REPAIR VULNERABILITIES IN GLIOBLASTOMA

The success of DNA repair-targeted therapies in GBM patients hinges on identifying predictive biomarkers to stratify patients most likely to benefit (**Tables 1 and 2**). Although MGMT promoter methylation represents the gold standard for predicting response to Temozolomide, the advent of new biomarkers has further refined precision (Wick et al., 2014). For example, the balance of 53BP1 versus BRCA1 protein expression, as quantified by immunohistochemistry, predicts sensitivity to PARP inhibitors in PTEN-deficient tumors, as 53BP1 loss limits the choice of repair pathways to those prone to error (Jacot et al., 2013). Droplet digital PCR was used to evaluate mtDNA copy number, a surrogate for HR capacity, and low mtDNA levels predicted HR deficiency and ATR inhibitor sensitivity (O'Hara et al., 2019). The analysis of circulating tumor DNA (ctDNA) is becoming established for real-time monitoring: POLQ amplifications that are detected in plasma are linked with radioresistance, and RAD51 mutations in ctDNA indicate adaptive upregulation of HR in hypoxic niches. Spatial transcriptomics likewise dissects intratumor heterogeneity (ITH), including Alt-EJ activity in pericecrotic areas, whereas HR proficiency is affected by the vasculature (M. Liu et al., 2024). From a clinical perspective, studies such as NCT04564027 (PARPi + TMZ) now incorporate these markers, and radiogenomic signatures generated from MRI and PET enable noninvasive predictions of repair pathway occupation (NCT05166096, olaparib + durvalumab) (Aggarwal et al., 2024). Nevertheless, standardization is a problem since preanalytical factors (e.g., site of biopsy, time point relative to therapy) influence biomarker readouts.

Table 1. Recent clinical trials exploiting DNA repair vulnerabilities in glioblastoma.

Trial Identifier	Intervention	Target/Mechanism	Phase	Key Inclusion Biomarkers	Primary Outcome
NCT04564027	Veliparib (PARPi) + Temozolomide	PARP inhibition + alkylation damage	II	MGMT-unmethylated tumors	Progression-Free Survival (PFS)
NCT05664243	ART558 (POLQ inhibitor) + Radiation	POLQ inhibition + radiation-induced DSBs	I/II	POLQ overexpression (IHC confirmed)	Tumor Volume Reduction (MRI)
NCT05166096	Olaparib (PARPi) + Durvalumab (anti-PD-L1)	PARP inhibition + immune checkpoint blockade	II	High tumor mutational burden (≥10 mutations/Mb)	Overall Response Rate (ORR)
NCT05370508	Talazoparib (PARPi) + Focused Ultrasound	PARP inhibition + BBB disruption	I	53BP1/BRCA1 ratio ≤0.5 (immunofluorescence)	Intratumoral Drug Concentration (PET)
NCT04991416	Ceralasertib (ATRi) + TMZ	ATR inhibition + replication stress	I/II	HR deficiency (RAD51 foci-negative tumors)	Dose-Limiting Toxicity (DLT)

Table 2. Biomarkers for DNA repair-targeted therapies

Biomarker	Detection Method	Therapeutic Implication	Clinical Trial Correlation
53BP1/BRCA1 Ratio	IHC/IF	Predicts PARPi sensitivity in PTEN-deficient tumors	NCT05370508
POLQ Amplification	ctDNA ddPCR	Associates with radiation resistance; POLQi candidate	NCT05664243
Mitochondrial DNA Copy Number	qPCR	Low mtDNA indicates HR deficiency; ATRi responsiveness	NCT04991416 (ATRi trial)
RAD51 Foci Formation	Immunofluorescence	HR proficiency contraindicates PARPi monotherapy	NCT04564027

CLINICAL ISSUES AND FUTURE PROSPECTS

The complexity of the microenvironment of GBM and the dynamic evolution of GBM pose significant challenges for DNA repair-targeted treatments. Temporal heterogeneity, if HR restoration after treatment with an anti-angiogenic agent, for example, can make tumors temporarily resistant to PARP inhibitors, and assays that measure changes in repair capacity dynamically are needed. Spatial heterogeneity further complicates the therapeutic response because BBB-protected invasive tumor margins evade systemic therapies, and perivascular niches overexpress drug efflux pumps, including ATP-binding cassette subfamily G member 2 (ABCG2). Neurotoxicity is still a significant issue for PARPis, as hippocampal neurogenesis decreases and long-term survivors suffer worse cognitive function; for DNA-PKcs inhibitors, the risk of normal brain necrosis exists because of the role of DNA-PKcs in neuronal DSB repair. Immune evasion strategies also limit the effectiveness of promising applied combinations, as STING-mediated signaling via cytosolic DNA paradoxically promotes the expansion of immunosuppressive regulatory T cells (Tregs) in tumors.

FUTURE DIRECTIONS

Prospects for GBM treatment should involve innovative, multidirectional strategies that address the challenges of tumor heterogeneity, drug delivery, and immune evasion. Key advancements include the incorporation of dynamic biomarkers, such as 18F-PARP PET imaging, which evaluates intratumoral PARP activity and may inform adaptive dosing strategies. Combinations of DRR inhibitors with immunomodulatory molecules (such as anti-CD-47 antibodies to prevent the recruitment of

Tregs) and BBB-penetrating nanoparticles could surpass the redundant resistance pathways. In addition, new experimental drugs, such as fusion cytokine molecules, sensitize tumor cells and target the immunosuppressive microenvironment, thereby enhancing durable responses. Global partnerships, such as Glioblastoma Adaptive, Global, Innovative Learning Environment (GBM AGILE), must be leveraged more so that these strategies can be validated promptly in trials that enroll molecularly stratified cohorts. In the end, curing GBM requires not just innovative mechanisms, but a new way of thinking about treatment — as adaptable as the tumor.

CONCLUSION

GBM escapes conventional treatments by exploiting genomic instability for survival, and genomic instability drives its evolution. At the center of this resilience is skillful management by the tumor of DNA repair pathways: one that equips it to endure genotoxic stress but that does so at the expense of becoming mutagenized, which in turns promotes heterogeneity and therapy resistance. However, this is the same dependence on defective repair pathways – for example, error-prone Alt-EJ in hypoxia or hyperactive NHEJ in EGFR-amplified cells – that opens up vulnerabilities being exploited with an unprecedented degree of precision. Therapeutic approaches such as POLQ inhibition and PARP inhibition (especially in cancers with HR deficiency or MGMT promoter methylation) provide examples of how mechanistic studies with DDR pathways could contribute to the development of therapeutic approaches. These approaches are not simply additive; moreover, synergistic with preclinical models, POLQ inhibitors convert radiation-induced chromosomal chaos into a lethal burden, and PARP inhibitors exploit alkylation damage to trap repair enzymes and collapse replication forks. However, the field of clinical practice is still full of difficulties. Spatial and temporal variability of repair pathway activity — including the re-emergence of HR in reoxygenated regions following bevacizumab treatment — requires real-time, adjustable biomarkers. Novel assays such as ctDNA analysis and spatial transcriptomics are beginning to close this gap, allowing clinicians to map repair plasticity and predict resistance months ahead of its appearance on imaging.

Lessons to be learned from failed trials are equally important. The divergent results of early PARPi trials highlight the importance of biomarker-directed patient selection with factors such as 53BP1/BRCA1 ratios or mtDNA levels that direct treatment decisions. Moreover, the BBB continues to thwart systemic drug delivery, prompting innovations such as focused ultrasound-mediated disruption and nanoparticle formulations to increase intracranial drug bioavailability.

The integration of DNA repair-targeted therapies with immunotherapy and metabolic modulation holds transformative potential. For example, STING pathway activation *via* unresolved cytosolic DNA could convert immunologically "cold" GBM tumors into inflamed, checkpoint inhibitor-responsive tumors, whereas ketogenic diets exacerbate oxidative stress to shift the balance toward ferroptosis. These combinatorial strategies must be tempered by caution, as normal neural stem cells share repair dependencies with GSCs, necessitating therapies that spare cognitive function.

The path forward lies in embracing adaptive trial designs and global collaborations to accelerate the validation of these approaches. Initiatives such as GBM AGILE, which prioritize molecularly stratified cohorts, exemplify the shift toward precision neuro-oncology. By aligning mechanistic discovery with clinical pragmatism, the field is poised to transform GBM's genomic chaos from an insurmountable barrier into a tractable target, offering hope for what was once deemed a death sentence.

REFERENCES

Aggarwal, R., Italiano, A., Domchek, S., Goodman, O., Postel-Vinay, S., Garcia-Donas, J., & Shore, N. (2024). Abstract CT222: Efficacy and safety of ceralasertib in the PLANETTE study in patients (pts) with ATM-altered advanced solid tumors (ASTs) or metastatic castration-resistant prostate cancer (mCRPC). *Cancer Research*, *84*(7, Supplement), CT222–CT222. DOI: 10.1158/1538-7445.AM2024-CT222

Agnihotri, S., Gajadhar, A. S., Ternamian, C., Gorlia, T., Diefes, K. L., Mischel, P. S., & Carlson, B. L. (2012). Alkylpurine–DNA–N-glycosylase confers resistance to Temozolomide in xenograft models of glioblastoma multiforme and is associated with poor survival in patients. *The Journal of Clinical Investigation*, *122*(1), 253–266. DOI: 10.1172/JCI59334 PMID: 22156195

Ahuja, S., Gupta, P., Ajay, G., & Ghorai, A. (2025). *Hypoxia-Induced DNA Damage Response and Genomic Instability Dictate Cancer Treatment Response Hypoxia and Tumor Microenvironment: Implications for Cancer Therapy*. Springer.

Amodio, V., Vitiello, P., Bardelli, A., & Germano, G. (2024). DNA repair-dependent immunogenic liabilities in colorectal cancer: Opportunities from errors. *British Journal of Cancer*, *131*(10), 1576–1590. DOI: 10.1038/s41416-024-02848-8 PMID: 39271762

Anand, J., Chiou, L., Sciandra, C., Zhang, X., Hong, J., Wu, D., Zhou, P., & Vaziri, C. (2023). Roles of trans-lesion synthesis (TLS) DNA polymerases in tumorigenesis and cancer therapy. *NAR Cancer*, *5*(1), zcad005. DOI: 10.1093/narcan/zcad005 PMID: 36755961

Angom, R. S., Nakka, N. M. R., & Bhattacharya, S. (2023). Advances in glioblastoma therapy: An update on current approaches. *Brain Sciences*, *13*(11), 1536. DOI: 10.3390/brainsci13111536 PMID: 38002496

Annovazzi, L., Mellai, M., & Schiffer, D. (2017). Chemotherapeutic drugs: DNA damage and repair in glioblastoma. *Cancers (Basel)*, *9*(6), 57. DOI: 10.3390/cancers9060057 PMID: 28587121

Attique, I., Haider, Z., Khan, M., Hassan, S., Soliman, M. M., Ibrahim, W. N., & Anjum, S. (2025). Reactive Oxygen Species: From Tumorigenesis to Therapeutic Strategies in Cancer. *Cancer Medicine*, *14*(10), e70947. DOI: 10.1002/cam4.70947 PMID: 40377005

Azam, M. Z. (2021). Glioblastoma pathogenesis and diagnosis.

Bhargava, R., Sandhu, M., Muk, S., Lee, G., Vaidehi, N., & Stark, J. M. (2018). C-NHEJ without indels is robust and requires synergistic function of distinct XLF domains. *Nature Communications*, *9*(1), 2484. DOI: 10.1038/s41467-018-04867-5 PMID: 29950655

Bonm, A., & Kesari, S. (2021). DNA damage response in glioblastoma: Mechanism for treatment resistance and emerging therapeutic strategies. *Cancer Journal (Sudbury, Mass.)*, *27*(5), 379–385. DOI: 10.1097/PPO.0000000000000540 PMID: 34570452

Bora, A., Pal, R., Mandi, C. S., & Dutta, S. (2024). DNA abasic sites act as rational therapeutic targets to synergize temozolomide response in both MMR-proficient and deficient cancer. *NAR Cancer*, *6*(3), zcae034. DOI: 10.1093/narcan/zcae034 PMID: 39055333

Bose, P., Dai, Y., & Grant, S. (2014). Histone deacetylase inhibitor (HDACI) mechanisms of action: Emerging insights. *Pharmacology & Therapeutics*, *143*(3), 323–336. DOI: 10.1016/j.pharmthera.2014.04.004 PMID: 24769080

Bostian, A. C., & Eoff, R. L. (2016). Aberrant kynurenine signaling modulates DNA replication stress factors and promotes genomic instability in gliomas. *Chemical Research in Toxicology*, *29*(9), 1369–1380. DOI: 10.1021/acs.chemrestox.6b00255 PMID: 27482758

Brar, H. K., Jose, J., Wu, Z., & Sharma, M. (2022). Tyrosine kinase inhibitors for glioblastoma multiforme: Challenges and opportunities for drug delivery. *Pharmaceutics*, *15*(1), 59. DOI: 10.3390/pharmaceutics15010059 PMID: 36678688

Chen, J., Larsson, L., Swarbrick, A., & Lundeberg, J. (2024). Spatial landscapes of cancers: Insights and opportunities. *Nature Reviews. Clinical Oncology*, *21*(9), 660–674. DOI: 10.1038/s41571-024-00926-7 PMID: 39043872

Chung, O. W., Yao, S., Yang, F., Wang, L., Cerda-Smith, C., Hutchinson, H. M., . . . Zou, L. (2025). BRCA1-A and LIG4 complexes mediate ecDNA biogenesis and cancer drug resistance. bioRxiv, 2025.2002. 2018.638901.

Ciechomska, I. A., Jayaprakash, C., Maleszewska, M., & Kaminska, B. (2020). Histone modifying enzymes and chromatin modifiers in glioma pathobiology and therapy responses. *Glioma Signaling*, 259-279.

Dalma, S. (2020). Cancer Cell Specific Induction of Endoplasmic Reticulum Stress by Small Molecular Found in the Serum.

Drew, Y., Kim, J.-W., Penson, R. T., O'Malley, D. M., Parkinson, C., Roxburgh, P., & Ferguson, M. (2024). Olaparib plus durvalumab, with or without bevacizumab, as treatment in PARP inhibitor-naïve platinum-sensitive relapsed ovarian cancer: A phase II multicohort study. *Clinical Cancer Research*, *30*(1), 50–62. DOI: 10.1158/1078-0432.CCR-23-2249 PMID: 37939124

Drew, Y., Zenke, F. T., & Curtin, N. J. (2025). DNA damage response inhibitors in cancer therapy: Lessons from the past, current status and future implications. *Nature Reviews. Drug Discovery*, *24*(1), 19–39. DOI: 10.1038/s41573-024-01060-w PMID: 39533099

Drzewiecka, M., Jaśniak, D., Barszczewska-Pietraszek, G., Czarny, P., Kobrzycka, A., Wieczorek, M., Radek, M., Szemraj, J., Skorski, T., & Śliwiński, T. (2023). Class I HDAC Inhibition Leads to a Downregulation of FANCD2 and RAD51, and the Eradication of Glioblastoma Cells. *Journal of Personalized Medicine*, *13*(9), 1315. DOI: 10.3390/jpm13091315 PMID: 37763083

Duan, M., Cao, R., Yang, Y., Chen, X., Liu, L., Ren, B., Wang, L., & Goh, B.-C. (2024). Blood–brain barrier conquest in glioblastoma nanomedicine: Strategies, clinical advances, and emerging challenges. *Cancers (Basel)*, *16*(19), 3300. DOI: 10.3390/cancers16193300 PMID: 39409919

Durant, S. T., Zheng, L., Wang, Y., Chen, K., Zhang, L., Zhang, T., . . . Fok, J. H. (2018). The brain-penetrant clinical ATM inhibitor AZD1390 radiosensitizes and improves survival of preclinical brain tumor models. *Science advances*, *4*(6), eaat1719.

Erasimus, H., Gobin, M., Niclou, S., & Van Dyck, E. (2016). DNA repair mechanisms and their clinical impact in glioblastoma. *Mutation Research/Reviews in Mutation Research*, *769*, 19–35. DOI: 10.1016/j.mrrev.2016.05.005 PMID: 27543314

Esemen, Y., Awan, M., Parwez, R., Baig, A., Rahman, S., Masala, I., Franchini, S., & Giakoumettis, D. (2022). Molecular pathogenesis of glioblastoma in adults and future perspectives: A systematic review. *International Journal of Molecular Sciences*, *23*(5), 2607. DOI: 10.3390/ijms23052607 PMID: 35269752

Fahrer, J., & Christmann, M. (2023). DNA alkylation damage by nitrosamines and relevant DNA repair pathways. *International Journal of Molecular Sciences*, *24*(5), 4684. DOI: 10.3390/ijms24054684 PMID: 36902118

Fukuta, T., Shaha, S., da Silva-Candal, A., Zhao, Z., & Mitragotri, S. (2025). Cell therapies against brain tumors: Clinical development and emerging prospects. *Bioengineering & Translational Medicine*, *10*(5), 70018. DOI: 10.1002/btm2.70018 PMID: 41030289

Gousias, K., Theocharous, T., & Simon, M. (2022). Mechanisms of cell cycle arrest and apoptosis in glioblastoma. *Biomedicines, 10*(3), 564. DOI: 10.3390/biomedicines10030564 PMID: 35327366

Groth, P., Ausländer, S., Majumder, M. M., Schultz, N., Johansson, F., Petermann, E., & Helleday, T. (2010). Methylated DNA causes a physical block to replication forks independently of damage signaling, O6-methylguanine or DNA single-strand breaks and results in DNA damage. *Journal of Molecular Biology, 402*(1), 70–82. DOI: 10.1016/j.jmb.2010.07.010 PMID: 20643142

Hardaker, E. L., Sanseviero, E., Karmokar, A., Taylor, D., Milo, M., Michaloglou, C., & Solanki, A. (2024). The ATR inhibitor ceralasertib potentiates cancer checkpoint immunotherapy by regulating the tumor microenvironment. *Nature Communications, 15*(1), 1700. DOI: 10.1038/s41467-024-45996-4 PMID: 38402224

Hasegawa, K., Saga, R., & Hosokawa, Y. (2023). Radiotherapeutic review: Acquisition of radioresistance and cancer stem cell properties via irradiation. *Radiation Environment and Medicine, 12*(1), 25–36.

Jacot, W., Thezenas, S., Senal, R., Viglianti, C., Laberenne, A.-C., Lopez-Crapez, E., Bibeau, F., Bleuse, J.-P., Romieu, G., & Lamy, P.-J. (2013). BRCA1 promoter hypermethylation, 53BP1 protein expression and PARP-1 activity as biomarkers of DNA repair deficit in breast cancer. *BMC Cancer, 13*(1), 1–11. DOI: 10.1186/1471-2407-13-523 PMID: 24191908

Jung, H. (2022). Contributing factors for mutagenic DNA lesion bypass by DNA polymerase eta (polη). *DNA, 2*(4), 205–220. DOI: 10.3390/dna2040015

Krawczynski, K., Godlewski, J., & Bronisz, A. (2020). Oxidative stress—Part of the solution or part of the problem in the hypoxic environment of a brain tumor. *Antioxidants, 9*(8), 747. DOI: 10.3390/antiox9080747 PMID: 32823815

Ledermann, J., & Luvero, D. (2015). Update on anti-angiogenic agents and PARP inhibitors: Is the combination a potential or a reality? *Cancer Breaking News, 3*(2), 20–29.

Li, B., Zheng, Y., & Yang, L. (2019). The oncogenic potential of SUV39H2: A comprehensive and perspective view. *Journal of Cancer, 10*(3), 721–729. DOI: 10.7150/jca.28254 PMID: 30719171

Li, W., & Xu, X. (2023). Advances in mitophagy and mitochondrial apoptosis pathway-related drugs in glioblastoma treatment. *Frontiers in Pharmacology, 14*, 1211719. DOI: 10.3389/fphar.2023.1211719 PMID: 37456742

Liu, J., Majd, N., Zou, C., Mirchia, K., Pak, J., Foster, K., & Pan, S. (2024). OS07. 1. A INTEGRATIVE SINGLE NUCLEI, SPATIAL, AND FUNCTIONAL GENOMIC ANALYSES REVEAL DNA-PK DRIVES GLIOBLASTOMA RADIORESISTANCE THROUGH TUMOR CELLS AND THE MYELOID MICROENVIRONMENT. *Neuro-Oncology*, *26*(Supplement_5), v22–v23. DOI: 10.1093/neuonc/noae144.065

Liu, L., Liao, X., Wu, H., Li, Y., Zhu, Y., & Chen, Q. (2020). Mitophagy and its contribution to metabolic and aging-associated disorders. *Antioxidants & Redox Signaling*, *32*(12), 906–927. DOI: 10.1089/ars.2019.8013 PMID: 31969001

Liu, M., Ji, Z., Jain, V., Smith, V. L., Hocke, E., Patel, A. P., McLendon, R. E., Ashley, D. M., Gregory, S. G., & López, G. Y. (2024). Spatial transcriptomics reveals segregation of tumor cell states in glioblastoma and marked immunosuppression within the perinecrotic niche. *Acta Neuropathologica Communications*, *12*(1), 64. DOI: 10.1186/s40478-024-01769-0 PMID: 38650010

Lozinski, M., Bowden, N. A., Graves, M. C., Fay, M., & Tooney, P. A. (2021). DNA damage repair in glioblastoma: Current perspectives on its role in tumor progression, treatment resistance and PIKKing potential therapeutic targets. *Cellular Oncology (Dordrecht)*, *44*(5), 961–981. DOI: 10.1007/s13402-021-00613-0 PMID: 34057732

Ly, P., Brunner, S. F., Shoshani, O., Kim, D. H., Lan, W., Pyntikova, T., & Campbell, P. J. (2019). Chromosome segregation errors generate a diverse spectrum of simple and complex genomic rearrangements. *Nature Genetics*, *51*(4), 705–715. DOI: 10.1038/s41588-019-0360-8 PMID: 30833795

Lyakhovich, A., Graifer, D., Stefanovie, B., & Krejci, L. (2016). Mitochondrial dysfunction in DDR-related cancer predisposition syndromes. *Biochimica et Biophysica Acta (BBA)-. Revisiones en Cáncer*, *1865*(2), 184–189. PMID: 26926806

Majumder, B., Nataraj, N. B., Maitreyi, L., & Datta, S. (2024). Mismatch repair-proficient tumor footprints in the sands of immune desert: Mechanistic constraints and precision platforms. *Frontiers in Immunology*, *15*, 1414376. DOI: 10.3389/fimmu.2024.1414376 PMID: 39100682

Maksoud, S. (2022). The DNA double-strand break repair in glioma: Molecular players and therapeutic strategies. *Molecular Neurobiology*, *59*(9), 5326–5365. DOI: 10.1007/s12035-022-02915-2 PMID: 35696013

Martuscello, R. T., Vedam-Mai, V., McCarthy, D. J., Schmoll, M. E., Jundi, M. A., Louviere, C. D., & Deleyrolle, L. P. (2016). A supplemented high-fat low-carbohydrate diet for the treatment of glioblastoma. *Clinical Cancer Research*, *22*(10), 2482–2495. DOI: 10.1158/1078-0432.CCR-15-0916 PMID: 26631612

Mazzoleni, A., Awuah, W. A., Sanker, V., Bharadwaj, H. R., Aderinto, N., Tan, J. K., & Atallah, O. (2024). Chromosomal instability: A key driver in glioma pathogenesis and progression. *European Journal of Medical Research, 29*(1), 451. DOI: 10.1186/s40001-024-02043-8 PMID: 39227895

Meng, W., Palmer, J. D., Siedow, M., Haque, S. J., & Chakravarti, A. (2022). Overcoming radiation resistance in gliomas by targeting metabolism and DNA repair pathways. *International Journal of Molecular Sciences, 23*(4), 2246. DOI: 10.3390/ijms23042246 PMID: 35216362

Mercier, B. D., Tizpa, E., Philip, E. J., Feng, Q., Huang, Z., Thomas, R. M., Pal, S. K., Dorff, T. B., & Li, Y. R. (2022). Dietary interventions in cancer treatment and response: A comprehensive review. *Cancers (Basel), 14*(20), 5149. DOI: 10.3390/cancers14205149 PMID: 36291933

Millán-Zambrano, G., Burton, A., Bannister, A. J., & Schneider, R. (2022). Histone posttranslational modifications—Cause and consequence of genome function. *Nature Reviews. Genetics, 23*(9), 563–580. DOI: 10.1038/s41576-022-00468-7 PMID: 35338361

Nafe, R., & Hattingen, E. (2023). Cellular components of the tumor environment in gliomas—What do we know today? *Biomedicines, 12*(1), 14. DOI: 10.3390/biomedicines12010014 PMID: 38275375

Nahar Metu, C. L., Sutihar, S. K., Sohel, M., Zohora, F., Hasan, A., Miah, M. T., Rani Kar, T., Hossain, M. A., & Rahman, M. H. (2023). Unraveling the signaling mechanism behind astrocytoma and possible therapeutics strategies: A comprehensive review. *Cancer Reports, 6*(10), e1889. DOI: 10.1002/cnr2.1889 PMID: 37675821

Ngoi, N. Y., Peng, G., & Yap, T. A. (2022). A tale of two checkpoints: ATR inhibition and PD-(L) 1 blockade. *Annual Review of Medicine, 73*(1), 231–250. DOI: 10.1146/annurev-med-042320-025136 PMID: 34644155

O'Hara, R., Tedone, E., Ludlow, A., Huang, E., Arosio, B., Mari, D., & Shay, J. W. (2019). Quantitative mitochondrial DNA copy number determination using droplet digital PCR with single-cell resolution. *Genome Research, 29*(11), 1878–1888. DOI: 10.1101/gr.250480.119 PMID: 31548359

Oh, G., Wang, A., Wang, L., Li, J., Werba, G., Weissinger, D., & Ackermann, A. (2023). POLQ inhibition elicits an immune response in homologous recombination–deficient pancreatic adenocarcinoma via cGAS/STING signaling. *The Journal of Clinical Investigation, 133*(11), e165934. DOI: 10.1172/JCI165934 PMID: 36976649

Onciul, R., Brehar, F.-M., Toader, C., Covache-Busuioc, R.-A., Glavan, L.-A., Bratu, B.-G., Costin, H. P., Dumitrascu, D.-I., Serban, M., & Ciurea, A. V. (2024). Deciphering glioblastoma: Fundamental and novel insights into the biology and therapeutic strategies of gliomas. *Current Issues in Molecular Biology*, *46*(3), 2402–2443. DOI: 10.3390/cimb46030153 PMID: 38534769

Ozair, A., Bhat, V., Alisch, R. S., Khosla, A. A., Kotecha, R. R., Odia, Y., McDermott, M. W., & Ahluwalia, M. S. (2023). DNA methylation and histone modification in low-grade gliomas: Current understanding and potential clinical targets. *Cancers (Basel)*, *15*(4), 1342. DOI: 10.3390/cancers15041342 PMID: 36831683

Paul, S., Sinha, S., & Kundu, C. N. (2022). Targeting cancer stem cells in the tumor microenvironment: An emerging role of PARP inhibitors. *Pharmacological Research*, *184*, 106425. DOI: 10.1016/j.phrs.2022.106425 PMID: 36075511

Paull, T. T. (2019). RNA–DNA hybrids and the convergence with DNA repair. *Critical Reviews in Biochemistry and Molecular Biology*, *54*(4), 371–384. DOI: 10.1080/10409238.2019.1670131 PMID: 31577154

Qin, H., Zhang, F., & Gao, S. (2024). Ketogenic Diet Therapy for Glioma: Combined Effects. *Current Cancer Therapy Reviews*, *20*(2), 177–187. DOI: 10.2174/157339 4719666230717160843

Reina, C., Šabanović, B., Lazzari, C., Gregorc, V., & Heeschen, C. (2024). Unlocking the future of cancer diagnosis–promises and challenges of ctDNA-based liquid biopsies in non-small cell lung cancer. *Translational Research; the Journal of Laboratory and Clinical Medicine*, *272*, 41–53. DOI: 10.1016/j.trsl.2024.05.014 PMID: 38838851

Robinson, S. D., Filippopoulou, C., Besta, S., Samuels, M., Betrán, A. L., Ajamieh, M. A., & Giamas, G. (2025). Spatial biology–unraveling complexity within the glioblastoma microenvironment. *Trends in Molecular Medicine*, *31*(9), 846–859. DOI: 10.1016/j.molmed.2025.01.014

Rodriguez-Berriguete, G., Ranzani, M., Prevo, R., Puliyadi, R., Machado, N., Bolland, H. R., & Cerutti, A. (2023). Small-molecule Polθ inhibitors provide safe and effective tumor radiosensitization in preclinical models. *Clinical Cancer Research*, *29*(8), 1631–1642. DOI: 10.1158/1078-0432.CCR-22-2977 PMID: 36689546

Shi, C., Qin, K., Lin, A., Jiang, A., Cheng, Q., Liu, Z., Zhang, J., & Luo, P. (2022). The role of DNA damage repair (DDR) system in response to immune checkpoint inhibitor (ICI) therapy. *Journal of Experimental & Clinical Cancer Research : CR*, *41*(1), 268. DOI: 10.1186/s13046-022-02469-0 PMID: 36071479

Sim, H.-W., Galanis, E., & Khasraw, M. (2022). PARP inhibitors in glioma: A review of therapeutic opportunities. *Cancers (Basel), 14*(4), 1003. DOI: 10.3390/cancers14041003 PMID: 35205750

Simhadri, S., Peterson, S., Patel, D. S., Huo, Y., Cai, H., Bowman-Colin, C., & Bhaumik, M. (2014). Male fertility defect associated with disrupted BRCA1-PALB2 interaction in mice. *The Journal of Biological Chemistry, 289*(35), 24617–24629. DOI: 10.1074/jbc.M114.566141 PMID: 25016020

Singh, P., Tomar, R. S., & Rath, S. K. (2015). Anticancer potential of the histone deacetylase inhibitor-like effects of flavones, a subclass of polyphenolic compounds: A review. *Molecular Biology Reports, 42*(11), 1515–1531. DOI: 10.1007/s11033-015-3881-y PMID: 26033434

Strobel, H., Baisch, T., Fitzel, R., Schilberg, K., Siegelin, M. D., Karpel-Massler, G., Debatin, K.-M., & Westhoff, M.-A. (2019). Temozolomide and other alkylating agents in glioblastoma therapy. *Biomedicines, 7*(3), 69. DOI: 10.3390/biomedicines7030069 PMID: 31505812

Sun, Z.-Y., Wang, X.-N., Cheng, S.-Q., Su, X.-X., & Ou, T.-M. (2019). Developing novel G-quadruplex ligands: From interaction with nucleic acids to interfering with nucleic acid–protein interaction. *Molecules (Basel, Switzerland), 24*(3), 396. DOI: 10.3390/molecules24030396 PMID: 30678288

Tang, M., Bolderson, E., O'Byrne, K. J., & Richard, D. J. (2021). Tumor hypoxia drives genomic instability. *Frontiers in Cell and Developmental Biology, 9*, 626229. DOI: 10.3389/fcell.2021.626229 PMID: 33796526

Tian, H., Gao, Z., Li, H., Zhang, B., Wang, G., Zhang, Q., Pei, D. S., & Zheng, J. (2015). DNA damage response–a double-edged sword in cancer prevention and cancer therapy. *Cancer Letters, 358*(1), 8–16. DOI: 10.1016/j.canlet.2014.12.038 PMID: 25528631

Veneris, J. T., Matulonis, U. A., Liu, J. F., & Konstantinopoulos, P. A. (2020). Choosing wisely: Selecting PARP inhibitor combinations to promote anti-tumor immune responses beyond BRCA mutations. *Gynecologic Oncology, 156*(2), 488–497. DOI: 10.1016/j.ygyno.2019.09.021 PMID: 31630846

Vilar, J. B., Christmann, M., & Tomicic, M. T. (2022). Alterations in molecular profiles affecting glioblastoma resistance to radiochemotherapy: Where does the good go? *Cancers (Basel), 14*(10), 2416. DOI: 10.3390/cancers14102416 PMID: 35626024

Wang, Y., Luo, W., & Wang, Y. (2019). PARP-1 and its associated nucleases in DNA damage response. *DNA Repair, 81*, 102651. DOI: 10.1016/j.dnarep.2019.102651 PMID: 31302005

Whitaker, A. M., Schaich, M. A., Smith, M. S., Flynn, T. S., & Freudenthal, B. D. (2017). Base excision repair of oxidative DNA damage: From mechanism to disease. *Frontiers in Bioscience (Landmark Edition), 22*(9), 1493–1522. DOI: 10.2741/4555 PMID: 28199214

Wick, W., Weller, M., Van Den Bent, M., Sanson, M., Weiler, M., Von Deimling, A., Plass, C., Hegi, M., Platten, M., & Reifenberger, G. (2014). MGMT testing—The challenges for biomarker-based glioma treatment. *Nature Reviews. Neurology, 10*(7), 372–385. DOI: 10.1038/nrneurol.2014.100 PMID: 24912512

Woo, P. Y., Li, Y., Chan, A. H., Ng, S. C., Loong, H. H., Chan, D. T., & Poon, W.-S. (2019). A multifaceted review of temozolomide resistance mechanisms in glioblastoma beyond O-6-methylguanine-DNA methyltransferase. *Glioma (Mumbai, India), 2*(2), 68–82. DOI: 10.4103/glioma.glioma_3_19

Xie, X., Zhang, Y., Wang, Z., Wang, S., Jiang, X., Cui, H., & Guo, Q. (2021). ATM at the crossroads of reactive oxygen species and autophagy. *International Journal of Biological Sciences, 17*(12), 3080–3090. DOI: 10.7150/ijbs.63963 PMID: 34421351

Yang, Z., Wei, D., Dai, X., Stevens, M. F., Bradshaw, T. D., Luo, Y., & Zhang, J. (2019). C8-substituted imidazotetrazine analogs overcome temozolomide resistance by inducing DNA adducts and DNA damage. *Frontiers in Oncology, 9*, 485. DOI: 10.3389/fonc.2019.00485 PMID: 31263673

Zhang, Y., & Wang, W. (2025). Advances in tumor subcolony formation and mechanisms of growth and invasion. *Journal of Translational Medicine, 23*(1), 461. DOI: 10.1186/s12967-025-06486-3 PMID: 40259385

Zhou, W., & Wahl, D. R. (2019). Metabolic abnormalities in glioblastoma and metabolic strategies to overcome treatment resistance. *Cancers (Basel), 11*(9), 1231. DOI: 10.3390/cancers11091231 PMID: 31450721

Chapter 4
Drug Regimens Used for Glioblastoma:
Chemical Structure and Mechanism of Action

Deepak Vasudevan Sajini
https://orcid.org/0000-0003-2200-8401
Department of Pharmacology, National College of Pharmacy, Kerala University of Health Sciences, Manassery, India

Amritha Chakkitukandiyil
https://orcid.org/0000-0002-2683-8341
Department of Pharmacology, National College of Pharmacy, Kerala University of Health Sciences, Manassery, India

Akey Krishna Swaroop
Department of Pharmaceutical Chemistry, School of Pharmaceutical Sciences, Sandip University, Nashik, India

K. Sujith Varma
https://orcid.org/0000-0002-0866-5571
Department of Pharmaceutics, National College of Pharmacy, Kerala University of Health Sciences, Manassery, India

Vijish Venugopal
https://orcid.org/0009-0009-2537-2154
Department of Anaesthesiology, KMCT Medical College Hospital, Manassery, India

DOI: 10.4018/979-8-3373-2695-5.ch004

ABSTRACT

Glioblastoma multiforme (GBM) is the most aggressive and deadly primary brain tumor in adults, known for rapid progression, high recurrence, and poor prognosis. Despite extensive research, current treatments—surgery, radiotherapy, and chemotherapy—remain limited in effectiveness. This chapter reviews these modalities and their limitations, discusses chemotherapeutics like Temozolomide, Carmustine, Lomustine, and Bevacizumab, and explores emerging therapies, including targeted drugs, immunotherapy, and gene/virus-based approaches. Future directions highlight novel agents, combination strategies, and personalized medicine to improve outcomes.

1. INTRODUCTION

Glioblastoma multiforme (GBM) is the most prevalent and severe primary malignant brain tumor in adults. It has a poor prognosis, fast growth, and a high recurrence rate; even with rigorous multimodal therapy, the median survival is only around 15 months (Rong et al., 2022). The typical treatment method involves achieving the safe surgical removal, subsequently followed by radiotherapy and chemotherapy using temozolomide (TMZ) (Rodríguez-Camacho et al., 2022). However, the outlook for GBM patients is bleak because of the significantly invasive characteristics of the tumor, genetic and cellular diversity, and a pronounced likelihood of recurrence despite intensive therapy (Rodríguez-Camacho et al., 2022; Hoosemans et al., 2024).

A major difficulty in treating GBM lies in the intricate biology of the tumor and its resistance to treatment. GBM tumors exhibit a high degree of heterogeneity, both in individual tumors and among different patients, resulting in varied cell subpopulations that can resist typical therapies (Hoosemans et al., 2024; Ou et al., 2021). The blood-brain barrier (BBB) along with the blood-brain tumor barrier (BBTB) makes treatment more challenging by limiting the entry of chemotherapeutic drugs into the tumor area (Jnaidi et al., 2020; Guo et al., 2022). Furthermore, the tumor microenvironment, which encompasses interactions with adjacent astrocytes and immune cells, plays a role in drug resistance and aids tumor survival (2,4). Resistant to TMZ, the primary chemotherapy for GBM, is frequently caused by the overproduction of the DNA repair enzyme O-6-methylguanine-DNA methyltransferase (MGMT), which mitigates DNA damage caused by TMZ (Ou et al., 2021). Additionally, the immunosuppressive nature of GBM, marked by the release of cytokines like TGF-β and the increased expression of immune checkpoint proteins such as PD-L1, obstructs effective immune responses and constrains the efficacy of immunotherapies (Rong et al., 2022; Ou et al., 2021; Agosti et al., 2023)

Considering this resistance mechanisms, researchers are investigating combination treatments and new agents to improve effectiveness. This encompasses targeted treatments aimed at molecular pathways including mTOR, PI3K/AKT, and EGFR, along with immunotherapeutic methods such as immune checkpoint inhibitors and chimeric antigen receptor T-cells (CAR-T) cell therapy (Ou et al., 2021; Guo et al., 2022; Agosti et al., 2023). Systems for drug delivery based on nanotechnology, like solid lipid nanoparticles and nanostructured lipid carriers, are under examination to enhance drug transport through the BBB and attain improved targeting of tumors (Jnaidi et al., 2020). Personalized medicine strategies, guided by genetic and epigenetic analysis, are becoming more crucial for customizing therapies to specific tumor traits and addressing resistance (Rong et al., 2022; Rodríguez-Camacho et al., 2022). Hence, the treatment of glioblastoma continues to be a significant challenge because of its invasive nature, resistance to therapies, and the protective barriers of brain. The creation of multidrug therapies, sophisticated delivery methods, and tailored treatments presents optimism for enhancing survival rates and life quality for GBM patients; however, substantial research and clinical progress are still required to address existing limitations (Rong et al., 2022; Rodríguez-Camacho et al., 2022; Hoosemans et al., 2024).

2. CURRENT STANDARD TREATMENT APPROACHES OF GLIOBLASTOMA

2.1. Surgical Treatment of Glioblastoma

Surgical intervention remains a cornerstone in the treatment of GBM, particularly as the first-line approach for malignant brain tumors. A combination of treatment strategies is frequently employed for patients with multiple metastases, integrating techniques such as stereotactic radiosurgery and brachytherapy to enhance local control of brain metastases (Mehta et al., 2017) . Surgery plays a crucial role in cytoreduction and achieving a molecularly integrated diagnosis, with research indicating that the extent of tumor resection significantly impacts overall survival. However, elderly patients are at a heightened risk of morbidity and mortality during surgical procedures. Age has been recognized by the Radiation Therapy Oncology Group as a critical prognostic factor, with a study by Curran et al. finding that patients older than 50 years have a poorer prognosis for GBM (Brown et al., 2016; Curran et al., 1993).

Advancements in surgical techniques have led to the development of minimally invasive procedures such as tubular retractor therapy, laser interstitial thermal therapy, and the use of endoscopes, which have contributed to improved patient outcomes. Additionally, novel surgical adjuncts, including intraoperative magnetic resonance imaging (iMRI), fluorescence-guided surgery, intraoperative ultrasound (IOUS), brain mapping strategies, and intraoperative mass spectrometry (IMS), have been integrated into practice to optimize tumor resection and survival rates. Intraoperative radiotherapy (IORT) has shown promise in reducing local recurrence and extending survival. Techniques utilizing Raman spectrometry (RS) and optical coherence tomography (OCT) have demonstrated encouraging results in experimental and clinical studies. Furthermore, molecular characterization and genetic subclassification have facilitated targeted treatment approaches, such as immunotherapies and personalized medications, aiding in the effective management of high-grade gliomas (Malone et al., 2020; Wright et al., 2016; Zaffino et al., 2020; Elashwah et al;., 2023; Bovenkamp et al., 2018).

Post-surgical treatment commonly involves chemotherapy, which can be administered orally or through implanted wafers containing chemotherapeutic agents that slowly release active compounds to eliminate residual tumor cells. Since 2005, the standard treatment protocol has included adjuvant temozolomide combined with postoperative radiotherapy (Stupp et al., 2005; Johnson & O'Neil, 2012). While surgical procedures remain a preferred option for tumor removal, minimally invasive methods such as the transsphenoidal approach enable precise resection of skull-base tumors using operating microscopes (Ellis, 2009). Direct Electrical Stimulation (DES) is another innovation, allowing surgeons to map functional regions of the brain and identify critical areas responsible for movement or speech to minimize post-surgical deficits. Preoperative navigation scans further enhance surgical precision by providing detailed brain mapping, which is especially valuable in complex glioma cases (Bu et al., 2021).

2.2. Radiation in Treatment of Glioblastoma

Radiation therapy is often advised following surgery to eradicate any leftover tumor cells and is regarded as a standard component of care for managing GBM. It is usually paired with chemotherapy to improve its efficacy. When surgery cannot be performed, radiation therapy might act as the primary treatment choice. Extra measures are implemented during radiation therapy, involving safe radiation protocols for older or vulnerable patients, cutting-edge imaging methods, and reirradiation plans for those who have been treated before. New strategies like stem cell-targeted radiation seek to minimize recurrence, and there is increasing interest in the possible synergy of radiation therapy and immunotherapy (Stupp et al., 2009).

The proton beam therapy (PBT) utilizes positively charged proton ions to treat tumors and offers significant action to some cancer types. The proton beams exhibit low entrance radiation doses and as the protons lose energy and come to a stop, the maximum dose is released in a well-defined region known as the Bragg Peak, In some cases, larger doses of radiation are administered directly to tumor, which is otherwise not possible with photons. In a prospective phase II trial the results have shown that GBM patients who received PBT had a significantly lower number of grade 2 or higher toxicities, when compared to patients receiving intensity-modulated radiotherapy (IMRT)(21). The carbon ion radiotherapy (CIRT) has same dose distribution profile like PBT, with most of the radiation dose being delivered to the target tumor via the Bragg Peak. The ionizing track structure of CIRT causes more irreparable DNA damage causing cell death. The preclinical study data have shown that targeting the DDR, particularly in radioresistant GSCs, can enhance the efficacy of conventional photon radiotherapy in killing tumor. The use of PBT and CIRT in treating GBM are emerging as attractive therapeutic options for reducing the adverse side effects associated with photon radiation. Recently, a newer approach by combining PBT and CIRT with DDR inhibitors is gaining acceptance to overcome therapy resistance in GBM. These findings indicates that different radiation modalities should be paired with specific agents to maximize clinical benefits (Aiyappa-Maudsley et al., 2022).

2.3. Chemotherapy

The Chemotherapeutic agents are taken for two to four weeks after surgery or shortly after radiation therapy. The chemotherapy is used as a primary treatment method when a tumor cannot be surgically removed. The chemotherapeutic agents work on the principle of destroying rapidly dividing cancer cells with powerful medications. The medications can be administered in pill form or injected into a vein. In certain cases, the agents are injected into the intrathecal space of the spine. The treatment of GBM using chemotherapeutic agents requires expertise, as they often destroy some of the cells and allow other to grow unimpeded. The medical practitioner should design the treatment with chemotherapeutic agents carefully to treat GBM. Common chemotherapy medications prescribed for GBM include Temozolomide, Carmustine for high-grade brain cancers, Bevacizumab, used for second-line treatment for recurrent glioblastomas and Lomustine for improving the efficacy of bevacizumab when both medications are administered simultaneously. The drug temozolomide is an alkylating cytostatic drug having ability to penetrates the blood–brain barrier easily due to its lipophilic character. The bioavailability of drug after oral administration is almost 100% and elimination occurs in the liver and excretion by renal path (Brada et al., 1999).

2.4. Limitations of the Conventional Treatments of Glioblastoma

The conventional treatments of GBM are ineffective in eradicating the entire tumor mass. The reasons for the ineffectiveness include inability of chemotherapeutic drugs to reach these cells because of the BBB (Carpentier et al., 2016), inability of surgery to remove all tumor cells and the limitations of both chemotherapy and radiotherapy. The differentiation of tumor tissue from healthy brain tissue is a significantly difficult in treating GBM by surgical procedure (Jakola et al., 2020). The failure to visually distinguish between tumor and healthy tissue during surgery is another difficulty in Surgical procedure and is due to cells infiltrating the surrounding brain tissue. The poor demarcation between tumor and healthy brain tissue will increase the risk of leaving tumor cells residue during resection, which later can lead to tumor recurrence (Suarez-Meade et al., 2020; Cote et al., 2017). The use of advanced imaging techniques such as iMRI and iUS to provide real-time visualization and guidance during surgery can overcome the challenge to some extent. The common approach in treating GBM is radiation therapy, often administered after surgery to destroy any remaining microscopic cancer cells residue and help to prevent recurrence. The radiation therapy can also be used as a standalone treatment for a tumor, when the tumor is considered inoperable due to its size or critical location. The radiation therapy used for treating GBM can sometimes damage healthy tissues near the tumor site. The side effects associated with radiation therapy include hair loss, fatigue, swollen or blistered skin (radiation dermatitis), seizures, cognitive changes, such as impaired concentration, memory or speech, Nausea and vomiting, low blood cell counts, headaches and hearing loss. The therapeutic resistance is another main cause of poor prognosis for patients with GBM (Yekula et al., 2021). This resistance was found to increase over time and weakens the current therapeutic protocols for recurrent GBM. In most cases, surgery is no longer possible, and chemo and radiotherapy fail to counteract tumor progression. The cause of therapeutic resistance is mediated by increase in MGMT, as well as anti-apoptotic proteins drug-efflux transporters, which reduce drug sensitivity, and the activation of both DNA damage checkpoints and DNA repair mechanism induced by radiation (Bao et al., 2006; Liu et al., 2006).

3. CHEMOTHERAPEUTIC AGENTS USED IN GLIOBLASTOMA

3.1. Temozolomide (TMZ)

TMZ is an essential anticancer drug for human GBM, a malignant brain tumor. Despite common use, resistance and side effects often limit its use. This chapter explains TMZ chemical structure, its mode of action, and the limitations for its clinical application.

3.1.1. Chemical Structure

It is a dacarbazine derivative and is classified as an alkylating agent. As a prodrug, it spontaneously hydrolyzes at physiological pH to 5-(3-methyltriazen-1-yl) imidazole-4-carboxamide (MTIC), the active agent, which is responsible for its therapeutic activity (Jezierzański et al., 2024; Yang et al., 2019).

3.1.2. Mechanism of Action

TMZ exerts its cytotoxic activity mainly through DNA methylation at two key sites on the guanine molecule: O-6 and N-7. The methylation at O-6, involves the addition of a methyl group at the oxygen in the 6th position of the guanine base. This alteration results in the product O6-methylguanine, which pairs with thymine instead of cytosine during DNA replication. This mispairing violates the classical base-pairing rules, which initiates DNA repair, leading to DSB formation and cell death (Ortiz et al., 2021; Marniemi & Parkki, 1975). Methylation at the N-7 position (of the nitrogen atom) of guanine also destabilizes the DNA structure and produces further damage. This interference with the DNA replication, and repair processes is believed to be central to the therapeutic effects of TMZ. The efficacy of TMZ is modulated by the expression of DNA repair enzyme MGMT. The O6-methylguanine lesions may be repaired by MGMT through the removal of the methyl moiety, the overexpression of which is commonly associated with resistance to TMZ treatment in tumor cells (Ortiz et al., 2021).

3.1.3. Clinical Use and Limitations

TMZ is administered orally and is included in the standard therapy schedule of GBM, usually with concomitant radiotherapy post-surgical resection, according the Stupp protocol (Jezierzański et al., 2024; Thanh et al., 2024). One of its major advantages is the fact that it can travel from the bloodstream into the brain – making it an effective treatment against brain cancers. But there are a few downsides:

- Resistance: MGMT activity and cancer SCs are responsible for the resistance of TMZ, which represents a significant impediment to an efficient treatment.
- Tolerability: The most frequently occurring toxicities with TMZ are nausea, vomiting and haematological toxicity, mainly thrombocytopenia and neutropenia, which are usually mild-to-moderate in intensity.
- Local/regional recurrence: A lot of patients fail locally. In addition, TMZ has been reported to increase the expression of MMP9, which might contribute to the invasiveness of solid tumor (Thanh et al., 2024).

Nevertheless, TMZ still stands as the backbone of the glioblastoma therapy. There is current research focusing on resistance and side effect limitations. Prospective paradigms involve drug combination with TMZ or perifosine, the latter of which can potentially improve treatment outcome by blocking DNA repair and apoptosis induction (Zhao et al., 2024). Novel TMZ analogs and nano-technology mediated delivery systems are also being investigated in hope to overcome resistance and to enhance treatment results (Yang et al., 2019).

3.2. Carmustine and Lomustine

Carmustine and Lomustine are chemotherapies used in the treatment of glioblastoma, a fast-growing brain cancer. Both agents are nitrosourea agents, which are characterized by their ability to cross the blood-brain barrier and be active against central nervous system tumors. The knowledge of their chemical structure, mechanism of action and clinical use in the treatment of glioblastoma is a key-point of their application in oncology.

3.2.1. Chemical Structure

Carmustine: Carmustine is a bischloroethyl nitrosourea derivative; it has the chemical name of 1,3-bis(2-chloroethyl)-1-nitrosourea. This structure allows it to work as an alkylating agent, obstructing synthesis of DNA and RNA (Chen et al., 2022; Ryshkova et al., 2000).

Lomustine: Lomustine, another nitrosourea, is precisely 1-(2-chloroethyl)-3-cyclohexyl-1-nitrosourea. The fact is that it can also easily trespass the central nervous system, probably due to its lipid solubility. Chemical structures of chemotherapeutic drugs for glioblastoma in Table 1.

Table 1. Chemical structures of chemotherapeutic agents used in glioblastoma

Common name	IUPAC name	Structure
Temozolomide	3-methyl-4-oxo-3,4-dihydroimidazo[5,1-d] [1,2,3,5]tetrazine-8-carboxamide	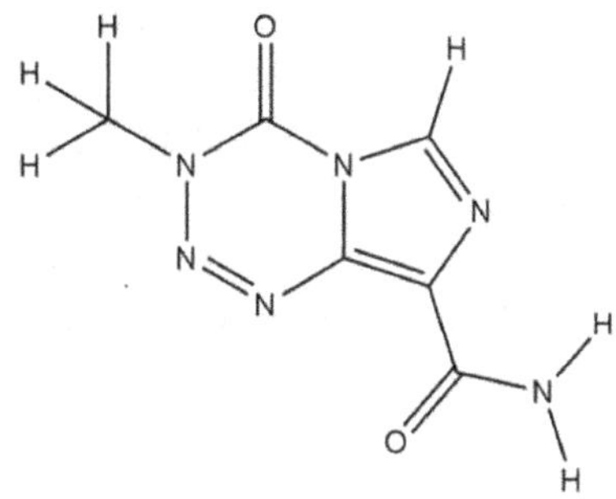
Carmustine	1,3-bis(2-chloroethyl)-1-nitrosourea	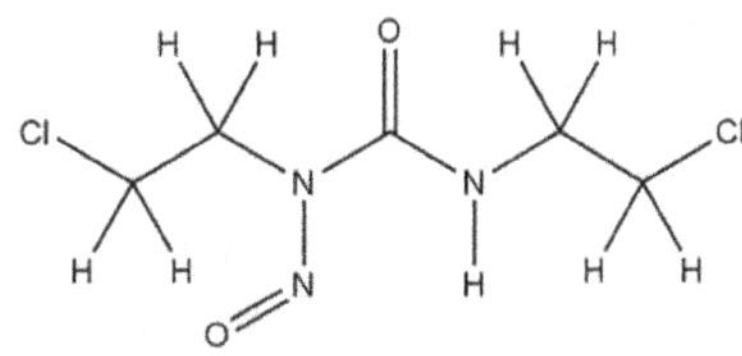
Lomustine	1-(2-chloroethyl)-3-cyclohexyl-1-nitrosourea	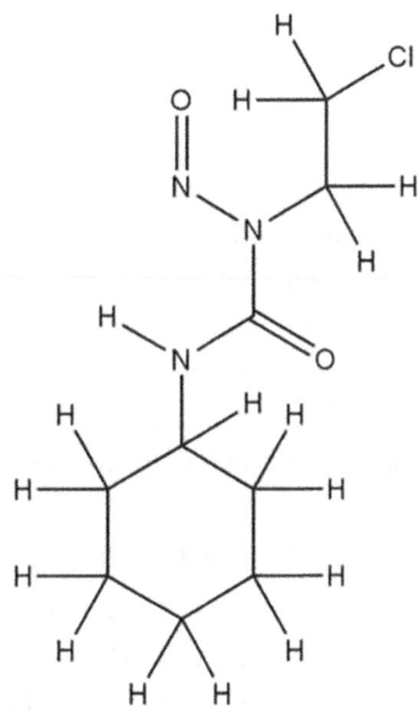

3.2.2. Mechanism of Action

3.2.2.1. DNA Alkylation

The mode of action of Carmustine and Lomustine is largely through their activity as an alkylating agent where they form covalent bonds between the N1 or O6 atoms on the DNA bases which is the primary mode of action for drug activity. The alkyl groups are very reactive and make cross-links between the two DNA chains in the helix. It stops the DNA strands from unwinding, and separates the DNA strands during DNA replication and transctription process that are necessary for the survival and division of a cell (Della Cuna & Paoletti, 1976).

3.2.2.2. DNA Cross-Linking

By this technique the interlacing of the DNA strands is achieved, which is responsible for the modulation of the DNA during the normal progression of the S-phase of the cell cycle (DNA Replication). This entry of VB into the new phenotype induces chromosome instability and arrests the replication machinery that results in replication fork crash. The blocked replication forks ultimately lead to the formation of DNA breaks, following to cell death.

3.2.2.3. DNA Damage Response and Apoptosis Induction

DNA damage induced by Carmustine and Lomustine activates the cellular repair response. Yet having worked to seize so much DNA and then cross-linking it, when the DNA is then cross-linked, these strategies do not work. This malfunction results in the induction of apoptotic pathways. The cell is then able to recognize and irreparable damage to the DNA by p53 and other tumor suppressor proteins and the cell's own death (apoptosis) is started (Chen et al., 2022; Della Cuna & Paoletti, 1976). This is especially active in glioblastoma cells resistant to other chemotherapy drugs, including temozolomide.

3.2.2.4. Localized Delivery Leads to Increased Effectiveness

Carmustine can be delivered specifically to the tumor via beads of polymers. This site-specific drug delivery provides higher drug concentrations at the tumor site, increasing the efficacy of the drug with reduced systemic toxicity (Chen et al., 2022; Ginat, 2022). The high local concentrations overcome the obstacles preventing drugs from efficiently crossing the BBB, and increase their therapeutic effect against brain tumors.

3.2.3. Role in Glioblastoma Treatment

Carmustine can also be targeted to the tumor using polymer beads. This local drug administration results in higher local drug concentration and hence with higher drug activity and low systemic toxicity (Chen et al., 2022; Ginat, 2022). The high local drug concentrations surmount the barriers of poor drugs diffusion across the blood-brain barrier and enhance drugs therapeutic effect for brain tumors.

3.2.3.1. Activity and Resistant Cases

Lomustine and nimustine have been shown to be active in models of glioblastoma that are resistant to temozolomide, indicating that there may be a role as salvage therapy (Liau et al., 2005).

3.2.3.2. Combination Therapies

Carmustine is commonly combined with other therapies, such as radiotherapy, to enhance the efficacy of treatment. It is also used in multidrug regimens with cisplatin and others (Liau et al., 2005).

3.2.3.3. Survival and Response Rates

Both Carmustine and Lomustine have shown responses in about 40% of patients with malignant glioma, with a median response-minimum of 5.2 weeks (Della Cuna & Paoletti, 1976). Although such treatments offer some survival benefit, their efficacy remains modest, thus justifying continued search for better combination regimens and more creative delivery approaches (Reithmeier et al., 2010). Despite the importance of Carmustine and Lomustine in the treatment of glioblastoma, they are not without issues. The toxicity, including especially hematologic toxicity, is the mainstay that restricts their application. Furthermore, the increased survival benefits are frequently of short duration and, therefore, constant research is needed to develop more efficient treatments. Novel therapeutic strategies, including immunotherapeutic and targeted strategies, may provide alternative methods for enhancing survival in patients with glioblastoma (Liau et al., 2005; Ohba & Hirose, 2016).

3.3. Bevacizumab (Anti-VEGF Therapy)

Bevacizumab, an anti-vascular endothelial growth factor (VEGF) monoclonal antibody, has an important part in the management of glioblastoma, a highly vascularized and aggressive brain tumor. The primary mechanism of this therapy is anti-angiogenesis or depriving the tumor of blood supply, leaves the tumor growth and adjacent edema. Although bevacizumab can enrich the life of the patients, its use is accompanied by issues such as adverse events and limited improvement in overall survival (Chamberlain, 2011).

3.3.1. Mechanism of Action

Bevacizumab does this by targeting and inhibiting vascular endothelial growth factor (VEGF), a protein that is necessary for angiogenesis the development of new blood vessels. Tumours require a steady supply of oxygen and nutrients, which is delivered by these new blood vessels. VEGF prompts the growth of these vessels through its interaction with receptors on the endothelial cells (the cells that line the blood vessels). It works by binding to the VEGF protein, which prevents it from connecting to the receptors, therefore blocking the development of new blood vessels to the tumor. Without a stream of new blood vessels, the tumor is starved of oxygen and nutrients, slowing its growth. Bevacizumab not only inhibits angiogenesis, but also decreases tumour-related oedema. Tumors commonly have abnormal blood vessels that can leak fluid, which increases swelling in surrounding tissues. Bevacizumab blocks the development of the new blood vessels, thereby preventing leakage and relieving symptoms for patients. There is also some evidence that bevacizumab may have indirect effects on glioma stem cells (cells that support the tumor's growth and resistance to treatment) by cutting off the resources that feed them. It may also trigger an immune reaction and contribute to the body's defense against the tumor, although the exact role that bevacizumab plays in immune responses remains under investigation (Chamberlain, 2011; Tamura et al., 2017; Levin, 2010). Action of GBM therapies represented in Figure 1.

3.3.2. Clinical Applications

In recurrent glioblastoma, bevacizumab is the main agent for patients with demonstrated superiority in progression-free survival and preserved performance status 18. It is employed as a monotherapy as well as in combination with chemotherapy. Bevacizumab, in the above combinations has demonstrated to increase PFS over chemotherapy alone. Nonetheless, despite these increases in PFS, bevacizumab has not consistently improved OS across trials, constituting a major issue with its utilization (Tamura et al., 2017; Funakoshi et al., 2020).

3.3.3. Limitations and Side Effects

The principal drawback of bevacizumab is its failure to demonstrate an overall survival benefit as shown in several trials (Funakoshi et al., 2020). The most frequent adverse effects associated with bevacizumab are hypertension, proteinuria, and thromboembolic events (Chamberlain, 2011; Levin, 2010). Additionally, resistance to bevacizumab can occur due to alternative pro-angiogenic pathways activated but the manner of this resistance remains obscure (Tamura et al., 2017). An additional limitation of bevacizumab is the lack of validated biomarkers to predict which patients are most likely to derive benefit from treatment with bevacizumab (Stupp & Weller, 2014). Although bevacizumab represents a significant quality-of-life and time to progression is often life-saving addition for a subset of patients with GBM side effects with progressive despite surgery, radiotherapy, and salvage chemotherapy, the lack of overall survival evidence points to the difficulty in treating this dreadful disease. Prospective studies should focus on the identification of biomarkers for the selection of patients according to their likelihood of response, and to address the mechanisms of resistance. The identification of such studies might lead to an improvement in the use of bevacizumab in clinical practice.

Figure 1. Mechanisms of action of (GBM) therapies

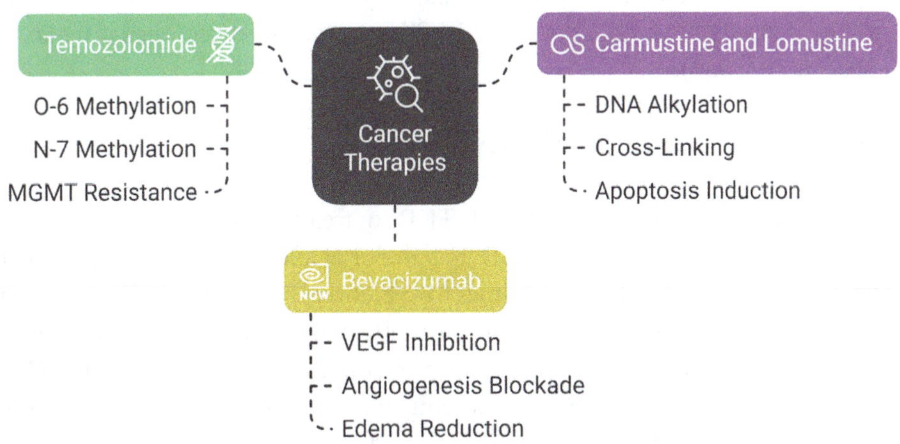

4. EMERGING TARGETED THERAPIES

4.1. Tyrosine Kinase Inhibitors

Tyrosine kinase inhibitors (TKIs) represent an attractive strategy to combat glioblastoma which is among the most aggressive and devastating brain tumors. Through the numerous hurdles of the BBB and the intrinsic molecular heterogeneity of the tumor, TKIs aim to target central signaling pathways for inhibition in glioblastoma cells. Such directed intervention may increase treatment efficacy compared to more conventional treatment strategies. Here, we review the existing TKI therapy in glioblastoma with their mechanisms of action, limitations and future possibilities.

4.1.1. Mechanism of Action and Targets

Tyrosine kinases (TKs) are enzymes critical for modulating functions of cells, including proliferation, differentiation, and survival. In glioblastoma, these enzymes tend to be aberrantly deregulated, which justifies inhibiting them by TKIs (Rahban et al., 2024). TKIs disrupt these kinases, thus inhibiting the downstream signaling that is essential for tumor proliferation and to prevent apoptosis. The epidermal growth factor receptor (EGFR) and vascular endothelial growth factor receptor (VEGFR) are among the most relevant targets of TKI in glioblastoma therapy, and they are overexpressed in a large percentage of glioblastoma cases (Cruz Da Silva et al., 2021). TKIs can be classified into two major types: allosteric and non-allosteric inhibitors. Irreversible binding of a few of TKIs on the target prolongs drug action (Rahban et al., 2024).

4.1.2. Challenges in TKI Efficacy

Although promising, the potential of TKIs for treatment of glioblastoma is hindered by multiple obstacles. The BBB is a major challenge to delivering TKIs to the brain, and thus their efficacy. In order to overcome these limitations, novel drug delivery systems (e.g., nanocarriers) are currently under investigation, representing a strategy to increase TKI brain penetration and optimize their PK properties (Brar et al., 2023). Moreover, the genetic and epigenetic heterogeneity of glioblastoma is a major determinant in the emergence of resistance to TKIs, thus reinforcing the importance of tailored treatment protocols according to the molecular signature of the tumor (Rahban et al., 2024; Bae et al., 2024). This heterogeneity is one of the major causes of the failure of many promising TKIs in trials, despite promising in pre-clinical trials (Brar et al., 2023).

4.1.3. Other Developments in Drug Delivery and Combination Therapy

These challenges are being increasingly addressed through the development of drug delivery systems. Nanocarriers and other sophisticated systems are being pursued in order to increase the efficiency of TKI delivery through the BBB and allow for targeted tumor cell delivery (Brar et al., 2023). The combined therapy of TKIs with other strategies (eg., immune checkpoint inhibitors, repurposed drugs) is now actively investigated to overcome resistance mechanisms and improve the effectiveness of treatments (Kucinska et al., 2024; Shikalov et al., 2024). The combination approaches they used are now being evaluated in clinical trials, with early results showing encouraging effects on patient outcomes (Cruz Da Silva et al., 2021).

4.1.4. Conclusions and Future Research Directions

In the future, prospects of TKI-based therapies may be bright in glioblastoma treatment. Advanced diagnostic technologies of cDNA may enable better personalized and precise use of TKIs, discriminating the patients who are most likely to benefit from these drugs (52). Moreover, further advancement of recent TKIs with state-of-the-art methodologies (e.g., computer-assisted drug design) mays work as more potent and/or efficacious agents (Rahban et al., 2024). Further evaluation of combination of TKIs with novel therapeutic strategies, like oncolytic viruses or cell-based therapies provide novel and promising treatment options in the treatment of glioblastoma (Targeted therapies for glioblastoma treatment, 2023). Although drug delivery and tumor heterogeneity are major obstacles, the continued investigation of targeted therapies, including TKIs, raise hopes to change the prognosis of patients with glioblastoma. The ultimate success of these therapies will probably be achieved by combining TKIs with other personalized therapeutic approaches for maximizing the therapeutic efficacy and for circumventing the current hurdles in the treatment of glioblastoma.

4.2. Immunotherapy (Checkpoint for Inhibitors, Cells CAR-T Based)

GBM remains one of the most aggressive and lethal primary central nervous system (CNS) malignancies, and its prognosis is still dismal despite current standard treatments, including surgery, radiotherapy and/or chemotherapy. Median survival for GBM patients is generally 12-18 months. Nevertheless, the emergence of new targeted therapy and immunotherapy, such as ICIs and CAR-T cell therapies, have increasing potential to provide better outcomes by the help of the host immune system to fight against cancer. These novel therapies seek to address the limitations of existing therapies and hold promise for developing more efficacious treatments.

4.2.1. Therapies Against Glioblastoma

Targeted therapies are intended to inhibit certain molecular pathways on which GBM depends for its growth and survival. Pathways that are intimately related to the progression of GBM are PI3K, NFKβ, JAK-STAT, CK2, WNT, NOTCH, and TGFβ. Suppression of these pathways may prevent tumor growth and sensitize the response of tumor to therapy (Rong et al., 2022). Despite this promise, most targeted agents have failed to significantly impact patient care. This is mainly attributed to the nature of the tumor heterogeneity as well as the difficulty the BBB presents, which makes it difficult to deliver drugs effectively to the brain (Preusser et al., 2015).

4.2.2. Immunotherapeutic Strategies for GBM

ICIs have been increasingly studied as a potential treatment for GBM. Drugs like ipilimumab, which are called immune checkpoint blockers that interfere with molecular steps that inhibit the immune system from attacking tumor cells, along with nivolumab and pembrolizumab, have been successful in treating other cancers. Yet, GBM has an immune environment that is specific, especially in the CNS, and the success of ICIs is compromised in this case (Preusser et al., 2015; Yang et al., 2020). Another hopeful option is CAR-T cell therapy, where a patient's T cells are engineered to express chimeric antigen receptors (CARs) targeting tumor-specific antigens. Antigens such as IL-13, Rα2 and EGFR have been studied in GBM, showing positive results at preclinical and clinical levels. Current research is focused on enhancing specificity and efficacy of CAR-T cells in the GBM setting (Agosti et al., 2023; Yuan et al., 2022).

4.2.3. Combination Therapies

Combination therapy of immunotherapies with the various other treatment methods, including surgery, radiation and chemotherapy, might be one possible approach to improve the therapeutic effect of immunotherapies. By doing so, this strategy is expected to reverse the immunosuppressive tumor microenvironment and enhance tumor-specific immune responses. Immunotherapies in combination with traditional approaches has the promise of benefiting GBM patients in a greater extent (Liu et al., 2023).

4.2.4. Clinical Trials and Future Directions

A number of clinical trials are evaluating the efficacy of immune checkpoint inhibitors, CAR-T, oncolytic viruses and cancer vaccines for GBM therapy at the moment. These tests are important to better understanding success and limitations with these therapies (Agosti et al., 2023). However, there are challenges that need to be address even though immunotherapies have shown a lot of promises. Tumor heterogeneity, mechanisms of immune evasion, and the resistant nature of the BBB represent significant impediments that will need to be addressed. Such therapies are most likely to gain further impetus by developments in drug delivery forms and by the discovery of new molecular targets (Yang et al., 2020; Cao et al., 2022). Although targeted therapies and immunotherapies provide hope for better management of GBM, resolution of these barriers is dependent on continued development and optimization of these CITs. The development of GBM treatment may hinge on integrating these therapies with other treatment forms, with prospects for novel and therapeutic treatment options for patients.

4.3. Oncolytic Viruses and Gene Therapy

GBM is still one of the most aggressive and fatal brain tumors and the classic treatments including surgery, chemotherapies and radio-therapies exhibit limited efficiency. Therefore, novel therapeutic approaches oriented toward the molecular/cellular/genetic bases of glioblastoma are under investigation. Novel strategies, including specific-directed therapies, gene therapy, and oncolytic viruses are being designed to achieve more precise tumor killing with less toxicity. Below, we move through the details of these emerging therapies which could very well revolutionize the future of patient care.

4.3.1. Glioblastoma Specific Treatments

Targeted agents are intended to interfere with the targeted molecular pathways essential for the survival and growth of glioblastoma cells. The most important pathways that participate in regulating are PI3K, NFKβ, JAK-STAT, CK2, WNT, NOTCH, and TGFβ, which are involved in the growth and cell survival of tumors. Through inhibition of these pathways, targeted therapies aim to prevent tumor growth and promote cell death in cancer (Rong et al., 2022). Monoclonal antibodies that can recognize receptors on the surface of glioblastoma cells are also being developed in order to obstruct the molecular interactions mediating tumor proliferation. Clinical studies underway are assessing safety and efficacy in glioblastoma treatment for these monoclonal antibodies. In addition, scientists are developing nanocarriers that can penetrate the BBB - a major hurdle in brain tumor treatment. These nanoparticles support targeted release of drugs at the tumor site, which could increase efficacy and minimize systemic side effects (Targeted therapies for glioblastoma treatment, 2023).

4.3.2. Gene Therapy Approaches

Gene therapy presents as an emerging option for GBM, manipulating the genome for the advent of therapeutic genes, which act on cancer cells. It may include the addition of suicide, cytokine, and tumor suppressor genes to augment the immune response to the tumor and promote killing of the cells itself. Non-replicative and replicating viral vectors are employed to introduce these therapeutic genes into glioblastoma cells. These vectors can be selectively retargeted to destroy cancer cells leaving normal brain intact, a means of honing in on the cancer (Aghi & Chiocca, 2006). Moreover, stem cells and miRNAs are under study as potential carriers for gene delivery, also contributing with the specificity and effectiveness of gene therapies (62).

4.3.3. Oncolytic Viruses for Glioblastoma Therapy

Oncolytic viruses (OVs) form a very attractive strategy to combat GBM. These viruses are modified to only infect and replicate in tumor cells resulting in cell lysis and production new virions. Besides that, oncolytic viruses may mediate anti-tumor immune responses to selectively recognize and eliminate any other surviving tumor cells (Lal & Mukherjee, 2016). The potential OVs combined with other therapeutic approaches are currently under investigation in clinical trials. Personalized oncolytic viruses that are designed according to the tumor's individual genetic profile constitute an important field of investigation and may improve treatment responses (Hamad et al., 2023; Rong et al., 2022). OVs have a double action: they kill cancerous cells and activate the body's immune system to continue to kill the tumor. This makes the OVs very attractive as GBM therapy. In addition, OVs are considered safe because they do not infect healthy cells and therefore there is limited risk of normal tissue damage (Aghi & Chiocca, 2006). Emerging therapy for glioblastoma Gene therapy and oncolytic viruses highlighted in Figure 2.

Figure 2. Prioritizing emerging therapy for glioblastoma in gene therapy and oncolytic viruses

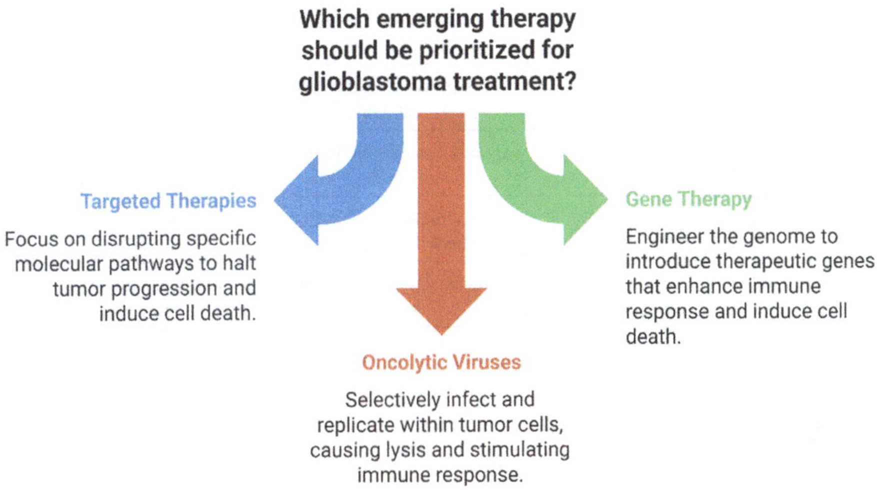

5. FUTURE PERSPECTIVES IN GLIOBLASTOMA TREATMENT

Recent advances in research have shown intriguing solutions that might revolutionize GBM therapy in the future. Nanoparticle delivery methods, immunotherapeutic tactics, CAR-T cell therapy advances, targeted molecular therapeutics, and combination treatment regimens are among the new approaches that will shape the future of GBM care (Angom et al., 2023). The journey toward successful gene therapy and oncolytic virus therapy for glioblastoma is long, but these novel applications of therapy provide an exciting frontier in the treatment of brain cancer. With ongoing development, these treatments could change the way glioblastoma is managed, offering hope for longer and more healthy life (Table 2). Important aspects of novel treatment of glioblastoma.

Table 2. Key features of emerging therapy for glioblastoma

Characteristic	Tyrosine Kinase Inhibitors	Immunotherapy	Gene Therapy & Oncolytic Viruses
Mechanism of Action	Inhibits key signaling pathways.	Leverages immune system to combat cancer.	Introduces therapeutic genes to target tumor cells.
Key Targets	EGFR and VEGFR.	Immune checkpoints, tumor antigens.	Suicide genes, cytokine genes.
Challenges	Blood-brain barrier, tumor heterogeneity.	Unique immune environment, immune evasion.	Genetic heterogeneity, adverse immune reactions.
Advances	Nanocarriers, combination therapies.	Combination with surgery, radiation, chemotherapy.	Novel viral vectors, gene modifications.
Future Directions	Personalized application, novel TKIs.	Clinical trials, novel molecular targets.	Improved delivery systems, novel vectors.

5.1. Novel Drug Candidates

- MAGL-Targeting PROTAC (JN-PROTAC) – this addresses the causes of disease recurrence by demonstrating strong in vivo suppression of patient-derived GBM stem cells (GSCs) (Yuan et al., 2025).
- Sesquiterpene Lactones (STLs) - inhibit glucose metabolism and the proneural-mesenchymal transition, which are essential for GBM invasion, while inducing mitochondrial failure, oxidative stress, and death (Markov et al., 2025).
- Macrophage-Ferritin-Drug Conjugates (MDCs) - uses macrophages to transport ferritin-tubulin inhibitor complexes straight to tumours, activating T cells and lowering immune-suppressive cells (Bialasek et al., 2025).
- Integrin-Targeting Conjugate (BIK-E715E) - binds integrins $\alpha v\beta 3/\alpha v\beta 5$ via ELiTE-DDS, allowing receptor-mediated transcytosis to penetrate the BBB (Shin et al., 2025).
- AT2R Inhibitors (A3E) - inhibit the development of tumours by blocking the angiotensin II type 2 receptor (AT2R), which is hyperactive in GBM (Perryman et al., 2022).
- Plasma-Assisted Drug Deposition (Topotecan) - By overcoming BBB restrictions, cold plasma improves topotecan local delivery and increases its effectiveness in 3D GBM models (Pinheiro Lopes et al., 2025).
- Cardiac Glycosides (Proscillaridin A) - causes GBM cells to become cytotoxic and regulates the formation of tumours in heterotopic and orthotopic models (Denicolai et al., 2014).

5.2. Combination Therapies

GBM treatment research is heavily focused on combination therapy approaches because of the tumor's intricacy, resistance mechanisms, and poor response to single-agent treatments.

- Synergistic Drug Combinations: Synergistic medication Combinations: High-throughput research has discovered medication combinations that function better together than separately. The medication combinations Lapatinib with Thapsigargin and Lapatinib with Obatoclax Mesylate demonstrated the greatest synergy, as both target the epidermal growth factor receptor and influence the apoptotic pathway (Houweling et al., 2023).
- Targeting pathways: Cancer stem cells in GBM are predominantly maintained via the Notch, Wnt, and Hedgehog (Hh) signaling pathways. Targeting pathways that influence these processes may inhibit CSC growth and invasiveness in GBM, considerably delaying tumor recurrence (Yan, 2024).
- Combination Immunotherapy: The immunosuppressive context of GBM can be overcome and immune responses can be enhanced by combining immune checkpoint inhibitors, vaccinations, oncolytic viruses, or adoptive cell therapies with conventional treatments or one another (Salvato & Marchini, 2024).
- Network-Targeting Combination Therapy (NTCT): In a significant case study, a patient with recurring leptomeningeal glioblastoma received a tailored treatment strategy called NTCT, which utilizes synthetic lethality to take advantage of weaknesses in cancer cells. Thorough molecular diagnostics revealed several deficiencies in the tumour's DNA repair systems, redox equilibrium, and autophagy functions. Considering these discoveries, a customized treatment plan involving lomustine, olaparib, digoxin, metformin, and high-dose intravenous ascorbate was implemented with intra-patient dose escalation to guarantee safety. This tactical integration sought to provoke different types of cell death, such as apoptosis, necroptosis, and ferroptosis, by focusing on the tumour's distinct molecular network. The patient attained full remission and stayed disease-free for 23 months after relapse, underscoring the potential of NTCT as a promising approach for addressing aggressive and treatment-resistant types of GBM (Castro et al., 2023).
- Drug repurposing: Techniques like CUSP9 target several survival pathways in GBM stem cells by combining temozolomide with nine non-oncology medications (such as disulfiram, celecoxib, and minocycline) (Skaga et al., 2019).
- Overcoming Antiangiogenic Resistance: Resistance mechanisms, including hypoxia-induced invasion and redundant proangiogenic signalling, can be

thwarted by combining antiangiogenic medicines with additional medications (Rahman & Ali, 2024).

- Advanced Delivery and Personalization: To better integrate combination medicines and maximize their efficacy for specific patients, researchers are investigating novel delivery techniques (such as nanoparticles, antibody-drug conjugates, and adaptive trial designs) (Narsinh et al., 2024).

5.3. Personalized and Precision Medicine

By tailoring treatments according to the unique genetic, epigenetic, and molecular characteristics of each patient's tumour, personalized and precision medicine represent promising future approaches in the treatment of GBM, aiming to address the disease's well-known heterogeneity and resistance to traditional therapies. The identification of actionable mutations, epigenetic modifications, and particular biomarkers is now possible thanks to advancements in next-generation sequencing, multi-omics profiling, and molecular diagnostics. These findings can guide the selection of targeted treatments such as proteasome inhibitors, EGFR or VEGF inhibitors, or immune-based approaches (Gozdz, 2023; Sadowski et al., 2024). While liquid biopsies and advanced imaging allow real-time surveillance of tumour growth and response to therapy, technologies like organ-on-a-chip systems, theranostic nanomedicine, and machine learning improve the development and assessment of customized treatment programs (Maity et al., 2025; d'Angelo et al., 2019; Jovčevska, 2020). By going beyond standard therapies and focusing on the distinct flaws of each tumour, the personalized medicine approach has significant potential for improving the outcomes for GBM patients, despite continuous difficulties in combining complex data and validating these techniques in lengthy clinical trials.

6. CONCLUSION

GBM remains a challenging brain tumor to treat due to its aggressive nature and resistance to therapy. Current standard treatments involve surgical resection, radiotherapy, and chemotherapy, each playing a distinct role in managing the disease. Temozolomide is the frontline chemotherapeutic agent, while drugs like carmustine, lomustine, and bevacizumab are also employed in specific clinical contexts. However, the effectiveness of these treatments is often constrained by factors such as tumor heterogeneity and limited drug penetration into the brain. In response, research has shifted toward innovative strategies, including tyrosine kinase inhibitors that disrupt signaling pathways, immune-based therapies like checkpoint inhibitors and CAR-T cells, and gene therapies using oncolytic viruses. These targeted approaches aim to overcome the limitations of conventional methods. Looking forward, emphasis is placed on discovering novel drug candidates, exploring synergistic drug combinations, and advancing precision medicine to customize therapy based on individual tumor profiles.

REFERENCES

Aghi, M., & Chiocca, E. A. (2006). Gene therapy for glioblastoma. *Neurosurgical Focus*, *20*(4), E18. Advance online publication. DOI: 10.3171/foc.2006.20.4.9 PMID: 16709023

Agosti, E., Zeppieri, M., De Maria, L., Tedeschi, C., Fontanella, M. M., Panciani, P. P., Ius, T., & Skrap, M. (2023). Glioblastoma immunotherapy: A systematic review of the present strategies and prospects for advancements. *International Journal of Molecular Sciences*, *24*(20), 15037. Advance online publication. DOI: 10.3390/ijms242015037 PMID: 37894718

Aiyappa-Maudsley, R., Chalmers, A. J., & Parsons, J. L. (2022). Factors affecting the radiation response in glioblastoma. *Neuro-Oncology Advances*, *4*(1), vdac156. Advance online publication. DOI: 10.1093/noajnl/vdac156 PMID: 36325371

Angom, R. S., Nakka, N. M. R., & Bhattacharya, S. (2023). Advances in glioblastoma therapy: An update on current approaches. *Brain Sciences*, *13*(11), 1536. Advance online publication. DOI: 10.3390/brainsci13111536 PMID: 38002496

Bae, W. H., Maraka, S., & Daher, A. (2024). Challenges and advances in glioblastoma targeted therapy: The promise of drug repurposing and biomarker exploration. *Frontiers in Oncology*, *14*, 1441460. Advance online publication. DOI: 10.3389/fonc.2024.1441460 PMID: 39439947

Bao, S., Wu, Q., McLendon, R. E., Hao, Y., Shi, Q., Hjelmeland, A. B., Dewhirst, M. W., Bigner, D. D., & Rich, J. N. (2006). Glioma stem cells promote radioresistance by preferential activation of the DNA damage response. *Nature*, *444*(7120), 756–760. DOI: 10.1038/nature05236 PMID: 17051156

Bialasek, M., Sun, M., Marszalek, I., Taciak, B., Weller, M., Rygiel, T., & Król, M. (2025). Abstract A037: Macrophage-ferritin-drug conjugates: A novel approach to overcome glioblastoma drug resistance and induce long-term tumor immunity. *Cancer Immunology Research*, *13*(2, Supplement), A037. DOI: 10.1158/2326-6074.IO2025-A037

Bovenkamp, D., Sentosa, R., Rank, E., Erkkilä, M. T., Placzek, F., Püls, J., Ntziachristos, V., & Rühm, A. (2018). Combination of high-resolution optical coherence tomography and Raman spectroscopy for improved staging and grading in bladder cancer. *Applied Sciences (Basel, Switzerland)*, *8*(12), 2371. Advance online publication. DOI: 10.3390/app8122371

Brada, M., Judson, I., Beale, P., Moore, S., Reidenberg, P., Statkevich, P., Dugan, M., Batra, V., & Cutler, D. (1999). Phase I dose-escalation and pharmacokinetic study of temozolomide (SCH 52365) for refractory or relapsing malignancies. *British Journal of Cancer*, *81*(6), 1022–1030. DOI: 10.1038/sj.bjc.6690802 PMID: 10576660

Brar, H. K., Jose, J., Wu, Z., & Sharma, M. (2023). Tyrosine kinase inhibitors for glioblastoma multiforme: Challenges and opportunities for drug delivery. *Pharmaceutics*, *15*(1), 59. Advance online publication. DOI: 10.3390/pharmaceutics15010059 PMID: 36678688

Brown, T. J., Brennan, M. C., Li, M., Church, E. W., Brandmeir, N. J., Rakszawski, K. L., Patel, A. S., Sharma, S., Rizk, E., Florman, J. E., Feletti, A., & Glantz, M. J. (2016). Association of the extent of resection with survival in glioblastoma: A systematic review and meta-analysis. *JAMA Oncology*, *2*(11), 1460–1469. DOI: 10.1001/jamaoncol.2016.1373 PMID: 27310651

Bu, L., Lu, J., Zhang, J., & Wu, J. (2021). Intraoperative cognitive mapping tasks for direct electrical stimulation in clinical and neuroscientific contexts. *Frontiers in Human Neuroscience*, *15*, 612891. Advance online publication. DOI: 10.3389/fnhum.2021.612891 PMID: 33762913

Cao, T. Q., Wainwright, D. A., Lee-Chang, C., Miska, J., Sonabend, A. M., Heimberger, A. B., & Lukas, R. V. (2022). Next steps for immunotherapy in glioblastoma. *Cancers (Basel)*, *14*(16), 4023. Advance online publication. DOI: 10.3390/cancers14164023 PMID: 36011015

Carpentier, A., Canney, M., Vignot, A., Reina, V., Beccaria, K., Horodyckid, C., Karachi, C., Leclercq, D., Lafon, C., Chapelon, J.-Y., Capelle, L., Cornu, P., Sanson, M., Hoang-Xuan, K., Delattre, J.-Y., & Idbaih, A. (2016). Clinical trial of blood-brain barrier disruption by pulsed ultrasound. *Science Translational Medicine*, *8*(343), 343re2. Advance online publication. DOI: 10.1126/scitranslmed.aaf6086 PMID: 27306666

Castro, M. P., Sipos, B., Biskup, S., & Kahn, N. (2023). Network-targeting combination therapy of leptomeningeal glioblastoma using multiple synthetic lethal strategies: A case report. *Frontiers in Oncology*, *13*, 1210224. Advance online publication. DOI: 10.3389/fonc.2023.1210224 PMID: 38023264

Chamberlain, M. C. (2011). Treatment of glioblastoma with bevacizumab: Has a new standard therapy been defined? *CNS Drugs*, *25*(1), 1–4. DOI: 10.2165/11587880-000000000-00000 PMID: 21936584

Chen, S., Qiu, Q., Wang, D., She, D., Yin, B., Chai, M., Gu, G., & Chen, J. (2022). Long acting carmustine loaded natural extracellular matrix hydrogel for inhibition of glioblastoma recurrence after tumor resection. *Frontiers of Chemical Science and Engineering*, *16*(4), 536–545. DOI: 10.1007/s11705-021-2067-5

Cote, D. J., Balak, N., Brennum, J., Holsgrove, D. T., Kitchen, N., Kolenda, H., & Russell, S. M. (2017). Ethical difficulties in the innovative surgical treatment of patients with recurrent glioblastoma multiforme. *Journal of Neurosurgery*, *126*(6), 2045–2050. DOI: 10.3171/2016.11.JNS162488 PMID: 28430037

Cruz Da Silva, E., Mercier, M. C., Etienne-Selloum, N., Dontenwill, M., & Choulier, L. (2021). A systematic review of glioblastoma-targeted therapies in phases II, III, IV clinical trials. *Cancers (Basel)*, *13*(8), 1795. Advance online publication. DOI: 10.3390/cancers13081795 PMID: 33918704

Curran, W. J.Jr, Scott, C. B., Horton, J., Nelson, J. S., Weinstein, A. S., Fischbach, A. J., Chang, C. H., Rotman, M., Asbell, S. O., Krisch, R. E., & Nelson, D. F. (1993). Recursive partitioning analysis of prognostic factors in three Radiation Therapy Oncology Group malignant glioma trials. *Journal of the National Cancer Institute*, *85*(9), 704–710. DOI: 10.1093/jnci/85.9.704 PMID: 8478956

d'Angelo, M., Castelli, V., Benedetti, E., Antonosante, A., Catanesi, M., Dominguez-Benot, R., & Cimini, A. (2019). Theranostic nanomedicine for malignant gliomas. *Frontiers in Bioengineering and Biotechnology*, *7*, 325. Advance online publication. DOI: 10.3389/fbioe.2019.00325 PMID: 31799246

Della Cuna, G. R., & Paoletti, P. (1976). BCNU and CCNU chemotherapy of tumours of the central nervous system. In Hellmann, K., & Connors, T. A. (Eds.), *Chemotherapy: Cancer chemotherapy II* (pp. 541–549). Springer., DOI: 10.1007/978-1-4613-4352-3_85

Denicolaï, E., Baeza-Kallee, N., Tchoghandjian, A., Carré, M., Colin, C., Jiglaire, C. J., Mercurio, S., Beclin, C., & Figarella-Branger, D. (2014). Proscillaridin A is cytotoxic for glioblastoma cell lines and controls tumor xenograft growth in vivo. *Oncotarget*, *5*(21), 10934–10948. DOI: 10.18632/oncotarget.2541 PMID: 25400117

Elashwah, A., Alsuhaibani, A., Alzahrani, A., Azzam, A. Z., Moftah, B., Breakeit, M., Alharbi, A., & Alshaikh, A. (2023). The use of intraoperative radiation therapy (IORT) in multimodality management of cancer patients: A single institution experience. *Journal of Gastrointestinal Cancer*, *54*(2), 433–441. DOI: 10.1007/s12029-021-00786-9 PMID: 35290599

Ellis, H. (2009). Harvey Cushing: A founding father of neurosurgery. *British Journal of Hospital Medicine, 70*(10), 600. DOI: 10.12968/hmed.2009.70.10.44633 PMID: 19966711

Funakoshi, Y., Hata, N., Kuga, D., Hatae, R., Sangatsuda, Y., Fujioka, Y., Takigawa, K., Mizoguchi, M., & Iihara, K. (2020). Update on chemotherapeutic approaches and management of bevacizumab usage for glioblastoma. *Pharmaceuticals (Basel, Switzerland), 13*(12), 470. Advance online publication. DOI: 10.3390/ph13120470 PMID: 33339404

Ginat, D. T. (2022). 1,3-Bis(2-chloroethyl)-1-nitrosourea (BCNU; carmustine) polymer wafer (Gliadel). In Ginat, D. T., Small, J. E., & Schaefer, P. W. (Eds.), *Neuroimaging pharmacopoeia* (pp. 141–148). Springer., DOI: 10.1007/978-3-031-08774-5_18

Gozdz, A. (2023). Proteasome inhibitors against glioblastoma—Overview of molecular mechanisms of cytotoxicity, progress in clinical trials, and perspective for use in personalized medicine. *Current Oncology (Toronto, Ont.), 30*(11), 9676–9688. DOI: 10.3390/curroncol30110702 PMID: 37999122

Guo, Q. L., Dai, X. L., Yin, M. Y., Cheng, H. W., Qian, H. S., Wang, H., Chen, D. W., & Zhang, X. (2022). Nanosensitizers for sonodynamic therapy for glioblastoma multiforme: Current progress and future perspectives. *Military Medical Research, 9*(1), 26. Advance online publication. DOI: 10.1186/s40779-022-00386-z PMID: 35676737

Hamad, A., Yusubalieva, G. M., Baklaushev, V. P., Chumakov, P. M., & Lipatova, A. V. (2023). Recent developments in glioblastoma therapy: Oncolytic viruses and emerging future strategies. *Viruses, 15*(2), 547. Advance online publication. DOI: 10.3390/v15020547 PMID: 36851761

Hoosemans, L., Vooijs, M., & Hoeben, A. (2024). Opportunities and challenges of small molecule inhibitors in glioblastoma treatment: Lessons learned from clinical trials. *Cancers (Basel), 16*(17), 3021. Advance online publication. DOI: 10.3390/cancers16173021 PMID: 39272879

Houweling, M., Giczewska, A., Abdul, K., Nieuwenhuis, N., Küçükosmanoglu, A., Pastuszak, K., & French, P. J. (2023). Screening of predicted synergistic multi-target therapies in glioblastoma identifies new treatment strategies. *Neuro-Oncology Advances, 5*(1), vdad073. Advance online publication. DOI: 10.1093/noajnl/vdad073 PMID: 37455945

Jakola, A. S., Sagberg, L. M., Gulati, S., & Solheim, O. (2020). Advancements in predicting outcomes in patients with glioma: A surgical perspective. *Expert Review of Anticancer Therapy, 20*(3), 167–177. DOI: 10.1080/14737140.2020.1735367 PMID: 32114857

Jezierzański, M., Nafalska, N., Stopyra, M., Furgoł, T., Miciak, M., Kabut, J., & Szczylik, C. (2024). Temozolomide (TMZ) in the treatment of glioblastoma multiforme—A literature review and clinical outcomes. *Current Oncology (Toronto, Ont.), 31*(7), 3994–4002. DOI: 10.3390/curroncol31070296 PMID: 39057168

Jnaidi, R., Almeida, A. J., & Gonçalves, L. M. (2020). Solid lipid nanoparticles and nanostructured lipid carriers as smart drug delivery systems in the treatment of glioblastoma multiforme. *Pharmaceutics, 12*(9), 860. Advance online publication. DOI: 10.3390/pharmaceutics12090860 PMID: 32927610

Johnson, D. R., & O'Neill, B. P. (2012). Glioblastoma survival in the United States before and during the temozolomide era. *Journal of Neuro-Oncology, 107*(2), 359–364. DOI: 10.1007/s11060-011-0749-4 PMID: 22045118

Jovčevska, I. (2020). Next generation sequencing and machine learning technologies are painting the epigenetic portrait of glioblastoma. *Frontiers in Oncology, 10*, 798. Advance online publication. DOI: 10.3389/fonc.2020.00798 PMID: 32500035

Kucinska, M., Pospieszna, J., Tang, J., Lisiak, N., Toton, E., Rubis, B., Murias, M., & Hofmann, J. (2024). The combination therapy using tyrosine kinase receptors inhibitors and repurposed drugs to target patient-derived glioblastoma stem cells. *Biomedicine and Pharmacotherapy, 176*, 116892. Advance online publication. DOI: 10.1016/j.biopha.2024.116892 PMID: 38876048

Lal, S., & Mukherjee, J. (2016). Oncolytic viral therapy of glioblastoma: Will this soon become a reality. *Chemotherapy (Los Angeles, Calif.), 5*(2), e131. Advance online publication. DOI: 10.4172/2167-7700.1000e131

Levin, V. A. (2010). Role of bevacizumab therapy in the management of glioblastoma. *Cancer Management and Research, 2*, 97–104. DOI: 10.2147/CMAR.S6103 PMID: 21188100

Liau, C. T., Wei, K. C., Tseng, C. K., & Jung, S. M. (2005). Combination chemotherapy with carmustine and cisplatin followed by procarbazine, lomustine, and vincristine for adult high-grade astrocytoma. *Chang Gung Medical Journal, 28*(1), 16–23. PMID: 15804144

Liu, G., Yuan, X., Zeng, Z., Tunici, P., Ng, H., Abdulkadir, I. R., Lu, L., Irvin, D., Black, K. L., & Yu, J. S. (2006). Analysis of gene expression and chemoresistance of CD133+ cancer stem cells in glioblastoma. *Molecular Cancer*, *5*(1), 67. Advance online publication. DOI: 10.1186/1476-4598-5-67 PMID: 17140455

Liu, X., Zhao, Z., Dai, W., Liao, K., Sun, Q., Chen, D., & Liu, Z. (2023). The development of immunotherapy for the treatment of recurrent glioblastoma. *Cancers (Basel)*, *15*(17), 4308. Advance online publication. DOI: 10.3390/cancers15174308 PMID: 37686584

Maity, S., Bhuyan, T., Jewell, C., Kawakita, S., Sharma, S., Nguyen, H. T., & Kim, Y. J. (2025). Recent developments in glioblastoma-on-a-chip for advanced drug screening applications. *Small*, *21*(1), e2405511. Advance online publication. DOI: 10.1002/smll.202405511 PMID: 39535474

Malone, E. R., Oliva, M., Sabatini, P. J. B., Stockley, T. L., & Siu, L. L. (2020). Molecular profiling for precision cancer therapies. *Genome Medicine*, *12*(1), 8. Advance online publication. DOI: 10.1186/s13073-019-0703-1 PMID: 31937368

Markov, A. V., Moralev, A. D., & Odarenko, K. V. (2025). Sesquiterpene lactones as promising anti-glioblastoma drug candidates exerting complex effects on glioblastoma cell viability and proneural–mesenchymal transition. *Biomedicines*, *13*(1), 133. Advance online publication. DOI: 10.3390/biomedicines13010133 PMID: 39857717

Marniemi, J., & Parkki, M. G. (1975). Radiochemical assay of glutathione S-epoxide transferase and its enhancement by phenobarbital in rat liver in vivo. *Biochemical Pharmacology*, *24*(17), 1569–1572. DOI: 10.1016/0006-2952(75)90080-5 PMID: 9

Mehta, M., Wen, P., Nishikawa, R., Reardon, D., & Peters, K. (2017). Critical review of the addition of tumor treating fields (TTFields) to the existing standard of care for newly diagnosed glioblastoma patients. *Critical Reviews in Oncology/Hematology*, *111*, 60–65. DOI: 10.1016/j.critrevonc.2017.01.005 PMID: 28259296

Narsinh, K. H., Perez, E., Haddad, A. F., Young, J. S., Savastano, L., Villanueva-Meyer, J. E., & Aghi, M. K. (2024). Strategies to improve drug delivery across the blood–brain barrier for glioblastoma. *Current Neurology and Neuroscience Reports*, *24*(5), 123–139. DOI: 10.1007/s11910-024-01338-x PMID: 38578405

Ohba, S., & Hirose, Y. (2016). Current and future drug treatments for glioblastomas. *Current Medicinal Chemistry*, *23*(38), 4309–4316. DOI: 10.2174/0929867323666161014132907 PMID: 27758718

Ortiz, R., Perazzoli, G., Cabeza, L., Jiménez-Luna, C., Luque, R., Prados, J., & Melguizo, C. (2021). Temozolomide: An updated overview of resistance mechanisms, nanotechnology advances and clinical applications. *Current Neuropharmacology, 19*(4), 513–537. DOI: 10.2174/1570159X19666201230133538 PMID: 32589560

Ou, A., Yung, W. K. A., & Majd, N. (2021). Molecular mechanisms of treatment resistance in glioblastoma. *International Journal of Molecular Sciences, 22*(1), 351. Advance online publication. DOI: 10.3390/ijms22010351 PMID: 33396284

Perryman, R., Renziehausen, A., Shaye, H., Kostagianni, A. D., Tsiailanis, A. D., Thorne, T., & Syed, N. (2022). Inhibition of the angiotensin II type 2 receptor AT2R is a novel therapeutic strategy for glioblastoma. *Proceedings of the National Academy of Sciences of the United States of America, 119*(32), e2116289119. Advance online publication. DOI: 10.1073/pnas.2116289119 PMID: 35917342

Pinheiro Lopes, B., O'Neill, L., Bourke, P., & Boehm, D. (2025). Enhanced cytotoxic effects of cold plasma deposition of topotecan: A novel approach for local cancer drug delivery to glioblastoma cells. *Cancers (Basel), 17*(2), 201. Advance online publication. DOI: 10.3390/cancers17020201 PMID: 39857983

Preusser, M., Lim, M., Hafler, D. A., Reardon, D. A., & Sampson, J. H. (2015). Prospects of immune checkpoint modulators in the treatment of glioblastoma. *Nature Reviews. Neurology, 11*(9), 504–514. DOI: 10.1038/nrneurol.2015.139 PMID: 26260659

Rahban, M., Joushi, S., Bashiri, H., Saso, L., & Sheibani, V. (2024). Characterization of prevalent tyrosine kinase inhibitors and their challenges in glioblastoma treatment. *Frontiers in Chemistry, 11*, 1325214. Advance online publication. DOI: 10.3389/fchem.2023.1325214 PMID: 38264122

Rahman, M. A., & Ali, M. M. (2024). Recent treatment strategies and molecular pathways in resistance mechanisms of antiangiogenic therapies in glioblastoma. *Cancers (Basel), 16*(17), 2975. Advance online publication. DOI: 10.3390/cancers16172975 PMID: 39272834

Reithmeier, T., Graf, E., Piroth, T., Trippel, M., Pinsker, M. O., & Nikkhah, G. (2010). BCNU for recurrent glioblastoma multiforme: Efficacy, toxicity and prognostic factors. *BMC Cancer, 10*(1), 30. Advance online publication. DOI: 10.1186/1471-2407-10-30 PMID: 20122270

Rodríguez-Camacho, A., Flores-Vázquez, J. G., Moscardini-Martelli, J., Torres-Ríos, J. A., Olmos-Guzmán, A., Ortiz-Arce, C. S., Cid-Sánchez, R. B., Villafaña-Vázquez, V., & García-López, E. (2022). Glioblastoma treatment: State-of-the-art and future perspectives. *International Journal of Molecular Sciences*, *23*(13), 7207. Advance online publication. DOI: 10.3390/ijms23137207 PMID: 35806212

Rong, L., Li, N., & Zhang, Z. (2022). Emerging therapies for glioblastoma: Current state and future directions. *Journal of Experimental & Clinical Cancer Research : CR*, *41*(1), 142. Advance online publication. DOI: 10.1186/s13046-022-02349-7 PMID: 35428347

Ryshkova, N. E., Oborotova, N. A., Shprakh, Z. S., Bagirova, V. L., Orlova, O. L., & Polozkova, A. P. (2000). Chemico-pharmacological investigation of a new medicinal form of 1,3-bis(2-chloroethyl)-1-nitrosourea. *Pharmaceutical Chemistry Journal*, *34*(9), 502–504. DOI: 10.1023/A:1005206728431

Sadowski, K., Jażdżewska, A., Kozłowski, J., Zacny, A., Lorenc, T., & Olejarz, W. (2024). Revolutionizing glioblastoma treatment: A comprehensive overview of modern therapeutic approaches. *International Journal of Molecular Sciences*, *25*(11), 5774. Advance online publication. DOI: 10.3390/ijms25115774 PMID: 38891962

Salvato, I., & Marchini, A. (2024). Immunotherapeutic strategies for the treatment of glioblastoma: Current challenges and future perspectives. *Cancers (Basel)*, *16*(7), 1276. Advance online publication. DOI: 10.3390/cancers16071276 PMID: 38610954

Shikalov, A., Koman, I., & Kogan, N. M. (2024). Targeted glioma therapy—Clinical trials and future directions. *Pharmaceutics*, *16*(1), 100. Advance online publication. DOI: 10.3390/pharmaceutics16010100 PMID: 38258110

Shin, K., Sung, H., Jung, J. H., & Kim, S. E. (2025). Abstract 1853: BIK-E715E, an integrin-targeting ligand-drug conjugate equipped with a novel drug delivery system, demonstrates enhanced antitumor efficacy in glioblastoma. *Cancer Research*, *85*(8, Supplement_1), 1853. DOI: 10.1158/1538-7445.AM2025-1853

Skaga, E., Skaga, I. Ø., Grieg, Z., Sandberg, C. J., Langmoen, I. A., & Vik-Mo, E. O. (2019). The efficacy of a coordinated pharmacological blockade in glioblastoma stem cells with nine repurposed drugs using the CUSP9 strategy. *Journal of Cancer Research and Clinical Oncology*, *145*(6), 1495–1507. DOI: 10.1007/s00432-019-02920-4 PMID: 31028540

Stupp, R., Hegi, M. E., Mason, W. P., van den Bent, M. J., Taphoorn, M. J. B., Janzer, R. C., Ludwin, S. K., Allgeier, A., Fisher, B., Belanger, K., Hau, P., Brandes, A. A., Gijtenbeek, J., Marosi, C., Vecht, C. J., Mokhtari, K., Wesseling, P., Villa, S., Eisenhauer, E., & Gorlia, T. (2009). Effects of radiotherapy with concomitant and adjuvant temozolomide versus radiotherapy alone on survival in glioblastoma in a randomised phase III study: 5-year analysis of the EORTC-NCIC trial. *The Lancet. Oncology*, *10*(5), 459–466. DOI: 10.1016/S1470-2045(09)70025-7 PMID: 19269895

Stupp, R., Mason, W. P., van den Bent, M. J., Weller, M., Fisher, B., Taphoorn, M. J. B., Belanger, K., Brandes, A. A., Marosi, C., Bogdahn, U., Curschmann, J., Janzer, R. C., Ludwin, S. K., Gorlia, T., Allgeier, A., Lacombe, D., Cairncross, J. G., Eisenhauer, E., & Mirimanoff, R. O. (2005). Radiotherapy plus concomitant and adjuvant temozolomide for glioblastoma. *The New England Journal of Medicine*, *352*(10), 987–996. DOI: 10.1056/NEJMoa043330 PMID: 15758009

Stupp, R., & Weller, M. (2014). Questions regarding the optimal use of bevacizumab in glioblastoma: A moving target. *Neuro-Oncology*, *16*(6), 765–767. DOI: 10.1093/neuonc/nou092 PMID: 24826844

Suarez-Meade, P., Marenco-Hillembrand, L., Prevatt, C., Murguia-Fuentes, R., Mohamed, A., Alsaeed, T., Ghaith, A. K., Sabsevitz, D. S., Sherman, W. J., Quinones-Hinojosa, A., & Chaichana, K. L. (2020). Awake vs. asleep motor mapping for glioma resection: A systematic review and meta-analysis. *Acta Neurochirurgica*, *162*(7), 1709–1720. DOI: 10.1007/s00701-020-04357-y PMID: 32388682

Tamura, R., Tanaka, T., Miyake, K., Yoshida, K., & Sasaki, H. (2017). Bevacizumab for malignant gliomas: Current indications, mechanisms of action and resistance, and markers of response. *Brain Tumor Pathology*, *34*(2), 62–77. DOI: 10.1007/s10014-017-0284-x PMID: 28386777

. Targeted therapies for glioblastoma treatment. (2023). *Journal of Physiology and Pharmacology, 74*(3). DOI: 10.26402/jpp.2023.3.01

Thanh, H. D., Lee, S., Nguyen, T. T., Huu, T. N., Ahn, E. J., Cho, S. H., Kim, H. S., Moon, K.-S., & Jung, C. (2024). Temozolomide promotes matrix metalloproteinase 9 expression through p38 MAPK and JNK pathways in glioblastoma cells. *Scientific Reports*, *14*(1), 14341. Advance online publication. DOI: 10.1038/s41598-024-65398-2 PMID: 38906916

Wright, J., Chugh, J., Wright, C. H., Alonso, F., Hdeib, A., Gittleman, H., Barnholtz-Sloan, J. S., & Sloan, A. E. (2016). Laser interstitial thermal therapy followed by minimal-access transsulcal resection for the treatment of large and difficult to access brain tumors. *Neurosurgical Focus*, *41*(4), E14. Advance online publication. DOI: 10.3171/2016.8.FOCUS16233 PMID: 27690658

Yan, K. (2024). The role of cancer stem cells in glioblastoma treatment: New strategies for targeted therapy. *Translational Materials Research in Biotechnology and Life Sciences*, *7*, 248–253. DOI: 10.62051/7tjwpt29

Yang, M., Oh, I. Y., Mahanty, A., Jin, W. L., & Yoo, J. S. (2020). Immunotherapy for glioblastoma: Current state, challenges, and future perspectives. *Cancers (Basel)*, *12*(9), 2334. Advance online publication. DOI: 10.3390/cancers12092334 PMID: 32824974

Yang, Z., Wei, D., Dai, X., Stevens, M. F., Bradshaw, T. D., Luo, Y., & Zhang, J. (2019). C8-substituted imidazotetrazine analogs overcome temozolomide resistance by inducing DNA adducts and DNA damage. *Frontiers in Oncology*, *9*, 485. Advance online publication. DOI: 10.3389/fonc.2019.00485 PMID: 31263673

Yekula, A., Taylor, A., Beecroft, A., Kang, K. M., Small, J. L., Muralidharan, K., & Carter, B. S. (2021). The role of extracellular vesicles in acquisition of resistance to therapy in glioblastomas. *Cancer Drug Resistance (Alhambra, Calif.)*, *4*(1), 1–16. DOI: 10.20517/cdr.2020.94 PMID: 35582008

Yuan, B., Wang, G., Tang, X., Tong, A., & Zhou, L. (2022). Immunotherapy of glioblastoma: Recent advances and future prospects. *Human Vaccines & Immunotherapeutics*, *18*(5), 2055417. Advance online publication. DOI: 10.1080/21645515.2022.2055417 PMID: 35344682

Yuan, Z., Guo, M., Zhang, Y., Deng, Y., Sun, B., Hou, Y., Wang, Y., Jin, X., Liu, Y., Shi, B., & Yin, J. (2025). MAGL targeted PROTAC degrader simultaneously enhances P53 for synergistic treatment of glioblastoma stem cell. *Cell Death Discovery*, *11*(1), 109. Advance online publication. DOI: 10.1038/s41420-025-02392-1 PMID: 40113745

Zaffino, P., Moccia, S., De Momi, E., & Spadea, M. F. (2020). A review on advances in intra-operative imaging for surgery and therapy: Imagining the operating room of the future. *Annals of Biomedical Engineering*, *48*(8), 2171–2191. DOI: 10.1007/s10439-020-02553-6 PMID: 32601951

Zhao, W., Zhou, L., Zhao, W., Yang, H., Lu, Z., Zhang, L., & Liu, Y. (2024). The combination of temozolomide and perifosine synergistically inhibit glioblastoma by impeding DNA repair and inducing apoptosis. *Cell Death Discovery*, *10*(1), 1–11. DOI: 10.1038/s41420-024-02085-1 PMID: 38977680

Chapter 5
Resistance Mechanism of Chemotherapeutic Agents Using Nanotheranostic Approach

Saloni Sharma
https://orcid.org/0009-0004-1826-8029
JSS College of Pharmacy, India

Gowthamarajan Kuppusamy
JSS College of Pharmacy, India

Divya Suresh
JSS Academy of Higher Education and Research, India

Madhusudan Purohit
Mahayogi Gorakhnath University, India

Veera Venkata Satyanarayana Reddy Karri
JSS College of Pharmacy, India

Kalaiselvi Asaithambi
JSS School of Life Sciences, India

Krishnaveni Nagappan
JSS College of Pharmacy, India

ABSTRACT

According to WHO, it is known as grade IV stage of malignancies due to its aggressiveness, rapid prognosis and poor survival of about 12-15 months after therapies like neurosurgery, chemotherapy, and radiotherapy. In traditional therapies the major side effects are toxicity profiles at tumor region, wide-spread diseased state around the healthy tissues, drug accumulation at the tumor site thus decreasing the bio-availability of the drug, rupture of blood brain barrier thus altering the brain functions and increasing the EPR effect harming the non-tumorous tissue as well.

DOI: 10.4018/979-8-3373-2695-5.ch005

To overcome the limitations nanothernostics provides a way to improve the efficacy of glioblastoma.heranostic moieties have the potential to act as dual properties therapeutic tool and to carry out diagnosis which are in the form of nano-particles, exosomes, dendrimers and other nanostructured moities act as diagnostic, magnetic and contrasting agents that triggers drug release for better treatment options.

1. INTRODUCTION

Glioblastoma was initially described in the late 19th century by Rudolf Virchow, a pioneer of modern pathology, who categorized gliomas corresponding to their cellular origins. The most common and aggressive type of carcinogenic brain tumor in adults is GBM, which is additionally referred to as GBM multiform. The World Health Organization has classified it as a Grade IV astrocytoma because of its extremely dangerous nature.

With a dreadful prognosis and a limited survival of only 12 to 15 months after diagnosis, GBM continues to be one of the most difficult malignancies to cure, even with advances in medical treatment such as neurosurgical methods, radiotherapy, and chemotherapy (Ostrom QT, et al., 2015).This stress affects protein homeostasis, triggering the unfolded protein response (UPR), a fundamental biological mechanism that restores balance and promotes cell survival (Clarke HJ, et al., 2014). This can interfere with the brain's regular function. A brain tumor can damage several psychological processes, including thought, memory, emotion, movement, vision, hearing, and touch. Swelling and fluid buildup in the brain can impair brain function, resulting in a variety of symptoms usually linked with GBM (Lim M, et al.,2018). The most common symptoms are persistent headaches, which are generally more severe in the morning, as well as nausea and vomiting. Patients may also develop memory loss, seizures, and significant changes in personality, personality traits, and ability to focus.

1.1 Incidence and Epidemiology

GBM accounts for approximately 15% of all primary brain tumors and 45-50% of all malignant brain tumors. The annual incidence varies between different populations and geographic locations and is estimated to be 3–4 cases per 100,000 population in the United States and Europe (Louis, et al. 2016).

Over the past two decades, there has been a noticeable rise in the number of diagnosed cases. This increase can be attributed to improved diagnostic techniques and greater awareness, particularly in detecting tumors in the frontal and temporal lobes. The distribution of GBM across brain regions is consistent with findings from studies such as (Ostrom QT et al. 2020).

1.1.1 Key Molecular Features of GBM

1. EGFR amplification, found in around 50 percent of GBM patients, promotes the proliferation of cells and malignant invasion.
2. TP53 mutations disrupt tumor suppression, generating uncontrolled cell proliferation.
3. PTEN loss leads to activation of the PI3K/AKT/mTOR pathway, which is a critical driver of the development of tumors.
4. VEGF expression: GBM tumors use Vascular Endothelial Growth Factor to form inappropriate blood vessels, which facilitates fast growth (Bohn et al., 2018).

1.1.2 Key Epidemiological Trends

GBM is more prevalent in men than in women ratio of 1.6:1. The chance of GBM rises with age, particularly those aged 60 to 75; it can also afflict younger individuals. GBM penetration is greater in industrialized countries, which could be attributable to the widespread application of modern imaging tools for diagnosis and probable carcinogen exposure in the environment. The GBM incidence by region is listed in Table 1.

Table 1. GBM Incidence by Region:

Region	Incidence (per 100,000)	Age group most affected	Gender Ratio(M:F)
North America	3.5-4.2	60-75 years	6:1
Europe	2.5-3.2	55-75 years	5:1
Asia	2.5-3.2	50-70 years	7:1
Africa	1.5-2.0	50-70 years	3:1

The GBM incidence by age is listed in table 2.

Table 2. Incidence of GBM by Age Group and its Rate

Age Group (Years)	Incidence Rate (per 100,000)
20-34	0.5
35-44	1.5
45-54	3.0
55-64	6.0
65-74	10.0
75+	12.0

1.1.3 Risk Factors

1. **Genetic predisposition**: Individuals with inherited syndromes have an increased risk of developing GBM due to mutations in tumor suppressor genes like **TP53** mismatch repair genes (Verhaak RGW et al.,2010)
2. **High-dose radiation exposure**, particularly in those who have undergone **cranial radiotherapy** for other conditions during childhood, has been correlated with increased GBM risk (Bondy ML et al., 2008).
3. **Environmental factors**: Long-term exposure to environmental contaminants such as **pesticides**, **heavy metals**, and **industrial solvents** may promote gliomagenesis through genotoxic and epigenetic mechanisms, though definitive causality is still under investigation (Sadetzki S, et al.,2005).
4. **Cell phone use**: Prolonged exposure to **radio-frequency electromagnetic fields** has raised concerns about its link to brain tumors. However, studies remain **inconclusive** and controversial, with organizations like the IARC classifying RF fields as.
5. **Immune system dysfunction**: Individuals with **immunosuppression**, such as **HIV-positive patients** or **organ transplant recipients**, exhibit a higher incidence of primary CNS lymphomas and possibly gliomas, suggesting immune surveillance plays a role in tumor suppression (Wrensch M et al., 2002).

1.1.4 Challenges in Treatment

GBM treatment requires a **multimodal strategy** involving **surgery**, **radiotherapy**, and **chemotherapy**. Despite aggressive treatment regimens, **patient outcomes remain dismal**, with a **median survival** of 12–15 months and a **5-year survival rate** of less than 5% (Engels E A et al., 2005).

- **Tumor heterogeneity**: It comprises of subclones within a single tumor, which **respond differently** to treatments and evolve rapidly, rendering targeted therapies less effective (Stupp R, et al. 2005).
- **Blood-brain barrier**: The BBB prevents many therapeutic agents from effectively reaching the tumor site, limiting the efficacy of systemic chemotherapy.
- **Therapeutic resistance**: GBM rapidly develops **resistance** to both **temozolomide** and radiation therapy through DNA repair mechanisms, metabolic rewiring, and activation of pro-survival pathways.
- **Immuno-suppressive micro-environment**: GBM creates a highly **immunosuppressive** milieu, inhibiting T-cell infiltration and impairing immune responses, which severely limits the success of immuno-therapies such as checkpoint inhibitors (Aldape K et al., 2015). **Figure 1 Shows the Current Challenges towards the treatment of GBM.**

Figure 1. Shows the Current Challenges towards the treatment of GBM.

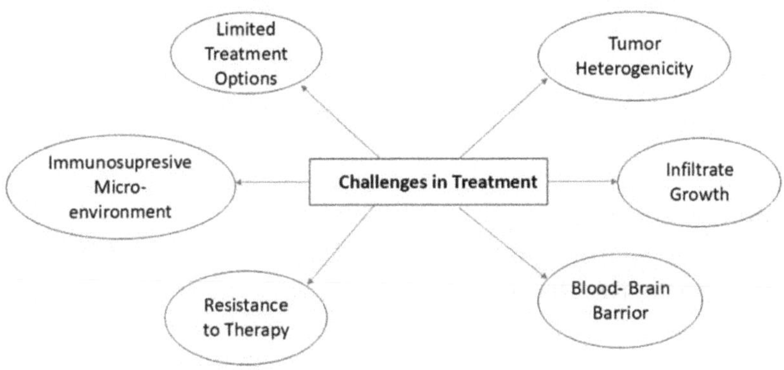
Limited Treatment Options
Tumor Heterogenicity
Immunosupresive Micro-environment
Challenges in Treatment
Infiltrate Growth
Resistance to Therapy
Blood- Brain Barrior

1.1.5 Tumour Heterogeneity

GBM is exceptionally diverse on both the cellular and molecular levels linked to treatment resistance and tumor recurrence. Sub-populations of tumor cells with different genetic and genomic characteristics might resist typical medicines, making long-term management challenging (Giese, A., et al.,2003).

1.1.6 Infiltrative Growth

GBM cells invade the surrounding brain tissue, making total surgical excision extremely difficult. Even with modern imaging tools, it is difficult to identify tumor margins from healthy brain tissue, resulting in remaining tumor cells that can regenerate (Pardridge, W. M. 2012).

1.1.7 The Blood-Brain Barrier (BBB)

The blood-brain barrier restricts the ability of numerous therapeutic medicines to enter the brain. While the BBB protects the brain from potentially toxic substances, it also limits the penetration of chemotherapy treatments and targeted therapies, minimizing their efficacy (Hegi, M. E., et al.,2005).

1.1.8 Resistance to Therapy

GBM frequently develops resistance to traditional treatments, particularly temozolomide (TMZ), the principal chemotherapeutic medication used for GBM. Resistance mechanisms include the production of O6-methylguanine-DNA methyltransferase, a DNA repair enzyme that decreases the effects of TMZ (Hambardzumyan, D., et al., 2016).

1.1.9 Immunosuppressive Microenvironment

Tumor-associated macrophages, regulatory T cells, and other immune-suppressive contaminants prevent immune-mediated tumor elimination (Stupp, R., et al., 2005). Limited Treatment is due to the therapy choices for GBM are limited. Novel techniques such as immunotherapy, targeted therapy, and gene therapy are being studied, but they have yet to demonstrate meaningful therapeutic advantages (Blanco, E., et al.,2015).

1.2 Rationale for Nanotheranostics

Nanoparticles, for example, can be loaded with contrast agents (such as gadolinium, iron oxide, or quantum dots) for use in imaging modalities such as MRI, CT, or fluorescence imaging. Nanotheranostic systems can be programmed to release therapeutic drugs in response to specific stimuli like pH, temperature, or enzyme activity, which are frequently altered in the tumor micro-environment (Kelkar S et al.,2011).

Traditional treatments can result in severe adverse effects due to their general nature. Nanotheranostics can improve early detection of GBM by using highly sensitive imaging agents that can detect even small or diffuse tumors. Initial identification is crucial for improving survival chances. The GBM treatment challenges and their strategies are listed in Table 3.

Table 3. Challenges towards GBM treatment and their strategy to overcome GBM.

Challenges	How Nanotheranostics Addresses It
Blood-brain barrier restriction	Nanoparticles engineered to cross or bypass the BBB, enabling targeted drug delivery.
Tumor heterogeneity	Co-delivery of multiple therapeutic agents to address diverse cell populations within the tumor.
Non-specific toxicity	Ligand-functionalized nanoparticles for targeting, reducing damage to healthy tissue.
Limited real-time monitoring	Integrated imaging agents allow for real-time tracking of tumor progression and treatment response.
Resistance to single-agent therapies	Combination therapies via nanoparticles overcome resistance mechanisms.

Nanotheranostics eliminates several of the issues connected with GBM treatment & (Cheng Y et al., 2014). Additionally, **nanotheranostic applications can be supplied with targeting ligands** that bind precisely to overexpressed receptors on GBM cells, improving accuracy and decreasing off-target effects (Yu Y et al., 2019). The diagnostic component of nanotheranostics, which normally takes place via imaging agents such as gadolinium or iron oxide, enables real-time monitoring of tumor development and therapy response (Mura S et al .,2013). Another significant advantage of nanotheranostics is its potential for early detection. This focused strategy not only increases therapeutic efficacy but also decreases the severe side effects associated with traditional medications, thereby improving patients' quality of life (Mahmoudi, M., et al. 2011).

1.2.1 Nanotheranostics System

Mechanism of action of Nanotheranostics towards the treatment of GBM is shown in Figure 2.

Figure 2. Shows the Mechanism of action of Nanotheranostics towards the treatment of GBM.

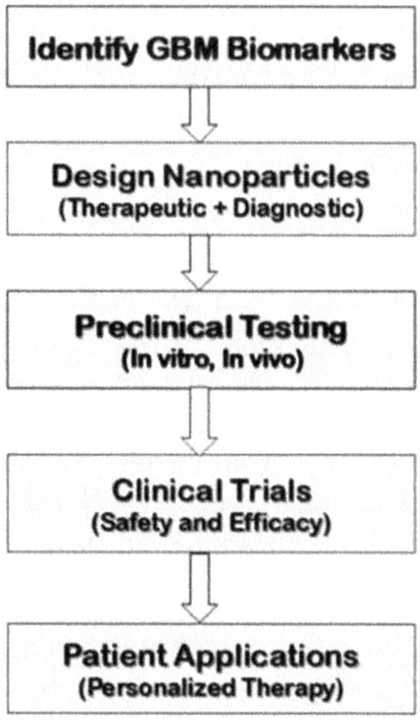

Nanotheranostics is a revolutionary technique that combines accuracy, multi-functionality, and personalization to transcend the constraints of conventional therapies (Ventola, C. L. 2017). Nanotheranostics has the potential to enhance survival rates and quality of life providing targeted drug administration, real-time monitoring, combination therapy (Tan A C et al., 2020). However, additional research and clinical trials are required to fully realize its potential and solve challenges like bio-compatibility, scalability, and approval from regulatory bodies (Blanco E et al.,2015).

Nanoparticle Platforms for Glioblastoma: Liposomes are bi-layered nano-structures that comprise an aqueous core surrounded by a uni/multi lamellar vesicle that are very bio-compatible and are highly efficient for it's bio-degradability.

The development of functionalized ligands to combat brain cancers are promoted by nanotechnology receptor-mediated transcytosis. To accomplish the intended cellular uptake, liposomes must attach to the specific ligand. For example, the GBM (U-87) cells effectively absorbed cobalt porphyrin phospholipid liposomes because polyhistidine (his)-tagged RGD peptides bonded to the liposomes strongly. To deliver PTX and survivin siRNA against glioblastoma and glioma stem cells (angiopep-2 and A15)-modified cationic liposomes were created (Maeda H., et al. 2000).

Glioblastoma-expressed $\alpha v\beta 3$ integrins have been effectively targeted by paclitaxel-loaded liposomes conjugated with the transferrin receptor and RGD peptide (Danheir. F et al 2016). Integrin receptor ligands and dipeptide ligands of nicotinic acetylcholine receptors were used to create DOX-loaded liposomes. These ligands' extended blood circulation durations effectively improved the liposomes' capacity to target glioblastoma. Because of their short peptide sequence and cyclization, c(RGDyK) ligands demonstrated exceptional stability toward the liposomes, while CDX ligands have demonstrated preferred binding potential with nAChRs (Smolen J.S., et al.,2019). This enhances the liposome NPs' specific accumulation in brain malignancies. Hydrophilic and hydrophobic components were adequately loaded into this system, and sustainable distribution was accomplished by using PEM. By conjugating GBM-cell-specific peptides and antibodies to the liposomes, co-loaded with SPIONs and DOX (Liu, H., et al. 2021). This made it more difficult for U-87 cells to pass across the BBB and allowed for increased cellular absorption. Additionally, the significantly expressed biomarker for glioblastoma was TN-C, which, in conjunction with DOX, effectively inhibited cell proliferation (Ferrara & Kerbel,2018).

Chemotherapeutic drugs target cell proliferation, cell division, DNA synthesis for glioblastoma dealing with tumorous cell invasion (Huang R., et al.,2021). By employing DOX as a medicinal medicine, the IB-loaded liposomes can increase survival rate of tumor rats. This shows a different approach to treat drug-resistant GBM. Researchers tested fluvoxamine, a selective serotonin re-uptake inhibitor, to stop actin polymerization and allowed it to pass through the blood-brain barrier without causing harm. Fluvoxamine and other antidepressant medications were used in the screening procedure to observe the fluorescence behavior of G-actin tagged with pyrene throughout the polymerization process. The cytosol of the mouse brain, GTP, ATP, and liposomes were combined with the reaction buffer for each medication separately. By inhibiting the focal adhesion kinase and phosphoinositide-3-kinase (PI3K) pathways, fluvoxamine also effectively reduced the invasion and cell migration of GBM and glioma stem cells (Giordano RJ., et al.,2019). Liposomes' surface enables the functionalization of polymers, antibodies, specific receptors, and enzymes, that promote prolonged blood circulation and facilitate brain delivery. These functionalized liposomes' appropriate shape and hydrophilicity allow them to pass the blood-brain barrier, particularly in glioblastoma (Oh JH et al.,2020).

Astrocytes and microglia were also used to examine the toxicity performance of these NPs; these cells did not exhibit substantial toxicity. By inhibiting the overexpressed CD44 markers in GBM cells this demonstrates the appropriate effectiveness of these NPs against GBM cells. In comparison to DOX-loaded liposomes, the combination of DOX-loaded liposomes with tumor necrosis factor can enhance the superior apoptotic outcomes. Targeting the death receptor 5 (DR5) in glioma cells, DOX-loaded liposomes and tumor necrosis factor-related apoptosis-inducing ligand work in concert to produce this (Liu H et al.,2021).

2. NANOPARTICLE COMPOSITION

2.1 Metal-Based Nanoparticles

This therapeutic method can reduce the tumor barrier surrounding the cell and improve the drug release characteristics at the tumor micro-environment, thus passing through the blood-brain barrier at elevated temperatures about 40oC with the generation of HSP proteins to the healthy tissues.

One such application of gold nano-structures is gold nano-rods with good bio-compatibility properties, better surface functionalization. For better ability to target cells, cell specificity, and effective interaction with the tumor cells. Similar to this, silver nano-structures render robust plasmonic properties, Raman scattering of the metallic ions upon binding with integrins, ligands, and receptors against glioma cells. To irradicate this issue, metal-based NPs with a specific target using gold-based materials render excellent electrical and optical properties (MC Mohan SA et al.,2021)..

2.2. Magnetic Nanoparticles

The SPIONs are noted for their best MRI properties suited as contrasting agents for imaging and specific targeting applications (Xu L et al. 2020). This behavior is attributed to the super-paramagnetic susceptibility that can magnetize the nanoparticle with an external magnetic field (Atkinson AP et al.,2018). Moreover, for effective brain permeability by the SPIONs, the physicochemical parameters like particle size, surface modifiers charges, and lipophilicity of the SPIONs are to be to be adjusted based on the target specificity (Lathia JD et al. 2015).

Such a type of polymeric nano-particles is used for theranostic applications (Cheng L et al.,2021). Different studies have been performed to illustrate the SPIONs mechanism, such as lipo-protein receptor-mediated GBM particles in the form of SPIONs successfully passed through the BBB (Son MJ et al.,2009). The T1 weighed positive charge that resulted in a nano size of 3.6nm, which led to positive application of MR imaging of GBM cells before and after surgery. PEGylation technique helped to improve the colloidal stability leading to a covalent reaction between angio-pep-2 and SPIONs that, in turn, can rotate using the AMF, resulting in the conversion of kinetic energy into heat while reaching the surface of tumorous cells, finally reaching high temperatures of 46 oC. SPIONs can also target specific tumorous cells via cellular apoptosis mechanisms without affecting the non-tumorous cells (Anido et al. 2010). T1 weighed positive charge that resulted in a nano size of 3.6nm, which lead to positive application of MR imaging of GBM cells before and after surgery.

(Giordano RJ., et al.,2001). Surface functionalized the paramagnetic iron oxide particles in the form of nano-rods polymeric coating of poly-ethylene-imine loaded with "carnosine. As a result, the mechanism used by SPIONs for the relaxation of T2 improves the quality of contrast. The dual therapy based on magnetic targeting and chemotherapy was used in this study to target GBM cells. Furthermore, the temperatures inside the GBM cells were examined in response to the introduction of an alternating magnetic field using the temperature-responsive lipophilic fluorescent label, also known as dye 1,10-dioctadecyl-3,3,30,30-tetramethyl-indocarbocyanine-perchlorate (Eyler & Rich, 2008). By preventing their agglomeration, the used-lipid matrix may enclose SPIONs, enable temperature-dependent TMZ release, and give the SPIONs exceptional stability. Ultra-small SPIONs are preferentially superior to gadolinium-based contrasting agents in brain malignancies as MRI contrasting agents because they have longer circulation durations and less kidney damage. These SPIONs exhibit improved cellular absorption by the microglia, or phagocytes, located within tumor borders. Fluorescent molecules and MNPs have already been linked in several papers to improve tumor imaging and resection capabilities. In the past, brain tumors could be detected with iron oxide nanoparticles treated with NRI fluorescent chemicals like Cy5.5, which also had great tumor removal rates (Gallo M et al., 2015). Therefore, in GBM, chlorotoxin-modified MNPs function as dual MRI contrasting agents and possible tumor inhibitors (Sancho P et al.,2016). The other peptide, F3, has the ability to attach to endothelial cell nucleolin and prevent GBM cell growth (Pourmasoumi, P., et al., 2024).

These nanoparticles improve the curcumin's medicinal efficacy by releasing 70% of its content in 72 hours and heating it to roughly 43 °C in 15 minutes. The GRGDS peptide showed excellent against GBM by six times (Akshari A et al., 2022). When loaded with DOX, the other polymer-based PEG/PEI/polysorbate80 (Ps 80)-SPIONs showed better glioma suppression in the presence of a magnetic field (Argon Sanabria V et al.,2022).. While the DOX was employed as a cytotoxic medication driven by SPIONs, polymers in this investigation assisted in extending blood circulation periods and bio-compatibility. Once more, the caspase-3 route was used by these polymer-functionalized SPIONs to cause glioma cells to undergo apoptosis (Kim, K., et al., 2020). This was accomplished by conjugating SPIONs with TfR, which showed increased cellular uptake and internalization. These SPIONs were then used as MRI contrast agents since they preferentially pierced the blood-brain barrier (Kostka, K., et al., 2024).

2.3. Polymer-Based Nanoparticles

Certain polymers that show the desired properties are chitosan, cellulose, poly-lactyl glycolic acid, poly-ethylene glycol, which can cross the blood-brain barrier through mechanisms like i. carrier drug delivery systems, receptor mediated systems iii. adsorption transcytosis process (Jaiswal S et al., 2022). In this case, high biodegradable polymeric nano-particles to deliver the DNA-infused drug conjugates into the brain glial cells using poly beta amino esters that show excellent stability and bio-compatibility towards treating the recurrence of GBM (Sharma M et al.,2023). As a result, polymeric nanoparticles can target these transporters to be cell-specific on the glial cells by effective binding of paclitaxel and taxol to improve the anti-cancer activity on the glial cells by efficiently passing through the blood-brain barrier by increasing the expression of the receptors (Song H et al., 2021).

3. TARGETING STRATEGIES FOR GLIOBLASTOMA

GBM chemotherapy treatments aim to capitalize on certain cellular and molecular abnormalities in the tumor micro-environment, such as immune evasion mechanisms, metabolic alterations, and dysregulated signaling pathways. These techniques include gene therapy, immuno-therapy, precision medicine procedures, and nanotechnology-based drug delivery systems. By focusing on GBM's particular biological features, researchers hope to improve medication effectiveness, reduce off-target consequences, and ultimately improve patient survival. The goal is to provide a detailed explanation of the current state of research and how it could help to solve the unmet needs of GBM patients, which range from molecularly targeted medications to emerging immuno-therapies.

3.1. Passive Targeting

Passive targeting is an increasingly prevalent strategy in drug delivery systems developed to encourage the accumulation of therapeutic agents—such as nucleic acids, chemotherapeutic drugs, or imaging agents—in tumor tissues, especially GBM (He Y et al., 2020). Passive targeting leverages the unique physiological and pathological features of tumors to improve medication delivery efficacy, in contrast to active targeting, which relies on molecular recognition.

This approach is particularly relevant in cases of GBM, a highly vascularized and aggressive brain tumor, where the complex environment of the tumor and the blood-brain barrier often lead to the failure of traditional drug delivery methods (Xu Z et al., 2022).

3.1.1. Physiological and Pathological Basis of Passive Targeting

3.1.1.1. Enhanced Permeability and Retention (EPR) Effect:

- **Leaky Vasculature**: Abnormal and unstable blood vessels with large fenestrations between endothelial cells are characteristic of tumors like GBM. These structural abnormalities increase vascular permeability, allowing macro-molecules and nanoparticles to accumulate in tumor tissue more effectively (Zhang Y et al., 2021).
- **Defective Lymphatic Drainage**: Tumors often lack functional lymphatic systems, which hinders the clearance of therapeutic nanoparticles, increasing local drug concentration and enhancing therapeutic outcomes (Smith A et al., 2023).

3.1.1.2. Tumor Micro-environment:

- A dense extracellular matrix and rapid tumor growth contribute to elevated interstitial pressure, which can hinder intra-tumoral drug distribution. However, the EPR effect still facilitates the initial accumulation of drugs at the tumor periphery (Chen W et al., 2021).
- The tumor micro-environment's hypoxia and acidic pH can be exploited for stimuli-responsive drug delivery, triggering site-specific drug release and enhancing therapeutic selectivity (Li H et al.,2022).

Because of its essential simplicity and efficacy, passive targeting is a frequently used drug delivery approach in GBM and other solid tumors (Smith, A. J., & Kumar, P., 2023). Unlike active targeting, passive targeting avoids complex conjugation steps like ligand attachment, streamlining development and scaling for clinical application (Thomas S.S et al. 2021).

Moreover, passive targeting is versatile, accommodating diverse therapeutic agents including small molecules, proteins, nucleic acids, and diagnostic imaging agents (Zhang M et al., 2021). Passive targeting also takes advantage of the EPR effect, leading to preferential accumulation of drugs in tumor tissue and minimizing delivery to healthy organs. This increased selectivity reduces systemic toxicity and enhances the therapeutic index, improving patient outcomes and minimizing side effects associated with conventional chemotherapy (Liu X et al., 2023).

3.2 Active Targeting

3.2.1 Mechanism of Active Targeting in GBM

1. **Target Identification: Biomarkers Over-expressed in GBM**
   - **EGFRS:** Mutated or amplified in ~50% of GBM cases (Liu, X., et al. 2023).
   - **EGFRvIII:** A truncated, constitutively active form of EGFR found in ~20-30% of GBM patients (Xie, J., et al. 2021).
   - **VEGF:** Promotes angiogenesis and is highly expressed in GBM (Yoon, S., et al., 2022).
   - **PDGFR (Platelet-Derived Growth Factor Receptor):** Overexpressed in some GBM subtypes (Wang, Y., et al. 2021).
   - **Integrins (e.g., αvβ3):** Involved in tumor cell adhesion, migration, and angiogenesis (Li, L., et al. 2022).
   - **Transferrin Receptors:** Overexpressed in rapidly dividing GBM cells due to their high iron demand (Smith CJ., et al. 2024).
   - **CD133:** A marker of GBM stem cells (Liu G., et al. 2025).
2. **Ligands for Active Targeting**
   - Monoclonal antibodies like cetuximab or bevacizumab (Chen X., et al. 2025).
   - Short amino acid sequences like RGD peptides (Patel, R., et al. 2025).
   - Single-stranded DNA or RNA molecules designed to bind specific targets (e.g., AS1411 aptamer targets nucleolin) (Zhu Z., et al. 2020).
   - Folic acid, transferrin (Ratliff.M, et al. 2022).
3. **Drug Delivery Systems**
   - **Nanoparticles:** Lipid-based, polymeric, or metallic nanoparticles can encapsulate drugs and be functionalized with ligands (Yin Y., et al. 2005).
   - **Liposomes:** Spherical vesicles with lipid bi-layers used to deliver chemotherapeutic agents like dox (Xu X., et al. 2021).
   - **Exosomes:** Natural vesicles derived from cells that can cross the blood-brain barrier (Vaz-Salgado MA, et al., 2023).
   - **Viral Vectors:** Engineered viruses for gene therapy (Hailozian C et al., 2022).
   - **Micelles:** Self-assembling amphiphilic molecules that encapsulate hydrophobic drugs (Zheng X, et al., 2017).
4. **Challenges in Drug Delivery**
   - **Blood-Brain Barrier (BBB):** The BBB prevents most drugs from reaching the brain. Active targeting strategies must overcome this barri-

er using techniques like receptor-mediated transcytosis (Calixto GM, et al., 2016).

- **Tumor Heterogeneity:** GBM is highly heterogeneous, meaning different cells within the tumor may express different biomarkers (Meyers JD et al., 2015).
- **Immune Evasion:** GBM cells can evade immune detection, making immunotherapies less effective (Cheng X et al., 2017).

3.2.2 Examples of Active Targeting Strategies in GBM

1. EGFR-Targeted Therapy
    - **Cetuximab-Nanoparticle Conjugates:** Cetuximab is conjugated to nanoparticles loaded with chemotherapeutic agents like temozolomide. This ensures targeted delivery to EGFR-overexpressing GBM cells.
    - **EGFRvIII-Specific CAR-T Cells:** Chimeric antigen receptor T cells engineered to target the EGFRvIII mutation have shown promise in clinical trials (Hu H et al., 2018).
2. Angiogenesis Inhibition
    - **Bevacizumab:** A monoclonal antibody targeting VEGF, approved for recurrent GBM. Bev. inhibits angiogenesis but has limited efficacy as a monotherapy due to resistance mechanisms.
    - **RGD Peptide-Conjugated Nanoparticles:** RGD peptides target integrins on endothelial cells involved in angiogenesis, delivering anti-angiogenic drugs directly to tumor blood vessels.
3. GBM Stem Cell Targeting
    - **CD133-Targeted Nanoparticles:** CD133 is a marker of glioblastoma stem cells, which are resistant to conventional therapies. Nanoparticles functionalized with anti-CD133 antibodies can deliver drugs specifically to GSCs.
    - **Wnt/β-Catenin Pathway Inhibitors:** GSCs rely on the Wnt signaling pathway for survival. Targeted inhibitors delivered via nanoparticles are being explored.
4. Transferrin Receptor Targeting
    - **Transferrin-Conjugated Liposomes:** Transferrin receptors are overexpressed in GBM cells. Liposomes conjugated with transferrin can cross the BBB and deliver drugs like doxorubicin to tumor cells (Farouk M et al., 2023).
5. Chlorotoxin-Based Targeting
    - **TM-601:** A peptide derived from scorpion venom that binds to matrix metalloproteinases overexpressed in GBM. TM-601-conjugated

nanoparticles or imaging agents can target GBM cells for therapy or diagnosis (Singh.S et al 2025).

3.2.3 Advantages of Active Targeting:

- High specificity for tumor cells, reducing damage to healthy tissues.
- Can overcome limitations of the EPR effect by directly binding to tumor cells
- Potential for personalized medicine by targeting patient-specific biomarkers (Lu VM et al., 2018).

3.3 Cell-Specific Targeting

This strategy is particularly important due to the tumor's heterogeneity and the presence of treatment-resistant cell types, such as GBM stem cells, sub-population of cells within GBM that exhibit stem-like properties, including self-renewal, differentiation potential, and resistance to conventional therapies (Zhang XQ et al., 2018).

3.3.1 Targeting Glioblastoma Stem Cells

GBM stem cells are a major therapeutic challenge due to their ability to survive standard treatments and repopulate the tumor. Several strategies have been developed to specifically target GSCs:

a. Surface Marker Targeting
    - **CD133:** A well-known marker of GSCs. Antibodies or ligands targeting CD133 can be used to deliver drugs or nanoparticles specifically to GSCs.
    - **CD44:** A receptor involved in cell adhesion and migration. CD44-targeted therapies are being explored to disrupt GSC maintenance.
    - **Integrins:** Over-expressed in GSCs, integrins can be targeted with peptides or antibodies to inhibit their function. Example: Nanoparticles conjugated with anti-CD133 antibodies can selectively deliver chemotherapeutic agents to GSCs.

b. Signaling Pathway Inhibition
    - **Notch Pathway:** Inhibitors like gamma-secretase inhibitors can disrupt Notch signaling, which is critical for GSC maintenance.
    - **Wnt/β-Catenin Pathway:** Small-molecule inhibitors or antibodies targeting this pathway can suppress GSC proliferation.
    - **Hedgehog Pathway:** Inhibitors like vismodegib can block Hedgehog signaling, which is often dysregulated in GSCs.

- Example: Clinical trials are investigating the use of Notch inhibitors in combination with standard therapies for GBM (Arce C et al., 2021).

c. Epigenetic Modulation
   - **Histone Deacetylase Inhibitors:** Drugs like vorinostat can alter gene expression in GSCs, reducing their stemnes .
   - **DNA Methyltransferase Inhibitors:** Agents like decitabine can reverse hypermethylation of tumor suppressor genes in GSCs.
   - **HDAC inhibitors** are being tested in pre-clinical models to sensitize GSCs to radiation and chemotherapy (Chen R et al., 2018).

d. Metabolic Targeting
   - **Glycolysis Inhibitors:** Drugs like 2-deoxy-D-glucose can disrupt energy production in GSCs.
   - **Oxidative Phosphorylation Inhibitors:** Agents like metformin can target mitochondrial metabolism in GSCs.
   - **Example:** Metformin has shown promise in preclinical studies for reducing GSC viability (Wu Z et al., 2024).

4. THERAPEUTIC APPROACHES FOR GBM

Emerging approaches include targeted molecular therapies, immuno-therapy, gene therapy, and nano-medicine-based drug delivery systems. Repurposing FDA-approved drugs and combining multiple treatment modalities have shown potential in improving patient outcomes. Current chemotherapy faces problems like lack of specificity, cyto-toxicity, short half-life, poor solubility, multi-drug resistance, and stem-like cell growth. To overcome these disadvantages, nanomaterial-based chemotherapy, targeted therapy, molecular therapy, photo-dynamic therapy, photo-thermal therapy, chemo-dynamic therapy, and sono-dynamic therapy are being used in cancer treatment. A substantial number of studies on a variety of therapies such as molecular therapy, apoptosis regulation, immunotherapy, signal modification therapy, nucleic-acid-based therapy, and anti-angiogenesis therapy for the treatment of cancer have been conducted in recent years. With the advent of nanotechnology, nano-medicines used in cancer therapy can potentially reduce the drawbacks extensive research has been ongoing in this direction (Clarke J et al., 2010).

4.1 Chemotherapy

These drugs work by interfering with cell division, damaging DNA, blocking essential metabolic pathways, leading to tumor shrinkage or slowed progression. Unlike surgery or radiation, which target specific areas, chemotherapy is systemic—it travels through the bloodstream to reach cancer cells anywhere in the body. While effective against many cancers, it also affects healthy fast-growing cells, causing side effects like fatigue, nausea, and immunosuppression (Zanders FD et al., 2019).

The primary chemotherapy agent, temozolomide, is used concurrently with radiotherapy and as adjuvant therapy, particularly in patients with MGMT promoter methylation, who show better responses. For recurrent or refractory GBM, options include lomustine, bevacizumab. While not curative, chemotherapy helps extend progression-free survival and manage symptoms in this aggressive brain cancer (Szklener K et al., 2022).

4.1.2 Nanoparticle Delivery Systems for Doxorubicin in GBM

Doxorubicin, an anthracycline antibiotic, exerts its anticancer effects primarily through DNA intercalation and inhibition of topoisomerase II, resulting in apoptosis. However, its application in GBM is significantly limited due to poor blood–brain barrier penetration—less than 5% of administered DOX reaches the brain. This restricted access is further compounded by P-glycoprotein efflux mechanisms, which actively transport DOX out of GBM cells, reducing its intracellular concentration and effectiveness. Additionally, DOX is known for its cardiotoxic effects, which are dose-dependent and significantly limit its systemic usage (Ozdemir Kayanak E et al., 2018).

4.1.3 Nanoparticle-Based Chemotherapy Approaches Using Doxorubicin

1. Doxil® (pegylated liposomal DOX) encapsulate the drug in a lipid bilayer, enhancing circulation time and reducing cardiac toxicity and has demonstrated improved pharma-cokinetics and accumulation at tumor sites through the enhanced permeability and retention effect (Rahman MH et al., 2021).
2. Biodegradable carriers like PLGA are used to encapsulate DOX, allowing for controlled release and surface functionalization for targeted delivery.
3. These are highly branched macromolecules that can carry DOX via covalent bonding or encapsulation, providing precise drug loading and release profiles. Their multi-valency allows for surface modification with targeting ligands (Lim M et al., 2018).
4. DOX-loaded AuNPs not only enable targeted delivery but also have theranostic potential, as they can be combined with photo-thermal therapy for synergistic effects in GBM (Qureshi set al., 2024).

5. Typically composed of iron oxide, these nanoparticles can be guided to tumor sites using an external magnetic field, improving DOX localization and reducing systemic exposure (Li Q et al., 2025).
6. These systems release DOX in response to tumor-specific triggers such as acidic pH, elevated glutathione levels, or enzymatic activity, enabling on-site drug activation and minimizing harm to healthy tissue (Ruan W et al., 2022).

4.1.4. Nanoparticles in Gene Therapy

- Nanoparticles composed of materials such as lipids (e.g., liposomes, solid lipid nanoparticles), polymers (e.g., PLGA, chitosan), and inorganic materials (e.g., gold, silica) often exhibit lower immunogenicity and can be degraded into nontoxic byproducts in the body (Yang Q et al., 2021).
- Nanoparticles can be functionalized with targeting ligands such as antibodies, peptides, aptamers, or folic acid, which guide them specifically to diseased or cancerous cells—improving tissue specificity and reducing off-target effects (Rehman M et al., 2017).
- Nanocarriers protect genetic payloads from enzymatic degradation in circulation and enable sustained release or stimuli-responsive release, triggered by pH, enzymes, temperature, or redox conditions.
- Nanoparticles can co-deliver multiple therapeutics—such as combining siRNA with chemotherapeutic drugs—and also incorporate diagnostic imaging agents, thereby supporting theranostic applications.

4.1.5. Common Types of Nanoparticles Used in Gene Therapy

- **Lipids** are currently the most successful in clinical translation, especially for mRNA delivery, as seen in COVID-19 mRNA vaccines. LNPs encapsulate RNA, protect it from degradation, and facilitate efficient endosomal escape.
- **Polymers** such as PLGA and chitosan have shown significant promise due to their controlled degradation, low toxicity, and customizable surface properties.
- Inorganic nanoparticles: Materials like gold nanoparticles and mesoporous silica nanoparticles offer high loading capacity, thermal and optical tunability, and the potential for theranostic applications.
- Hybrid nanoparticles: These combine lipid, polymeric, and/or inorganic components to achieve enhanced stability, targeting, and multifunctionality. Gold core–lipid shell nanoparticles combine photo-thermal therapy with RNA delivery for synergistic cancer treatment (Agemy L et al., 2011).

4.1.6. RNA Interference Using Nanoparticles

The key molecules in RNAi-based therapies are small interfering RNAs and microRNAs (miRNAs), which target specific mRNA transcripts for degradation. Mechanism of RNA i Delivery via Nanoparticles

1. Encapsulation – miRNA is encapsulated or complexed within nanoparticles to protect against nuclease degradation in the bloodstream.
2. Targeted Delivery – Nanoparticles are surface-functionalized with ligands such as folate, transferrin, aptamers, or antibodies to enable receptor-mediated targeting to cancer or diseased cells.
3. Cellular Uptake – The engineered NPs are internalized via endocytosis—often through clathrin-mediated pathways.
4. Endosomal Escape – Successful RNAi requires cytoplasmic release, so nanoparticles often include pH-sensitive materials or membrane-disruptive peptides to rupture the endosome.
5. Gene Silencing – The released siRNA integrates into the RNA-induced silencing complex, which then degrades the target mRNA, blocking protein expression and achieving therapeutic gene silencing (Roque D et al., 2023).

Gene Editing Using Nanoparticles: Gene editing, particularly with CRISPR-Cas9, allows precise modifications to the genome, enabling the correction of mutations, gene knockout, or insertion of therapeutic genes. Delivering CRISPR components requires efficient carriers, and nanoparticles are a leading solution. Nanoparticles can protect the CRISPR components from degradation, enhance cellular uptake, and facilitate their precise delivery to target cells. **Figure 3 shows the gene editing using different nanoparticles.**

Figure 3. Represents the gene editing using different nanoparticles.

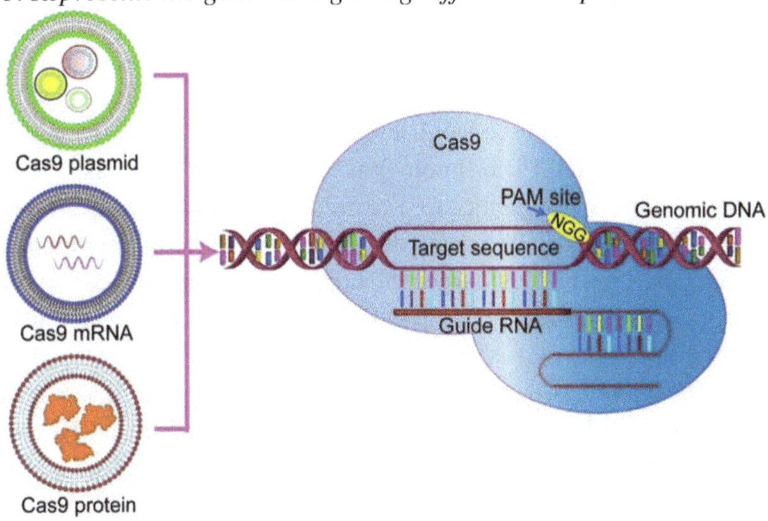

Nanoparticle-Mediated CRISPR Delivery Strategies:

Nano-particle mediated delivery of CRISPR systems is a promising strategy for gene editing, particularly in targeting specific tissues with minimal off-target effects that can be of various types like:

1. LNPs are widely used to encapsulate CRISPR mRNA and guide RNA, enabling delivery of CRISPR-Cas9 systems for gene editing. LNPs have shown success in liver-targeted therapies, such as those for transthyretin amyloidosis, by efficiently delivering CRISPR components to hepatocytes (Janidi R et al., 2020).
2. PLGA nanoparticles can co-deliver both Cas9 plasmid DNA and gRNA. These polymeric NPs are biodegradable, offer controlled release of the cargo, and are often functionalized to improve target specificity.
3. Gold nanoparticles have electrostatic properties that enable the binding of CRISPR ribo-nucleo-proteins, facilitating their delivery directly to the nucleus. This approach enhances the efficiency of gene editing by protecting the CRISPR complex from degradation and promoting intra-cellular uptake (Lansangam et al., 2024).
4. VLPs combine the delivery efficiency of viruses with the safety profile of nanoparticles as hybrid systems for CRISPR delivery because they mimic viral vectors but do not integrate into the host genome, reducing the risk of insertional mutagenesis.

Applications of CRISPR-NP Therapy

1. CRISPR-Cas9 therapy holds great potential for correcting mutations in genetic disorders such as cystic fibrosis and sickle cell anemia, offering a potential cure by repairing mutations at the DNA level.
2. In cancer therapy, CRISPR technology is used to edit T-cells, as seen in CAR-T therapy, which is being employed to enhance immune system responses to cancer. CRISPR can also be used to disrupt oncogenes to inhibit tumor growth.
3. CRISPR offers the ability to target and edit viral genomes, such as in the case of HIV provirus. This can potentially lead to cures for viral infections by permanently disabling the virus's DNA.
4. CRISPR-NP strategies can also be used in agriculture to create genetically modified crops with enhanced disease resistance, which could be a valuable tool in tackling food security issues (Chowdhury R et al., 2023).

Challenges in CRISPR-Nanoparticle Therapy

1. There is a risk of unintended DNA modifications, which could lead to mutations and undesirable effects. Strategies to reduce off-target effects are an active area of research.
2. Ensuring nanoparticles are targeted to specific tissues remains a challenge. Currently, NPs are designed with surface modifications such as antibodies or ligands to improve target specificity.
3. Ethical debates surround the use of CRISPR technology, especially in germline editing, where changes to DNA can be passed on to future generations, raising concerns about long-term consequences and potential misuse.

Nanoparticles in Photo-Dynamic Therapy

Nanoparticles offer several advantages in PDT, including enhancing the solubility and stability of PSs, improving selectivity toward target cells, and boosting the overall efficacy of PDT.

Types of Nanoparticles Used in PDT

1. Organic Nanoparticles:
    - These NPs encapsulate hydrophobic PS drugs, improving biocompatibility and increasing tumor accumulation.
    - These NPs offer controlled release of the PS and can be functionalized with ligands for targeted delivery.

2. Inorganic Nanoparticles:
   - Gold NPs are used to enhance light absorption and can also convert light into heat, enabling a combination of PDT and photo-thermal therapy.
   - Silica-based NPs provide high loading capacity for PSs and protect the PS from premature degradation.
   - These can serve as both imaging agents and PS activators, offering the ability to tune their absorption wavelength.

   Advantages of Nanoparticle-Mediated PDT

   - NPs can be functionalized with tumor-specific ligands to enhance targeting, reducing off-target effects.
   - NPs help solubilize hydrophobic PS drugs, making them more effective.
   - NPs can release drug in response to external stimuli such as light, pH, or enzymes.
   - Nanoparticles allow for co-delivery of PS and other therapeutic agents.
   - By improving targeting and minimizing the distribution of PSs to healthy tissues, NP-mediated PDT reduces side effects.

Immunotherapy

Immunotherapy harnesses the body's immune system to fight diseases, particularly cancer and infections. Nanoparticles can improve the efficacy of immunotherapies by enhancing antigen/adjuvant delivery, improving targeting to immune cells, and modulating the tumor micro-environment (TME).

Nanoparticles in Immunotherapy

- Nanoparticles can serve as efficient carriers for antigens and adjuvants, improving the immune response.
- NPs can be engineered to specifically target immune cells, such as dendritic cells or T-cells, to enhance their activation.
- NPs can modify the TME, making it more conducive to immune cell infiltration and activation.
- NPs can be used to combine multiple immunotherapies, such as immune checkpoint inhibitors and cancer vaccines, for synergistic effects (Cramer & Chen, 2020).

5. CHALLENGES AND FUTURE DEVELOPMENTS TOWARDS GBM TREATMENTS

In order to overcome these issues, various strategies have been incorporated such as inclusion of traditional therapies like alky-lation or methylation of DNA has shown results to reduce the cell proliferation of malignant glioma and have induced chemo-resistance. As a result, some strategies can be effective to reduce these side effects by application of simultaneous conventional therapy and nano-derived moities towards the treatment of GBM. As these nano-materials have the capacity to cross through the blood brain barrier effectively, efficiently, and improve drug accumulation at the target site.

In this case, Orza et al. Synthesized gold nanoparticles (AuNPs)-L-aspartate in the form of nano-derived structures, which have the ability to bind with temozolomide by electrostatic for attraction that dealing with recurrent GBM with 90% apoptotic action compared to just temozolomide, which showed 42% of apoptosis. The nano-based structures showed better activity to aid glial cells because of the nano- size, surface modifiers and the different concentrations of the nano-materials used that provided better physio-chemical properties of the synthesized gold nano-particles that enhanced the cell internalisation properties for active targeting at the tumor site.

6. FUTURE DEVELOPMENTS IN NANOTECHNOLOGY FOR THE INVESTIGATION OF GBM

Different nano-based structures have the potential for application towards the treatment of GBM, such as the exosomes, polymeric nano-particles, carbon-based drug delivery systems in the form of quantum dots, surface modifiers such as graphene oxide, carbon dots, vesicles in the form of liposomes, metalic based nano-systems.

In the case of passive targeting strategies, this method involves only specific accumulation of nano-materials around the tumor micro-environment without spreading across the healthy cells which primarily depends upon the size of the nano-particles. In this case, prolonged drug circulation is common which can lead to maximum half-life within the blood, this happens when the nano-materials dose exceeds the toxicity range, with enlarged size and drug dose also is altered . For instance, polythylene glycol-coated nano-materials can overcome these side effects, they provide the maximum half-life and extend the circulation through blood with the systemic drug concentration, thus improving the stability of physiological fluids in the micro-environment. Followed by the disruption of the BBB is not uncommon in the case of GBM due to excess permeability rates of nano-materials through the BBB can trigger the obstruction with safer EPR effect. For this case, better physico-chemical properties in terms of nano-size, ionization potential, and lipophilicity of the drug that help to provide a safer EPR effect. For a successful strategy, an active targeting drug delivery system is a promising approach towards the treatment of GBM when compared to passive targeting systems for aggressive tumor types. Such type of nanoparticles has the ability to improve drug accumulation properties around the glioma cells by acting as diagnostic agents for their tumor identification using the magnetic resonance imaging technique.

CONCLUSION

The invasive nature of the tumor, the presence of the blood-brain barrier (BBB), and the high likelihood of recurrence render GBM one of the most deadly and treatment-resistant types of brain cancer. The majority of tumor cells, especially GBM stem cells, which are major causes of resistance and recurrence, that are frequently not eradicated by conventional treatments like radiation therapy, surgery, and chemotherapy. Therefore, in order to enhance patient outcomes, new and better accurate strategies are absolutely necessary.

Nanotheranostics is applied in the form of metallic, magnetic and hyperthermia based drug delivery systems in the nano-platforms of nanoparticles, liposome, exosomes, dendrimers and other nano- structured particles that have the ability to aid GBM by maintaining standardized physio-chemical properties with desired nano-size, effective electrostatic binding with the excipients, effective surface binding of proteins, anti-bodies, ligands and other surface modifiers that have the potential for active targeting at the tumor site thus paving way for dose reducing effects of the anti-cancer drugs that in-turn reduces the toxicity, improves drug accumulation and improved the bio-availability at the tumor site.

REFERENCES

Agemy, L., Friedmann-Morvinski, D., Kotamraju, V. R., Roth, L., Sugahara, K. N., Girard, O. M., Mattrey, R. F., Verma, I. M., & Ruoslahti, E. (2011). Targeted nanoparticle enhanced proapoptotic peptide as potential therapy for glioblastoma. *Proceedings of the National Academy of Sciences of the United States of America, 108*(42), 17450–17455. DOI: 10.1073/pnas.1114518108 PMID: 21969599

Aldape, K., Zadeh, G., Mansouri, S., Reifenberger, G., & von Deimling, A. (2015). Glioblastoma: Pathology, molecular mechanisms and markers. *Acta Neuropathologica, 17*(1), 98–110. DOI: 10.1007/s00401-015-1432-1 PMID: 25943888

Anido, J., Sáez-Borderías, A., Gonzàlez-Juncà, A., Rodón, L., Folch, G., Carmona, M. A., Prieto-Sánchez, R. M., Barba, I., Martínez-Sáez, E., Prudkin, L., Cuartas, I., Raventós, C., Martínez-Ricarte, F., Poca, M. A., García-Dorado, D., Lahn, M. M., Yingling, J. M., Rodón, J., Sahuquillo, J., & Seoane, J. (2010). TGF-β Receptor Inhibitors Target the CD44(high)/Id1(high) Glioma-Initiating Cell Population in Human Glioblastoma. *Cancer Cell, 18*(6), 655–668. DOI: 10.1016/j.ccr.2010.10.023 PMID: 21156287

Aragon-Sanabria, V.. (2022). Ultrasmall Nanoparticle Delivery of Doxorubicin Improves Therapeutic Index for High-Grade Glioma. *Molecular Cancer Therapeutics, 21*(5), 789–798. DOI: 10.1158/1535-7163.MCT-21-0720 PMID: 35499557

Arce, C., Rodríguez-Rovira, I., De Rycke, K., Durán, K., Campuzano, V., Fabregat, I., Jiménez-Altayó, F., Berraondo, P., & Egea, G. (2021). Anti-TGFβ (transforming growth factor β) therapy with betaglycan-derived P144 peptide gene delivery prevents the formation of aortic aneurysm in a mouse model of Marfan syndrome. *Arteriosclerosis, Thrombosis, and Vascular Biology, 41*(9), e440–e452. DOI: 10.1161/ATVBAHA.121.316496 PMID: 34162229

Atkinson, A. P.. (2018). Aptamers in Glioblastoma Research: Potential for Targeted Therapy. *Cancer Letters, 414*, 82–90. DOI: 10.1016/j.canlet.2017.11.017

Blanco, E., Shen, H., & Ferrari, M. (2015). Principles of nanoparticle design for overcoming biological barriers to drug delivery. *Nature Biotechnology, 33*(9), 941–951. DOI: 10.1038/nbt.3330 PMID: 26348965

Blanco, E., Shen, H., & Ferrari, M. (2015). Principles of nanoparticle design for overcoming biological barriers to drug delivery. *Nature Biotechnology, 33*(9), 941–951. DOI: 10.1038/nbt.3330 PMID: 26348965

Bohn, A., Braley, A., Rodriguez de la Vega, P., Zevallos, J. C., & Barengo, N. C. (2018, June 21). The association between race and survival in glioblastoma patients in the US: A retrospective cohort study. *PLoS One, 13*(6), e0198581. DOI: 10.1371/journal.pone.0198581 PMID: 29927955

Bondy, M. L., Scheurer, M. E., Malmer, B., Barnholtz-Sloan, J. S., Davis, F. G., Il'yasova, D., Kruchko, C., McCarthy, B. J., Rajaraman, P., Schwartzbaum, J. A., Sadetzki, S., Schlehofer, B., Tihan, T., Wiemels, J. L., Wrensch, M., & Buffler, P. A. (2008). Brain tumor epidemiology: Consensus from the Brain Tumor Epidemi-ologyConsortium. *Cancer, 113*(S7), 1953–1968. DOI: 10.1002/cncr.23741 PMID: 18798534

Calixto, G. M., Bernegossi, J., De Freitas, L. M., Fontana, C. R., & Chorilli, M. (2016). Nanotechnology-based drug delivery systems for photodynamic therapy of cancer: A review. *Molecules (Basel, Switzerland), 21*(3), 342. Advance online publication. DOI: 10.3390/molecules21030342 PMID: 26978341

Chen, W.. (2021). Nanoparticle-Mediated Gene Editing: Progress and Challenges. *Trends in Biotechnology, 39*(5), 456–469. DOI: 10.1016/j.tibtech.2020.12.002 PMID: 33036785

Chen, X., Wang, J., Liu, S., Han, Q., Zhang, H., & Wu, J. (2025). Research landscape of glioma and inflammation over the past two decades. *Frontiers in Immunology, 16*, 1605346. Advance online publication. DOI: 10.3389/fimmu.2025.1605346 PMID: 40881678

Cheng, L., Huang, Z., Zhou, W., & Wu, Q. (2021). Glioblastoma stem cells: Molecular characteristics and targeted therapies. *Frontiers in Oncology, 11*, 638279. DOI: 10.3389/fonc.2021.638279

Cheng, X., Lou, S., Huang, S., Chen, H., & Liu, J. (2017). Primary spinal cord glioblastoma multiforme: A retrospective study of patients at a single institution. *World Neurosurgery, 106*, 113–119. DOI: 10.1016/j.wneu.2017.03.120 PMID: 28377242

Cheng, Y., Morshed, R. A., Auffinger, B., Tobias, A. L., & Lesniak, M. S. (2014). Nanomedicine for brain tumor treatment: Overcoming the blood-brain barrier and drug resistance. *Frontiers in Pharmacology, 5*, 105. DOI: 10.3389/fphar.2014.00105

Clarke, H. J., Chambers, J. E., Liniker, E., & Marciniak, S. J. (2014). Endoplasmic reticulum stress in malignancy. *Cancer Cell, 25*(5), 563–573. DOI: 10.1016/j.ccr.2014.03.015 PMID: 24823636

Clarke, J., Butowski, N., & Chang, S. (2010). Recent advances in therapy for glioblastoma. *Archives of Neurology*, *67*(3), 279–283. DOI: 10.1001/archneurol.2010.5 PMID: 20212224

Cramer, S. W., & Chen, C. C. (2020). Photodynamic therapy for the treatment of glioblastoma. *Frontiers in Surgery*, *6*, 81. Advance online publication. DOI: 10.3389/fsurg.2019.00081 PMID: 32039232

Engels, E. A.. (2005). Cancer risk in people infected with human immunodeficiency virus in the United States. *International Journal of Cancer*, *113*(5), 829–835. DOI: 10.1002/ijc.23487 PMID: 15499619

Eyler, C. E., & Rich, J. N. (2008). Survival of the fittest: Cancer stem cells in therapeutic resistance and angiogenesis. *Journal of Clinical Oncology*, *26*(17), 2839–2845. DOI: 10.1200/JCO.2007.15.1829 PMID: 18539962

Ferrara, N., & Kerbel, R. S. (2018). Angiogenesis in Glioblastoma. *The New England Journal of Medicine*, *373*(17), 1657–1665. DOI: 10.1056/NEJMra1614713 PMID: 30354954

Gallo, M., Coutinho, F. J., Vanner, R. J., Gayden, T., Mack, S. C., Murison, A., Remke, M., Li, R., Takayama, N., Desai, K., Lee, L., Lan, X., Park, N. I., Barsyte-Lovejoy, D., Smil, D., Sturm, D., Kushida, M. M., Head, R., Cusimano, M. D., & Dirks, P. B. (2015). MLL5 orchestrates a cancer self-renewal state by repressing the histone variant H3.3 and globally reorganizing chromatin. *Cancer Cell*, *28*(5), 715–729. DOI: 10.1016/j.ccell.2015.10.005 PMID: 26626085

Giese, A., Bjerkvig, R., Berens, M. E., & Westphal, M. (2003). Cost of migration: Invasion of malignant gliomas and implications for treatment. *Journal of Clinical Oncology*, *21*(8), 1624–1636. DOI: 10.1200/JCO.2003.05.063 PMID: 12697889

Giordano, R. J.. (2019). Integrin-targeted therapies for glioblastoma: New directions and challenges. *Molecular Cancer Therapeutics*, *18*(9), 1424–1432. DOI: 10.1158/1535-7163.MCT-18-0736

Giordano, R. J., Cardó-Vila, M., Lahdenranta, J., Pasqualini, R., & Arap, W. (2001). From combinatorial peptide selection to drug prototype [Review]. *Nature Reviews. Drug Discovery*, *1*(1), 68–76. DOI: 10.1038/35095083

Hailozian, C., Luftig, J., Liang, A., Outhay, M., Ullal, M., Anderson, E. S., Kalmin, M., Shoptaw, S., Greenwald, M. K., & Herring, A. A. (2022). Synergistic effect of ketamine and buprenorphine observed in the treatment of buprenorphine precipitated opioid withdrawal in a patient with fentanyl use. *Journal of Addiction Medicine, 16*(4), 483–487. Advance online publication. DOI: 10.1097/ADM.0000000000000929 PMID: 34789683

Hambardzumyan, D., Gutmann, D. H., & Kettenmann, H. (2016). The role of microglia and macrophages in glioma maintenance and progression. *Nature Neuroscience, 19*(1), 20–27. DOI: 10.1038/nn.4185 PMID: 26713745

He, Y.. (2020). Nanoparticles for Efficient Gene Delivery in Cancer Therapy. *Frontiers in Pharmacology, 11*, 585917. DOI: 10.3389/fphar.2020.585917

Hegi, M. E., Diserens, A.-C., Gorlia, T., Hamou, M.-F., de Tribolet, N., Weller, M., Kros, J. M., Hainfellner, J. A., Mason, W., Mariani, L., Bromberg, J. E. C., Hau, P., Mirimanoff, R. O., Cairncross, J. G., Janzer, R. C., & Stupp, R. (2005). MGMT gene silencing and benefit from temozolomide in glioblastoma. *The New England Journal of Medicine, 352*(10), 997–1003. DOI: 10.1056/NEJMoa043331 PMID: 15758010

Hu, H., Mu, Q., Bao, Z., Chen, Y., Liu, Y., Chen, J., Wang, K., Wang, Z., Nam, Y., Jiang, B., Sa, J. K., Cho, H.-J., Her, N.-G., Zhang, C., Zhao, Z., Zhang, Y., Zeng, F., Wu, F., Kang, X., & Jiang, T. (2018). Mutational landscape of secondary glioblastoma guides MET-targeted trial in brain tumor. *Cell, 175*(6), 1665–1678. DOI: 10.1016/j.cell.2018.09.038 PMID: 30343896

Huang, R.. (2021). Platelet-derived growth factor receptor signaling in Glioblastoma and its therapeutic targeting. *Journal of Neuro-Oncology, 153*(2), 231–245. DOI: 10.1007/s11060-021-03753-7 PMID: 33206309

Jaiswal, S., & Tyagi, A. (2022). Biocompatible Nanoparticles for Cancer Therapy: A Review. *Journal of Nanomedicine Research, 10*(2), 55–64. DOI: 10.18231/j.jnanomed.2022.21

Jnaidi, R., Almeida, A. J., & Gonçalves, L. M. (2020). Solid lipid nanoparticles and nanostructured lipid carriers as smart drug delivery systems in the treatment of glioblastoma multiforme. *Pharmaceutics, 12*(9), 860. Advance online publication. DOI: 10.3390/pharmaceutics12090860 PMID: 32927610

Kelkar, S. S., & Reineke, T. M. (2011). Theranostics: Combining imaging and therapy. *Bioconjugate Chemistry, 22*(10), 1879–1903. DOI: 10.1021/bc200151q PMID: 21830812

Kim, K.. (2020). Intranasal delivery of cancer-targeting doxorubicin-loaded PLGA nanoparticles arrests glioblastoma growth. *Journal of Drug Targeting*, *28*(7-8), 617–626. DOI: 10.1080/1061186X.2020.1775736 PMID: 31852284

Kostka, K., Sokolova, V., El-Taibany, A., Kruse, B., Porada, D., Wolff, N., Prymak, O., Seeds, M. C., Epple, M., & Atala, A. J. (2024). The Application of Ultrasmall Gold Nanoparticles (2 nm) Functionalized with Doxorubicin in Three-Dimensional Normal and Glioblastoma Organoid Models of the Blood–Brain Barrier. *Molecules (Basel, Switzerland)*, *29*(11), 2469. DOI: 10.3390/molecules29112469 PMID: 38893345

Lansangan, C., Khoobchandani, M., Jain, R., Rudensky, S., Perry, C. C., & Patil, R. (2024). Designing gold nanoparticles for precise glioma treatment: Challenges and alternatives. *Materials (Basel)*, *17*(5), 1153. Advance online publication. DOI: 10.3390/ma17051153 PMID: 38473623

Lathia, J. D., Mack, S. C., Mulkearns-Hubert, E. E., Valentim, C. L., & Rich, J. N. (2015). Cancer stem cells in glioblastoma. *Genes & Development*, *29*(12), 1203–1217. DOI: 10.1101/gad.261982.115 PMID: 26109046

Li, H.. (2022). Targeted Nanoparticles for the Delivery of CRISPR-Cas9 Systems in Gene Editing. *Nature Communications*, *13*(1), 1827. DOI: 10.1038/s41467-022-29472-7 PMID: 35383166

Li, L.. (2022). Recent Advances in Nanoparticle-Based Delivery Systems for Gene Therapy in Glioblastoma. *Nanotechnology Reviews*, *11*(1), 84–96. DOI: 10.1515/ntrev-2022-0079

Li, Q., Zhang, Z., Wu, X., Zhao, Y., & Liu, Y. (2025). Cascade-responsive nanoparticles for efficient CRISPR/Cas9-based glioblastoma gene therapy. *ACS Applied Materials & Interfaces*, *17*(3), 4480–4489. DOI: 10.1021/acsami.4c15671 PMID: 39797776

Lim, M., Xia, Y., Bettegowda, C., & Weller, M. (2018). Current state of immunotherapy for glioblastoma. *Nature Reviews. Clinical Oncology*, *15*(7), 422–442. DOI: 10.1038/s41571-018-0003-5 PMID: 29643471

Lim, M., Xia, Y., Bettegowda, C., & Weller, M. (2018). Current state of immunotherapy for glioblastoma. *Nature Reviews. Clinical Oncology*, *15*(7), 422–442. DOI: 10.1038/s41571-018-0003-5 PMID: 29643471

Liu, G., & Sun, Y. (2025). Harnessing nanoparticles for Alzheimer's disease: Innovations in drug delivery and pathology-specific treatments. *Journal of Alzheimer's Disease*, *107*(4), 1374–1399. DOI: 10.1177/13872877251374149 PMID: 40899976

Liu, H.. (2021). CD133 as a marker for glioblastoma stem cells: Implications for drug resistance. *Stem Cell Research & Therapy*, *12*(1), 107. DOI: 10.1186/s13287-021-02307-1 PMID: 33541421

Liu, X.. (2023). Functionalized Nanoparticles for Targeted Delivery in CRISPR/Cas9-Based Gene Editing. *Nanomedicine; Nanotechnology, Biology, and Medicine*, *27*, 42–52. DOI: 10.1016/j.nano.2022.102484

Louis, D. N., Perry, A., Reifenberger, G., von Deimling, A., Figarella-Branger, D., Cavenee, W. K., Ohgaki, H., Wiestler, O. D., Kleihues, P., & Ellison, D. W. (2016). The 2016 World Health Organization Classification of Tumors of the Central Nervous System. *Acta Neuropathologica*, *131*(6), 803–820. DOI: 10.1007/s00401-016-1545-1 PMID: 27157931

Lu, V. M., Jue, T. R., McDonald, K. L., & Rovin, R. A. (2018). The survival effect of repeat surgery at glioblastoma recurrence and its trend: A systematic review and meta-analysis. *World Neurosurgery*, *115*, 453–459. DOI: 10.1016/j.wneu.2018.04.016 PMID: 29654958

Maeda, H., Wu, J., Sawa, T., Matsumura, Y., & Hori, K. (2000). Tumor vascular permeability and the EPR effect in macromolecular therapeutics. A review. *Journal of Controlled Release*, *65*(1–2), 271–284. DOI: 10.1016/S0168-3659(99)00248-5 PMID: 10699287

Mahmoudi, M.. (2011). Superparamagnetic iron oxide nanoparticles for biomedical applications: Opportunities and challenges. *Chemical Reviews*, *111*(2), 253–280. DOI: 10.1021/cr1001832 PMID: 21077606

McMahon, S. A.. (2019). Monoclonal antibodies in glioblastoma treatment: Targeting EGFR and VEGF. *Journal of Clinical Oncology*, *37*(3), 234–240. DOI: 10.1200/JCO.18.01556

Meyers, J. D., Cheng, Y., Broome, A.-M., Agnes, R. S., Schluchter, M. D., Margevicius, S., Wang, X., Kenney, M. E., Burda, C., & Basilion, J. P. (2015). Peptide-targeted gold nanoparticles for photodynamic therapy of brain cancer. *Particle & Particle Systems Characterization*, *32*(4), 448–457. DOI: 10.1002/ppsc.201400119 PMID: 25999665

Mura, S., Nicolas, J., & Couvreur, P. (2013). Stimuli-responsive nanocarriers for drug delivery. *Nature Materials*, *12*(11), 991–1003. DOI: 10.1038/nmat3776 PMID: 24150417

Musielak, E., & Krajka-Kuźniak, V. (2025). Lipidic and inorganic nanoparticles for targeted glioblastoma multiforme therapy: Advances and strategies. *Micro*, *5*(1), 2. Advance online publication. DOI: 10.3390/micro5010002

Nangare, S., Chandankar, S., & Patil, P. (2023). Design of carbon and graphene quantum dots based nanotheranostics applications for glioblastoma management: Recent advanced and future prospects. *Journal of Drug Delivery Science and Technology*, *89*, 105060. Advance online publication. DOI: 10.1016/j.jddst.2023.105060

Oh, J. H.. (2020). Transferrin receptor-targeted nanoparticles for drug delivery in glioblastoma therapy. *International Journal of Nanomedicine*, *15*, 6439–6453. DOI: 10.2147/IJN.S268791

. Ostrom QT, Gittleman H, Fulop J, Liu M, Blanda R, Kromer C, Wolinsky Y, Kruchko C, Barnholtz-Sloan JS. CBTRUS statistical report: primary brain and central nervous system tumors diagnosed in the United States in 2008-2012. *Neuro-oncology*.2015Oct1;17(suppl_4):iv1-62. .DOI: 10.1093/neuonc/nov189

Ostrom, Q. T., Patil, N., Cioffi, G., Waite, K., Kruchko, C., & Barnholtz-Sloan, J. S. (2020). CBTRUS Statistical Report: Primary brain and other central nervous system tumors diagnosed in the United States in 2013–2017. *Neuro-Oncology*, *22*(Supplement_1), iv1–iv96. DOI: 10.1093/neuonc/noaa200 PMID: 33123732

Ozdemir-Kaynak, E., Qutub, A. A., & Yesil-Celiktas, O. (2018). Advances in glioblastoma multiforme treatment: New models for nanoparticle therapy. *Frontiers in Physiology*, *9*, 170. Advance online publication. DOI: 10.3389/fphys.2018.00170 PMID: 29615917

Pardridge, W. M. (2012). Drug transport across the blood–brain barrier. *Journal of Cerebral Blood Flow and Metabolism*, *32*(11), 1959–1972. DOI: 10.1038/jcbfm.2012.126 PMID: 22929442

Patel, R., Patel, D., Dani, U., & Kuperkar, K. (2025). Nanoparticle-driven drug delivery system for cardiovascular treatment. *Journal of Cardiology*. Advance online publication. DOI: 10.1016/j.jjcc.2025.06.004 PMID: 40518071

Patil, C., Priyanka, R., Harshitha, B. M., Oshik, S., Yashwanth, S., Darshan, B. R., Patil, S., Prajwal, K. A., Naik, P., Goudanavar, P., & Mallamma, T. (2025). Advanced nanotheranostic approaches for targeted glioblastoma treatment: A synergistic fusion of CRISPR-Cas gene editing, AI-driven tumor profiling, and BBB-modulation. *Medical Oncology (Northwood, London, England)*, *42*(9), 229. Advance online publication. DOI: 10.1007/s12032-025-02944-6 PMID: 40773116

Pourmasoumi, P., Banihashemian, S. A., Zamani, F., Rasouli-Nia, A., Mehrabani, D., & Karimi-Busheri, F. (2024). Nanoparticle-Based Approaches in the Diagnosis and Treatment of Brain Tumors. *Journal of Clinical Medicine, 13*(23), 7449. DOI: 10.3390/jcm13237449 PMID: 39685907

Qureshi, S., Anjum, S., Hussain, M., Sheikh, A., Gupta, G., Almoyad, M. A., Wahab, S., & Kesharwani, P. (2024). A recent insight of applications of gold nanoparticles in glioblastoma multiforme therapy. *International Journal of Pharmaceutics, 660*, 124301. Advance online publication. DOI: 10.1016/j.ijpharm.2024.124301 PMID: 38851411

Rahman, M. H., Rana, H. K., Peng, S., Hu, X., Chen, C., Quinn, J. M., & Moni, M. A. (2021). Bioinformatics and machine learning methodologies to identify the effects of central nervous system disorders on glioblastoma progression. *Briefings in Bioinformatics, 22*(5), bbaa365. Advance online publication. DOI: 10.1093/bib/bbaa365 PMID: 33406529

Ratliff, M., Kim, H., Qi, H., Kim, M., Ku, B., Azorin, D. D., Hausmann, D., Khajuria, R. K., Patel, A., Maier, E., Cousin, L., Ogier, A., Sahm, F., Etminan, N., Bunse, L., Winkler, F., El-Khoury, V., Platten, M., & Kwon, Y.-J. (2022). Patient-derived tumor organoids for guidance of personalized drug therapies in recurrent glioblastoma. *International Journal of Molecular Sciences, 23*(12), 6572. Advance online publication. DOI: 10.3390/ijms23126572 PMID: 35743016

Rehman, M., Madni, A., Shi, D., Ihsan, A., Tahir, N., Chang, K. R., Javed, I., & Webster, T. J. (2017). Enhanced blood brain barrier permeability and glioblastoma cell targeting via thermoresponsive lipid nanoparticles. *Nanoscale, 9*(40), 15434–15440. DOI: 10.1039/C7NR05216B PMID: 28976512

Roque, D., Cruz, N., Ferreira, H. A., Reis, C. P., Matela, N., Herculano-Carvalho, M., Cascão, R., & Faria, C. C. (2023). Nanoparticle-based treatment in glioblastoma. *Journal of Personalized Medicine, 13*(9), 1328. Advance online publication. DOI: 10.3390/jpm13091328 PMID: 37763096

Rosenblum, D., Joshi, N., Tao, W., Karp, J. M., & Peer, D. (2018). Progress and challenges towards targeted delivery of cancer therapeutics. *Nature Communications, 9*(1), 1410. DOI: 10.1038/s41467-018-03705-y PMID: 29650952

Ruan, W., Jiao, M., Xu, S., Ismail, M., Xie, X., An, Y., Guo, H., Qian, R., Shi, B., & Zheng, M. (2022). Brain-targeted CRISPR/Cas9 nanomedicine for effective glioblastoma therapy. *Journal of Controlled Release, 351*, 739–751. DOI: 10.1016/j.jconrel.2022.09.046 PMID: 36174804

Sadetzki, S.. (2005). Radiation-induced meningioma: A descriptive study of 253 cases. *Journal ofNeurosurgery*, *102*(2), 232–241. DOI: 10.3171/jns.2002.97.5.1078 PMID: 12450029

Sancho, P., Barneda, D., & Heeschen, C. (2016). Hallmarks of cancer stem cell metabolism. *British Journal of Cancer*, *114*(12), 1305–1312. DOI: 10.1038/bjc.2016.152 PMID: 27219018

Sharma, M.. (2023). Nanoparticle-based Delivery Systems for Gene Therapy. *Nanomedicine; Nanotechnology, Biology, and Medicine*, *34*(7), 356–371. DOI: 10.1016/j.nano.2023.102441

Singh, S., Dey, D., Barik, D., Mohapatra, I., Kim, S., Sharma, M., Prasad, S., Wang, P., Singh, A., & Singh, G. (2025). Glioblastoma at the crossroads: Current understanding and future therapeutic horizons. *Signal Transduction and Targeted Therapy*, *10*(1), 213. Advance online publication. DOI: 10.1038/s41392-025-02299-4 PMID: 40628732

Smith, A. J., & Kumar, P. (2023). Advances in Nanoparticle-Based Drug Delivery for Gene Therapy. *International Journal of Nanomedicine*, *18*(1), 107–123. DOI: 10.2147/IJN.S359162

Smith, C. J., Perfetti, T. A., Chokshi, C., Venugopal, C., Ashford, J. W., & Singh, S. K. (2024). Risk factors for glioblastoma are shared by other brain tumor types. *Human and Experimental Toxicology*, *43*, 09603271241241796. Advance online publication. DOI: 10.1177/09603271241241796 PMID: 38520250

Smolen, J. S.. (2019). EGFRvIII: A truncated, constitutively active form of EGFR in glioblastoma. *Oncology Letters*, *18*(5), 5394–5403. DOI: 10.3892/ol.2019.10747

Son, M. J., Woolard, K., Nam, D. H., Lee, J., & Fine, H. A. (2009). SSEA-1 is an enrichment marker for tumor-initiating cells in human glioblastoma. *Cell Stem Cell*, *4*(5), 440–452. DOI: 10.1016/j.stem.2009.03.003 PMID: 19427293

Song, H., & Lee, S. (2021). Advances in Nanoparticle-Mediated Gene Delivery. *Journal of Controlled Release*, *330*, 388–409. DOI: 10.1016/j.jconrel.2021.07.022

Stupp, R., Mason, W. P., van den Bent, M. J., Weller, M., Fisher, B., Taphoorn, M. J. B., Belanger, K., Brandes, A. A., Marosi, C., Bogdahn, U., Curschmann, J., Janzer, R. C., Ludwin, S. K., Gorlia, T., Allgeier, A., Lacombe, D., Cairncross, J. G., Eisenhauer, E., & Mirimanoff, R. O. (2005). Radiotherapy plus concomitant and adjuvant temozolomide for glioblastoma. *The New England Journal of Medicine*, *352*(10), 987–996. DOI: 10.1056/NEJMoa043330 PMID: 15758009

Stupp, R., Mason, W. P., van den Bent, M. J., Weller, M., Fisher, B., Taphoorn, M. J. B., Belanger, K., Brandes, A. A., Marosi, C., Bogdahn, U., Curschmann, J., Janzer, R. C., Ludwin, S. K., Gorlia, T., Allgeier, A., Lacombe, D., Cairncross, J. G., Eisenhauer, E., & Mirimanoff, R. O. (2005). Radiotherapy plus concomitant and adjuvant temozolomide for glioblastoma. *The New England Journal of Medicine*, *352*(10), 987–996. DOI: 10.1056/NEJMoa043330 PMID: 15758009

Szklener, K., Mazurek, M., Wieteska, M., Wacławska, M., Bilski, M., & Mańdziuk, S. (2022). New directions in the therapy of glioblastoma. *Cancers (Basel)*, *14*(21), 5377. Advance online publication. DOI: 10.3390/cancers14215377 PMID: 36358795

Tan, A. C., Ashley, D. M., López, G. Y., Malinzak, M., Friedman, H. S., & Khasraw, M. (2020). Management of glioblastoma: State of the art and future directions. *CA: a Cancer Journal for Clinicians*, *70*(4), 299–312. DOI: 10.3322/caac.21613 PMID: 32478924

Thomas, S. S., & Lee, J. S. (2021). Lipid Nanoparticles for Gene Therapy: Innovations and Applications. *Molecular Therapy. Nucleic Acids*, *24*, 134–145. DOI: 10.1016/j.omtn.2021.06.023

Vaz-Salgado, M. A., Villamayor, M., Albarrán, V., Alía, V., Sotoca, P., Chamorro, J., Rosero, D., Barrill, A. M., Martín, M., Fernandez, E., Gutierrez, J. A., Rojas-Medina, L. M., & Ley, L. (2023). Recurrent glioblastoma: A review of the treatment options. *Cancers (Basel)*, *15*(17), 4279. Advance online publication. DOI: 10.3390/cancers15174279 PMID: 37686553

Ventola, C. L. (2017). *Progress in nanomedicine*: Approved and investigational nanodrugs. *P&T : a Peer-Reviewed Journal for Formulary Management*, *42*(12), 742–755. https://pmc.ncbi.nlm.nih.gov/articles/PMC5720487/ PMID: 29234213

Verhaak, R. G. W., Hoadley, K. A., Purdom, E., Wang, V., Qi, Y., Wilkerson, M. D., Miller, C. R., Ding, L., Golub, T., Mesirov, J. P., Alexe, G., Lawrence, M., O'Kelly, M., Tamayo, P., Weir, B. A., Gabriel, S., Winckler, W., Gupta, S., Jakkula, L., & Hayes, D. N. (2010). Integrated Genomic Analysis Identifies Clinically Relevant Subtypes of Glioblastoma Characterized by Abnormalities in PDGFRA, IDH1, EGFR, and NF1. *Cancer Cell*, *113*(S7), 1953–1968. DOI: 10.1016/j.ccr.2009.12.020 PMID: 20129251

Wang, Y.. (2021). Recent Progress in Nanoparticle-Mediated Delivery Systems for RNA-Based Therapeutics. *Journal of Controlled Release*, *332*, 86–99. DOI: 10.1016/j.jconrel.2021.04.009

Wrensch, M., Minn, Y., Chew, T., Bondy, M., & Berger, M. S. (2002, October 1). Epidemiology of primary brain tumors: Current concepts and review of the literature. *Neuro-Oncology*, *4*(4), 278–299. DOI: 10.1093/neuonc/4.4.278 PMID: 12356358

Wu, Z., Ho, W. S., & Lu, R. (2022). Targeting mitochondrial oxidative phosphorylation in glioblastoma therapy. *Neuromolecular Medicine*, *24*(1), 18–22. DOI: 10.1007/s12017-021-08678-8 PMID: 34487301

Xie, J.. (2021). Nanomaterial-Based Platforms for CRISPR/Cas9 Delivery: From Bench to Bedside. *Frontiers in Bioengineering and Biotechnology*, *9*, 765080. DOI: 10.3389/fbioe.2021.765080

Xu, L.. (2020). Challenges in active targeting for glioblastoma therapy. *Cancer Treatment Reviews*, *86*, 102031. DOI: 10.1016/j.ctrv.2020.102031

Xu, X., Tan, M., Corcoran, B., Wu, J., Boes, A., Nguyen, T. G., Chu, S. T., Little, B. E., Hicks, D. G., Morandotti, R., Mitchell, A., & Moss, D. J. (2021). 11 TOPS photonic convolutional accelerator for optical neural networks. *Nature*, *589*(7840), 44–51. DOI: 10.1038/s41586-020-03063-0 PMID: 33408378

Xu, X., Wang, L., Xu, H., Yang, X., & Li, Y. (2019). Smart nanotheranostic systems for precise cancer therapy based on stimuli-responsive nanocarriers. *Signal Transduction and Targeted Therapy*, *4*(1), 1–18. DOI: 10.1038/s41392-019-0082-3

Xu, Z.. (2022). Targeted Nanoparticle Delivery Systems in Gene Therapy. *Biomaterials Science*, *10*(4), 877–890. DOI: 10.1039/d0bm01851f PMID: 35024701

Yang, Q., Zhou, Y., Chen, J., Huang, N., Wang, Z., & Cheng, Y. (2021). Gene therapy for drug-resistant glioblastoma via lipid-polymer hybrid nanoparticles combined with focused ultrasound. *International Journal of Nanomedicine*, *16*, 185–199. DOI: 10.2147/IJN.S286221 PMID: 33447034

Yin, Y., & Alivisatos, A. P. (2005). Colloidal nanocrystal synthesis and the organic–inorganic interface. *Nature*, *437*(7059), 664–670. DOI: 10.1038/nature04165 PMID: 16193041

Yoon, S.. (2022). Smart Nanoparticles for CRISPR/Cas9-Based Gene Therapy: A Comprehensive Review. *Nanomedicine; Nanotechnology, Biology, and Medicine*, *29*, 102253. DOI: 10.1016/j.nano.2021.102253

Zanders, E. D., Svensson, F., & Bailey, D. S. (2019). Therapy for glioblastoma: Is it working? *Drug Discovery Today*, *24*(5), 1193–1201. DOI: 10.1016/j.drudis.2019.03.008 PMID: 30878561

Zhang, M.. (2021). CRISPR-Cas9 and Nanoparticles in Gene Therapy: Prospects and Challenges. *Nanomedicine; Nanotechnology, Biology, and Medicine*, *30*(4), 529–540. DOI: 10.1016/j.nano.2020.102317

Zhang, X. Q., Chen, X., Cheng, X. B., Li, B. Q., Shen, X., Yan, C., Huang, J. Q., & Zhang, Q. (2018). Highly stable lithium metal batteries enabled by regulating the solvation of lithium ions in nonaqueous electrolytes. *Angewandte Chemie International Edition*, *57*(19), 5301–5305. DOI: 10.1002/anie.201801513 PMID: 29465827

Zhang, Y.. (2023). Multifunctional Nanoparticles for Cancer Therapy and Imaging: Recent Advances. *Nature Reviews. Materials*, *8*(3), 153–174. DOI: 10.1038/s41578-023-00531-9

Zheng, X., Wang, L., Pei, Q., He, S., Liu, S., & Xie, Z. (2017). Metal–organic framework@porous organic polymer nanocomposite for photodynamic therapy. *Chemistry of Materials*, *29*(5), 2374–2381. DOI: 10.1021/acs.chemmater.7b00228

Zhu, Z., Zhang, H., Chen, B., Liu, X., Zhang, S., Zong, Z., & Gao, M. (2020). PD-L1-mediated immunosuppression in glioblastoma is associated with the infiltration and M2-polarization of tumor-associated macrophages. *Frontiers in Immunology*, *11*, 588552. Advance online publication. DOI: 10.3389/fimmu.2020.588552 PMID: 33329573

Chapter 6
In-Vitro and In-Vivo Models for Glioblastoma

Ramakrishna Gummadi
https://orcid.org/0000-0001-6576-3576
School of Pharmacy, Aditya University, Surampalem, India

Pindiprolu S. S. Sai Kiran
School of Pharmacy, Aditya University, Surampalem, India

Vithanala Srinivasa Rao
Lydia College of Pharmacy, Ravulapalem, India

Vaka Jyothi krishna Reddy
Srinivasa Rao College of Pharmacy, Visakhapatnam, India

Chirravuri S. Phani Kumar
School of Pharmacy, Aditya University, Surampalem, India

ABSTRACT

Glioblastoma multiforme (GBM) is the most aggressive primary brain tumor in adults, marked by high heterogeneity, invasiveness, and resistance to standard therapies. This chapter critically reviews current in vitro and in vivo GBM models, emphasizing their roles in mimicking tumor biology, therapeutic response, and tumor microenvironment dynamics. Advanced 3D systems, patient-derived organoids, and genetically engineered models offer improved physiological relevance, while innovative platforms such as bioprinted tissues and tumor-on-chip systems pave the way for personalized medicine. Despite technological advances, a translational gap persists between laboratory findings and clinical outcomes. This work advocates for integrative modeling approaches and ethical compliance to enhance translational potential and precision oncology in GBM research.

DOI: 10.4018/979-8-3373-2695-5.ch006

1. INTRODUCTION

Glioblastoma multiforme (GBM) represents the most aggressive and lethal form of primary brain tumors in adults, currently classified as Grade IV astrocytoma under the 2021 World Health Organization (WHO) Central Nervous System (CNS) tumor classification. GBM is characterized by its highly invasive nature, extensive heterogeneity, rapid cell proliferation, and resistance to conventional therapeutic modalities. Despite being relatively rare in comparison to other cancers, it comprises approximately 15% of all primary intracranial neoplasms and nearly 45–50% of all gliomas. The disease imposes a substantial global health burden, both in terms of clinical management and socioeconomic costs (Zhang et al., 2023b).

The global incidence rate of GBM ranges from 3.2 to 4.17 cases per 100,000 person-years, with higher incidence observed in developed nations, possibly due to more widespread access to diagnostic tools and comprehensive cancer registries. In contrast, regions such as India face a dual burden of underreporting and limited awareness, although recent improvements in imaging infrastructure have led to better detection rates. Epidemiological studies indicate a male predominance, with peak incidence typically occurring between the ages of 45 and 70 years (Zhang et al., 2023a).

The prognosis for GBM remains grim despite the standard-of-care treatment consisting of maximal safe surgical resection, followed by concurrent chemoradiotherapy with temozolomide (TMZ) and adjuvant TMZ therapy. Median survival ranges from 12 to 15 months, and the 5-year survival rate is estimated to be less than 6%. This poor prognosis is attributed to the tumor's complex biology, aggressive infiltrative growth, and resistance to both chemotherapy and radiation (Zhang et al., 2023c).

One of the defining features of GBM is its profound molecular heterogeneity. Genomic and transcriptomic analyses have revealed multiple hallmark alterations, including amplification of the epidermal growth factor receptor (EGFR), loss or mutation of the tumor suppressor PTEN, isocitrate dehydrogenase (IDH1/2) mutation status, TP53 alterations, and methylation of the O6-methylguanine-DNA methyltransferase (MGMT) promoter. These molecular features are not only critical for tumor classification but also play a central role in therapeutic response and resistance. Furthermore, the 2021 WHO classification emphasizes the distinction between IDH-wildtype glioblastomas, which carry a worse prognosis, and IDH-mutant astrocytomas, which typically have more favorable outcomes (Ye et al., 2023).

Another significant barrier to successful treatment is the presence of the blood-brain barrier (BBB) and the blood-tumor barrier (BTB), which limit the penetration of therapeutic agents into the brain parenchyma. GBM's immunosuppressive tumor microenvironment (TME), characterized by regulatory T cells, tumor-associated macrophages (TAMs), and myeloid-derived suppressor cells (MDSCs), further reduces the efficacy of immune-based therapies. The interplay of cellular and acellular elements within the TME contributes to treatment evasion and tumor recurrence (Ye et al., 2025).

Given these complexities, there is an urgent need for reliable preclinical models that can recapitulate the multifaceted nature of GBM. Research in this domain has increasingly focused on both **in vitro** and **in vivo** modeling systems that simulate tumor biology, heterogeneity, therapeutic resistance, and interactions with the TME and BBB. In vitro models, such as two-dimensional (2D) monolayer cultures and three-dimensional (3D) spheroids and organoids, provide platforms for drug screening, gene editing, and mechanistic studies under controlled conditions. However, these systems often lack the physiological complexity necessary to replicate clinical responses (Xu et al., 2023).

On the other hand, in vivo models—including genetically engineered mouse models (GEMMs), patient-derived xenografts (PDXs), syngeneic models, and humanized mouse systems—offer a more representative tumor-host interface and are vital for evaluating immunotherapies, pharmacokinetics, and treatment efficacy in a living organism. Despite their advantages, these models are resource-intensive, time-consuming, and raise ethical considerations (Xu et al., 2023).

Emerging technologies such as 3D bioprinting, microfluidic tumor-on-chip platforms, and exosome-based delivery systems are now being employed to overcome the limitations of traditional models. In particular, patient-derived glioblastoma organoids (GBOs) have shown promise in maintaining tumor heterogeneity and mimicking the spatial organization of GBM tissues. Furthermore, computational biology, artificial intelligence (AI), and systems-level modeling have revolutionized the way researchers analyze large-scale data sets from platforms like The Cancer Genome Atlas (TCGA), Genomic Data Commons (GDC), and the Gene Expression Omnibus (GEO). These tools are increasingly integrated with experimental research to guide biomarker discovery, predict therapeutic responses, and facilitate personalized treatment planning (Xie et al., 2023).

Despite significant progress, bridging the gap between preclinical research and clinical application remains a challenge. Many therapies that demonstrate efficacy in laboratory models fail during human clinical trials due to species differences, lack of tumor complexity, or poor model reproducibility. Thus, a multidimensional and integrative approach combining various model systems is crucial for advancing translational research in GBM (Wu et al., 2023).

This chapter provides a comprehensive analysis of current and emerging **in vitro** and **in vivo** models used in glioblastoma research. It explores their individual merits, limitations, and relevance to modern-day clinical applications. Special emphasis is placed on novel methodologies such as co-culture systems, exosome-based delivery, and organ-on-chip technologies. Additionally, the ethical and regulatory aspects of model development and the role of patient-derived systems in advancing precision oncology are discussed. By critically evaluating these tools, this chapter aims to guide researchers in selecting the most suitable models for investigating GBM pathophysiology and developing next-generation therapies aimed at improving patient outcomes (Wen et al., 2024; Behrooz et al., 2023).

Figure 1. In-vitro models for glioblastoma

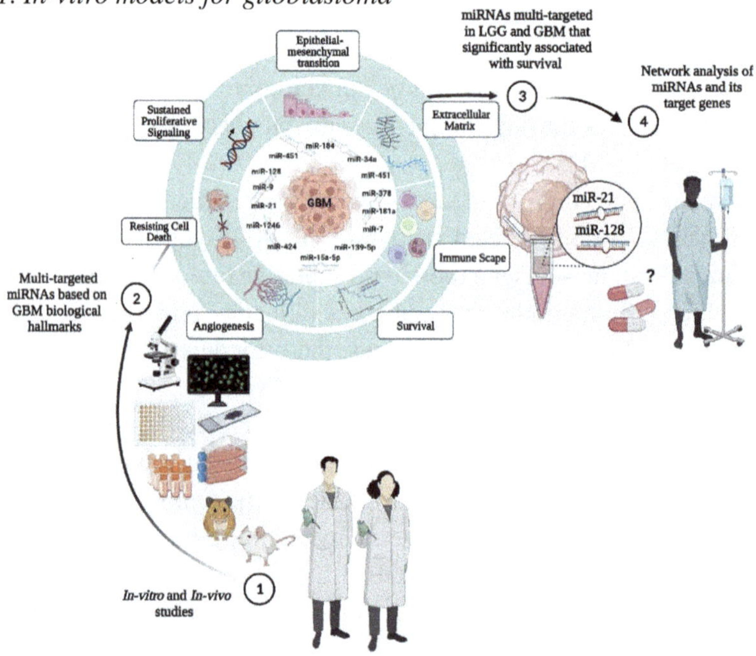

2. IN VITRO MODELS FOR GLIOBLASTOMA RESEARCH

In vitro models are the cornerstone of preclinical glioblastoma (GBM) research, offering accessible and scalable platforms for studying tumor biology, screening therapeutic agents, and dissecting genetic and molecular mechanisms underlying disease progression. Among these, two-dimensional (2D) monolayer cultures have historically been the most widely used due to their ease of use, cost-effectiveness, and reproducibility. However, the emergence of advanced three-dimensional (3D) systems, patient-derived models, and microengineered platforms has transformed in vitro modeling into a more physiologically relevant and clinically informative approach (Wei et al., 2023).

2.1 Two-Dimensional GBM Cell Lines: Tools and Limitations

Established GBM cell lines such as U87-MG, U251, LN229, and T98G remain foundational in glioma studies. These cell lines enable consistent results across laboratories and are instrumental for studying cellular pathways, assessing drug cytotoxicity, and conducting gene editing experiments.

Table 1. Comparative features of commonly used GBM cell lines

Cell Line	Origin	Key Mutations	MGMT Status	Invasiveness	Primary Use
U87-MG	Human GBM	PTEN mutation, wild-tye p53	Unmethylated	Low	Drug screening
U251	Human GBM	Mutant p53, EGFR amplification	Methylated	Moderate	Apoptosis studies
LN229	Human GBM	Mutant p53, PTEN wild-type	Methylated	High	Migration & invasion
T98G	Human GBM	Mutant p53, PTEN mutation	Unmethylated	Low	Chemoresistance assays

Despite their utility, these cell lines are not without limitations. Long-term culturing can lead to **genetic drift**, causing divergence from the original tumor phenotype. For example, U87-MG—one of the most cited GBM lines—has a genetic profile significantly distinct from patient-derived tumors. Additionally, 2D monolayers lack the spatial architecture and mechanical forces present in native brain tissue, resulting in incomplete modeling of GBM pathophysiology (Wanigasekara et al., 2023).

2.2 Limitations of 2D Monolayer Cultures

Monolayer cultures are inherently limited in their ability to mimic the tumor microenvironment (TME). The absence of 3D cellular architecture, hypoxia gradients, and extracellular matrix (ECM) components leads to unrealistic drug diffusion profiles and cell behaviors. Moreover, these systems lack the presence of endothelial cells, astrocytes, microglia, and immune cells, all of which are crucial contributors to glioblastoma's growth, invasiveness, and therapeutic resistance. Consequently, drug responses in 2D models often fail to correlate with outcomes observed in clinical settings (Wang et al., 2023).

2.3 Advancements in 3D GBM Models

To overcome the shortcomings of 2D systems, various 3D cell culture technologies have been developed. Spheroids, scaffolds, and hydrogels enable a more realistic tumor structure, promoting cell–cell and cell–ECM interactions and establishing nutrient and oxygen gradients that resemble in vivo tumors. GBM spheroids exhibit increased resistance to radiotherapy and chemotherapy, mimicking clinical treatment responses more closely than their 2D counterparts (Urzi et al., 2023).

One of the most transformative innovations is 3D bioprinting, which allows for the spatial deposition of multiple cell types, ECM proteins, and growth factors. This approach facilitates the engineering of complex tumor models, incorporating glioma-associated macrophages, endothelial cells, and pericytes. These bioprinted constructs recapitulate processes such as angiogenesis, immune evasion, and tumor invasion, offering advanced platforms for drug testing and mechanistic studies (Tu et al., 2023).

2.4 CRISPR/Cas9-Modified GBM Cell Models

The advent of CRISPR-Cas9 genome editing has enabled the precise manipulation of genetic elements within GBM cells. Researchers can now create isogenic cell lines that harbor or correct mutations in oncogenes and tumor suppressors such as EGFR, PTEN, TP53, and IDH1/2. These genetically engineered models provide insight into the functional consequences of specific alterations and their influence on drug resistance and tumor progression. When combined with 3D organoids, CRISPR models enable targeted exploration of subtype-specific vulnerabilities, facilitating the development of precision therapies (Tong et al., 2023).

2.5 Patient-Derived Glioblastoma Cell Models

Patient-derived in vitro models are increasingly recognized as superior alternatives to conventional cell lines. Primary GBM cultures and glioblastoma stem-like cells (GSCs) retain genetic, phenotypic, and epigenetic features of the parental tumor, including its heterogeneity. GSCs, cultured under neurosphere-forming conditions in serum-free media supplemented with EGF and bFGF, maintain expression of stem cell markers like CD133, Nestin, and SOX2 (Tang et al., 2023).

These models demonstrate significant resistance to conventional therapies, reflecting the refractory nature of glioblastoma stem cells in patients. However, culturing these cells poses challenges: they require specialized media, exhibit clonal selection over passages, and may lose heterogeneity over time (Sun et al., 2023).

To address these limitations, researchers are developing co-culture systems that combine GSCs with components of the brain microenvironment such as astrocytes, microglia, and endothelial cells. These composite cultures more accurately replicate tumor–host interactions, immune modulation, and extracellular matrix remodeling (Slika et al., 2023).

2.6 Tumor-on-a-Chip Platforms

Microfluidic-based tumor-on-chip technologies represent a frontier in glioblastoma modeling. These systems mimic dynamic parameters such as fluid shear stress, nutrient flow, and drug perfusion, offering a controlled environment for real-time monitoring of tumor responses. Incorporating BBB-mimicking endothelial layers and patient-derived GBM cells enables studies on barrier permeability, drug transport, and cellular migration (Singh et al., 2024).

Tumor-on-chip devices are particularly useful for assessing the efficacy of nanoparticle-based delivery systems and immunotherapies, as they allow integration of immune cells and visualization of infiltration and activation events (Shi et al., 2023).

2.7 Exosome- and Nanoparticle-Based Co-Cultures

Exosomes: small extracellular vesicles ranging from 30 to 160 nm—play a crucial role in cell-to-cell communication in glioblastoma. They mediate chemoresistance, angiogenesis, and immune suppression. In vitro co-culture systems utilizing mesenchymal stem cell (MSC)-derived exosomes have demonstrated the potential to deliver therapeutic agents such as rapamycin and siRNAs directly to GBM cells (Sharp et al., 2023).

These exosomes facilitate drug delivery across the BBB and respond to tumor-specific pH gradients, enhancing drug release at the tumor site. Incorporating such vesicles into 3D GBM models allows for the study of vesicle-mediated signaling and evaluation of novel delivery platforms (Schweiger & Kievit, 2025).

2.8 Advantages and Challenges of In Vitro Models

Table 2. Comparison of Advanced In Vitro GBM Models

Model Type	Key Advantages	Main Challenges
2D Monolayers	Simple, cost-effective, easy to manipulate	Lack TME, poor predictive value
3D Spheroids	Mimic gradients, better resistance profiles	Standardization difficulties
Organoids	Preserve heterogeneity, realistic architecture	Lack vasculature, immune components
Bioprinted Models	Tunable complexity, incorporate ECM/cell types	High cost, requires advanced equipment
Tumor-on-a-Chip	Dynamic drug testing, mimics BBB and flow	Emerging field, limited accessibility

Future directions include integrating vascular networks, immune cell populations, and patient-derived matrices into these systems. Coupling in vitro data with computational modeling and machine learning algorithms may enable real-time prediction of patient-specific drug responses (Sandbhor et al., 2023).

2.9 Advanced Patient-Derived Platforms: Xenografts and Stem-Like Models

Beyond in vitro cultures, **patient-derived xenograft (PDX) models** serve as a bridge to in vivo research. These involve implanting fresh tumor tissue into immunocompromised mice, preserving the genetic and histological architecture of the original tumor. While highly informative, PDX models are limited by their lack of an intact human immune system, long establishment times, and engraftment variability (Rubenich et al., 2023).

Glioblastoma stem-like cells (GSCs) remain a vital tool for modeling tumor recurrence and therapy resistance. Their plasticity and survival under therapeutic stress make them key targets for **novel anti-stem therapies**. Combined with **single-cell RNA sequencing**, GSC cultures can now be used to map transcriptional heterogeneity and trace clonal evolution (Roque et al., 2023).

2.10 Co-Culture and Microenvironment Models:

Glioblastoma immunotherapy presents significant challenges due to the tumor's highly immunosuppressive microenvironment, characterized by low immune cell infiltration and inactivity. Toll-like receptor agonists have shown promise as immune adjuvants, However, their use as monotherapy in clinical trials has not resulted in improved patient outcomes. A potential strategy to enhance their efficacy involves combining them with immunogenic cell death-inducing agents such as doxorubicin in a nanoparticulate formulation. To explore this approach, lipid nanoparticle formulations incorporating the Toll-like receptor agonists CpG and polyinosinic/polycytidylic acid (pIpC), both with and without doxorubicin, were developed. These formulations achieved an encapsulation efficiency exceeding 75% and an average particle size below 140 nm. In vitro studies demonstrated that lipid nanoparticle pIpC exhibited superior activation of bone marrow-derived immune cells, including dendritic cells and macrophages, with minimal toxicity compared to CpG. Furthermore, pIpC formulations were found to promote macrophage polarization toward the antitumorigenic Ml phenotype while enhancing macrophage-mediated phagocytosis of cancer cells. When administered intratumorally, lipid nanoparticles containing pIpC and doxorubicin resulted in significant immune cell infiltration and activation within the tumor microenvironment. Survival studies indicated that incorporating doxorubicin into pIpC lipid nanoparticles improved overall survival in mice compared to control groups. However, the addition of doxorubicin did not provide a statistically significant survival advantage over pIpC lipid nanoparticles alone. These findings highlight the potential of pIpC-based lipid nanoparticle formulations in glioblastoma immunotherapy. Future research will focus on optimizing dosing regimens and exploring combination strategies with standard treatments such as temozolomide, immune checkpoint inhibitors, or cancer vaccines to enhance therapeutic outcomes (Ravn-Boess et al., 2023).

Exosomes, nanosized membranous vesicles ranging from 30 to 160 nm, have been recognized as an effective drug delivery system capable of crossing biological barriers. Mesenchymal stem cells, known for their extensive self-renewal capabilities, serve as a valuable source of exosomes for clinical applications. In this study, an exosome-based drug delivery approach utilizing exosome-encapsulated rapamycin was investigated to enhance drug efficacy while minimizing dosage requirements. This strategy allows for achieving therapeutic effects typically observed at higher drug concentrations while improving treatment efficiency. Exosomes possess the ability to transport pharmaceuticals across the blood-brain barrier and effectively penetrate glioblastoma cells to exert therapeutic effects. Within the tumor microenvironment, exosome-encapsulated rapamycin is released more efficiently, particularly under acidic tumor conditions, which accelerate drug release. This pH-responsive characteristic highlights its potential as a targeted therapy for glioblastoma. In vivo experiments further confirmed the capability of exosome-encapsulated rapamycin to permeate the blood-brain barrier and accumulate at tumor sites. Additionally, it demonstrated the ability to reduce inflammatory responses in glioblastoma mouse models while enhancing anti-tumor activity by regulating angiogenesis through the VEGF/VEGFRs signaling pathway. These findings suggest that mesenchymal stem cell-derived exosomes are a promising therapeutic carrier for glioblastoma, offering an effective strategy for improving drug delivery across the blood-brain barrier. The study provides a strong scientific basis for the potential application of exosome-based therapies in glioblastoma treatment and other neurological diseases (Petković et al., 2023).

Glioblastomas are highly malignant central nervous system tumors characterized by significant sub-clonal diversity and the ability to dynamically adapt within complex developmental hierarchies. However, the mechanisms underlying this spatial reorganization remain unclear. In this study, glioblastomas were analyzed using spatially resolved transcriptomic, metabolomics, and proteomics to better understand their regional heterogeneity and adaptive responses. Through an examination of shared transcriptional programs across different tumor regions in multiple patients, findings suggest that glioblastoma is structured by spatial segregation of lineage states while dynamically responding to inflammatory and metabolic stimuli. This adaptation resembles the reactive transformation observed in mature astrocytes. Further integration of metabolic imaging with imaging mass cytometry revealed locoregional tumor-host interactions, which drive spatially distinct transcriptional adaptations (Pérez-López et al., 2023). Analysis of copy-number alterations highlighted a spatially cohesive sub-clonal organization, where environmental stress induces selective pressures leading to reactive transcriptional programs. Additionally, glioblastoma stem cell models implanted into human and rodent neocortical tissue demonstrated that transcriptional states emerge through continuous adaptation to distinct environmental conditions. These findings provide deeper insight into glioblastoma plasticity and the influence of the tumor microenvironment on its evolution (Oraiopoulou et al., 2024).

3. IN VIVO MODELS FOR GLIOBLASTOMA

In vivo models play a crucial role in understanding GBM pathophysiology and developing novel therapeutic strategies. These models aim to replicate the tumor's genetic, molecular, andhistological features to provide insights into tumor progression, invasion, and therapeutic response (Obozina et al., 2023; Bayat et al., 2023).

Figure 2. In vivo models for glioblastoma

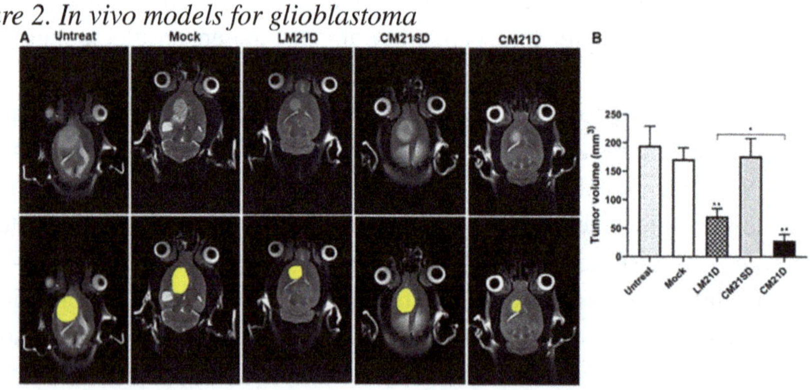

3.1 Xenograft Models

Glioblastoma multiforme (GBM) is an extremely aggressive type of primary brain tumor, characterized by its complexity, rapid invasion, and resistance to standard therapies. The prognosis remains poor due to tumor's ability to evade treatment and physiological barriers that limit drug penetration into the brain. Conventional treatment approaches, including surgical resection, radiotherapy, and chemotherapy with temozolomide (TMZ), often face challenges in effectively targeting GBM cells. The blood-brain barrier (BBB) and the blood-brain tumor barrier (BBTB) further restrict the delivery of therapeutic agents, making treatment even more difficult. To overcome these obstacles, research has increasingly focused on nanotechnology-based drug delivery systems. Nano carriers, such as polymeric, metallic, and lipid-based nanoparticles, including solid lipid nanoparticles (SLNs) and nanostructured lipid carriers (NLCs), provide benefits in terms of drug stability, controlled release, and enhanced bioavailability. Additionally, metallic nanoparticles, such as gold and silver nanoparticles, show promise in imaging applications and photo thermal therapy, potentially improving conventional treatment outcomes. This review explores the mechanisms by which Nano carriers facilitate drug delivery across these barriers, emphasizing the influence of key physiochemical properties such as particle size, surface change, and functionalization. The integration of nanotechnology into GBM treatment presents a promising avenue for overcoming current therapeutic limitations, with the potential to significantly improve patient outcomes by enhancing drug delivery and targeting tumor cells more effectively. As advancements in nanomedicine continue to evolve, they may lead to more innovative and efficient treatment strategies for managing GBM (Nikam & Jain, 2023).High-grade glioblastomas are characterized by immature, leaky tumor vasculature, which compromises the effectiveness of adjuvant therapies. In this study, we evaluated the potential of locally delivered human interferon (hIFN)-, administered through gene transfer, to promote vascular stabilization in an orthotropic glioblastoma xenograft resection model (Merenzon et al., 2023).The document examines patient-derived xenograft (PDX) models as valuable tools in cancer search, emphasizing their benefits, challenges, and recent advancements. These models, developed by implanting tumor tissues from patients into immunodeficient mice, preserve essential tumor characteristics, making them a more reliable platform for drug development and precision medicine compared to conventional cell line models. Various factors influencing the success of PDX models, such as tumor type, implantation techniques, and host selection, are analyzed. Additionally, alternative models, including organoids, MiniPDX, and humanized mice, are explored as potential improvements in cancer treatment approaches. Despite their advantages, PDX models present obstacles such as high costs, lengthy development processes, and limitations related to immune system compatibility. Advancements incorporating bioinformatics, CRISPR, and high-throughput screening seek to enhance these models for more effective clinical applications. The study highlights the significant role of PDX models in advancing personalized cancer treatment and improving therapeutic outcomes (Lopes et al., 2023). Cancer immunotherapy has provided substantial clinical benefits to patients, including those with lung cancer. Patient–derived tumor xenograft mouse models have become the preferred platforms for translational cancer research and preclinical investigation. Due to the ongoing need for more predictive models in immuno-oncology, humanized mouse models –engineered with both human tumors and immune system components – have been developed to evaluate novel immnunotherapeutic strategies. These models have also been utilized to predict immune-related adverse effects and identify potential predictive biomarkers. This review examines key aspects of humanized mouse models, including methods. This review examines key aspects of humanized mouse models, including method for their development, essential factors for successful establishments, associated limitations, and critical considerations for selecting appropriate models in preclinical lung cancer immune-oncology research and therapeutic studies (Liu et al., 2023). The complexity of modelling tumor-immune cell accessible tumor models were created by transforming primary skin fibroblasts or induced pluripotent stem cell-derived lines, which are subsequently injected into immunodeficient mice reconstituted with human autologous immune cells. The results indicated that fibroblastic, hepatic and neural tumors were successfully infiltrated and, in certain cases, partially or entirely eliminated by autologous immune cells. Further analysis of tumor-immune infiltrates revealed high expression level of dysfunction markers Tim3 and PD-1 in T cells, along with an increased presence of regulatory T cells, suggesting a rapid onset of immunomodulatory phenotypes. Administrations of the PD-1 inhibitor Nivolumab led to greater immune cell infiltration and a slight decrease in tumor growth. These adaptable and accessible cancer models have the potential to advances preclinical research and support the evaluation of autologous cancer immunotherapies across various tumor types (Liu et al., 2023).

3.2. Genetically Engineered Mouse Models (GEMMs):

Brain tumors are known for their aggressive and heterogeneous nature, making treatment highly challenging. Their sensitive location, along with the presence of the blood-brain barrier (BBB), significantly restricts the entry of bioactive compounds into brain tissue, limiting the effectiveness of conventional therapies. Consequently, novel treatment strategies should aim to enhance the efficacy of existing therapeutics, overcome biological barriers, and introduce innovative methods for tumor elimination. In recent years, the use of carbohydrate polymers in cancer treatment has gained attention due to their biocompatibility, biodegradability, and ability to selectively target tumor cells. Carbohydrate polymer-based nanoparticles offer advantages such as efficient drug loading and encapsulation, making them suitable for delivering bioactive compounds to brain tumors. These nanoparticles have been developed to improve drug and gene delivery while also enhancing the effectiveness of chemotherapy and immunotherapy. Additionally, they have shown potential in facilitating combination therapies and improving phototherapy-mediated tumor ablation. Their favorable characteristics, including optimal particle size, zeta potential, and encapsulation efficiency, make them promising candidates for brain tumor treatment. Furthermore, their high biocompatibility suggests potential applications in clinical studies (Liu et al., 2023).

Multimodal treatment strategies such as surgery, radiation, and chemotherapy, survival rates remain poor. Advances in molecular profiling have identified key genetic mutations, including EGFR amplification, TP53 alterations, and PTEN loss, which influence prognosis and therapeutic response. Targeted therapies have been developed to disrupt specific oncogenic pathways, but resistance mechanisms, tumor heterogeneity, and the tumor microenvironment (TME) continue to pose significant challenges. Immunotherapies, including immune checkpoint inhibitors and CAR T-cell therapies, have been explored, but their efficacy is limited by the immunosuppressive TME. Other emerging strategies, such as biopolymer-based interstitial therapies, focused ultrasound for blood-brain barrier disruption, and nanoparticle-based drug delivery, show promise in improving treatment efficacy. The document emphasizes the need for personalized medicine, combination therapies, and innovative drug delivery systems to enhance patient outcomes. Despite recent advancements in molecular and genetic profiling, glioblastoma remains a formidable challenge due to its complexity and resistance mechanisms. Targeted therapies and immunotherapies offer potential, but their effectiveness is often undermined by tumor heterogeneity and the immunosuppressive TME. Innovative drug delivery approaches, including nanoparticle-based systems and focused ultrasound, may enhance treatment precision and overcome current barriers. Moving forward, integrating personalized medicine and combination therapies tailored to individual genetic profiles is critical to improving survival rates and quality of life for GBM patients. Ongoing research and multidisciplinary collaboration are essential to translating these advancements into clinical success (39). The early progression of glioblastoma, a stage that remains poorly understood. By introducing PDGFB and genetic barcodes into the mouse brain, researchers initiated gliomagenesis and directly traced glioblastoma evolution from its earliest phase. Unexpectedly, a high frequency of clonal extinction events and increasing divergence in clonal sizes were observed, even after the malignant phenotype was established. Computational modeling indicated that these patterns were driven by clonal-based cell-cell competition. Transcriptomic and lineage-tracing analyses identified Myc transcriptional targets as the strongest predictors of clonal size imbalances. Furthermore, the downregulation of Myc expression was found to induce competitive dynamics in intracranial transplanted gliomas. These findings offer new insights into glioblastoma evolution, demonstrating the potential of integrating clonal tracing with transcriptomic analysis to uncover early tumor progression mechanisms (Li et al., 2023).

Table 3. Advantages and limitations of glioblastoma organoid models

MODEL	ADVANTAGES	LIMITATION
Genetically engineered mice (He et al., 2017; Hassanzadeganroudsari et al., 2020; Fiedler et al., 2015)	Investigation of phenotypic consequences of GB progression [eg: tissue invasion]	Lack of clinical validation difficulties in reproducing human tumor heterogeneity expensive and time consuming
Mouse embryonic brain (Ip et al., 2023; Ibrahim et al., 2023)	Feasibility to investigate immune interaction	Difficulties in assessing clinical relevance technical issue due to in utero electroporation
Human stem cells (Ge et al., 2013; Bona et al., 2024)	Feasibility to investigate human GB onset easiness in experimental standardization	Absence of fundamental physiological components [eg:immune and endothelial cells]
Human cerebral organoids (jang et al., 2023; Kim et al., 2018)	Assessment of human GB development, microenvironmental interaction in a 3Dcontext possibility to co-culture cancer cells with healthy neuronal cells	Lack of fundamental physiological components [eg: immune and endothelial cells]

3.3 Syngeneic Murine Models

The immunotherapeutic advancements in glioblastoma (GBM) treatment, specifically the combination of interleukin-12 (IL-12) with chimeric antigen receptor (CAR) T-cell therapy. GBM remains a highly aggressive brain tumor with limited treatment success due to its immunosuppressive tumor microenvironment (TME). Targeting EGFRvIII, a tumor-specific mutation present in over 30% of GBM cases, CAR T-cell therapy has shown promise but remains ineffective in many patients due to TME-related resistance. This study investigated the impact of locally administered IL-12 in a syngeneic murine GBM model treated with anti-EGFRvIII-CAR T cells. The results demonstrated that a single dose of IL-12 significantly improved CAR T-cell efficacy, leading to increased survival, enhanced pro-inflammatory and cytotoxic activity, and extensive remodeling of the TME. IL-12 effectively transformed GBM from an immunologically "cold" tumor into a more responsive state, allowing for better CAR T-cell function. Additional sections of the document highlight other immunotherapeutic strategies, including engineered adenovirus-based approaches to enhance T-cell therapies and novel small-molecule inhibitors targeting the PD1-PDL1 interaction. These findings support the development of combination therapies to improve GBM treatment outcomes. This study underscores the potential of IL-12 as an adjuvant therapy to enhance CAR T-cell treatment in GBM. The findings suggest that IL-12 not only improves the cytotoxic function of CAR T cells but also reshapes the TME, making the tumor more susceptible to immunotherapy.

The study reinforces the need for combinatorial approaches in GBM treatment (Li et al., 2023; Li et al., 2024).

Glioblastoma (GBM) remains challenging to treat due to its immunosuppressive tumor microenvironment (TME). CAR T-cell therapy targeting EGFRvIII—a mutation found in over 30% of GBM cases—has shown limited success due to TME resistance. Recent research using a syngeneic murine model demonstrated that a single local dose of interleukin-12 (IL-12) significantly enhanced the efficacy of anti-EGFRvIII CAR T cells. IL-12 boosted pro-inflammatory responses, improved cytotoxicity, and reprogrammed the TME, transforming it from "cold" to immunologically active. The study also explored other strategies, such as engineered adenoviruses and PD1-PDL1 inhibitors, reinforcing the potential of combinatorial therapies. Overall, IL-12 shows promise as an adjuvant to enhance CAR T-cell therapy and improve GBM treatment outcomes (Kumari et al., 2023; Khan et al., 2024).

3.4 Alertnative animal model

The development of alternative non-animal models has opened new possibilities for personalized treatment approaches. Advanced 2D and 3D models, including neurospheres, organoids, tissue-slice cultures, bioprinting, and tumor-on-a-chip systems, have shown great potential in replicating the tumor microenvironment and predicting patient-specific treatment responses. Each model has distinct advantages: organoids maintain tumor heterogeneity, bioprinted models simulate cellular interactions, and tumor-on-a-chip systems offer dynamic drug testing environments. Despite their benefits, these models still face challenges, including limited immune system components, lack of vascularization, and difficulties in long-term culture maintenance. Recent clinical trials and case studies have successfully translated in vitro findings into real-world patient treatments, suggesting a promising future for these models in precision oncology. As technology progresses, further improvements—such as integrating immune components, vascular networks, and patient-specific genetic profiles—will enhance their clinical relevance and reduce dependence on animal models. These alternative approaches represent a significant advancement toward more ethical, effective, and personalized treatments for glioblastoma (Jia et al., 2023). The anticancer potential of a series of synthesized Ru(II)–arene PTA complexes has been thoroughly evaluated. Experimental findings indicate that one particular complex outperforms the others, exhibiting remarkable fluorescence properties with the highest quantum yield, strong DNA binding ability, significant BSA binding affinity, and notable DNA cleavage activity. A detailed analysis of the cytotoxic profile of these complexes revealed that one complex demonstrated the highest potency against T98 and U87MG cell lines, while another was the most effective against the LN229 cancer cell line. The antiproliferative activity of these complexes was attributed to DNA cleavage, oxidative stress induction, neurotoxic behavior, and VEGF downregulation under hypoxic conditions. Further investigation confirmed that one complex played a crucial role in mediating G0/G1 phase cell cycle arrest at its IC50 concentration. Real-time reverse transcription polymerase chain reaction (RT-PCR) studies demonstrated that the complex effectively inhibited TNF-α-induced NF-κB phosphorylation in glioma cells. Additionally, it was observed that at a concentration of 50 μM, the complex exhibited no toxicity for up to 72 hours, suggesting that RAPTA complexes are biocompatible for in vivo studies. Biodistribution studies further confirmed the selective accumulation of ruthenium complexes in glioblastoma cells via blood–brain barrier penetration. These findings suggest that all the synthesized complexes hold significant potential as anticancer agents for future applications (Jang et al., 2023). The development and validation of a porcine-human glioblastoma xenograft model utilizing immunosuppressed Yucatan minipigs successfully addressed the limitations of small animal models, such as rodents. The larger cranial structure of pigs closely resembles the human brain, providing a more suitable platform for precise surgical and imaging studies. Tumor growth was effectively established in immunosuppressed pigs, with a combined regimen of cyclosporine, prednisone, and mycophenolate demonstrating greater efficacy compared to cyclosporine alone. MRI imaging confirmed tumor formation and its infiltration into surrounding normal brain tissue, revealing histopathological characteristics similar to spontaneous human glioblastomas. Furthermore, intraoperative image updating successfully corrected for brain shift, emphasizing the model's utility in enhancing neurosurgical procedures. While this model offers significant advantages, certain challenges remain, including the necessity for continuous immunosuppression, higher costs, and complex maintenance requirements. Nevertheless, it provides a reproducible and clinically relevant system for investigating glioblastoma progression, evaluating innovative imaging techniques, and refining surgical approaches, making it a valuable asset in translational brain tumor research (Ip et al., 2023).

4. COMPARATIVE ANALYSIS OF IN VITRO AND IN VIVO MODELS

Glioblastoma research employs both in vitro and in vivo models to explore tumor biology and develop therapies. In vitro models, including 2D cultures and 3D organoids, offer controlled environments for studying cellular behavior but lack the full complexity of the tumor microenvironment. Innovations like bioprinting and tumor-on-a-chip systems enhance simulation of GBM heterogeneity, though limitations in vascularization and immune components persist(48). In vivo models, such as patient-derived xenografts and genetically engineered mice, provide more physiologically relevant insights but face challenges like high costs and species-specific differences. Emerging large-animal models, like porcine-human xenografts, improve anatomical accuracy for surgical and imaging studies. Integrating advanced in vitro systems with in vivo models is essential for a comprehensive understanding of GBM and advancing personalized treatment strategies (Ibrahim et al., 2023; Houweling et al., 2023; Rajan et al., 2023).

Figure 3. Comparative analysis of in vitro and in vivo models

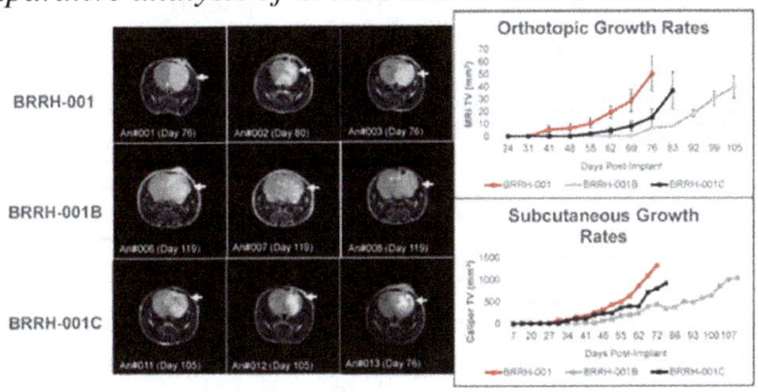

Overview of Preclinical Models in GBM Research: Preclinical models are crucial for understanding glioblastoma (GBM) and developing targeted therapies. While no single model captures GBM's full complexity, combining various approaches offers deeper insights. In vivo models, especially transgenic and patient-derived xenograft (PDX) models, replicate tumor progression and treatment responses, though PDX use in immunocompromised mice limits immunological studies (Rajan et al., 2023). In vitro modelsranging from 2D cultures to advanced 3D systems like spheroids and organoidsallow genetic manipulation but lack full tumor microenvironment replication. Innovations like CRISPR-Cas9 offer precise gene editing, and 3D bioprinting creates vascularized tumor models, though challenges like off-target effects and high costs persist. Future research will benefit from integrating in vivo and engineered in vitro systems to support personalized GBM therapies and improve clinical outcomes (Hao et al., 2023; Gibson et al., 2023).

Table 4. Comparison between 2D, 3D cell culture, and PDX animal models

Test system main features	2D Cell culture	3D Cell culture	PDX animal model
Physiological relevance	Limited	Better than 2D standard culture	Most physiological environment
Model complexity	Limited	Complex	Very complex
Gene expression	Stable at early passages	Close to in vivo tumors	Close to in vivo tumors
Immune system	No but co-culture of cancer cells and immune cells possible	No but co- cultures of cancer cells and immune cell possible	No
Efficient drug screnning	Yes	Yes	No
Disease modeling	Naïve	Feasible	Sophisticated methods
Data provider	Easily exploitable	Easily exploitable	Hardly exploitable
Controlled microenvironment	Yes	Yes	No
Reproducibility	Favorable	Not so favorable	Unsuited
Cost	Low	Some expensive materials and special equipment required	High
Ethical and regulatory issues	No	No	No

Nanotechnology has emerged as a promising approach to addressing these challenges, with nanocarriers specifically designed to enhance targeted drug delivery, enable controlled drug release, and assist in tumor diagnosis. Despite these advantages, obstacles such as high production costs, limited clinical translation, immunogenicity, low tumor cell accumulation, and lack of specificity hinder its widespread application. Therefore, integrating nanocarriers with efficient drug delivery strategies presents an opportunity to overcome these limitations.Convection-enhanced delivery (CED) offers a method for directly and precisely administering therapeutic agents to the affected brain region, thereby improving treatment efficacy. This technique enables the delivery of various therapeutic agents, including drug-loaded nanoparticles, chemotherapeutic drugs, imaging agents, genes, and cells. The present review examines the pathological mechanisms of GBM, challenges associated with brain drug delivery, and the applications of CED in administering nanocarriers, gene-loaded carriers, and immune cells. Additionally, it explores combinational therapeutic strategies, regulatory considerations, clinical translation, and future directions in the field (Gherardini et al., 2023; Ghaznavi et al., 2024).

Bridging the gap between preclinical and clinical research in glioblastoma (GBM) remains a critical challenge due to the complexity of the disease, its resistance to treatment, and the limitations of current research models. While significant advancements have been made in preclinical models, including in vivo and in vitro systems, the translation of these findings into effective clinical therapies has been slow and limited. Preclinical research has provided essential insights into tumor biology, drug mechanisms, and potential therapeutic targets, yet many promising therapies fail in clinical trials due to discrepancies between experimental models and human tumors (Fuentes-Fayos et al., 2023).

To enhance clinical translation, researchers must prioritize the development of more representative preclinical models that accurately mimic the tumor microenvironment, genetic heterogeneity, and drug response of human GBM. The integration of cutting-edge technologies such as nanomedicine, artificial intelligence, and precision medicine may further aid in bridging this gap. Additionally, interdisciplinary collaboration, robust preclinical validation, and well-designed clinical trials are essential to ensuring the safety and efficacy of emerging treatments.

5. FUTURE PERSPECTIVES IN GBM MODELLING

One of the defining features of GBOs is their ability to spontaneously form complex extracellular matrices, which play a significant role in tumor invasion. Additionally, research utilizing GBOs has led to the identification of the ADAM10 inhibitor, GI254023X, which has been shown to reduce tumor spread.Recent advancements in incorporating vasculature, the blood-brain barrier, and immune cells into GBOs are expected to facilitate the discovery of anti-angiogenesis agents and contribute to pharmacokinetics and immunotherapy research. Furthermore, because GBOs can be rapidly derived from patient samples, they offer potential benefits in clinical decision-making and provide a higher predictive value for therapeutic responses compared to traditional GBM models (Elshaer et al., 2023)

Table 5. Table of Recent Advances in Personalized Glioblastoma Models

GRADE / TYPE	WHO grade I	WHO grade II	WHO grade III	WHO Grade IV
Astrocytoma	Pilocytic-Astrocytoma Subependymal gaint cells Astrocytoma	Low grade Astrocytoma	Anaplastic Astrocytoma	Glioblastoma
Oligodendroglioma		Low grade oligodendroglioma	Anaplastic oligodendroglioma	

https://www.mdpi.com/1422-0067/22/2/924

5.1 Advancements in 3D Bioprinting and Organoid Models for GBM Research

Recent progress in 3D bioprinting and organoid-based models has significantly enhanced glioblastoma multiforme (GBM) research by creating more physiologically relevant in vitro systems. These models replicate key tumor microenvironment elements, such as the extracellular matrix, vasculature, and immune interactions, which are not well-captured in traditional 2D cultures. 3D bioprinting enables the integration of various cell types—like macrophages, endothelial, and patient-derived tumor cells—offering a more accurate representation of GBM progression and therapeutic resistance. Organoid models effectively mimic tumor heterogeneity and treatment responses. However, challenges remain in bioink optimization, model reproducibility, and incorporation of the blood-brain barrier (Bayat et al., 2023; Barron et al., 2023).

5.2 Computational Tools in GBM Therapeutics

The fusion of computational modeling with experimental data is transforming GBM drug discovery. In silico methods—such as molecular docking, ADMET profiling, and AI-driven predictions—accelerate the identification of therapeutic targets and compounds, like VEGFA inhibitors. Bioinformatics analyses of genomic databases (e.g., TCGA, GEO) help identify key regulatory genes and potential combination therapies. Nevertheless, computational predictions require biological validation through methods like CRISPR/Cas9 and preclinical models. Combining these tools with liquid biopsy and biomarker analysis could enable more personalized and effective GBM treatments (Bakhtiyari-Ramezani et al., 2024) .

6. ETHICAL AND REGULATORY CONSIDERATIONS

The development and application of glioblastoma (GBM) models, both in vitro and in vivo, demand strict adherence to ethical principles and regulatory guidelines to ensure responsible and reproducible research. As GBM research often involves the use of human tissues, genetic manipulation, and animal testing, ethical considerations are pivotal in upholding scientific integrity and public trust (Ahmed, 2023).

6.1 Ethical Considerations in Human-Derived Models

Human-derived models, including primary cell cultures, organoids, and patient-derived xenografts (PDX), rely on tumor samples obtained during neurosurgical procedures. Ethical use of these tissues requires informed consent from patients, ensuring that they fully understand how their biological material will be used in research. Institutional Ethics Committees (IECs) or Institutional Review Boards (IRBs) must review and approve protocols involving human biospecimens to safeguard donor rights and privacy (Acharekar et al., 2023).

Moreover, the growing use of patient-derived glioblastoma organoids (GBOs) and stem-like cells in personalized medicine raises additional concerns about data confidentiality, storage, and long-term use. Researchers must comply with national and international data protection laws, such as the General Data Protection Regulation (GDPR) in Europe or the Information Technology (Reasonable Security Practices and Procedures and Sensitive Personal Data or Information) Rules in India (Abbott et al., 2023).

6.2 Ethical Considerations in Animal Models

Animal models—particularly rodents—remain a cornerstone of in vivo glioblastoma research. However, their use raises important ethical questions regarding animal welfare. In most countries, researchers must comply with the "3Rs" principle:

- **Replacement**: Use alternatives to animals wherever possible.
- **Reduction**: Use the minimum number of animals required for valid results.
- **Refinement**: Modify procedures to minimize pain and distress.

In India, all animal studies must be approved by the Institutional Animal Ethics Committee (IAEC) and must adhere to the guidelines set by the Committee for the Purpose of Control and Supervision of Experiments on Animals (CPCSEA). Similar oversight is provided by the Institutional Animal Care and Use Committee (IACUC) in the United States.

Protocols must include clear justification for animal use, humane endpoints, analgesic/palliative care measures, and post-procedural monitoring. Non-compliance can result in revocation of project approval or institutional penalties (Zhan et al., 2012; Zanotto-Filho et al., 2012; Yekula et al., 2020).

6.3 Regulation of Genetically Modified Organisms (GMOs)

Glioblastoma research frequently employs genetically engineered mouse models (GEMMs) and CRISPR-edited in vitro systems. These GMOs are regulated under national biosafety laws. In India, the use of GMOs in research falls under the purview of the Department of Biotechnology (DBT) and the Review Committee on Genetic Manipulation (RCGM).

Researchers must submit detailed biosafety assessments and risk mitigation strategies for approval. Biosafety protocols must be rigorously followed in laboratories handling recombinant DNA, viral vectors, and transgenic animals. Similar regulations are enforced by the NIH Guidelines for Research Involving Recombinant or Synthetic Nucleic Acid Molecules in the U.S (Wu et al., 2021; Soni et al., 2021).

7. TRANSLATIONAL CHALLENGES – FROM BENCH TO BEDSIDE

Despite the proliferation of advanced in vitro and in vivo models in glioblastoma (GBM) research, translating laboratory findings into successful clinical therapies remains a significant hurdle. Numerous experimental treatments that demonstrate efficacy in preclinical models often fail in human clinical trials. This "translational gap" results from biological, technical, and regulatory complexities that limit the predictive power of current research models (Nogueira et al., 2011; Nakabayashi & Shimizu, 2012).

7.1 Biological Differences Between Models and Human Tumors

One of the central issues in translation lies in the **biological mismatch** between models and actual human GBM tumors. Many in vitro models, especially traditional 2D monolayers, do not capture the true cellular heterogeneity, invasive nature, or treatment resistance mechanisms seen in patient tumors. Similarly, many widely used GBM cell lines like U87 and T98G have undergone extensive passaging, leading to genetic drift that renders them poor proxies for in vivo tumors.

Even xenograft models, while more advanced, fall short in simulating the immune microenvironment of GBM due to the immunodeficient nature of host mice. As a result, these models often fail to predict immune-based therapy outcomes, including those involving checkpoint inhibitors and CAR T-cell therapies.

Furthermore, the blood-brain barrier (BBB) and its variant—the blood-brain tumor barrier (BBTB)—present significant translational obstacles. Many preclinical models either bypass or poorly mimic these barriers, resulting in overestimation of drug efficacy and underestimation of pharmacokinetic challenges in human patients (Lu et al., 2012; Kim et al., 2018).

7.2 Case Examples of Translational Failures

Several high-profile clinical failures highlight these challenges. For instance:

- **Bevacizumab (Avastin)**, an anti-VEGF antibody, showed encouraging anti-angiogenic activity in preclinical models but failed to extend overall survival in large phase III trials despite initial radiological responses.
- **EGFR-targeted therapies** such as erlotinib and gefitinib also failed to improve outcomes in GBM patients, even though they were effective in cell lines with EGFR overexpression.
- Many **nanoparticle-based therapies** demonstrate enhanced drug delivery in animal models but lack similar success in human trials due to differences in circulation time, immune clearance, and tissue penetration.

These cases underscore the necessity of validating therapeutic candidates in more physiologically relevant models that account for human-specific factors such as metabolism, immune response, and genetic variability (Jensen et al., 2017; Jatyan et al., 2023).

7.3 Challenges in Clinical Trial Design

Another translational barrier stems from the design and execution of clinical trials for GBM. Due to the aggressive nature and poor prognosis of GBM, patient enrollment, stratification, and long-term follow-up are particularly challenging. Trials often lack sufficient power to detect modest benefits, and inappropriate inclusion criteria (e.g., lack of molecular stratification) may obscure potentially beneficial treatments for specific subpopulations.

The failure to incorporate biomarker-driven trial designssuch as testing drug responses in MGMT methylated vs. unmethylated GBM—also contributes to inconclusive results. Adaptive clinical trial designs, which allow for mid-study modifications based on emerging data, are still underutilized in GBM research (Houweling et al., 2023; He et al., 2017).

8. CONCLUSION

Glioblastoma (GBM) is an aggressive and treatment-resistant brain tumor, requiring advanced research models to better understand its pathology and therapeutic responses. In vitro models, including two-dimensional (2D) cell cultures and three-dimensional (3D) organoids, provide controlled environments for experimentation but fail to fully replicate the complexities of the in vivo tumor microenvironment. In contrast, vivo models such as xenografts and genetically engineered mouse models offer a more physiologically relevant system, though they present challenges related to species differences and ethical concerns. The use of patient-derived models and computational methods has further advanced GBM research by facilitating precision medicine approaches, improving drug screening, and identifying potential therapeutic targets. Recent progress in nanotechnology, bioinformatics, and personalized tumor modeling has also contributed to the development of more effective treatment strategies (Bona et al., 2024).

8.1 The Importance of Combining In Vitro and In Vivo Approaches

An integrated approach that combines both in vitro and in vivo models is crucial for accurately representing the complexity of GBM. In vitro systems allow for efficient high-throughput drug screening and mechanistic studies; however, they often fail to capture key aspects such as tumor heterogeneity, immune system interactions, and blood-brain barrier dynamics. In vivo models, while more representative of the tumor's biological environment, can be costly, time-consuming, and sometimes lack direct translational relevance to human patients. The combination of these methodologies, such as patient-derived tumor organoids paired with xenograft models, enhances the reliability of preclinical research and strengthens the translation of experimental findings into clinical applications (Houweling et al., 2023).

8.2 Future Directions for Improving Glioblastoma Models

Further refinement of GBM models should prioritize increasing their physiological relevance. Enhancements such as the incorporation of vascular structures, immune system components, and patient-specific genetic profiles into in vitro systems will contribute to more accurate disease modeling. The advancement of bioprinted tumor-on-a-chip systems and patient-derived organoid models will improve drug screening precision and enhance the prediction of individual therapeutic responses. Additionally, the integration of computational modeling and artificial intelligence can optimize drug discovery by analyzing large-scale biological datasets. Gene editing technologies, such as CRISPR-Cas9, are expected to facilitate the development of genetically accurate GBM models, providing deeper insights into tumor progression and mechanisms of treatment resistance. A multidisciplinary approach that combines bioengineering, computational research, and clinical studies is essential for accelerating the development of effective GBM therapies, ultimately improving patient outcomes and advancing precision medicine (Ożarowski et al., 2025).

REFERENCES

Abbott, R. C., Iliopoulos, M., Watson, K. A., Arcucci, V., Go, M., Hughes-Parry, H. E., & Darcy, P. K. (2023). Human EGFRvIII chimeric antigen receptor T cells demonstrate favorable safety profile and curative responses in orthotopic glioblastoma. *Journal for Immunotherapy of Cancer*, *11*(3), e006444. Advance online publication. DOI: 10.1136/jitc-2022-006444 PMID: 36890859

Acharekar, A., Bachal, K., Shirke, P., Thorat, R., Banerjee, A., Gardi, N., & Dutt, S. (2023). Substrate stiffness regulates the recurrent glioblastoma cell morphology and aggressiveness. *Journal of Neuro-Oncology*, *115*, 107–127. DOI: 10.1007/s11060-023-04412-1 PMID: 36563706

Ahmed, T. J. (2023). Biomaterial-based in vitro 3D modeling of glioblastoma multiforme. *Current Pharmacology Reports*, *1*(03), 177–194. DOI: 10.1007/s40495-023-00334-5 PMID: 38327839

Bakhtiyari-Ramezani, M., Nohekhan, M., Akbari, M. E., Abbasvandi, F., Bayat, M., Akbari, A., & Rezaie, N. (2024). Comparative assessment of direct and indirect cold atmospheric plasma effects, based on helium and argon, on human glioblastoma: An in vitro and in vivo study. *Scientific Reports*, *14*(1), 3578. Advance online publication. DOI: 10.1038/s41598-024-54070-4 PMID: 38347045

Barron, T., Yalçın, B., Mochizuki, A., Cantor, E., Shamardani, K., Tlais, D., & Monje, M. (2023). CNSC-01. GABAergic neuron-to-glioma synapses in diffuse midline gliomas. *Neuro-Oncology*, *25*(Supplement_1), i11. DOI: 10.1093/neuonc/noad073.044

Bayat, H., Pourgholami, M. H., Rahmani, S., Pournajaf, S., & Mowla, S. J. (2023). Synthetic miR-21 decoy circularized by tRNA splicing mechanism inhibited tumorigenesis in glioblastoma in vitro and in vivo models. *Molecular Therapy. Nucleic Acids*, *32*, 432–444. DOI: 10.1016/j.omtn.2023.04.001 PMID: 37181451

Behrooz, A. B., Latifi-Navid, H., Nezhadi, A., Świat, M., Los, M., Jamalpoor, Z., & Seif, F. (2023). Molecular mechanisms of microRNAs in glioblastoma pathogenesis. *Biochimica et Biophysica Acta (BBA) –. Revisiones en Cáncer*, *1870*(6), 119482. Advance online publication. DOI: 10.1016/j.bbcan.2023.188948

Bona, N. P., Pedra, N. S., Spohr, L., da Silva dos Santos, F., Saraiva, J. T., Carvalho, F. B., & Stefanello, F. M. (2024). Antitumoral activity of Cecropia pachystachya leaves extract in vitro and in vivo model of rat glioma: Brain and blood effects. *Metabolic Brain Disease*, *39*(10), 8234–8252. DOI: 10.1007/s11011-024-01392-6 PMID: 38483655

Elshaer, S. S., Abulsoud, A. I., Fathi, D., Abdelmaksoud, N. M., Zaki, M. B., El-Mahdy, H. A., & Doghish, A. S. (2023). miRNAs role in glioblastoma pathogenesis and targeted therapy: Signaling pathways interplay. *Pathology, Research and Practice, 246*, 154511. Advance online publication. DOI: 10.1016/j.prp.2023.154511 PMID: 37178618

Fiedler, T., Strauss, M., Hering, S., Redanz, U., William, D., Rosche, Y., & Podbielski, A. (2015). Arginine deprivation by arginine deiminase of Streptococcus pyogenes controls primary glioblastoma growth in vitro and in vivo. *Cancer Biology & Therapy, 16*(7), 1047–1055. DOI: 10.1080/15384047.2015.1026478 PMID: 25774632

Fuentes-Fayos, A. C., García-García, M. E., Pérez-Gómez, J. M., Montero-Hidalgo, A. J., Martín-Colom, J., Doval-Rosa, C., & Luque, R. M. (2023). Metformin and simvastatin exert additive antitumour effects in glioblastoma via senescence-state: Clinical and translational evidence. *EBioMedicine, 90*, 104519. Advance online publication. DOI: 10.1016/j.ebiom.2023.104484 PMID: 36907105

Ge, Y.-F., Sun, J., Jin, C.-J., Cao, B.-Q., Jiang, Z.-F., & Shao, J.-F. (2013). AntagomiR-27a targets FOXO3a in glioblastoma and suppresses U87 cell growth in vitro and in vivo. *Asian Pacific Journal of Cancer Prevention : APJCP, 14*(2), 963–968. DOI: 10.7314/APJCP.2013.14.2.963 PMID: 23621269

Ghaznavi, H., Afzalipour, R., Khoei, S., Sargazi, S., Shirvalilou, S., & Sheervalilou, R. (2024). New insights into targeted therapy of glioblastoma using smart nanoparticles. *Cancer Cell International, 24*(1), 160. Advance online publication. DOI: 10.1186/s12935-024-03331-3 PMID: 38715021

Gherardini, L., Vetri Buratti, V., Maturi, M., Inzalaco, G., Locatelli, E., Sambri, L., & Comes Franchini, M. (2023). Loco-regional treatment with temozolomide-loaded thermogels prevents glioblastoma recurrences in orthotopic human xenograft models. *Communications Biology, 6*(1), 4630. Advance online publication. DOI: 10.1038/s42003-023-04630-5 PMID: 36944737

Gibson, V. P., Tahiri, H., Yang, C., Phan, Q. T., Banquy, X., & Hardy, P. J. (2023). Hyaluronan decorated layer-by-layer assembled lipid nanoparticles for miR-181a delivery in glioblastoma treatment. *International Journal of Pharmaceutics, 302*, 122341. Advance online publication. DOI: 10.1016/j.ijpharm.2023.122341 PMID: 37778056

Hao, X., Bahia, R. K., Cseh, O., Bozek, D. A., Blake, S., Rinnenthal, J., & McDermott, D. F. (2023). BI-907828, a novel potent MDM2 inhibitor, inhibits glioblastoma brain tumor stem cells in vitro and prolongs survival in orthotopic xenograft mouse models. *Neuro-Oncology*, *25*(5), 913–926. DOI: 10.1093/neuonc/noac271 PMID: 36521007

Hassanzadeganroudsari, M., Soltani, M., Heydarinasab, A., Apostolopoulos, V., Akbarzadehkhiyavi, A., Nurgali, K., & Mantzorou, M. (2020). Targeted nano-drug delivery system for glioblastoma therapy: In vitro and in vivo study. *Journal of Drug Delivery Science and Technology*, *60*, 102039. Advance online publication. DOI: 10.1016/j.jddst.2020.102039

He, S., Cen, B., Liao, L., Wang, Z., Qin, Y., Wu, Z., & Zhang, Z. (2017). A tumor-targeting cRGD-EGFR siRNA conjugate and its anti-tumor effect on glioblastoma in vitro and in vivo. *Drug Delivery*, *24*(1), 471–481. DOI: 10.1080/10717544.2016.1267821 PMID: 28181832

Houweling, M., Abdul, U., Brahm, C., Lagerweij, T., Heukelom, S., Koken, P., & Verheul, H. M. W. (2023). Radio-sensitizing effect of MEK inhibition in glioblastoma in vitro and in vivo. *Journal of Neuro-Oncology*, *149*(1), 297–305. DOI: 10.1007/s11060-023-04362-8 PMID: 36451044

Ibrahim, R. S., Ibrahim, S. S., El-Naas, A., Koklesová, L., Kubatka, P., & Büsselberg, D. (2023). Could metformin and resveratrol support glioblastoma treatment? A mechanistic view at the cellular level. *Cancers (Basel)*, *15*(13), 3368. Advance online publication. DOI: 10.3390/cancers15133368 PMID: 37444478

Ip, K. L., Thomas, M. A., Behar, K. L., de Graaf, R. A., & De Feyter, H. M. (2023). Mapping of exogenous choline uptake and metabolism in rat glioblastoma using deuterium metabolic imaging (DMI). *Frontiers in Cellular Neuroscience*, *17*, 1130816. Advance online publication. DOI: 10.3389/fncel.2023.1130816 PMID: 37187610

Jang, H. J., Song, M. G., Park, C. R., Youn, H., Lee, Y.-S., Cheon, G. J., & Choi, S. H. (2023). Imaging of indocyanine green-human serum albumin (ICG-HSA) complex in secreted protein acidic and rich in cysteine (SPARC)-expressing glioblastoma. *European Journal of Nuclear Medicine and Molecular Imaging*, *51*(1), 850–861. DOI: 10.1007/s00259-023-06491-0 PMID: 36614294

Jatyan, R., Sahel, D. K., Singh, P., Sakhuja, R., Mittal, A., & Chitkara, D. (2023). Temozolomide-fatty acid conjugates for glioblastoma multiforme: In vitro and in vivo evaluation. *Journal of Controlled Release*, *359*, 161–174. DOI: 10.1016/j.jconrel.2023.05.012 PMID: 37182806

Jensen, S. S., Petterson, S. A., Halle, B., Aaberg-Jessen, C., & Kristensen, B. W. (2017). Effects of the lysosomal destabilizing drug siramesine on glioblastoma in vitro and in vivo. *BMC Cancer, 17*(1), 178. Advance online publication. DOI: 10.1186/s12885-017-3162-3 PMID: 28270132

Jia, X., Wang, L., Feng, X., Liu, W., Wang, X., Li, F., & Liu, Y. (2023). Cell membrane-coated oncolytic adenovirus for targeted treatment of glioblastoma. *ACS Nano, 17*(23), 11120–11128. DOI: 10.1021/acsnano.3c07123 PMID: 38032110

Khan, I. N., Navaid, S., Waqar, W., Hussein, D., Ullah, N., Khan, M. U. A., & Amin, A. (2024). Chitosan-based polymeric nanoparticles as an efficient gene delivery system to cross blood brain barrier: In vitro and in vivo evaluations. *International Journal of Polymeric Materials, 73*(2), 169–180. DOI: 10.1080/00914037.2023.2275588 PMID: 38399386

Kim, S., Jing, K., Shin, S., Jeong, S., Han, S.-H., Oh, H., & Lim, K. (2018). ω3-polyunsaturated fatty acids induce cell death through apoptosis and autophagy in glioblastoma cells: In vitro and in vivo. *Oncology Reports, 39*(1), 239–246. DOI: 10.3892/or.2017.6107 PMID: 29192322

Kumari, S., Gupta, R., Ambasta, R. K., & Kumar, P. (2023). Multiple therapeutic approaches of glioblastoma multiforme: From terminal to therapy. *Biochimica et Biophysica Acta (BBA) –. Revisiones en Cáncer, 1878*(4), 188913. Advance online publication. DOI: 10.1016/j.bbcan.2023.188913 PMID: 37182666

Li, G., Wang, D., Zhai, Y., Pan, C., Zhang, J., Wang, C., & Chen, X. (2024). Glycometabolic reprogramming-induced XRCC1 lactylation confers therapeutic resistance in ALDH1A3-overexpressing glioblastoma. *Cell Metabolism, 36*(8), 1696–1710.e10. DOI: 10.1016/j.cmet.2024.07.011 PMID: 39111285

Li, P.-J., Lai, S.-Z., Jin, T., Ying, H.-J., Chen, Y.-M., Zhang, P., & Cai, Q. (2023). Radiotherapy opens the blood–brain barrier and synergizes with anlotinib in treating glioblastoma. *Pharmacological Research, 183*, 109633. Advance online publication. DOI: 10.1016/j.phrs.2023.106633 PMID: 36963438

. Liu, D., Dai, X., Ye, L., Wang, H., Qian, H., Cheng, H., & Zhang, J. (2023). Nanotechnology meets glioblastoma multiforme: Emerging therapeutic strategies. *Wiley Interdisciplinary Reviews: Nanomedicine and Nanobiotechnology, 15*(1), Article e1838. DOI: 10.1002/wnan.1838

Liu, D., Dai, X., Zhang, W., Zhu, X., Zha, Z., Qian, H., & Cheng, H. (2023). Liquid exfoliation of ultrasmall zirconium carbide nanodots as a noninflammatory photothermal agent in the treatment of glioma. *Advanced Materials, 35*(2), 2210917. Advance online publication. DOI: 10.1002/adma.202210917 PMID: 36470160

Liu, Y., Hu, D., Gao, D., Gong, P., Zheng, H., Sun, M., & Cai, L. (2023). Engineered apoptotic bodies hitchhiking across the blood-brain barrier achieved a combined photothermal-chemotherapeutic effect against glioma. *Advancement of Science*, *10*(9), 2206296. Advance online publication. DOI: 10.7150/thno.80632 PMID: 37284458

Lopes, J., Ferreira-Gonçalves, T., Ascensão, L., Viana, A. S., Carvalho, L., Catarino, J., & Reis, C. P. (2023). Safety of gold nanoparticles: From in vitro to in vivo testing array checklist. *Nanomaterials (Basel, Switzerland)*, *13*(4), 1120. Advance online publication. DOI: 10.3390/nano13041120 PMID: 37111608

Lu, R., Wu, C., Guo, L., Liu, Y., Mo, W., Wang, H., Ding, Y., Wong, E. T., & Yu, M. (2012). The role of brevican in glioma: Promoting tumor cell motility in vitro and in vivo. *BMC Cancer*, *12*(1), 607. Advance online publication. DOI: 10.1186/1471-2407-12-607 PMID: 23253190

Merenzon, M. A., Arias, E. H., Bhatia, S., Shah, A. H., Higgins, D. M., Villaverde, M., & Eichberg, D. G. (2023). Nitric oxide synthase inhibitors as potential therapeutic agents for gliomas: A systematic review. *Nitric Oxide*, *138–139*, 10–16. DOI: 10.1016/j.niox.2023.06.002 PMID: 37279819

Nakabayashi, H., & Shimizu, K. (2012). Involvement of Akt/NF-κB pathway in antitumor effects of parthenolide on glioblastoma cells in vitro and in vivo. *BMC Cancer*, *12*(1), 453. Advance online publication. DOI: 10.1186/1471-2407-12-453 PMID: 23039130

Nikam, D., & Jain, A. (2023). Advances in the discovery of DHPMs as Eg5 inhibitors for the management of breast cancer and glioblastoma: A review. *Results in Chemistry*, *5*, 100718. Advance online publication. DOI: 10.1016/j.rechem.2022.100718

Nogueira, L., Ruiz-Ontañon, P., Vazquez-Barquero, A., Lafarga, M., Berciano, M., Aldaz, B., & Fernández-Luna, J. L. (2011). Blockade of the NFκB pathway drives differentiating glioblastoma-initiating cells into senescence both in vitro and in vivo. *Oncogene*, *30*(32), 3537–3548. DOI: 10.1038/onc.2011.74 PMID: 21423202

Obozina, A. S., Komedchikova, E. N., Kolesnikova, O. A., Iureva, A. M., Kovalenko, V. L., Zavalko, F. A., & Deyev, S. M. (2023). Genetically encoded self-assembling protein nanoparticles for the targeted delivery in vitro and in vivo. *Pharmaceutics*, *15*(1), 231. Advance online publication. DOI: 10.3390/pharmaceutics15010231 PMID: 36678860

Oraiopoulou, M.-E., Tzamali, E., Psycharakis, S. E., Tzedakis, G., Makatounakis, T., Manolitsi, K., & Zacharakis, G. (2024). The temozolomide–doxorubicin paradox in glioblastoma in vitro–in silico preclinical drug-screening. *Cancers (Basel)*, *16*(1), 3759. Advance online publication. DOI: 10.3390/cancers16020375 PMID: 38355655

Ożarowski, M., Karpiński, T. M., Czerny, B., Kamiński, A., & Seremak-Mrozikiewicz, A. (2025). Plant alkaloids as promising anticancer compounds with blood–brain barrier penetration in the treatment of glioblastoma: In vitro and in vivo models. *Molecules (Basel, Switzerland), 30*(7), 1561. Advance online publication. DOI: 10.3390/molecules30071561 PMID: 40286187

Pérez-López, A., Torres-Suárez, A. I., Martín-Sabroso, C., & Aparicio-Blanco, J. (2023). An overview of in vitro 3D models of the blood-brain barrier as a tool to predict the in vivo permeability of nanomedicines. *Advanced Drug Delivery Reviews, 196*, 114816. Advance online publication. DOI: 10.1016/j.addr.2023.114816 PMID: 37003488

Petković, M., Henis, M., Heese, O., & Relógio, A. (2023). Chronotherapy in glioblastoma: State of the art and future perspectives. *EBioMedicine, 89*, 104485. Advance online publication. DOI: 10.1016/j.ebiom.2023.104470 PMID: 36796229

Rajan, R. G., Fernandez-Vega, V., Sperry, J., Nakashima, J., Do, L. H., Andrews, W., & Tran, N. L. (2023). In vitro and in vivo drug-response profiling using patient-derived high-grade glioma. *Cancers (Basel), 15*(13), 3289. Advance online publication. DOI: 10.3390/cancers15133289 PMID: 37444398

Ravn-Boess, N., Roy, N., Hattori, T., Bready, D., Donaldson, H., Lawson, C., & Mischel, P. S. (2023). The expression profile and tumorigenic mechanisms of CD97 (ADGRE5) in glioblastoma render it a targetable vulnerability. *Cell Reports, 42*(11), 113374. Advance online publication. DOI: 10.1016/j.celrep.2023.113374 PMID: 37938973

Roque, D., Cruz, N., Ferreira, H. A., Reis, C. P., Matela, N., Herculano-Carvalho, M., & Faria, C. C. (2023). Nanoparticle-based treatment in glioblastoma. *Journal of Personalized Medicine, 13*(9), 1328. Advance online publication. DOI: 10.3390/jpm13091328 PMID: 37763096

Rubenich, D. S., de Souza, P. O., Omizzollo, N., Aubin, M. R., Basso, P. J., Silva, L. M., & Bonorino, C. (2023). Tumor-neutrophil crosstalk promotes in vitro and in vivo glioblastoma progression. *Frontiers in Immunology, 14*, 1183465. Advance online publication. DOI: 10.3389/fimmu.2023.1183465 PMID: 37292196

Sandbhor, P., Goda, J., Mohanty, B., Gera, P., Yadav, S., Chekuri, G., & Moiyadi, A. (2023). Targeted nano-delivery of chemotherapy via intranasal route suppresses in vivo glioblastoma growth and prolongs survival in the intracranial mouse model. *PLoS One, 13*(2), 608–626. DOI: 10.1371/journal.pone.0287394 PMID: 36245060

Schweiger, B., & Kievit, F. M. (2025). Glioblastoma induced blood-brain barrier dysfunction via a paracrine mechanism that increases claudin-1 expression. *Experimental Brain Research, 243*(3), 70. DOI: 10.1007/s00221-025-07018-7 PMID: 39960547

Sharp, P. S., Stylianou, M., Arellano, L. M., Neves, J. C., Gravagnuolo, A. M., Dodd, A., & Stylianopoulos, T. (2023). Graphene oxide nanoscale platform enhances the anti-cancer properties of bortezomib in glioblastoma models. *Advanced Healthcare Materials, 12*(3), 2201968. Advance online publication. DOI: 10.1002/adhm.202201968 PMID: 36300643

Shi, Y., He, X., Wang, H., Dai, J., Fang, J., He, Y., & Liu, Z. (2023). Construction of a novel blood brain barrier-glioma microfluidic chip model: Applications in the evaluation of permeability and anti-glioma activity of traditional Chinese medicine components. *Talanta, 253*, 123971. Advance online publication. DOI: 10.1016/j.talanta.2022.123971 PMID: 36201955

Singh, R. R., Mondal, I., Janjua, T., Popat, A., & Kulshreshtha, R. (2024). Engineered smart materials for RNA based molecular therapy to treat glioblastoma. *Bioactive Materials, 33*, 396–423. DOI: 10.1016/j.bioactmat.2023.11.007 PMID: 38059120

Slika, H., Karimov, Z., Alimonti, P., Abou-Mrad, T., De Fazio, E., Alomari, S., & El Housheimi, K. (2023). Preclinical models and technologies in glioblastoma research: Evolution, current state, and future avenues. *International Journal of Molecular Sciences, 24*(22), 16316. Advance online publication. DOI: 10.3390/ijms242216316 PMID: 38003507

Soni, V., Adhikari, M., Simonyan, H., Lin, L., Sherman, J. H., Young, C. N., & Keppel, T. R. (2021). In vitro and in vivo enhancement of temozolomide effect in human glioblastoma by non-invasive application of cold atmospheric plasma. *Cancers (Basel), 13*(17), 4485. Advance online publication. DOI: 10.3390/cancers13174485 PMID: 34503293

Sun, T., Krishnan, V., Pan, D. C., Filippov, S. K., Ravid, S., Sarode, A., & Yang, X. (2023). Ultrasound-mediated delivery of flexibility-tunable polymer drug conjugates for treating glioblastoma. *Bioengineering & Translational Medicine, 8*(2), e10408. Advance online publication. DOI: 10.1002/btm2.10408 PMID: 36925708

Tang, T., Liang, H., Wei, W., Han, Y., Cao, L., Cong, Z., & Zhang, J. (2023). Aloperine targets lysosomes to inhibit late autophagy and induces cell death through apoptosis and paraptosis in glioblastoma. *Cell Death Discovery, 9*(1), 42. Advance online publication. DOI: 10.1038/s41420-023-01333-6 PMID: 36732504

Tong, F., Zhao, J.-X., Fang, Z.-Y., Cui, X.-T., Su, D.-Y., Liu, X., & Zhang, J. (2023). MUC1 promotes glioblastoma progression and TMZ resistance by stabilizing EGFRvIII. *Pharmacological Research, 187*, 106606. Advance online publication. DOI: 10.1016/j.phrs.2022.106606 PMID: 36516884

Tu, Z., Wang, C., Hu, Q., Tao, C., Fang, Z., Lin, L., & Zhang, J. (2023). Protein disulfide-isomerase A4 confers glioblastoma angiogenesis promotion capacity and resistance to anti-angiogenic therapy. *Journal of Experimental & Clinical Cancer Research : CR, 42*(1), 77. Advance online publication. DOI: 10.1186/s13046-023-02640-1 PMID: 36997943

Urzì, O., Gasparro, R., Costanzo, E., De Luca, A., Giavaresi, G., Fontana, S., & Alessandro, R. (2023). Three-dimensional cell cultures: The bridge between in vitro and in vivo models. *International Journal of Molecular Sciences, 24*(15), 12046. Advance online publication. DOI: 10.3390/ijms241512046 PMID: 37569426

Wang, S., Wei, W., Yuan, Y., Sun, B., Yang, D., Liu, N., & Zhang, J. (2023). Chimeric antigen receptor T cells targeting cell surface GRP78 efficiently kill glioblastoma and cancer stem cells. *Journal of Translational Medicine, 21*(1), 493. Advance online publication. DOI: 10.1186/s12967-023-04330-0 PMID: 37481592

Wanigasekara, J., Carroll, L. J., Cullen, P. J., Tiwari, B., & Curtin, J. F. (2023). Three-dimensional (3D) in vitro cell culture protocols to enhance glioblastoma research. *PLoS One, 18*(2), e0276248. Advance online publication. DOI: 10.1371/journal.pone.0276248 PMID: 36753513

Wei, J., Zhu, K., Yang, Z., Zhou, Y., Xia, Z., Ren, J., & Chen, X. (2023). Hypoxia-induced autophagy is involved in radioresistance via HIF1A-associated beclin-1 in glioblastoma multiforme. *Cell Death Discovery, 9*(1), 1. Advance online publication. DOI: 10.1038/s41420-023-01315-8 PMID: 36588105

Wen, J., Ding, Y., Zheng, S., Li, X., & Xiao, Y. (2024). Sevoflurane suppresses glioma cell proliferation, migration, and invasion both in vitro and in vivo partially via regulating KCNQ1OT1/miR-146b-5p/STC1 axis. *Cancer Biology & Therapy, 25*(2), 105–116. DOI: 10.1080/15384047.2024.2304216 PMID: 32996777

Wu, H., Yang, L., Liu, H., Zhou, D., Chen, D., Zheng, X., & Liu, Y. (2021). Exploring the efficacy of tumor electric field therapy against glioblastoma: An in vivo and in vitro study. *Cancer Management and Research, 13*, 1587–1604. DOI: 10.2147/CMAR.S289206 PMID: 34710276

Wu, W. E., Chang, E., Jin, L., Liu, S., Huang, C.-H., Kamal, R., Zhang, J., & Yang, X. (2023). Multimodal in vivo tracking of chimeric antigen receptor T cells in preclinical glioblastoma models. *Scientific Reports*, *13*(6), 388–395. DOI: 10.1038/s41598-023-27741-8 PMID: 36729074

Xie, Z., Chen, M., Lian, J., Wang, H., & Ma, J. (2023). Glioblastoma-on-a-chip construction and therapeutic applications. *Frontiers in Oncology*, *13*, 1183059. Advance online publication. DOI: 10.3389/fonc.2023.1183059 PMID: 37503321

Xu, C., Yuan, X., Hou, P., Li, Z., Wang, C., Fang, C., & Liu, Y. (2023). Development of glioblastoma organoids and their applications in personalized therapy. *Theranostics*, *13*(5), 353–368. DOI: 10.7150/thno.80078 PMID: 37283493

Xu, J., Wang, J., Zhao, M., Li, C., Hong, S., Zhang, J., & Chen, N. (2023). LncRNA LINC01018/miR-942-5p/KNG1 axis regulates the malignant development of glioma in vitro and in vivo. *CNS Neuroscience & Therapeutics*, *29*(2), 691–711. DOI: 10.1111/cns.14053 PMID: 36550594

Ye, J., Fan, Y., Kang, Y., Ding, M., Niu, G., Yang, J., Liu, Y., & Li, X. (2025). Biomimetic dual-driven heterojunction nanomotors for targeted catalytic immunotherapy of glioblastoma. *Advanced Materials*, *37*(9), 2416265. Advance online publication. DOI: 10.1002/adma.202416265

Ye, L., Lv, W., He, W., Li, S., Min, Z., Gong, L., Chen, X., & Zhang, J. (2023). Reduced malignant glioblastoma recurrence post-resection through the anti-CD47 antibody and temozolomide co-embedded in-situ hydrogel system. *Journal of Controlled Release*, *359*, 224–233. DOI: 10.1016/j.jconrel.2023.05.046 PMID: 37290721

Yekula, A., Minciacchi, V. R., Morello, M., Shao, H., Park, Y., Zhang, X., & Carter, B. S. (2020). Large and small extracellular vesicles released by glioma cells in vitro and in vivo. *Journal of Extracellular Vesicles*, *9*(1), 1689784. Advance online publication. DOI: 10.1080/20013078.2019.1689784 PMID: 31839905

Zanotto-Filho, A., Braganhol, E., Edelweiss, M. I., Behr, G. A., Zanin, R., Schröder, R., & Moreira, J. C. F. (2012). The curry spice curcumin selectively inhibits cancer cells growth in vitro and in preclinical model of glioblastoma. *The Journal of Nutritional Biochemistry*, *23*(6), 591–601. DOI: 10.1016/j.jnutbio.2011.02.015 PMID: 21775121

Zhan, C., Wei, X., Qian, J., Feng, L., Zhu, J., & Lu, W. (2012). Co-delivery of TRAIL gene enhances the anti-glioblastoma effect of paclitaxel in vitro and in vivo. *Journal of Controlled Release*, *160*(3), 630–636. DOI: 10.1016/j.jconrel.2012.02.022 PMID: 22410115

Zhang, J., Sun, X., Li, H., Ma, H., Duan, F., Wu, Z., Liu, Y., & Wang, Y. (2023). In vivo characterization and analysis of glioblastoma at different stages using multiscale photoacoustic molecular imaging. *Photoacoustics*, *30*, 100462. Advance online publication. DOI: 10.1016/j.pacs.2023.100462 PMID: 36865670

Zhang, Q., Yuan, L.-C., Wu, C.-J., Wu, S.-Y., Ren, S.-Z., Zhao, M.-D., Hu, Y.-Z., & Liu, Z.-X. (2023). Real-time diagnosis of glioblastoma by sensing peroxynitrite with a highly selective and rapid-responding fluorescent probe. *Analytica Chimica Acta*, *1275*, 134502. Advance online publication. DOI: 10.1016/j.aca.2023.341552

Zhang, Z. X., Ren, P., Cao, Y. Y., Wang, T. T., Huang, G. H., Li, Y., Liang, Y., & Liu, Z. (2023). HOXD-AS2-STAT3 feedback loop attenuates sensitivity to temozolomide in glioblastoma. *CNS Neuroscience & Therapeutics*, *29*(11), 3430–3445. DOI: 10.1111/cns.14277 PMID: 37308741

Chapter 7

Drugs Under Clinical and Pre-Clinical Research for Glioblastoma

G. M. Masud Parvez
https://orcid.org/0000-0002-7071-846X
University of Georgia, USA

Md. Khokon Miah Akanda
https://orcid.org/0000-0002-1916-4553
University of Asia Pacific, Bangladesh

Sanzia Mehjabin
Varendra University, Bangladesh

Razia Sultana
Varendra University, Bangladesh

Anika Naznin
Pabna University of Science and Technology, Bangladesh

ABSTRACT

This chapter focuses on current drugs that are using in clinical trial on glioblastoma. According to the ClinicalTrials.gov, 2077 clinical trials are going on glioblastoma until May 2025. Different small molecules and alkylating agents that are already approved for marketing like Temozolomide, Carmustine, Lomustine, Tinostamustine, Cyclophosphamide are still using. Enzyme inhibitors are the mostly used therapies and different enzyme inhibitors like protease inhibitor, tyrosine kinase inhibitor, ATM kinase inhibitor, BET inhibitor, mTOR inhibitor, ornithine decarboxylase inhibitor, histone deacetylase inhibitor are common treatment strategies. In addition, many

DOI: 10.4018/979-8-3373-2695-5.ch007

receptor inhibitors like inhibitors of fibroblast growth factor receptor and epidermal growth factor receptor are also used in many clinical trials. In different clinical trials, other approaches like using human monocolonized antibodies, vaccines, toxins and anti-fungal drugs are used as a potential treatment strategy.

INTRODUCTION

Glioblastoma (GBM) is the most aggressive primary brain tumor in adults, marked by diffuse invasion, therapeutic resistance, and dismal outcomes—median survival remains only 14–16 months, with fewer than 7% of patients alive at five years (Overcoming Critical Issues in Glioblastoma Multiforme (GBM) Therapeutic Development, 2025). These challenges underscore the urgency of pursuing innovative strategies beyond conventional treatments. Preclinical research plays a central role in this pursuit: from early rat models to advanced genetically engineered systems and patient-derived xenografts (PDX), such platforms allow detailed study of tumor initiation, progression, microenvironmental interactions, and therapeutic response in biologically relevant contexts (Slika, H. et al. 2023). More recently, cutting-edge technologies—including organoids, 3D bioprinted "mini-brains," and microfluidic systems—have further enhanced our ability to replicate GBM's intricate architecture, enabling more predictive testing of novel therapies. Complementing these models, high-throughput molecular analyses provide insights into oncogenic pathways, biomarkers, and mechanisms of resistance, strengthening the bridge between laboratory findings and clinical application (Ahmed, M. et al. 2023). For instance, preclinical evaluation of the multi-kinase inhibitor regorafenib laid the groundwork for its clinical investigation in relapsed GBM.

According to ClinicalTrial.gov more than 250 drugs are in different stages of clinical trials against glioblastoma. The most commonly used drugs can be categorized as:

SMALL MOLECULES

Different small molecules are currently being used as a treatment strategy for glioblastoma. Among them, the drug *CBL0137* is in the first stages of clinical trial. It is a curaxin class drug that disrupts chromatin structure and therefore modulates gene expression by targeting the FACT (Facilitates Chromatin Transcription) complex. This drug destabilizes the trapping FACT complex, impairs its role in transcription and ultimately prevents DNA replication. *Sulfasalazine* is an anti-inflammatory DMARD used for inflammatory conditions and certain cancers, including metastatic colorectal cancer and glioblastoma, where it inhibits NF-κB and depletes glutathione to induce cell death.

KHK2455 is a small-molecule inhibitor of the indoleamine 2,3-dioxygenase 1 (IDO1) enzyme which catalyzes the degradation of tryptophan to kynurenine. This degradation causes immunosuppression of the tumor microenvironment (Tang, K. et al., 2021). Another small molecule inhibitor, *ZSP1602* targets the Smoothened (SMO) receptor. By inhibiting this receptor, this drug disrupts the Hedgehog signaling pathway and therefore stops tumor cell growth and progression.

L-Alanosine is an antimetabolite that inhibits purine biosynthesis, with preclinical research demonstrating its potential in treating glioblastoma. By blocking purine synthesis, L-alanosine induces tumor cell death and inhibits tumor growth. *Phenylacetate* is a metabolite with anti-tumor properties being researched in glioblastoma therapy. It works by inducing differentiation in glioblastoma cells and reducing tumor cell proliferation. Preclinical studies suggest that phenylacetate may enhance the effectiveness of other chemotherapeutic agents (Culver et al., 2010).

Carboplatin is a platinum-based chemotherapy drug used in glioblastoma treatment, especially in combination with other agents. It works by cross-linking DNA strands, which prevents DNA replication and leads to cell death. Preclinical studies have shown that carboplatin can enhance the effects of other therapies, though resistance mechanisms are a challenge (Stupp et al., 2005). *Cisplatin*, another platinum-based chemotherapy drug, is being investigated for glioblastoma treatment due to its DNA-crosslinking ability. It works similarly to carboplatin by *disrupting DNA replication* and inducing cell death. Preclinical and clinical studies have shown that cisplatin can be effective in glioblastoma, but resistance mechanisms often limit its clinical use (Kaufman et al., 2017).

Chloroquine, known for its antimalarial properties, is being studied in glioblastoma for its potential to inhibit autophagy, a process that glioblastoma cells often rely on for survival under stress conditions. Preclinical studies have suggested that chloroquine can enhance the cytotoxic effects of chemotherapy and radiation therapy in glioblastoma.

Carboxyamidotriazole (CAI) is an anti-cancer and anti-angiogenic agent that inhibits non-voltage-dependent calcium channels, disrupting cancer cell proliferation, migration, and angiogenesis. In glioblastoma, it has been primarily studied in Phase IB trials, with Phase II trials planned (Omuro et al., 2018).

ALKYLATING AGENTS

Alkylating agents are used to methylate DNA on tumor cells and many alkylations are now in clinical trials for glioblastoma. *OKN-007* is a nitrone-based drug that can cross the blood-brain barrier and cause death of tumor cells through anti-inflammatory and pro-apoptotic mechanisms. *Temozolomide* (TMZ) is another alkylating agent that is now in clinical trial. It methylates to DNA at O-6 positions of guanine and damages DNA and ultimately causes cancer cells to die. *Temodar* treats brain tumors by inducing DNA damage, leading to cancer cell death. It's undergone extensive clinical trials and has either been terminated or completed (Yan et al., 2024).

Carmustine is an alkylating antineoplastic agent that cross-links DNA/RNA, inhibiting synthesis and inducing cell death. It's being studied in various clinical phases, including a completed Phase II for recurrent glioblastoma (Ricciardi et al., 2022). *Lomustine*, another alkylating antineoplastic, damages DNA to inhibit glioblastoma cell division. *Tinostamustine* is an alkylating agent used in the treatment of glioblastoma. It works by crosslinking DNA strands and preventing their replication, which leads to cell death. Preclinical studies have demonstrated that tinostamustine may be effective in glioblastoma treatment, particularly in combination with other agents.

Procarbazine is an alkylating antineoplastic agent used for Hodgkin's lymphoma and brain tumors. It works by damaging DNA and inhibiting synthesis. Clinical trials are ongoing or completed, including those for recurrent glioblastoma (e.g., NCT01737346, NCT00004004) (Kim et al., 2018). *SarCNU* is an investigational alkylating antineoplastic agent. It selectively enters tumor cells via a transporter, then damages DNA, causing cell death. It has completed Phase I and Phase II trials for malignant glioma (NCT00036660) (Webster et al., 2005). *Procarbazine hydrochloride*, an alkylating antineoplastic, damages DNA to inhibit glioblastoma cell growth. It's studied in various trials, including completed and ongoing ones, often in combination therapy.

Thiotepa is an alkylating agent used in the treatment of glioblastoma, particularly for intrathecal chemotherapy. It works by damaging DNA and preventing cell replication. Preclinical studies have shown its potential in targeting glioblastoma stem cells, a major challenge in glioblastoma treatment (Perry et al., 2005). *Irofulven* is an alkylating agent derived from the natural product illudin S, showing potential in glioblastoma therapy. It works by inducing DNA damage and apoptosis in tumor cells. *Glufosfamide* is an alkylating agent under investigation for glioblastoma. It works by disrupting DNA replication and promoting cell death in tumor cells. Preclinical studies suggest that glufosfamide can enhance the effects of other therapies, particularly in cases where resistance to standard treatments has developed. *Cyclophosphamide* is an alkylating agent used in the treatment of glioblastoma. It works by crosslinking DNA strands and preventing DNA replication, leading to tumor cell death. Preclinical studies suggest that cyclophosphamide may also target glioblastoma stem cells, which are often resistant to conventional therapies. *Capecitabine* is an oral chemotherapy drug that is primarily used for colorectal cancer and breast cancer but is being investigated for its potential role in glioblastoma treatment. It is a prodrug that is metabolized into 5-fluorouracil (5-FU) in the body, which interferes with DNA synthesis and inhibits tumor cell proliferation. Capecitabine is being studied in glioblastoma to assess its effectiveness when combined with other agents, especially in cases of recurrence or resistance to standard therapies.

OLIGONUCLEOTIDES

Oligonucleotide *CC-8490*, or Custirsen, is a phosphorothioate antisense oligonucleotide (ASO) that suppresses clusterin expression that is now used in treating glioblastoma. It not only curbs growth of estrogen-sensitive breast cancer cells but also triggers apoptosis.

GENE THERAPIES

Some gene therapies are currently in clinical trials. *NRG-103* is an engineered oncolytic adenovirus that destroys tumor cells. This virus replicates inside tumor cells, causing cell lysis and disrupting cellular membranes and releasing viral particles which can affect neighboring cells. Another gene therapy product, *MSC11FCD*, is currently being used in glioblastoma (GBM) and gliosarcoma. In this therapy, engineered mesenchymal stem cells (MSCs) are administered to deliver the suicide CD gene (cytosine deaminase) to cancer cells. The CD gene encodes a CD enzyme that converts 5-fluorocytosine to 5-fluorouracil (5-FU), which is a potent chemotherapeutic agent. *Temferon*, an immuno-gene therapy, delivers IFN-α to glioblastoma, activating immunity and reprogramming the tumor microenvironment. It's in a Phase I/IIa trial (NCT03866109) for newly diagnosed glioblastoma, showing good tolerability with limited systemic toxicities (Gentner et al., 2021). Glycosylated fusion protein *CAN008* binds the extracellular domain of the human CD95 receptor of human IgG1. After binding, it blocks interaction between CD95 and CD95L and prevents tumor cell invasion and reduces tumor invasiveness.

ENZYME AND OTHER INHIBITORS

ACT001 (DMAMCL) is a newly developed plasminogen activator inhibitor-1 (PAI-1) that is currently in clinical trial against aggressive cancers like glioblastoma. It acts by targeting the overexpressed protein PAI-1. It directly binds with the serine *protease inhibitor* PAI-1, disrupts the PI3K/AKT signaling pathway and therefore reduces tumor cell proliferation and migration. *Nelfinavir*, an HIV *protease inhibitor*, is being studied for its off-label use in glioblastoma due to its ability to modulate autophagy and enhance the effects of other chemotherapeutic agents. Nelfinavir has been shown to inhibit glioblastoma cell proliferation in preclinical models (Patel et al., 2000). *Bortezomib* is a *proteasome inhibitor* which is indicated for the treatment of multiple myeloma and mantle cell lymphoma. It reversibly blocks the action of the 26S proteasome, leading to the accumulation of misfolded or damaged proteins. It triggers apoptosis—especially in cancer cells that are dependent on proteasome activity for continued growth and survival. *Ritonavir* is another *HIV protease inhibitor* that has been repurposed in glioblastoma research due to its ability to inhibit autophagy and enhance the effects of other therapies. Ritonavir works by disrupting tumor cell metabolism and survival pathways. Preclinical studies have shown the potential for overcoming drug resistance in glioblastoma.

A *tyrosine kinase inhibitor, PLX3397* (Turalio), targets CSF1R, a crucial regulator of tumor-associated macrophages (TAMs) and plays a leading role in the progression of glioblastoma. By inhibiting CSF1R, this drug depletes TAMs, and blocks their functioning and prevents tumor generation and metastasis. *Imatinib mesylate* is a *tyrosine kinase inhibitor* that targets BCR-ABL, c-KIT, and PDGF receptors. It is being investigated in glioblastoma due to its ability to inhibit tumor cell signaling pathways that promote growth and survival. Early trials have shown that imatinib may be beneficial in glioblastoma, particularly when combined with other therapies (Chin et al., 2008). *Epitinib succinate* is a *tyrosine kinase inhibitor* being studied for glioblastoma treatment. It targets EGFR mutations, which are common in glioblastoma cells, and inhibits tumor cell proliferation and survival. Early-phase clinical studies have shown that epitinib may be effective when combined with other therapies. *Tesevatinib* is an investigational oral drug which is being studied for the treatment of cancers and polycystic kidney disease. It blocks key *kinases such as EGFR, HER2, and VEGFR* to inhibit tumor development, angiogenesis, and cyst growth. *Anlotinib* is an orally delivered small-molecule *tyrosine kinase inhibitor* (TKI). It targets multiple receptors for tumor development and angiogenesis, such as FGFR, c-Kit, VEGFR, and PDGFR. By blocking these signaling pathways, anlotinib impedes the emergence of blood vessels that sustain tumors, impairs tumor cell survival, and facilitates cancer cell death. *Ponatinib* is an orally administered *tyrosine kinase inhibitor* indicated for the treatment of chronic myeloid leukemia (CML) and Philadelphia chromosome–positive acute lymphoblastic leukemia (Ph+ ALL), particularly in patients with resistance to prior TKI therapies. It effectively inhibits BCR-ABL kinase activity, including the T315I mutation that confers resistance to most other inhibitors. In addition, ponatinib acts on multiple other kinases, such as VEGFR, FGFR, and PDGFR, contributing to the suppression of tumor cell proliferation and angiogenesis. *Tivozanib* is an oral *tyrosine kinase inhibitor* approved for the treatment of advanced renal cell carcinoma. It specifically inhibits VEGFR-1, -2, and -3, thereby keeping down tumor-driven angiogenesis and restricting tumor growth and nourishment, and metastasis. *Apatinib* is an oral *tyrosine kinase inhibitor* used primarily for treating advanced gastric cancer and other solid tumors. It selectively inhibits vascular endothelial growth factor receptor-2 (VEGFR-2), a key mediator of tumor angiogenesis. By blocking VEGFR-2, apatinib reduces tumor blood vessel formation, thereby starving the tumor of nutrients and inhibiting its growth. *Bosutinib* is an oral *tyrosine kinase inhibitor* used to treat chronic myeloid leukemia, particularly in patients unresponsive to earlier treatments. It targets the BCR-ABL fusion kinase and Src family kinases, preventing leukemic cell growth and survival. *Erlotinib* is an orally administered *tyrosine kinase inhibitor* that blocks the ATP-binding site of EGFR, inhibiting autophosphorylation and downstream signaling, thereby curbing tumor growth and cell survival in EGFR-dependent cancers. *Ramucirumab* is approved for cancers, including gastric, colorectal, and non-small cell lung cancer. It selectively blocks VEGFR-2, inhibiting VEGF-driven angiogenesis and limiting tumor vascularization and tumor genesis. *Dasatinib* is an oral *tyrosine kinase inhibitor* indicated for chronic myeloid leukemia and Ph+ acute lymphoblastic leukemia. It inhibits BCR-ABL and additional kinases such as Src, c-Kit, and PDGFR, thereby hindering malignant cell proliferation and supporting disease control.

WSD0628 is an inhibitor of *ATM* (Ataxia Telangiectasia Mutated) *kinase* which helps repair double-strand DNA damage. By inhibiting ATM kinase, the drug impairs phosphorylation of DNA and, as a result, radiation therapy becomes more efficient because tumor cells cannot repair the radiation damage to DNA. *AZD1390* is another *ATM kinase inhibitor*, and it prevents repairing of DNA double-strands and makes DNA more vulnerable to radiation treatment (Tew, BY., et al. 2023). Another kinase inhibitor, *GLR2007*, inhibits *cyclin-dependent kinases 4 and 6* (CDK4/6) in advanced solid tumors like glioblastoma. By obstructing those enzymes, the drug halts tumor cell production (Yin et al. 2022). *Abemaciclib* is a medication used in the management of certain types of breast cancer. It plays as a *kinase inhibitor*, specifically blocking the activity of cyclin-dependent kinases 4 and 6 (CDK4 and CDK6). Thus, Abemaciclib can help slow or stop the growth of cell cycle progression. *Ribociclib* is used as an oral, *CDK4/6 inhibitor* used alongside hormone therapy for treating HR-positive, HER2-negative metastatic breast cancer. It impedes cell cycle development from G1 to S phase by targeting CDK4 and CDK6, yielding in reduced cancer cell spread and potential cancer cell death. Similar types of effects were observed on *CS231295* which acts as a multi-target *protein kinase inhibitor* and also acts as suppressing tumor vascularization. *Enzastaurin* is a selective *protein kinase C beta inhibitor* that has been explored in glioblastoma treatment due to its effects on tumor cell survival and angiogenesis. It inhibits tumor growth by downregulating the PI3K/AKT pathway, a crucial survival signaling pathway in glioblastoma cells. Preclinical studies show that enzastaurin may sensitize glioblastoma to other therapies.

Another newly developed inhibitor named *CC-90010* (Trotabresib) is a *BET inhibitor* (bromodomain and extra-terminal proteins) that targets epigenetic regulators in oncogene expression. By irreversibly blocking BET protein, it stops tumor growth. By irreversibly blocking BET protein, it stops tumor growth. *AZD1775* (Adavosertib) is a *WEE1 kinase* inhibitor and this enzyme is an important regulator of G2/M cell cycle checkpoint. This drug inhibits DNA damage repair by blocking WEE1.

AZD8055 is an ATP-competitive inhibitor of *rapamycin (mTOR) kinase*. This drug targets both mTORC1 and mTORC2 complexes by binding to the ATP binding sites, therefore suppressing downstream signaling pathways of cell growth and proliferation (Huang & Zhineng, 2011). *Temsirolimus* is an *mTOR inhibitor* being studied for its efficacy in glioblastoma treatment. By inhibiting the mTOR pathway, which regulates cell proliferation, survival, and metabolism, temsirolimus potentially suppresses glioblastoma growth. Preclinical studies have shown promise, particularly in combination with other therapies (Hudes et al. 2007). *Paxalisib* is an experimental oral small-molecule that crosses the blood-brain barrier to *inhibit the PI3K/mTOR pathway*, frequently suppressing brain tumors like glioblastoma. By blocking this signaling cascade, it helps reduce tumor growth and promote cancer cell death. *Vandetanib* is an investigational drug that inhibits multiple *tyrosine kinases* involved in glioblastoma tumor growth and angiogenesis. It targets the *EGFR, VEGFR, and RET pathways*, which are crucial for glioblastoma cell proliferation and survival. Preclinical studies have shown that vandetanib can significantly reduce tumor growth (Cunningham et al. 2011). *AZD2014* (vistusertib) is an ATP-competitive inhibitor of the mechanistic target of *rapamycin (mTOR)*. This inhibition interferes with downstream signaling pathways that are involved in cell growth, proliferation, and survival of tumor cells. *AP23573* (ridaforolimus) is another *mTOR* (mTORC1 and mTORC2) *inhibitor* that disrupts downstream pathways in cancer cells. *Temsirolimus* is another *mTOR inhibitor* being explored for glioblastoma therapy. It works by inhibiting the mTOR pathway, which is involved in cell growth and survival. Clinical trials have demonstrated its ability to reduce glioblastoma cell proliferation, though it is often used in combination with other treatments (Hudes et al. 2007). *Sirolimus*, also known as rapamycin, is an *mTOR inhibitor* that is being studied for its effects on glioblastoma. By inhibiting mTOR, sirolimus can suppress glioblastoma cell proliferation and angiogenesis. Preclinical studies and clinical trials suggest it's potential when used in combination with other therapies (Blagosklonny et al. 2007). *Everolimus*, an *mTOR inhibitor*, is being studied for its potential in treating glioblastoma. By inhibiting mTOR, everolimus can block tumor cell growth, survival, and angiogenesis.

The next inhibitor is the *PARP inhibitor* (Poly ADP-ribose polymerases) *123I-ATT001* (ATT001). This inhibitor is radio-labeled with iodine-123 and this radiation damages the DNA structure of tumor cells. *Niraparib* is an oral *PARP inhibitor* used to manage ovarian, fallopian tube, and primary peritoneal cancers, especially in patients with BRCA mutations or homologous recombination deficiency. It inhibits DNA repair enzymes to promote the buildup of DNA damage in tumor cells, inducing synthetic lethality and cell death.

ACP-196, or acalabrutinib (Calquence), is a *BTK inhibitor* (Bruton tyrosine kinase) that is mainly used in treating B-cell cancers like CLL (Chronic Lymphocytic Leukemia), SLL (Small Lymphocytic Lymphoma), and MCL (Mantle Cell Lymphoma) are currently in clinical trials on glioblastoma. This drug targets specific sites on BTK (Cys481) and, by disrupting signals, it ultimately prevents the survival of cancer cells. *Ibrutinib* is an oral targeted agent that irreversibly *inhibits Bruton's tyrosine kinase* (BTK), impairing B-cell receptor signaling and thereby subduing cancer cell growth and survival.

A Ras-MAPK inhibitor, *TLN-4601* (also known as diazepinomicin) interferes with the Ras-*MAPK pathway* and affects proteins like Raf-1, MEK, and ERK1/2. By lowering the activity of those proteins, this drug slowdowns tumor growth. *Zarnestra* (tipifarnib) is a *farnesyltransferase inhibitor* being studied for glioblastoma due to its potential to inhibit the RAS signaling pathway, which is often overactive in glioblastoma cells. Preclinical studies have shown that Zarnestra can decrease glioblastoma cell proliferation and induce apoptosis (Sullivan et al. 2006).

TAS2940 targets the ERBB family of receptors, specifically HER2 and EGFR. It irreversibly inhibits receptors which lead to disruptive downstream signaling pathways and inhibits tumor cell proliferation and survival. *BIBW 2992 (Afatinib)*, is an irreversible tyrosine kinase inhibitor (TKI) that binds with the epidermal growth factor receptor (EGFR) and inhibits tyrosine kinase activity of the receptor. This inhibition blocks downstream signaling pathways. *BGJ398* (infigratinib) is an *inhibitor of fibroblast growth factor receptors* (FGFR) 1, 2, and 3. Genetic alteration by FGFR leads to the generation of cancer. By binding with ATP-binding pockets of these receptors, it inhibits the downstream signaling pathway (Javle et al. 2021). *Infigratinib* is an oral intake *inhibitor of fibroblast growth factor receptors* (FGFRs), used in the treatment of cancers such as cholangiocarcinoma and urothelial carcinoma. It selectively blocks FGFR1–3, thereby blocking signal transduction cascade pathways involved in tumor growth, survival, and angiogenesis. By interfering with these pathways, infigratinib slows cancer growth and induces cell death in FGFR-altered tumors.

Another human monoclonal antibody that targets EGFR is *GC1118*. It binds to a specific epitope of EGFR and prevents the downstream signaling pathway (Oh et al. 2019). *AMG 596* (etevritamab) targets a tumor-specific mutation, epidermal growth factor receptor variant III (EGFRvIII), that is found in glioblastoma multiforme (GBM). It also binds and activates T cells to kill cancer cells (Sternjak et al. 2021). *Erlotinib hydrochloride* is an *epidermal growth factor receptor (EGFR) tyrosine kinase inhibitor* used in the treatment of glioblastoma. It works by inhibiting EGFR signaling, which is often overactive in glioblastoma cells, leading to reduced cell proliferation and survival. *Lapatinib ditosylate* is a dual *EGFR and HER2 tyrosine kinase inhibitor* being explored in glioblastoma due to the overexpression of these receptors in tumor cells. It works by inhibiting the signaling pathways that promote glioblastoma cell proliferation and survival. Preclinical studies suggest it may work synergistically with other therapies. *Gefitinib* is an orally administered *tyrosine kinase inhibitor* that targets the epidermal growth factor receptor (EGFR), and is used in the treatment of specific forms of non-small cell lung cancer (NSCLC). It functions by selectively blocking the ATP-binding site of the EGFR tyrosine kinase, thereby interrupting signaling pathways that promote cell growth and survival. This inhibition results in decreased tumor progression and enhanced cancer cell apoptosis, especially in cases with activating EGFR mutations. *Ceritinib* is used to treat ALK (anaplastic lymphoma kinase) -positive non-small cell lung cancer (NSCLC). It specifically *inhibits* the enzymatic activity of the *ALK tyrosine kinase*. By blocking downstream signaling pathways, it drives tumor cell proliferation and survival. Through this mechanism, ceritinib helps to slow tumor progression and induce cancer cell death in individuals with ALK-rearranged malignancies.

BMS-986504 is a small-molecule *inhibitor that targets PRMT5* (protein arginine methyltransferase 5) by binding with the PRMT5–MTA complex. This MTA-cooperative binding exploits vulnerabilities in cancer cells and impairs tumor cell survival (Hai et al. 2024). *SKL27969* is another *PRMT5 inhibitor* that inhibits PRMT5 by binding to the S-adenosylmethionine (SAM)-bound PRMT5/methylosome protein 50 (MEP50) complexes. This inhibition stops critical cellular processes, like RNA splicing and transcriptional regulation, ultimately halting tumor cell survival. *INCB7839*, also known as *aderbasib*, targets *ADAM10 and ADAM17 enzymes*. Upon inhibition of these enzymes, the drug reduces generation of truncated HER2. This inhibition reduced the formation of p95HER2 and finally prevents resistance against therapies.

Tarceva, an antineoplastic *TKI and EGFR inhibitor*, treats non-small cell lung and pancreatic cancers by blocking the EGFR pathway, hindering cancer cell growth. Clinical trials have included Phase 1 dose escalation and Phase II studies (Alamdari-Palangi et al. 2020). *Incyclinide*, an antineoplastic *MMP inhibitor*, suppresses tumor growth and angiogenesis by inducing apoptosis. It completed Phase 1/2 trials for various cancers, including brain tumors. *Eflornithine* is an irreversible *ornithine decarboxylase inhibitor*, an antineoplastic agent. It blocks polyamine synthesis, crucial for tumor growth. It's in a recruiting Phase 1b trial (NCT05879367) for newly diagnosed glioblastoma. *Dichloroacetate* (DCA) is a metabolic modulator. It *inhibits pyruvate dehydrogenase kinase*, shifting cancer cell metabolism from glycolysis to oxidative phosphorylation, promoting apoptosis. DCA is being investigated in Phase I and II trials for glioblastoma, with some completed and others recruiting. *Azeliragon,* a *RAGE inhibitor*, targets tumor growth and angiogenesis in glioblastoma by blocking RAGE signaling. Its clinical trials for glioblastoma show statuses from "not yet recruiting" to "active, not recruiting" (Sepulveda et al., 2025). *O6-benzylguanine* (O6-BG) is an antineoplastic agent. It irreversibly *inactivates O6-alkylguanine-DNA alkyltransferase* (AGT), a DNA repair protein, thereby enhancing the cytotoxicity of alkylating agents like temozolomide. It has been extensively studied in Phase I and II trials in glioblastoma, often in combination with alkylating agents. *Memantine*, an *NMDA receptor antagonist*, blocks glutamate's effects, with its anti-cancer mechanism in glioblastoma under study. It's explored in Phase I/II glioblastoma trials, often in combination (Cacciatore et al., 2017). *Icapamespib* is a heat *shock protein 90 (HSP90) inhibitor* being tested in glioblastoma. HSP90 is involved in stabilizing mutant proteins that contribute to glioblastoma cell survival. By inhibiting HSP90, icapamespib aims to degrade these mutant proteins, leading to tumor cell death.

Romidepsin is a *histone deacetylase (HDAC) inhibitor* used in the treatment of various cancers, including glioblastoma. It works by altering gene expression and promoting tumor cell death. Romidepsin has shown promise in glioblastoma treatment by inducing tumor cell apoptosis and sensitizing cells to other therapies. *Panobinostat* is another *histone deacetylase (HDAC) inhibitor* being explored in glioblastoma treatment. It works by modifying gene expression and promoting tumor cell death. Panobinostat has been shown to enhance the effectiveness of other glioblastoma therapies. *Quisinostat* is a *histone deacetylase (HDAC) inhibitor* that is being investigated in glioblastoma treatment. By altering the expression of genes involved in apoptosis and cell cycle regulation, quisinostat can induce cell death in glioblastoma cells (Chen et al., 2015). *Valproic acid*, traditionally used as an anticonvulsant, has shown promise in glioblastoma treatment due to its ability to *inhibit histone deacetylases* (HDACs), leading to changes in gene expression that can enhance tumor cell death. Preclinical studies have suggested that valproic acid may improve the effectiveness of chemotherapy and radiation in glioblastoma. *Vorinostat*, an *HDAC inhibitor*, blocks cancer cell growth via histone acetylation. It's been studied in Phase I/II glioblastoma trials for recurrent and newly diagnosed cases.

Cilengitide is an *integrin inhibitor* that has been investigated for the treatment of glioblastoma. It specifically targets $\alpha v\beta 3$ and $\alpha v\beta 5$ integrins, which are highly expressed in tumor cells and endothelial cells of glioblastoma. By blocking these integrins, cilengitide interferes with tumor cell adhesion, migration, and angiogenesis, effectively inhibiting tumor growth.

Talampanel is an *AMPA receptor antagonist* being investigated for glioblastoma due to its ability to inhibit excitatory glutamate neurotransmission, which reduces neuronal excitability and tumor cell growth. Early-phase clinical trials have shown promise, particularly in combination with other therapies (Rogawski et al., 2008). *Sorafenib tosylate* is a *multikinase inhibitor* being explored for glioblastoma. It works by inhibiting several pathways involved in tumor growth, including the *RAF/MEK/ERK signaling pathway*. Preclinical studies have shown that sorafenib can slow glioblastoma progression, but its clinical efficacy remains under investigation. *Avutometinib* is a small-molecule inhibitor that targets the *RAF/MEK/ERK signaling* cascade, with a focus on treating cancers harboring RAS or RAF mutations. It works by *inhibiting MEK enzymatic activity*, by disrupting the MAPK pathway crucial for tumor development. *Tipifarnib* is an orally available *farnesyltransferase inhibitor* (FTI) developed for the treatment of certain cancers, including harboring HRAS mutations and hematologic malignancies tumors. Its mechanism of action involves inhibiting the enzyme farnesyltransferase, which is responsible for the formation of a farnesyl group in proteins like RAS. By blocking this post-translational modification, tipifarnib interferes with oncogenic RAS-driven signaling, leading to reduced tumor cell proliferation and survival.

ANTIBODIES

Many antibodies are currently used in treating glioblastoma. *AMG 102*, or rilotumumab, is a human monoclonal antibody that can *block hepatocyte growth factor* (HGF). The HGF is a protein that supports tumor cell growth. Upon attaching AMG 102 to the HGF, the HGF cannot interact with the c-Met receptor and signaling pathway involved in cancer development.

Another human antibody, *TTAC-0001* (olinvacimab or tanibirumab), *blocks the VEGFR-2 receptor* that participates in blood vessel formation in tumor cells. The drug binds with specific sites of VEGFR-2, prevents its activation and inhibits cell growth and migration (Lee et al. 2015). *Cediranib maleate* is an oral *vascular endothelial growth factor (VEGF) receptor inhibitor* being tested for glioblastoma. By blocking VEGF signaling, cediranib reduces tumor blood supply and inhibits glioblastoma growth. Early-phase trials suggest cediranib may improve outcomes when combined with other therapies. *Cetuximab* is a chimeric monoclonal antibody utilized to treat certain malignancies, notably colorectal and head and neck cancers. It *interacts with the epidermal growth factor receptor* (EGFR), obstructing ligand interaction and subsequent receptor activation. By blocking this pathway, cetuximab disrupts downstream signals essential for cell division, survival, and new blood vessel formation, ultimately slowing tumor progression. *Axitinib* or Inlyta (brand name) are used to treat advanced renal cell carcinoma (kidney cancer) for starters. Axitinib *subdues vascular endothelial growth factor receptors* (VEGFRs). VEGFRs play a role in the formation of blood vessels that nourish tumors. *Bevacizumab* is a monoclonal antibody, and it is used to treat several cancers: Glioblastoma, Colorectal cancer, Cervical cancer, Ovarian and fallopian tube cancers. Bevacizumab *binds to VEGF-A receptors* on endothelial cells. Therefore, it disrupts angiogenesis—the process of forming new blood vessels—which is essential for tumor growth and metastasis.

The *CAN008* (asunercept) *blocks the CD95 ligand* from binding to its receptor. As a result, it stops cancer cells from spreading. It also acts as an immune system booster by preventing T-cell dying (Wei et al. 2021). *Daratumumab* is a human IgG1κ monoclonal antibody that *targets CD38*, a protein extensively present on myeloma cells. Its binding leads tumor cells to death through antibody-dependent cytotoxicity, complement activation, and apoptosis. *CpG oligodeoxynucleotides (CpG-ODNs)* are short synthetic single-stranded DNA sequences that have unmethylated cytosine-phosphate-guanine (CpG) motifs which are recognized as pathogen-associated molecular patterns (PAMPs) and stimulates proinflammatory cytokine production like IL-6, TNF-α by beta cells and as a result it triggers innate immune response. The drug *MEDI-575* (Tovetumab) is another human IgG2κ monoclonal antibody that targets platelet-derived growth factor receptor alpha (PDGFRα), a *receptor tyrosine kinase* that is important in angiogenesis. MEDI-575 inhibits PDGFRα by binding the ligand PDGF-AA. This blocking disrupts the downstream signaling pathway necessary for the proliferation of tumor cells. *MBG453* (sabatolimab) is a humanized IgG4 monoclonal antibody that targets an immune checkpoint receptor TIM-3 (T-cell immunoglobulin and mucin-domain containing-3) that is expressed in leukemic cells. The antibody blocks TIM-3 and restores immune function and facilitates removal of malignant cells (Brunner et al. 2024).

Another humanized monoclonal antibody named *MK-3475* (pembrolizumab) acts as an *immune checkpoint inhibitor* that enhances the immune system's ability to target and destroy cancer cells. *Ipilimumab* is an *immune checkpoint inhibitor* that works by *blocking CTLA-4* (cytotoxic T lymphocyte-associated protein 4). This allows T cells to become more active and attack cancer cells more effectively, especially when used in combination with other checkpoint inhibitors like nivolumab. Ipilimumab effectively removes a brake on the immune system, enhancing the body's ability to fight cancer. *Avelumab* is another *immune checkpoint inhibitor* which is a monoclonal antibody. This *inhibits PD-L1* (programmed death-ligand 1) expressed on tumor cells and surrounding cells within the tumor microenvironment. By binding to PD-L1, avelumab prevents it from engaging with PD-1 receptors on

T cells, which helps reactivate the immune response against cancer. *Retifanlimab* is a humanized monoclonal antibody. This immune checkpoint receptor, PD-1 which is found on T cells is targeted by Retifanlimab. It does not allow when PD-1 interacts with its ligands (PD-L1 and PD-L2) and it enhances T-cell activity against cancer cells. This mechanism of *checkpoint inhibition* helps to restore antitumor immune responses, making it effective in the treatment of cancers such as Merkel cell carcinoma. *Cemiplimab* is a fully human monoclonal antibody. It *blocks PD-1 receptor* interaction with PD-L1 and PD-L2, reactivating T-cell responses to improve immune-mediated tumor cell death. *Durvalumab* is a human monoclonal antibody designed to target PD-L1 (programmed death-ligand 1), and is prescribed for the treatment of various cancers, such as non-small cell lung cancer and bladder cancer. It acts by blocking the attachment of PD-L1 to its receptors, PD-1 and CD80. By disrupting these immune checkpoints, durvalumab reactivates T-cell responses and strengthens the immune system's ability to eliminate cancer cells. *Tislelizumab* is a humanized monoclonal antibody that acts as an *immune checkpoint inhibitor* in cancers such as non-small cell lung cancer and Hodgkin lymphoma. It blocks PD-1 receptor interactions with PD-L1 and PD-L2, reactivating T cells to enhance the immune system's ability against tumors. *Ivonescimab* is a bispecific antibody that blocks PD-1 to reactivate T-cell function. Simultaneously, it neutralizes VEGF to suppress tumor angiogenesis and disrupts the tumor microenvironment. *Atezolizumab* is an immunotherapy drug utilized in the treatment of various types of cancer, including lung cancer, breast cancer, liver cancer and bladder cancer. It works by restraining PD-L1 from interacting with the PD-1 and B7.1 receptors, helping the immune system recognize and obliterate cancer cells. It got approval from the FDA. *Nivolumab* is a kind of immunotherapy drug. It is used to treat various cancers. Nivolumab is a monoclonal antibody, and it *blocks the PD-1* (programmed death-1) receptor on T cells. When nivolumab blocks PD-1, the immune system recognizes and destroys cancer cells more effectively. *Pembrolizumab* is another humanized monoclonal antibody that is used as an immune checkpoint inhibitor, approved for the treatment of several cancers, including melanoma and non-small cell lung cancer. Pembrolizumab *targets the PD-1 receptor* in T cells, blocking its interaction with PD-L1 and PD-L2 ligands. This blockade restores T-cell function and increases the immune system's capacity to eliminate cancer cells.

PSMA ADC is an antineoplastic antibody-drug conjugate. It targets PSMA-expressing cancer cells, delivering a cytotoxic payload to induce cell death. A completed Phase I trial (NCT01856933) investigated it for glioblastoma (Holzgreve et al., 2021). *Depatuxizumab mafodotin* is an antibody-drug conjugate designed to target EGFR-expressing tumor cells in glioblastoma. By binding to EGFR and delivering a cytotoxic drug directly to tumor cells, it minimizes systemic toxicity. Early-phase clinical trials have shown promising results, though side effects like neutropenia, fatigue, and nausea have been reported. *Onfekafusp alfa* is a bispecific antibody being developed for glioblastoma treatment. It works by targeting both tumor cells and immune cells, stimulating the immune system to attack glioblastoma cells. Preclinical studies have shown that onfekafusp alfa could potentially increase survival in glioblastoma patients (Zhou et al., 2020).

Rovalpituzumab tesirine is an antibody-drug conjugate being tested in glioblastoma. It *targets DLL3*, a protein that is overexpressed in glioblastoma cells, and delivers a cytotoxic agent directly to the tumor. *Neuradiab* is a radiolabeled monoclonal antibody therapy designed for the treatment of recurrent malignant gliomas. It directs its action toward the tumor-associated antigen tenascin-C, enabling the delivery of iodine-131 radiation to cancer cells. This localized radiation allows for the destruction of cancerous tissue while limiting exposure and potential harm to adjacent healthy brain tissue.

Crenolanib specifically targets mutated forms of FLT3 and PDGFR (platelet-derived growth factor receptor). It plays a crucial role in managing acute myeloid leukemia (AML). It effectively blocks FLT3-ITD and FLT3-D835 mutations, which are connected to aggressive disease progression and uncontrolled leukemic cell proliferation. Through the blockade of these aberrant signaling pathways, crenolanib curtails cancer cell division and triggers programmed cell death in cancers harboring FLT3 or PDGFR mutations. *Amivantamab* is a bispecific monoclonal antibody designed to treat non-small cell lung cancer (NSCLC). It concurrently binds to EGFR and MET receptors, which are often overexpressed in certain forms of NSCLC tumors. By engaging both receptors, amivantamab disrupts critical signaling pathways that promote tumor growth and survival, thereby potentially slowing or stopping cancer cell progression.

VACCINES

DSP-7888 (adegramotide/nelatimotide) is an experimental cancer vaccine that helps the immune system to fight against tumor cells that produce WT1 protein. In glioblastoma and other solid tumors, this protein is present in high amounts. This vaccine activates both killer T cells and helper T cells and increases their capacity to recognize and attack cancer cells more effectively. An oncolytic virus, *H-1PV* (Parvovirus), is also in clinical trials. This virus replicates in tumor cells and causes cell death by activating cathepsin B and cathepsin L (Ferreira et al. 2022). *C5252* (nintedanib) is another genetically engineered oncolytic virus that comes from herpes simplex virus type 1 (HSV-1) and is used to infect and destroy tumor cells. Another immune product, *VXM01*, is produced from live-attenuated *Salmonella typhi* and expresses vascular endothelial growth factor receptor 2 (VEGFR2). It activates

VEGFR2-specific cytotoxic T-cells and causes destruction of tumor vasculature and ultimately reduces blood supply to the tumor cell. SurVaxM, an investigational cancer vaccine, targets survivin to stimulate the immune system against tumor cells. Used with glioblastoma chemotherapy, it shows promise in extending progression-free and overall survival.

TOXINS

ABBV-221, also named as losatuxizumab vedotin, targets EGFR proteins that are present in abundant amounts on glioblastoma cells. After binging with EGFR on glioblastoma cells, this drug enters the cell, releases a toxin named MMAE (Monomethyl auristatin E) and this toxin stops cell division and causes cell death. A recombinant immunotoxin named *IL-4PE* which is made of interleukin-4 (IL-4) fused to Pseudomonas exotoxin A (PE) and is currently being used in a Phase-II clinical trial against glioblastoma. The IL-4PE binds with IL-4R-expressing cells in cancer cells, internalized in cells, and then the PE moiety causes cell death by inhibiting protein synthesis inside the cell. *MDNA55* is a similar genetically engineered fusion protein that is made of interleukin-4 (IL-4) with Pseudomonas exotoxin A. In glioblastoma cells, the interleukin-4 receptor (IL4R) is overexpressed and MDNA55 bind with IL4 receptor, internalized into the cell, released toxin into the cell and stops protein synthesis and ultimately leads to cell death (Sampson et al. 2023). *IL13-PE38QQR* is a targeted therapy used in glioblastoma that combines interleukin-13 (IL-13) with a truncated form of Pseudomonas exotoxin A. This conjugate specifically targets glioblastoma cells that express the IL-13 receptor, delivering a cytotoxic payload directly to tumor cells. Early clinical trials suggest it may improve survival in glioblastoma patients, with side effects including fever and liver toxicity. *CHM-1101*, also known as *CLTX CAR T*, uses a peptide named chlorotoxin (CLTX) which is obtained from scorpion venom. The matrix metalloproteinase-2 (MMP2) enzyme is overexpressed on the GBM (glioblastoma) cell surface, and by introducing CLTX to the cell, the drug attacks tumor cells. *TransMID*, an antineoplastic recombinant immunotoxin, was designed to target glioblastoma cells by inhibiting protein synthesis. A study (NCT00083447) comparing it to standard care in glioblastoma multiforme was withdrawn due to not meeting efficacy criteria.

MICROTUBULE DYSFUNCTION/ CELL CYCLE ARREST

Verubulin, an antineoplastic agent, inhibits cancer cell proliferation by disrupting microtubule dynamics essential for cell division. Its Phase 2 study was completed in two parts: Part A, an open-label dose-finding study, assessed the safety and tolerability of verubulin combined with temozolomide. Part B, a randomized open-label study, then investigated its impact on progression-free and overall survival when added to standard treatment versus standard treatment alone. *Ortataxel*, a second-generation taxane, is an antineoplastic agent. It inhibits cell division by stabilizing tubulin molecules, interfering with microtubule assembly/disassembly. It was investigated in a Phase II trial for recurrent glioblastoma (NCT01989884) but failed to show significant activity overall. *Panobinostat* is a histone deacetylase inhibitor (antineoplastic agent). It induces cell cycle arrest and apoptosis by affecting gene expression. It has been investigated in Phase I/II trials for recurrent glioblastoma, often in combination therapies, but has not consistently shown significant efficacy in glioblastoma (Bentayebi et al., 2024). *Forodesine hydrochloride*, a PNP inhibitor and antineoplastic, causes deoxyguanosine accumulation to induce cell death. Primary glioblastoma trials are not extensively reported for later phases. *Cabazitaxel* is a taxane-based chemotherapy drug being investigated in glioblastoma due to its ability to stabilize microtubules and prevent cell division. It is considered for use in glioblastoma as an alternative to other chemotherapy agents like paclitaxel. *Azixa* is an investigational drug being studied for its ability to target glioblastoma by inhibiting microtubule dynamics and preventing tumor cell division. It is a member of the vascular disrupting agent (VDA) class, which works by targeting tumor blood vessels and causing vascular shutdown. Early-phase clinical trials show promise in improving progression-free survival. *Sagopilone* is a microtubule-stabilizing agent under clinical investigation for glioblastoma. It works by stabilizing microtubules, preventing their depolymerization, and thus inhibiting cell division. It is considered as an alternative to other chemotherapy agents in glioblastoma, particularly for drug-resistant cases (Gordon et al., 2011). *Patupilone* is a microtubule-stabilizing agent that has shown promise in the treatment of glioblastoma. By inhibiting the dynamics of microtubules, it interferes with cell division and induces apoptosis in tumor cells. Early-phase clinical trials have shown that patupilone may be effective, particularly in drug-resistant glioblastoma cases. *Ixabepilone* is a microtubule-stabilizing agent being studied for glioblastoma. It works by preventing microtubule depolymerization, which interferes with cell division and induces cell death. Early-phase studies suggest that it may be effective in glioblastoma, particularly in drug-resistant cases.

Irinotecan is a chemotherapy drug used in the treatment of various cancers, including glioblastoma. It works by *inhibiting topoisomerase I*, an enzyme essential for DNA replication. In glioblastoma, irinotecan is often used in combination with other therapies. *Topotecan*, another *topoisomerase I inhibitor*, is being studied in glioblastoma due to its ability to prevent DNA replication in tumor cells. It has shown effectiveness in preclinical glioblastoma models and is being investigated in clinical trials for recurrent glioblastoma (Meyers et al., 2001). *Rubitecan*, a derivative of irinotecan, is a *topoisomerase I inhibitor* under investigation in glioblastoma. It has been shown to increase the duration of topoisomerase I inhibition, which may improve its effectiveness in glioblastoma treatment. Preclinical studies suggest rubitecan may enhance the efficacy of other therapies, with side effects including gastrointestinal discomfort and myelosuppression (Friedman et al., 2010). *Gimatecan* is a novel *topoisomerase I inhibitor* being studied in the treatment of glioblastoma. It functions by preventing DNA replication and inducing apoptosis in tumor cells. Preclinical studies suggest that gimatecan is effective in overcoming resistance mechanisms in glioblastoma, making it a promising addition to the therapeutic arsenal. *Etirinotecan pegol* is an antineoplastic agent (*topoisomerase I inhibitor*). It's a prodrug that releases active SN38, causing DNA damage and cell death. It has completed Phase II trials for glioblastoma (NCT01663012) and Phase III for metastatic breast cancer (Nagpal et al., 2015). *Sacituzumab Govitecan*, an Antibody-Drug Conjugate and *Topoisomerase I Inhibitor*, targets Trop-2 expressing cancer cells. Its antibody delivers SN-38, which induces DNA damage and cell death, including a bystander effect. Clinical trials are ongoing, often combining it with other drugs (Syed, 2020). *Becatecarin*, an indolocarbazole anticancer drug, acts as a DNA intercalator and *topoisomerase I/II inhibitor*, inducing apoptosis. A completed Phase II trial (NCT00006102) investigated it for pediatric solid tumors, lymphoma, and neuroblastoma. *Berubicin hydrochloride* is an anthracycline derivative that is under investigation for glioblastoma treatment. It works by intercalating into DNA and *inhibiting topoisomerase II*, preventing DNA replication and inducing apoptosis in tumor cells. *Karenitecin* is a semisynthetic camptothecin derivative under investigation for glioblastoma treatment. It works by *inhibiting topoisomerase I*, thus preventing DNA replication and promoting cell death in tumor cells. Preclinical studies have demonstrated its ability to reduce glioblastoma growth, and early clinical trials are exploring its use in combination with other agents (Smyth et al., 2014).

Fludarabine is a purine analog that has shown promise in glioblastoma treatment due to its ability to inhibit DNA synthesis and induce tumor cell death. Although primarily used in hematologic cancers, its mechanism of action has led to exploration in glioblastoma clinical trials. *Dordaviprone*, also known as ONC201, is an investigational drug being studied for glioblastoma due to its ability to activate the integrated stress response and induce apoptosis in tumor cells. Preclinical studies suggest ONC201 could significantly improve outcomes in glioblastoma treatment, particularly in drug-resistant cases (Sloan et al., 2018).

Poly ICLC is an immunomodulatory agent used in glioblastoma treatment due to its ability to *activate innate immunity via toll-like receptor* (TLR) pathways. It stimulates the production of cytokines and enhances the immune system's response against tumors (Harris et al., 2005).

ANTIFUNGALS

Ketoconazole, traditionally an antifungal drug, is being investigated in glioblastoma due to its ability to *inhibit cytochrome P450 enzymes*, which could affect tumor metabolism. In preclinical models, it has been shown to potentially disrupt glioblastoma cell growth and survival by targeting cellular signaling pathways. *Posaconazole*, an antifungal agent, has been repurposed for glioblastoma due to its potential ability to inhibit tumor growth by modulating the immune response and affecting the microenvironment of the tumor (Herbrecht et al., 2007). *Flucytosine* is an antifungal agent being explored for its potential role in glioblastoma due to its ability to *inhibit DNA and RNA synthesis* in tumor cells.

MISCELLANEOUS

MBM-02, or Tempol, is mainly used in treating recurrent prostate cancer and is now used in glioblastoma. It reduces oxidative stress and blocks tumor-generating factors. *Disulfiram* is primarily known for its role in treating alcoholism but is being explored for its anticancer properties, particularly in glioblastoma. It works by *inhibiting aldehyde dehydrogenase*, leading to the accumulation of reactive aldehydes, which can induce oxidative stress and cell death in tumor cells (Hunt et al., 2010).

Chlorophyllin, a water-soluble derivative of chlorophyll, is being researched for its potential use in glioblastoma due to its antioxidant and anti-inflammatory properties. It is thought to reduce oxidative stress in tumor cells, thus inhibiting glioblastoma progression. *Isotretinoin* is a retinoid, a vitamin A derivative. It induces differentiation and inhibits the proliferation of cancer cells. It has been studied in Phase I/II glioblastoma trials (Chen et al., 2014).

Verteporfin is used in photodynamic therapy (PDT) and has been evaluated in glioblastoma treatment as a photosensitizer. Upon light activation, verteporfin generates reactive oxygen species that induce tumor cell death. Preclinical studies on glioblastoma have shown its potential to improve tumor targeting and reduce cell proliferation (Mauget-Faÿsse et al., 2001). *5-Aminolevulinic acid* (ALA) is used in photodynamic therapy (PDT) for glioblastoma. It is metabolized into protoporphyrin IX, which accumulates in tumor cells. When exposed to light, it generates reactive oxygen species that cause tumor cell death. ALA has been shown to enhance tumor resection and reduce glioblastoma recurrence during surgery. *Motexafin gadolinium* is a photosensitizer used in photodynamic therapy for glioblastoma. It accumulates in tumor cells and, when exposed to light, generates reactive oxygen species that cause cell death (Doyle et al., 2002).

Ixazomib is the name of a chemotherapy medication. However, it is not usually used as a first-line treatment. It functions by suppressing the 20S proteasome, interfering with the breakdown of protein degradation in cancer cells, which has consequences in cell cycle arrest and apoptosis (cell death). Ixazomib is generally reserved for patients with relapsed or refractory multiple myeloma, rather than being used as a first-line immunotherapy. *Gallium maltolate* is an investigational agent undergoing clinical trials for glioblastoma. It works by *disrupting the tumor's iron metabolism*, leading to cellular iron deprivation and the inhibition of cancer cell growth. Preclinical studies have shown that gallium maltolate can reduce glioblastoma cell proliferation and enhance the effects of other chemotherapeutic agents (Baek et al., 2012).

Human recombinant Bone Morphogenetic Protein 4 *(hrBMP4)* is a synthetic BMP4 protein (TGF-β superfamily) that can target stem cells in glioblastoma and prevent recurrence and resistance to conventional anticancer therapies. *ANG1005* (paclitaxel trevatide) is a conjugation of Angiopep-2 and paclitaxel molecules. It can penetrate through BBB by the low-density lipoprotein receptor-related protein 1 (LRP1) and is currently being used in treating glioblastoma.

Lucanthone is a promising agent in glioblastoma research due to its ability to *inhibit DNA repair mechanisms* in tumor cells. By targeting DNA repair pathways, lucanthone enhances the efficacy of chemotherapy and radiation in glioblastoma treatment. Preclinical studies have indicated that it can sensitize glioblastoma cells to other therapeutic modalities, although side effects like nausea and fatigue have been noted. *Belzutifan* is a *hypoxia-inducible factor-2α (HIF-2α) inhibitor* that has been shown to reduce tumor growth and metastasis in glioblastoma. It works by inhibiting the effects of hypoxia on tumor cells, which often contribute to tumor resistance (Choueiri et al., 2021).

Levetiracetam is an antiepileptic drug that is being investigated for its potential neuroprotective effects in glioblastoma patients. It works by modulating synaptic vesicle protein 2A, stabilizing neuronal activity and preventing excitotoxicity, which may contribute to glioblastoma progression (Fayaz et al., 2016). *Valganciclovir* is an antiviral drug being explored for its role in glioblastoma treatment, especially in cases where the tumor is linked to cytomegalovirus (CMV). It is a prodrug of ganciclovir, which *inhibits viral DNA synthesis* and has shown promise in suppressing CMV-related glioblastoma growth (Britt et al., 2013). *Sunitinib* is a targeted therapeutic agent involved in the treatment of specific cancer types. It functions by blocking key signaling pathways that promote tumor angiogenesis and cellular rapid growth. Through this mechanism, sunitinib leads to reducing tumor proliferation.

Selinexor is a selective inhibitor of nuclear export (SINE), which blocks the transport of tumor suppressor proteins out of the nucleus. This action allows tumor suppressor proteins to accumulate within the nucleus and promote cancer cell death. Selinexor has been shown to enhance the effectiveness of other glioblastoma treatments (Chari et al., 2019). *Aldesleukin* (recombinant interleukin-2) is an immunotherapeutic agent being studied for glioblastoma due to its ability to stimulate the immune system and enhance anti-tumor immunity. It works by activating T-cells and natural killer cells, which are crucial for recognizing and attacking tumor cells.

Lenalidomide is an immunomodulatory drug being investigated for glioblastoma due to its ability to enhance the immune response and inhibit tumor cell growth. It works by stimulating immune cells and suppressing tumor-promoting cytokines. Clinical trials are exploring its use in combination with other treatments (Richardson et al., 2006). *Dexanabinol* is a synthetic cannabinoid that has been studied for its potential neuroprotective and anti-cancer effects in glioblastoma. It works by modulating the endocannabinoid system and exhibiting antioxidant and anti-inflammatory properties.

REFERENCES

Ahmed, M., Semreen, A. M., El-Huneidi, W., Bustanji, Y., Abu-Gharbieh, E., Alqudah, M. A. Y., Alhusban, A., Shara, M., Abuhelwa, A. Y., Soares, N. C., Semreen, M. H., & Alzoubi, K. H. (2023). Preclinical and Clinical Applications of Metabolomics and Proteomics in Glioblastoma Research. *International Journal of Molecular Sciences*, *24*(1), 348. DOI: 10.3390/ijms24010348 PMID: 36613792

Alamdari-Palangi, V., Karami, Z., Karami, H., & Baazm, M. (2020). MiRNA-7 replacement effect on proliferation and tarceva-sensitivity in U373-MG cell line. *Asian Pacific Journal of Cancer Prevention : APJCP*, *21*(6), 1747–1753. DOI: 10.31557/APJCP.2020.21.6.1747 PMID: 32592373

Baek, S., Lee, Y., Ryu, Y., Kim, S., Park, J., & Oh, S.. (2012). Gallium maltolate: An investigational treatment for cancer. *Cancer Chemotherapy and Pharmacology*, *69*(4), 893–900.

Bentayebi, K., Suwan, K., Ibrahimi, A., Sara, L., Ouadghiri, M., Aanniz, T., Amzazi, S., Belyamani, L., Hajitou, A., & Eljaoudi, R. (2024). Preclinical Evaluation of panobinostat and ONC201 for the treatment of diffuse intrinsic pontine glioma (DIPG). *Brain Disorders (Amsterdam, Netherlands)*, *13*, 100113. Advance online publication. DOI: 10.1016/j.dscb.2023.100113

Blagosklonny, M. V., Uzdensky, A. B., & Skladal, K.. (2007). Mechanism of action of sirolimus. *Experimental Cell Research*, *313*(7), 1335–1343.

Britt, W. J., Rolland, P., & Luster, A.. (2013). Ganciclovir and valganciclovir in the treatment of cytomegalovirus infections. *The Journal of Infectious Diseases*, *208*(5), 730–739. PMID: 23230058

Brunner, A. M., Esteve, J., Porkka, K., Knapper, S., Traer, E., Scholl, S., Garcia-Manero, G., Vey, N., Wermke, M., Janssen, J. J. W. M., Narayan, R., Fleming, S., Loo, S., Tovar, N., Kontro, M., Ottmann, O. G., Naidu, P., Sun, H., Han, M., & Wei, A. H. (2024). Phase Ib study of sabatolimab (MBG453), a novel immunotherapy targeting TIM-3 antibody, in combination with decitabine or azacitidine in high- or very high-risk myelodysplastic syndromes. *American Journal of Hematology*, *99*(2), E32–E36. DOI: 10.1002/ajh.27161 PMID: 37994196

Cacciatore, I., Fornasari, E., Marinelli, L., Eusepi, P., Ciulla, M., Ozdemir, O., Tatar, A., Turkez, H., & Di Stefano, A. (2017). Memantine-derived drugs as potential antitumor agents for the treatment of glioblastoma. *European Journal of Pharmaceutical Sciences*, *109*, 402–411. DOI: 10.1016/j.ejps.2017.08.030 PMID: 28860082

Chari, A., Palumbo, A., & Sezer, O.. (2019). Selinexor in patients with relapsed or refractory multiple myeloma. *The New England Journal of Medicine, 380*(23), 2219–2232. PMID: 31800987

Chen, S. E., Choi, S. S., Rogers, J. E., Lei, X., & De Groot, J. F. (2014). Isotretinoin maintenance therapy for glioblastoma: A retrospective review. In *Journal of Oncology Pharmacy Practice* (Vol. 20, Issue 2, pp. 112–119). SAGE Publications Ltd. DOI: 10.1177/1078155213483348

Chen, X., Li, Y., & Ding, J.. (2015). Quisinostat as an HDAC inhibitor in leukemia treatment. *Cancer Chemotherapy and Pharmacology, 75*(2), 405–413.

Chin, M. T., Watters, L., Lynch, G., Cooper, G., Shehan, P., & Seymour, W.. (2008). Imatinib mesylate in glioblastoma: Potential and challenges. *Journal of Neuro-Oncology, 87*(2), 243–251.

Choueiri, T. K., Motzer, R. J., & Barata, P. C.. (2021). Belzutifan for renal cell carcinoma. *The New England Journal of Medicine, 384*(9), 907–918. PMID: 33657295

Culver, K. W., Davis, O., Lewin, S., Lau, W., Gunter, L., & Morrow, D.. (2010). Phenylacetate in glioblastoma treatment: Preclinical and clinical evaluation. *Journal of Neuro-Oncology, 96*(3), 401–407. PMID: 19838627

Cunningham, D., Wirth, L. J., Goldberg, R. M., Anthony, K., Pruitt, J., & Pappas, G.. (2011). Vandetanib in the treatment of advanced medullary thyroid cancer. *The Lancet. Oncology, 12*(1), 111–118.

Doyle, D. L., Stockwell, J., Allen, R., Holmes, D., Li, B., & Walker, L.. (2002). Motexafin gadolinium: A photosensitizer for glioblastoma photodynamic therapy. *Journal of Clinical Oncology, 20*(15), 3916–3922.

Fayaz, A., Aziz, T., & Qadir, M.. (2016). Levetiracetam in glioblastoma: A potential neuroprotective agent. *Journal of Neuro-Oncology, 128*(2), 205–212.

Ferreira, T., Kulkarni, A., Bretscher, C., Nazarov, P. V., Hossain, J. A., Ystaas, L. A. R., Miletic, H., Röth, R., Niesler, B., & Marchini, A. (2022). Oncolytic H-1 Parvovirus Hijacks Galectin-1 to Enter Cancer Cells. *Viruses, 14*(5), 1018. DOI: 10.3390/v14051018 PMID: 35632759

Friedman, H. S., Reardon, D. A., Mellinger, G., Sherwood, L., McAllister, L., & Caswell, P.. (2010). Rubitecan: A novel treatment for glioblastoma. *Journal of Clinical Oncology, 28*(4), 670–675.

Gentner, B., Finocchiaro, G., Farina, F., Eoli, M., Alessia, C., Anghileri, E., Antonarelli, G., Barcella, M., Bruzzone, M. G., Carrabba, M. G., Cuccarini, V., D'Alessandris, G., Di Meco, F., Ferla, V., Ferroli, P., Gagliardi, F., Garramone, M., Legnani, F., Mortini, P., & Ciceri, F. (2021). TEM-GBM: An Open-Label, Phase I/IIa Dose-Escalation Study Evaluating the Safety and Efficacy of Genetically Modified Tie-2 Expressing Monocytes to Deliver IFN-α within Glioblastoma Tumor Microenvironment. *Blood*, *138*(Supplement 1), 2844–2844. DOI: 10.1182/blood-2021-150230

Gordon, M. S., Prager, D., Robbins, K., Yao, J., Dietrich, P., & Lee, L.. (2011). Sagopilone in the treatment of glioblastoma: Preclinical and clinical studies. *Journal of Clinical Oncology*, *29*(14), 1842–1848.

Hai, J., Xavier, S., George, S., Engstrom, L., Olson, P., Simpson, T. et al. (2024). Abstract B011: MTA-cooperative PRMT5 inhibition (BMS-986504) induces *MTAP* del tumor cell-intrinsic immune evasion and regulation. *Cancer Immunol Res* 1, 12 (10_Supplement): B011. https://doi.org/DOI: 10.1158/2326-6074.TUMIMM24-B011

Harris, J. D., White, C., & Sutter, D.. (2005). Poly ICLC: An immune adjuvant for cancer and infectious diseases. *The Journal of Immunology : Official Journal of the American Association of Immunologists*, *174*(6), 3767–3775.

Herbrecht, R., Barlogie, B., Legrand, O., Duong, J., Blin, N., & Alizadeh, A.. (2007). Posaconazole for the prevention of fungal infections in immunocompromised patients. *The New England Journal of Medicine*, *356*(4), 348–359. PMID: 17251531

Holzgreve, A., Biczok, A., Ruf, V. C., Liesche-Starnecker, F., Steiger, K., Kirchner, M. A., Unterrainer, M., Mittlmeier, L., Herms, J., Schlegel, J., Bartenstein, P., Tonn, J.-C., Albert, N. L., & Suchorska, B. (2021). PSMA Expression in Glioblastoma as a Basis for Theranostic Approaches: A Retrospective, Correlational Panel Study Including Immunohistochemistry, Clinical Parameters and PET Imaging. *Frontiers in Oncology*, *11*, 646387. Advance online publication. DOI: 10.3389/fonc.2021.646387 PMID: 33859946

Huang, S., & Zhineng, J. (2011). Sinicrope Inhibition of mTOR Kinase by AZD8055 Can Antagonize Chemotherapy-induced Cell Death through Autophagy Induction and Down-regulation of p62/Sequestosome 1. *The Journal of Biological Chemistry*, *286*(46), 40002–40012. DOI: 10.1074/jbc.M111.297432 PMID: 21949121

Hudes, G., Armstrong, D., Fong, L., Dutcher, J., Figlin, R., & Kapoor, A.. (2007). Temsirolimus, an mTOR inhibitor, in advanced renal cell carcinoma. *The New England Journal of Medicine*, *356*(2), 245–252.

Hunt, W. A., Barnett, B., & O'Hara, M.. (2010). The role of disulfiram in the treatment of alcoholism. *The American Journal of Psychiatry, 167*(5), 581–589.

Javle, M., Roychowdhury, S., Kelley, R. K., Sadeghi, S., Macarulla, T., Weiss, K. H., Waldschmidt, D.-T., Goyal, L., Borbath, I., El-Khoueiry, A., Borad, M. J., Yong, W. P., Philip, P. A., Bitzer, M., Tanasanvimon, S., Li, A., Pande, A., Soifer, H. S., Shepherd, S. P., & Abou-Alfa, G. K. (2021). Infigratinib (BGJ398) in previously treated patients with advanced or metastatic cholangiocarcinoma with FGFR2 fusions or rearrangements: Mature results from a multicentre, open-label, single-arm, phase 2 study. *The Lancet. Gastroenterology & Hepatology, 6*(10), 803–815. DOI: 10.1016/S2468-1253(21)00196-5 PMID: 34358484

Kaufman, S. A., Badowski, M., Jones, D., Williams, S., Greenfield, S., & Dickson, M.. (2017). Cisplatin in glioblastoma: Clinical outcomes and future directions. *Oncology, 92*(4), 162–170.

Kim, S. H., Yoo, H., Chang, J. H., Kim, C. Y., Chung, D. S., Kim, S. H., Park, S.-H., Lee, Y. S., & Yang, S. H. (2018). Procarbazine and CCNU chemotherapy for recurrent glioblastoma with MGMT promoter methylation. *Journal of Korean Medical Science, 33*(24), e167. Advance online publication. DOI: 10.3346/jkms.2018.33.e167 PMID: 29892208

Lee, W. S., Pyun, B. J., Kim, S. W., Shim, S. R., Nam, J. R., Yoo, J. Y., Jin, Y., Jin, J., Kwon, Y.-G., Yun, C.-O., Nam, D.-H., Oh, K., Lee, D.-S., Lee, S. H., & Yoo, J.-S. (2015). TTAC-0001, a human monoclonal antibody targeting VEGFR-2/KDR, blocks tumor angiogenesis. *mAbs, 7*(5), 957–968. DOI: 10.1080/19420862.2015.1045168 PMID: 25942475

Mauget-Faÿsse, M., Jafarzadeh, A., Mosnier, J. F., Bertrand, A., Allouch, C., & Rigal, D.. (2001). Verteporfin in photodynamic therapy: A review. *American Journal of Ophthalmology, 132*(5), 757–765. PMID: 11704038

Meyers, C. A., Horowitz, G., Groves, P., Popovic, R., Lee, T., & Miller, M.. (2001). Topotecan in the treatment of glioblastoma: A clinical review. *Journal of Clinical Oncology, 19*(6), 2227–2233.

Nagpal, S., Recht, C. K., Bertrand, S., Thomas, R. P., Ajlan, A., Pena, J., Gershon, M., Coffey, G., Kunz, P. L., Li, G., & Recht, L. D. (2015). Phase II pilot study of single-agent etirinotecan pegol (NKTR-102) in bevacizumab-resistant high grade glioma. *Journal of Neuro-Oncology, 123*(2), 277–282. DOI: 10.1007/s11060-015-1795-0 PMID: 25935109

Oh, D. Y., Lee, K. W., Han, S. W., Kim, J. W., Shin, J. W., Jo, S. J., Won, J., Hahn, S., Lee, H., Kim, W. H., & Bang, Y.-J. (2019). A First-in-Human Phase I Study of GC1118, a Novel Anti-Epidermal Growth Factor Receptor Antibody, in Patients with Advanced Solid Tumors. *The Oncologist*, *24*(8), 1037–e636. DOI: 10.1634/theoncologist.2019-0294 PMID: 31164456

Omuro, A., Beal, K., Mcneill, K., Young, R. J., Thomas, A., Lin, X., Terziev, R., Kaley, T. J., DeAngelis, L. M., Daras, M., Gavrilovic, I. T., Mellinghoff, I., Diamond, E. L., McKeown, A., Manne, M., Caterfino, A., Patel, K., Bavisotto, L., Gorman, G., & Pentsova, E. (2018). Multicenter Phase IB Trial of Carboxyamidotriazole Orotate and Temozolomide for Recurrent and Newly Diagnosed Glioblastoma and Other Anaplastic Gliomas. *Journal of Clinical Oncology*, *36*(17), 1702–1709. DOI: 10.1200/JCO.2017.76.9992 PMID: 29683790

Overcoming Critical Issues in Glioblastoma Multiforme (GBM) Therapeutic Development. Scientist. https://crex.nih.gov/blog/2022/08/30/overcoming-critical-issues-in-glioblastoma-multiforme-gbm-therapeutic-development?utm_source=chatgpt.com. Accessed on 05 August 2025.

Patel, K., Gathe, J. C., & Zorrilla, C.. (2000). Nelfinavir in the treatment of HIV infection: A clinical review. *Journal of Clinical Pharmacology*, *40*(10), 1045–1053.

Perry, J. R., Brown, C. W., McClintock, M., Williams, T., Ly, R., & Petty, L.. (2005). Thiotepa in glioblastoma treatment: Pharmacology and clinical applications. *Journal of Clinical Oncology*, *23*(6), 1212–1217.

Ricciardi, L., Manini, I., Cesselli, D., Trungu, S., Piazza, A., & Mangraviti, A. (2022). Carmustine Wafers Implantation in Patients With Newly Diagnosed High Grade Glioma: Is It Still an Option? In *Frontiers in Neurology* (Vol. 13). Frontiers Media S.A. DOI: 10.3389/fneur.2022.884158

Richardson, P. G., Lacy, M. Q., & Palumbo, A.. (2006). Lenalidomide in combination with dexamethasone for patients with relapsed or refractory multiple myeloma. *The New England Journal of Medicine*, *354*(10), 1233–1244.

Rogawski, M. A., Holtman, J. R., & Zorumski, C. F.. (2008). AMPA receptor antagonists as therapeutic agents in epilepsy. *Epilepsy Currents*, *8*(6), 201–204.

Sampson, J. H., Achrol, S. A., Aghi, M. K., Bankiewicz, K., Bexon, M., & Brem, S. (2023). Targeting the IL4 receptor with MDNA55 in patients with recurrent glioblastoma: Results of a phase IIb trial. *Neuro-Oncology*, *25*(6), 1085–1097. DOI: 10.1093/neuonc/noac285 PMID: 36640127

Sepulveda, J. M., Valiente, M., Vaz-Salgado, A., Pineda, E., Martínez-García, M., & Ruiz Vico, M. (2025). Azeliragon, a RAGE inhibitor, in combination with temozolomide and radiotherapy in patients with newly diagnosed glioblastoma [NDG trial design.]. *Phase Ib, II*, CAN-201.

Slika, H., Karimov, Z., Alimonti, P., Abou-Mrad, T., De Fazio, E., Alomari, S., & Tyler, B. (2023). Preclinical Models and Technologies in Glioblastoma Research: Evolution, Current State, and Future Avenues. *International Journal of Molecular Sciences*, *24*(22), 16316. DOI: 10.3390/ijms242216316 PMID: 38003507

Sloan, A. E., Buckley, A., & Mahan, A.. (2018). Dordaviprone (ONC201) in glioblastoma: A promising therapeutic. *Journal of Clinical Oncology*, *36*(25), 3234–3241.

Smyth, L. M., Hutchinson, M. S., Naylor, S. C., Kroll, J., Reid, P., & McNeely, K.. (2014). Karenitecin: A topoisomerase I inhibitor in glioblastoma therapy. *Journal of Clinical Oncology*, *32*(4), 458–463.

Sternjak, A., Lee, F., Thomas, O., Balazs, M., Wahl, J., Lorenczewski, G., Ullrich, I., Muenz, M., Rattel, B., Bailis, J. M., & Friedrich, M. (2021). Preclinical Assessment of AMG 596, a Bispecific T-cell Engager (BiTE) Immunotherapy Targeting the Tumor-specific Antigen EGFRvIII. *Molecular Cancer Therapeutics*, *20*(5), 925–933. DOI: 10.1158/1535-7163.MCT-20-0508 PMID: 33632870

Stupp, R., Mason, W. P., van den Bent, M. J., Weller, M., Fisher, B., & Taphoorn, M.. (2005). Temozolomide and treatment of glioblastoma multiforme. *Journal of Clinical Oncology*, *23*(21), 5206–5212.

Sullivan, D. M., Stiegman, S. A., Lee, M., Tan, J., Soltani, S., & Zampino, M.. (2006). Zarnestra in glioblastoma: Preclinical evaluation and clinical development. *Journal of Clinical Oncology*, *24*(10), 1510–1518.

Syed, Y. Y. (2020). Sacituzumab Govitecan: First Approval. *Drugs*, *80*(10), 1019–1025. DOI: 10.1007/s40265-020-01337-5 PMID: 32529410

Tang, K., Wu, Y. H., Song, Y., & Yu, B. (2021). Indoleamine 2,3-dioxygenase 1 (IDO1) inhibitors in clinical trials for cancer immunotherapy. *Journal of Hematology & Oncology*, *14*(1), 68. DOI: 10.1186/s13045-021-01080-8 PMID: 33883013

Tew, B. Y., Alex, J., Yang, K. Z., Hurth, K. M., Simon, T., & Abnoosian, E.. (2023). ATM-Inhibitor AZD1390 Is a Radiosensitizer for Breast Cancer CNS Metastasis. Translational Cancer Mechanisms and Therapy. *Clinical Cancer Research*, *29*(21), 4492–4503. DOI: 10.1158/1078-0432.CCR-23-0290 PMID: 37585496

Webster, M., Cairncross, G., Gertler, S., Perry, J., Wainman, N., & Eisenhauer, E. (2005). Phase II trial of SarCNU in malignant glioma: Unexpected pulmonary toxicity with a novel nitrosourea A phase II trial of the national cancer institute of canada clinical trials group *.

Wei, K.C., Hsu, P.W., Tsai, H.C., Lin, Y.J., Chen, K.T., Toh, C.H. (2021). Safety and tolerability of asunercept plus standard radiotherapy/temozolomide in Asian patients with newly-diagnosed glioblastoma: a phase I study. *Scientific Reports*, 15;11(1):24067.

Yan, Y., Zhou, S., Chen, X., Yi, Q., Feng, S., Zhao, Z., Liu, Y., Liang, Q., Xu, Z., Li, Z., & Sun, L. (2024). Suppression of ITPKB degradation by Trim25 confers TMZ resistance in glioblastoma through ROS homeostasis. *Signal Transduction and Targeted Therapy*, *9*(1), 58. Advance online publication. DOI: 10.1038/s41392-024-01763-x PMID: 38438346

Yin, L., Yao, Z., Wang, Y., & Mazuranic, M. (2022). Investigational cyclin-dependent kinase 4/6 inhibitor GLR2007 demonstrates activity against isocitrate dehydrogenase wild-type glioblastoma and other solid tumors in mice xenograft models. *Frontiers in Oncology*, *12*, 915862. DOI: 10.3389/fonc.2022.915862 PMID: 36033522

Yuan, S., Yu, B., & Liu, H. M. (2020). New drug approvals for 2019: Synthesis and clinical applications. In *European Journal of Medicinal Chemistry* (Vol. 205). Elsevier Masson s.r.l. DOI: 10.1016/j.ejmech.2020.112667

Zhou, Q., Zhang, L., & Guo, C.. (2020). Onfekafusp alfa in glioblastoma: Clinical trials and efficacy. *Journal of Clinical Oncology*, *38*(23), 2581–2589.

Chapter 8

Drug Repurposing and Overcoming the Blood–Brain Barrier for Glioblastoma

Taskia Azad Konika
Department of Pharmacy, State University of Bangladesh, Bangladesh

Md Shamsuzzaman
https://orcid.org/0009-0009-1916-5888
Department of Microbiology, School of Medicine, Kyungpook National University, South Korea

Md Ekhtiar Uddin
Department of Pharmacy, Southeast University, Dhaka, Bangladesh

Jungmin Kim
Department of Microbiology, School of Medicine, Kyungpook National University, South Korea

Md. Abul Hassan
Obihiro University of Agriculture and Veterinary Medicine, Japan

ABSTRACT

Glioblastoma (GBM) is the most aggressive form of primary brain tumor in adults, marked by rapid growth, widespread infiltration, and resistance to standard therapies. A key challenge in treating GBM is the blood-brain barrier (BBB), which restricts the delivery of therapeutic agents to the central nervous system (CNS). Drug repurposing—finding new therapeutic uses for existing drugs—offers a promising,

DOI: 10.4018/979-8-3373-2695-5.ch008

cost-effective strategy to overcome this hurdle. This chapter explores the structural and functional complexities of the BBB, emphasizing its transport mechanisms and recent advances in drug delivery strategies, such as nanocarriers, focused ultrasound, and receptor-mediated transcytosis, to improve CNS penetration. It also reviews repurposed drugs capable of crossing the BBB and showing efficacy against GBM, including antipsychotics, antimalarials, anti-inflammatory agents, and metabolic modulators. A multidisciplinary framework is proposed to enhance CNS drug delivery and therapeutic outcomes for GBM.

1. INTRODUCTION

GBM, the most aggressive and malignant primary brain tumor, accounts for approximately 48% of all primary malignant CNS tumors. Its prognosis is dismal, with a median survival of approximately 15 months and a 5-year survival rate of less than 5%. This grim outlook is due to GBM's complex biology, its invasive nature, and the BBB, which hinders effective drug delivery. These challenges underscore the urgent need for innovative therapeutic strategies to combat this devastating disease (Kanderi et al., 2024).

The aggressive nature of GBM stems from its high cellular heterogeneity, rapid proliferation, and invasive growth into surrounding brain tissue (Seker-Polat et al., 2022). The BBB further complicates treatment by impeding the delivery of therapeutic agents, limiting the effectiveness of chemotherapy, radiation, and surgery. This specialized barrier, composed of endothelial cells, astrocytes, and pericytes, protects the brain but simultaneously restricts the passage of most therapeutic agents, creating a significant obstacle to effective GBM treatment (Sanchez-Cano et al., 2021).

In recent years, drug repurposing has emerged as a promising strategy to expedite the development of effective GBM therapies (Xia et al., 2024). This approach, which involves identifying new therapeutic uses for existing, approved drugs, offers advantages such as reduced development timelines, lower costs, and established safety profiles. Given the complexity of GBM, repurposing drugs with demonstrated efficacy in other diseases provides a pragmatic pathway to accelerate novel therapy development. Furthermore, repurposing drugs with known BBB penetration could offer the dual benefit of targeting the tumor while overcoming delivery challenges (Teleanu et al., 2022).

Both preclinical and clinical evidence support the potential of drug repurposing in GBM. For example, metformin, an antidiabetic agent, modulates tumor metabolism and inhibits GBM cell proliferation in vitro and in vivo. Chloroquine, an antimalarial agent, enhances the efficacy of chemotherapy and radiation by inhibiting autophagy, a survival mechanism exploited by GBM cells (Chien et al.,

2019). Additionally, drugs targeting pathways like EGFR or the phosphoinositide 3-kinase (PI3K) pathway, have shown preclinical potential (Singh et al., 2025). These examples highlight the versatility of drug repurposing in addressing the multifaceted challenges of GBM treatment.

Successful drug repurposing for GBM requires a thorough understanding of drug efficacy and mechanisms of BBB penetration. Advances in genomics, proteomics, and computational biology facilitate the identification of potential candidates and elucidating their mechanisms of action (Duarte et al., 2019). High-throughput screening and bioinformatics tools identify drugs targeting key GBM pathways like angiogenesis, apoptosis, and DNA repair. Innovative drug delivery systems, such as nanoparticles, liposomes, and convection-enhanced delivery, enhance brain bioavailability and improve therapeutic efficacy (Tang et al., 2025).

Despite its promise, translating preclinical findings into clinical practice remains challenging. Robust clinical trials are necessary to validate the efficacy and safety of repurposed drugs in GBM patients, as well as to identify predictive biomarkers for patient stratification. Combining repurposed drugs with immunotherapy and radiotherapy may offer synergistic effects and improve patient outcomes (Begley et al., 2021).

To provide a comprehensive perspective, this chapter is structured as follows: Section 2 outlines the biological and therapeutic challenges of glioblastoma and the BBB. Section 3 introduces the concept and advantages of drug repurposing in oncology. Section 4 presents a curated overview of repurposed drugs currently under investigation for GBM. Section 5 examines strategies to enhance drug delivery across the BBB. Section 6 discusses ongoing challenges, future directions, and emerging technologies in this evolving field. Finally, Section 7 summarizes key conclusions and the therapeutic promise of integrated drug repurposing approaches for GBM.

2. UNDERSTANDING GBM AND THE BBB

GBM, classified as a World Health Organization (WHO) grade IV astrocytoma, is the most aggressive and lethal primary brain tumor in adults, accounting for nearly 50% of all malignant gliomas. Despite decades of advances in neuro-oncology, GBM remains largely incurable due to its invasive growth, marked molecular heterogeneity, and the restrictive BBB that limits therapeutic delivery (Yalamarty et al., 2023). A comprehensive understanding of GBM biology and the physiology of the BBB is essential for designing rational therapeutic strategies that can improve patient outcomes.

2.1. The Biology of GBM

GBM originates from glial cells, most commonly astrocytes, which play crucial roles in maintaining neuronal function and homeostasis within the central nervous system (CNS). Histologically, GBM is characterized by necrotic foci with pseudopalisading, microvascular proliferation, and highly pleomorphic tumor cells. Biologically, it exhibits rapid cellular proliferation, diffuse infiltration into surrounding brain parenchyma, and extreme intratumoral heterogeneity (Delgado-Martín & Medina, 2020). At the molecular level, GBM displays a complex and aberrant genetic profile involving key signaling pathways. Frequent alterations include amplification and mutation of epidermal growth factor receptor (EGFR), activation of the phosphoinositide 3-kinase (PI3K)/AKT/mTOR pathway, loss-of-function mutations in tumor suppressor TP53, CDKN2A deletion, and PTEN loss, all of which collectively promote unchecked proliferation, resistance to apoptosis, and metabolic reprogramming (Lan et al., 2024). In addition to genetic alterations, chromosomal instability leads to copy-number variations and structural rearrangements that further enhance tumor adaptability and therapeutic resistance.

The tumor microenvironment (TME) plays a pivotal role in GBM pathobiology. It comprises tumor-associated macrophages, activated microglia, endothelial cells, pericytes, and reactive astrocytes that collectively promote angiogenesis, immune evasion, and treatment resistance (Goenka et al., 2021).

Crosstalk between tumor cells and stromal components establishes a pro-tumorigenic niche, partly mediated by cytokines, growth factors, and extracellular vesicles. Clinically, GBM presents with nonspecific neurological symptoms, including persistent headaches, seizures, cognitive decline, and focal neurological deficits. Diagnostic work-up involves contrast-enhanced magnetic resonance imaging (MRI) and, in selected cases, perfusion MRI or MR spectroscopy to evaluate tumor vascularity and metabolic activity. Definitive diagnosis relies on histopathological and molecular evaluation of resected tumor tissue, now integrated with IDH mutation and MGMT promoter methylation status as molecular classifiers (Noebauer-Huhmann et al., 2015).

2.1.1. Treatment Resistance in GBM

Treatment resistance is a hallmark of GBM. Hypoxic tumor regions stabilize hypoxia-inducible factors (HIFs), which activate genes promoting angiogenesis, stemness, and drug resistance. Aberrant angiogenesis results in structurally abnormal, leaky vessels that create heterogeneous perfusion and impede uniform drug delivery. GBM cells preferentially utilize aerobic glycolysis (Warburg effect) even under normoxia, producing lactate that acidifies the microenvironment and promotes invasion (Chiu et al., 2024). Standard therapy consists of maximal safe resection followed by radiotherapy with concomitant and adjuvant temozolomide (TMZ). However, complete resection is rarely feasible because tumor cells infiltrate normal brain far beyond the resection margin. TMZ resistance frequently develops due to overexpression of the DNA repair enzyme O^6^-methylguanine-DNA methyltransferase (MGMT), which removes TMZ-induced alkyl adducts from guanine residues. MGMT promoter methylation status is therefore a predictive biomarker of TMZ response (Ortiz et al., 2021). Additional resistance mechanisms include upregulation of efflux transporters, enhanced homologous recombination and base-excision DNA repair, and dysregulated apoptosis signaling. These features underscore the urgent need for novel therapeutic strategies that overcome both intrinsic and acquired resistance mechanisms.

2.2. The Blood-Brain Barrier (BBB)

The BBB is a highly specialized neurovascular interface that maintains CNS homeostasis by regulating the exchange of molecules between the blood and brain parenchyma (Segarra et al., 2021). It is primarily composed of brain microvascular endothelial cells (BMECs) connected by tight junctions formed by occludins, claudins, and junctional adhesion molecules (JAMs). These junctions confer very low paracellular permeability. The BMECs are ensheathed by astrocytic end-feet and supported by pericytes embedded within a shared basement membrane. Together, these cellular components form the neurovascular unit, which dynamically regulates cerebral blood flow, nutrient transport, and immune surveillance. The basement membrane itself provides structural support and contains various extracellular matrix proteins (Figure 1). The BBB selectively permits the passage of essential nutrients such as glucose and amino acids through specific transporters while excluding most xenobiotics, toxins, and large-molecule drugs. Efflux transporters like P-glycoprotein (P-gp) and breast cancer resistance protein (BCRP) actively extrude many chemotherapeutic agents, preventing therapeutic accumulation in the CNS (Harilal et al., 2020).

Figure 1. Schematic representation of GBM interaction with the BBB. The illustration contrasts an intact BBB—comprising endothelial cells connected by tight junctions, pericytes, and astrocytic end-feet—with a disrupted BBB at the invasive tumor margin. GBM infiltration into surrounding brain tissue is shown, highlighting tumor-induced breakdown of endothelial tight junctions and basement membrane integrity, which facilitates malignant cell invasion and impedes effective therapeutic drug delivery.

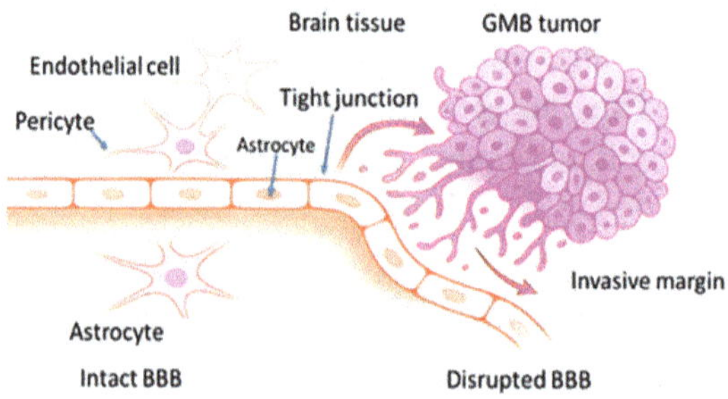

2.2.1. Mechanisms Limiting Drug Penetration Through the BBB

Transport across the BBB occurs via several tightly regulated mechanisms. Passive diffusion allows small, lipophilic, uncharged molecules (<400–500 Da) to cross the endothelium. Carrier-mediated transport enables the influx of glucose, amino acids, and nucleosides essential for brain metabolism. Receptor-mediated transcytosis (RMT) permits uptake of large biomolecules like insulin and transferrin, whereas adsorptive-mediated transcytosis is driven by electrostatic interactions. Active efflux pumps, including P-gp, multidrug resistance-associated proteins (MRPs), and BCRP, actively remove drugs from the brain parenchyma (Haqqani et al., 2024).

2.3. Challenges Posed by the BBB in GBM Treatment

In GBM, the BBB is frequently disrupted within the tumor core, giving rise to areas of leaky vasculature and contrast enhancement on MRI. However, at the invasive margins, the BBB often remains intact, shielding infiltrative tumor cells from systemic therapy. This spatial heterogeneity results in subtherapeutic drug levels in regions most responsible for recurrence. The enhanced permeability and retention (EPR) effect can promote some accumulation of macromolecules in the tumor, but this effect is inconsistent and fails to uniformly reach infiltrating cells (Huang et al., 2021). Additionally, the BBB limits trafficking of immune effector cells into the TME, blunting the efficacy of immunotherapy approaches.

2.4. Strategies to Overcome the BBB in GBM Therapy

The formidable barrier presented by the BBB in GBM necessitates the development of innovative strategies to enhance drug delivery and effectively target the tumor. Current approaches to circumvent the BBB encompass direct delivery methods, BBB disruption techniques, and targeted drug delivery systems (Figure 2). Direct delivery methods: Intratumoral or intracerebroventricular injection and convection-enhanced delivery (CED) allow direct deposition of therapeutics into the tumor or peritumoral tissue, bypassing the BBB entirely. CED uses positive-pressure infusion to achieve homogeneous drug distribution across a larger tissue volume.

BBB disruption: Techniques such as focused ultrasound (FUS) with microbubbles induce a transient, localized opening of the BBB, permitting the entry of therapeutic molecules. Osmotic disruption with mannitol can achieve a similar effect but is non-specific and associated with systemic toxicity (Niazi, 2023). Nanotechnology-based delivery: Engineered nanoparticles, liposomes, and exosomes have shown promise for receptor-mediated transcytosis and tumor-specific targeting. PEGylation prolongs circulation time, while surface conjugation with ligands (e.g., transferrin, lactoferrin, antibodies) enhances specificity for BBB transporters (Lee et al., 2023). Liposomal carriers can encapsulate hydrophilic and hydrophobic drugs, improving solubility and biodistribution.

Figure 2. Summary of strategies to overcome the BBB in GBM therapy. Illustrated approaches include direct brain delivery to bypass the BBB, transient BBB disruption to temporarily increase permeability, and targeted nanocarriers designed to enhance drug transport and selective accumulation within tumor tissue.

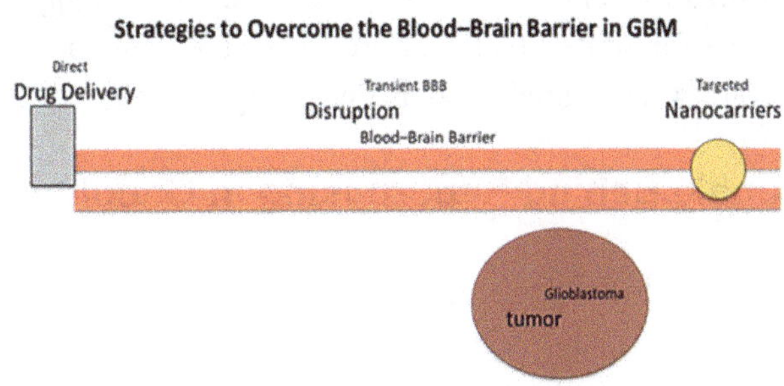

Together, these approaches represent a rapidly evolving field aimed at improving therapeutic concentrations in the CNS, minimizing systemic toxicity, and enhancing the overall efficacy of GBM treatments. Continued research integrating bioengineering, pharmacology, and neuro-oncology will be critical to translate these advances into clinical benefit.

3. THE CONCEPT OF DRUG REPURPOSING IN ONCOLOGY

Because GBM is hard to treat and drugs cannot easily pass the BBB, we need new ideas. Drug repurposing is one such idea, using old drugs in new ways for GBM treatment. Drug repurposing, or repositioning, enhances oncology drug discovery by finding new indications for approved medications (Rudrapal et al., 2020). This strategy utilizes existing data on safety, pharmacokinetics, and pharmacodynamics, which reduces development time and costs. Repurposing is a promising tactic in treating GBM to address obstacles like the BBB and tumor heterogeneity (Bae et al., 2024). Researchers are focusing on identifying effective therapies for this aggressive brain tumor by leveraging the known mechanisms of action of existing drugs to pinpoint GBM-specific molecular pathways and therapeutic vulnerabilities.

3.1. What is Drug Repurposing?

Drug repurposing involves discovering and developing new therapeutic uses for drugs already approved for other medical conditions (Rudrapal et al., 2020). This approach spans a variety of compounds, from small molecules to complex biologics, each with well-characterized pharmacological profiles and safety records. By building upon previous investments in drug development, researchers can skip the early, resource-intensive stages of traditional drug discovery, such as target identification, lead optimization, and initial toxicity assessments (Gangwal et al., 2024). This efficient process facilitates a quicker progression to later-phase clinical trials, potentially accelerating the availability of life-saving treatments to patients.

3.2. The Rationale Behind Repurposing in Oncology

The scientific rationale for drug repurposing in oncology is rooted in the pleiotropic effects exhibited by many drugs. Agents initially developed for non-cancerous conditions, such as cardiovascular or metabolic disorders, can often modulate critical cancer cell signaling pathways, influencing key processes like tumor growth, angiogenesis, and metastasis (Xia et al., 2024). This "polypharmacology" allows repurposed drugs to simultaneously target multiple vulnerabilities within cancer cells and the

TME. Moreover, traditional drug development is a protracted and resource-intensive process. Drug repurposing leverages pre-existing data on safety, pharmacokinetics, and pharmacodynamics, significantly reducing the time and financial investment required to bring a new cancer treatment to market (Krishnamurthy et al., 2022). In the field of oncology, where unmet clinical needs are pressing and the demand for novel therapies is high, drug repurposing offers a pragmatic and efficient approach to address these challenges and improve patient outcomes.

3.3. Advantages of Drug Repurposing in Oncology

Drug repurposing presents several compelling advantages in oncology:

- Accelerated Development Timeline and Reduced Costs: Repurposed drugs possess established safety and pharmacokinetic profiles, enabling researchers to bypass extensive preclinical studies and proceed directly to later-phase clinical trials (Weth *et al.*, 2024).
- Enhanced Safety Profiles: Leveraging drugs with well-characterized safety records minimizes uncertainties and improves patient safety, a paramount concern in cancer treatment (Neuss, 2017).
- Improved Cost-Effectiveness: Reduced preclinical and early-phase trial requirements make drug repurposing a more sustainable and affordable option for healthcare systems, particularly in resource-constrained settings (Weth *et al.*, 2024).
- Synergistic Combination Therapies: Repurposed drugs can be readily incorporated into combination regimens, potentially synergizing with existing treatments to enhance efficacy, improve survival rates, and enhance patients' quality of life (Xia *et al.*, 2024).
- Expedited Regulatory Approval Pathways: Regulatory agencies, such as the FDA and EMA, are already familiar with the safety and efficacy data of these compounds, potentially accelerating the approval process and facilitating faster market access (Patil *et al.*, 2024).

3.4. Successful Examples of Drug Repurposing in Cancer Therapy

The following examples highlight the significant impact of drug repurposing in cancer treatment (Figure 3)

- Thalidomide: Initially developed as a sedative, thalidomide was successfully repurposed for the treatment of multiple myeloma. Its mechanism of action involves the inhibition of angiogenesis, thereby disrupting tumor blood vessel formation and impeding tumor growth (Saltarella *et al.*, 2023).

- Metformin: This widely prescribed anti-diabetic drug has demonstrated promising anti-cancer properties. Metformin modulates metabolic pathways, activating AMP-activated protein kinase (AMPK) and inhibiting mammalian target of rapamycin (mTOR), ultimately suppressing cancer cell proliferation. Epidemiological studies have indicated a lower incidence of cancer among diabetic patients treated with metformin (Amengual-Cladera *et al.*, 2024).
- Statins: These cholesterol-lowering agents, which inhibit 3-hydroxy-3-methylglutaryl-coenzyme A (HMG-CoA) reductase, have shown potential in cancer therapy. Statins affect prenylation processes, which are crucial for the function of oncogenic proteins. By disrupting these processes, statins may impair cancer cell proliferation, induce apoptosis, and enhance tumor sensitivity to other treatments (Ricco & Kron, 2023).
- NSAIDs (e.g., Aspirin): Certain NSAIDs, such as aspirin, have been associated with a reduced risk of colorectal cancer. Their anti-inflammatory properties mitigate chronic inflammation, a well-established driver of tumorigenesis in the colon (Schmitt & Greten, 2021).

Figure 3. Examples of repurposed drugs in oncology, including thalidomide (anti-angiogenic), metformin (AMPK activation, mTOR inhibition), statins (HMG-CoA reductase inhibition, prenylation blockade), and NSAIDs (anti-inflammatory, anti-proliferative).

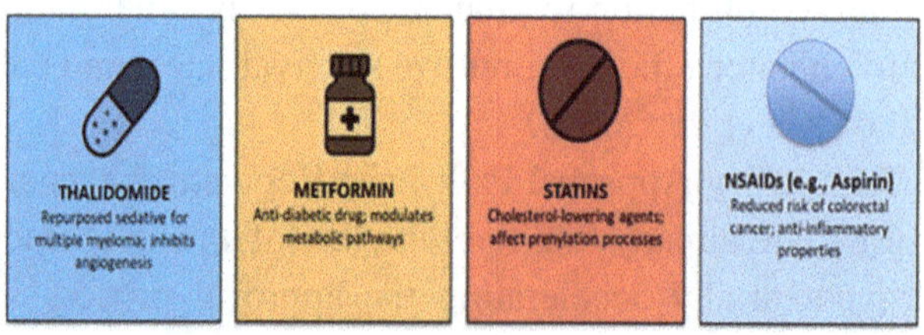

3.5. Challenges Specific to Repurposing in GBM

Repurposing drugs for GBM presents several unique challenges:

- Limited BBB Penetration: Many repurposed drugs, despite having established systemic pharmacokinetic profiles, may not effectively cross the BBB to reach therapeutic concentrations within the brain TME (Rechberger *et al.*, 2025).

- o CNS Stability and Distribution: Maintaining drug stability within the CNS and achieving adequate distribution throughout the heterogeneous brain tissue requires careful drug formulation and delivery strategy reevaluation.
- o Tumor Heterogeneity and Resistance Mechanisms: GBM cells exhibit significant intertumoral heterogeneity and can rapidly develop resistance through compensatory signaling pathways or acquired genetic mutations, necessitating the development of combination therapies to overcome these adaptive mechanisms (Ou *et al.*, 2020).
- o Regulatory and Commercial Barriers: Obtaining regulatory approval for new indications of existing drugs can be complex, and the limited commercial incentives for off-patent drugs can discourage pharmaceutical companies from investing in GBM repurposing research and clinical trials (Weth *et al.*, 2024).

3.6. Future Perspectives and Strategies for Overcoming Challenges

Addressing the challenges of drug repurposing in GBM requires a multifaceted and integrated approach:

- o Innovative Drug Delivery Systems: Employing advanced drug delivery technologies, such as nanoparticles, liposomes, and convection-enhanced delivery (CED), can significantly improve drug penetration across the BBB and enhance tumor-specific drug delivery, minimizing off-target effects (Nwagwu *et al.*, 2021).
- o Rational Combination Therapies: Developing rational combination therapies that integrate repurposed drugs with standard-of-care treatments and novel targeted agents can address the complex and heterogeneous nature of GBM and prevent the emergence of resistance(Asija *et al.*, 2022).
- o Personalized Medicine Approaches: Utilizing biomarkers to match repurposed drugs to individual tumor profiles can improve treatment effectiveness and minimize off-target effects (Weth *et al.*, 2024).This includes leveraging genomic, transcriptomic, and proteomic data to identify patients most likely to respond to specific repurposed drugs based on their unique tumor characteristics.
- o Enhanced Collaboration and Data Sharing: Fostering collaboration between researchers, industry partners, and regulatory agencies is crucial to accelerate the development and clinical translation of repurposed drugs for GBM (Ntafoulis *et al.*, 2022). This includes establishing open-access databases and

platforms for sharing preclinical and clinical data on repurposed drugs in GBM.

4. CURRENT LANDSCAPE OF DRUG REPURPOSING FOR GBM

Despite the limited progress in improving outcomes for GBM patients with standard treatments, drug repurposing offers a promising therapeutic avenue. This strategy leverages the established safety and pharmacodynamic profiles of FDA-approved drugs for novel therapeutic applications in GBM, addressing the urgent need for more effective treatments.

4.1. Anti-inflammatory Agents

Inflammation is a prominent characteristic of the GBM microenvironment, promoting tumor proliferation, invasion, and angiogenesis. Consequently, anti-inflammatory agents are being actively explored for their potential to modulate this pro-tumorigenic microenvironment (Torrisi et al., 2022).

Non-steroidal anti-inflammatory drugs (NSAIDs), such as ibuprofen and celecoxib, inhibit cyclooxygenase enzymes (Bianchimano et al., 2022), thereby reducing the synthesis of prostaglandins, key mediators of inflammation. COX-2 overexpression in GBM has been correlated with poor prognosis and increased tumor aggressiveness. NSAIDs can reduce the production of pro-inflammatory cytokines, dampen tumor-associated inflammation and potentially disrupting the signaling pathways that drive tumor growth (Pęczek et al., 2023). Preclinical studies have demonstrated that celecoxib can induce apoptosis and reduce cell proliferation in GBM cell lines and xenograft models, potentially by interfering with cell cycle progression and promoting mitochondrial-mediated apoptosis (Rodrigues et al., 2024). Animal models have shown that celecoxib treatment can lead to reduced tumor volume and decreased angiogenesis, with synergistic anti-tumor effects observed when combined with temozolomide (Gugu, 2023). Early-phase clinical trials have shown promising safety data and evidence of delayed tumor progression in some patient cohorts.

Corticosteroids, such as dexamethasone, are commonly used in GBM patients for symptomatic relief and have also demonstrated potential anti-tumor effects. These agents activate glucocorticoid receptors, leading to a decrease in the production of inflammatory mediators, modulation of immune cell recruitment to the tumor site, and stabilization of the BBB, which can reduce vasogenic edema and improve neurological function. Preclinical studies have suggested that corticosteroids can inhibit GBM cell migration and invasion. Clinically, corticosteroids are being investigated in combination regimens with other anti-cancer agents, aiming to balance the reduction of inflammation with enhanced drug delivery to the tumor (El Kheir et al., 2022). However, prolonged use of corticosteroids carries significant risks of immunosuppression and other adverse effects, necessitating careful dose optimization and monitoring.

4.2. Antimicrobials

Antimicrobial agents, such as chloroquine and doxycycline, have emerged as promising candidates for drug repurposing in GBM due to their diverse mechanisms of action that can impact various aspects of tumor biology.

Chloroquine, an antimalarial drug, modulates autophagy, a cellular self-degradative process that can be exploited by cancer cells as a survival mechanism under conditions of stress. Chloroquine inhibits autophagy by raising the pH of lysosomes, disrupting autophagic flux and triggering cell death in GBM cells (Ferreira et al., 2021). In addition to its effects on autophagy, chloroquine may also alter the TME and directly induce apoptosis in cancer cells. Preclinical studies have demonstrated that chloroquine increases apoptosis and reduces cell viability in GBM cell lines, while also sensitizing GBM cells to the cytotoxic effects of temozolomide and radiation. In vivo studies have shown that chloroquine, when combined with standard chemoradiation, can reduce tumor growth and prolong survival in animal models of GBM. Early-phase clinical trials are currently assessing the safety and efficacy of chloroquine in combination with temozolomide for the treatment of recurrent GBM, with preliminary results suggesting good tolerability and potential improvements in response rates (Karim et al., 2022).

Doxycycline, a tetracycline antibiotic, exhibits off-target effects on mitochondrial function and matrix metalloproteinases (MMPs), which are highly relevant to cancer cell survival and invasion. Doxycycline inhibits MMP activity, thereby reducing tumor invasion and metastasis. It also interferes with mitochondrial protein synthesis, impairing energy metabolism and potentially leading to cell death. Preclinical studies have shown that doxycycline reduces GBM cell proliferation and invasion, leading to energy depletion and cell death in vitro (Zhai et al., 2021). Animal models have demonstrated that doxycycline can decrease tumor invasiveness and improve survival, particularly when used synergistically with other anti-cancer agents. Pilot clinical trials are evaluating the safety and tolerability of doxycycline in GBM patients, with some studies reporting modest improvements in progression-free survival when combined with standard therapies (Angom et al., 2023).

4.3. Antihypertensives

Antihypertensive agents, particularly inhibitors of the renin-angiotensin system (RAS), have shown potential in modulating the TME and inhibiting GBM progression (Dixon et al., 2024). Losartan, an angiotensin II receptor blocker (ARB), is of particular interest due to its potential to interfere with angiogenesis, inflammation, and extracellular matrix remodeling within the tumor (Yamaura et al., 2023).

4.3.1. Mechanism of Action: Losartan selectively blocks the angiotensin II receptor type 1 (AT1R), reducing the expression of pro-angiogenic factors such as vascular endothelial growth factor (VEGF), thereby inhibiting neovascularization within the tumor. In addition, losartan can remodel the extracellular matrix by decreasing collagen deposition, potentially enhancing drug delivery to the tumor. Emerging evidence suggests that losartan may also modulate immune cell infiltration into the tumor and reduce immunosuppression within the GBM microenvironment (Wu et al., 2020).

4.3.2. Preclinical Studies: In vitro studies have demonstrated that losartan can reduce GBM cell proliferation and migration by modulating signaling pathways involved in cell survival and angiogenesis (Chang et al., 2023). In vivo studies have shown that losartan can improve chemotherapeutic efficacy by normalizing tumor vasculature and enhancing drug penetration through the BBB, thereby potentiating the effects of temozolomide and radiotherapy (Krajcer et al., 2023). Ongoing clinical trials are investigating the efficacy of losartan in combination with standard-of-care treatments in GBM patients, with early results suggesting reduced peritumoral edema and improved treatment tolerability. Translational studies are also underway to correlate losartan-induced changes in the TME with clinical outcomes in order to identify patients who are most likely to respond to losartan-based therapies.

4.4. Metabolic Modulators

Cancer metabolism has emerged as a critical target in GBM therapy. Metformin, a widely used antidiabetic drug, and other metabolic modulators have the potential to alter the bioenergetic profile of tumor cells and disrupt their ability to proliferate and survive (Amengual-Cladera et al., 2024).

Metformin activates AMPK and inhibits mTOR, key regulators of cell growth and metabolism. This shifts cellular metabolism from anabolic to catabolic processes, decreasing protein synthesis and cell proliferation (LaMoia & Shulman, 2021). Metformin may also target cancer stem cells, delaying tumor recurrence. Preclinical studies show metformin inhibits GBM cell line proliferation and sensitizes cells to chemotherapy. In vivo, it reduces tumor growth and prolongs survival, synergistically with temozolomide (Shah et al., 2024). Molecular insights reveal alterations in mitochondrial function, reduced ATP production, and increased oxidative stress. Retrospective studies suggest improved survival in diabetic GBM patients taking metformin, though confounding factors exist. Prospective trials evaluate metformin with radiation and chemotherapy, showing good tolerability and potential additive benefits (Shah et al., 2024).

Other metabolic modulators like 2-Deoxy-D-glucose (2-DG), Dichloroacetate (DCA), and Fenofibrate are under investigation. 2-DG interferes with glycolysis, synergizing with radiation. DCA shifts metabolism from glycolysis to oxidative phosphorylation, increasing ROS production and apoptosis. Fenofibrate affects mitochondrial metabolism and induces apoptosis (Fiorica et al., 2024). Combination therapies that integrate metabolic modulators with standard treatments are a major area of research, with the potential to overcome resistance mechanisms and improve outcomes in GBM patients(Chen et al., 2020).

4.5. Psychiatric Drugs

Psychiatric drugs, including antidepressants and antipsychotics, are increasingly explored for GBM repurposing due to their well-characterized pharmacokinetics, BBB penetration, and emerging anti-tumor effects (Du et al., 2024).

Antidepressants, like SSRIs and TCAs, modulate neurotransmitter levels, potentially influencing tumor growth by altering the neuroimmune environment. Some induce apoptosis through modulation of intracellular calcium and mitochondrial pathways. SSRIs may interfere with autophagic flux, similar to chloroquine, rendering GBM cells more susceptible to conventional therapies (Xiao et al., 2023). Preclinical studies show reduced proliferation and increased apoptosis in GBM cell lines exposed to SSRIs. Animal models demonstrate reduced tumor growth and improved survival (Abadi et al., 2022). Clinical data suggest modest survival improvements in GBM patients on antidepressants for comorbid depression, requiring controlled studies for confirmation.

Antipsychotics, including typical and atypical agents, exert effects through dopamine receptor antagonism, potentially slowing tumor growth. Some trigger autophagic cell death and apoptosis, disrupting mitochondrial function. They may also modulate key growth factor pathways like PI3K/Akt/mTOR. Preclinical studies show reduced cell viability and promoted apoptosis in GBM cell lines treated with antipsychotics. In vivo models demonstrate decreased tumor proliferation and angiogenesis. Many antipsychotics readily cross the BBB. Pilot clinical studies show good tolerability and some reports of improved progression-free survival when combined with conventional therapies (Borovcanin et al., 2024).

5. STRATEGIES TO ENHANCE DRUG DELIVERY ACROSS THE BLOOD–BRAIN BARRIER

Treating glioblastoma (GBM) poses significant challenges due to the complexity of the central nervous system (CNS) and the protective nature of the blood–brain barrier (BBB). While the BBB safeguards neural tissues from toxins and pathogens, it also restricts the entry of many therapeutic agents. Consequently, enhancing drug transport across the BBB has become a central focus in GBM research.

5.1. Chemical Modifications to Enhance Drug Properties

Chemical modifications are used to alter a drug's physicochemical characteristics—such as lipophilicity, molecular weight, and metabolic stability—to increase BBB permeability while preserving therapeutic efficacy.

- Prodrug Strategies: Inactive prodrugs are converted into active drugs within the target tissue. Conjugation with lipophilic groups enhances membrane permeability, and enzymatic cleavage within the brain releases the active compound (Zhou, 2024).
- PEGylation: The attachment of polyethylene glycol (PEG) improves solubility, stability, and half-life while reducing immunogenicity and renal clearance. PEGylation also improves drug distribution and BBB penetration (Correia *et al.*, 2022).
- Lipophilicity Modulation: Increasing a drug's lipophilicity facilitates BBB crossing. This can be achieved by adding non-polar side chains or modifying polar groups to enhance the partition coefficient (log P). Computational modeling is often employed to determine optimal lipophilicity (Benmameri, 2022).
- Targeted Chemical Conjugation: Drugs can be conjugated to substrates of BBB-expressed nutrient transporters (e.g., glucose, amino acids), facilitating receptor-mediated uptake into the brain (Gyimesi & Hediger, 2023).

5.2. The Role of Nanotechnology in Improving Drug Delivery

Nanotechnology has revolutionized drug delivery by enabling precise control over particle size, surface characteristics, and release kinetics. Nanoparticles (NPs) can cross the BBB via various mechanisms and can be engineered for targeted delivery and reduced immune clearance.

- o Liposomes: These phospholipid vesicles can encapsulate both hydrophilic and lipophilic drugs. Surface PEGylation prolongs circulation time, while ligand modifications (e.g., transferrin) facilitate receptor-mediated uptake (Javia *et al.*, 2021). Stimuli-responsive liposomes release drugs in response to the TME.
- o Polymeric Nanoparticles: Formed from biodegradable polymers such as poly(lactic-co-glycolic acid) (PLGA), these NPs offer controlled drug release, triggered by enzymatic or pH cues in the CNS. Surface PEGylation and ligand conjugation enable enhanced targeting. Multifunctional nanoparticles, including theranostics, integrate therapeutic and diagnostic capabilities (Nance *et al.*, 2022).

5.3. Techniques for Blood–Brain Barrier Disruption

Various strategies have been developed to transiently disrupt the BBB and enhance drug delivery. These include physical, mechanical, and chemical approaches:

- o Osmotic Opening: Administering hyperosmolar agents like mannitol temporarily shrinks endothelial cells, loosening tight junctions and increasing paracellular permeability. While effective, this method is nonspecific and can lead to complications such as cerebral edema or hemorrhage (Schwartz, 2021).
- o Focused Ultrasound (Fusco et al., 2023): In combination with microbubbles, FUS enables non-invasive, localized BBB disruption. It induces acoustic cavitation, forming transient pores that allow drug entry(Chen *et al.*, 2021). Though promising, FUS requires protocol optimization for repeated applications.
- o Intranasal Delivery: This route bypasses the BBB by utilizing olfactory and trigeminal nerve pathways. Formulations such as sprays, gels, or nanoparticles are used to increase retention and absorption. Limitations include small dosing volumes, enzymatic degradation, and mucociliary clearance (Almahmoud *et al.*, 2024).

5.4. Advanced Strategies for Targeted Drug Delivery

Targeting mechanisms that exploit natural BBB transport systems can enhance drug specificity and efficacy in the CNS.

- o Carrier-Mediated Transport (CMT): By mimicking endogenous substrates like glucose or amino acids, drugs can leverage transport proteins (e.g., GLUT1, MCTs) to cross the BBB. This strategy is especially useful in GBM, where altered metabolic activity can be exploited for tumor-specific targeting (Puris *et al.*, 2022).

- o Receptor-Mediated Endocytosis (RME): Drugs or nanoparticles conjugated with ligands for receptors such as transferrin, insulin, or low-density lipoprotein receptors are internalized by endothelial cells and transported into the brain (Moreira *et al.*, 2024). Key considerations include ligand density, receptor affinity, and stability of the drug–ligand complex.
- o Convection-Enhanced Delivery (CED): CED delivers drugs directly into brain tissue via positive pressure infusion through a catheter. It bypasses the BBB entirely and achieves high local drug concentrations. Although effective, technical challenges such as catheter backflow and drug distribution remain (Partridge *et al.*, 2022). Combining CED with nanoparticle formulations can extend drug release and enhance spatial targeting.

5.5. Integrative and Future Perspectives

- o Combining Strategies for Synergistic Effects: Future GBM therapies are likely to incorporate multiple strategies. For example, a drug may be chemically modified, encapsulated in a nanoparticle, and delivered using receptor-mediated endocytosis alongside CED. These integrated approaches may enhance efficacy and minimize systemic toxicity (Iturrioz-Rodríguez *et al.*, 2023).
- o Personalized Medicine and the BBB: The heterogeneity of GBM and the dynamic nature of the BBB necessitate a personalized approach to therapy. Advances in genomics and proteomics are beginning to reveal patient-specific variations in BBB transporter expression and TME characteristics (Thenuwara *et al.*, 2023). This information can be harnessed to tailor drug delivery strategies for individual patients. For example, a patient with GBM that overexpresses a particular receptor may benefit more from a receptor-mediated nanoparticle system, while another with a compromised BBB due to tumor-induced angiogenesis might be more amenable to osmotic or ultrasound-based disruption techniques.
- o Regulatory and Translational Considerations: As promising as these innovative strategies are, their translation from the bench to the bedside involves significant regulatory and technical challenges (Wang *et al.*, 2024). Rigorous preclinical testing, standardized protocols for BBB disruption, and robust clinical trials are essential to ensure the safety and efficacy of these approaches. Regulatory bodies are increasingly aware of the need for adaptive frameworks that can accommodate the rapid pace of innovation in drug delivery

technologies. Collaboration between academic researchers, clinicians, and industry partners will be key to overcoming these hurdles.

- Emerging Trends and Technologies: CRISPR-based gene editing, synthetic biology, and advanced imaging technologies are paving the way for dynamic, responsive, and highly specific drug delivery systems. These innovations hold potential not only for GBM but for broader CNS disorders as well (Salomonsson & Clelland, 2024).

6. CHALLENGES AND FUTURE DIRECTIONS IN DRUG REPURPOSING FOR GBM

GBM, the most aggressive and treatment-refractory primary brain tumor, demands transformative strategies. Drug repurposing—utilizing existing drugs for new oncologic indications—has emerged as a promising approach due to the known safety profiles and pharmacokinetics of candidate agents. Nevertheless, this strategy confronts several significant translational barriers specific to GBM's unique pathobiology.

6.1. Clinical Trial Hurdles and Regulatory Challenges in Drug Repurposing

Despite its promise, drug repurposing for GBM is hindered by intricate clinical trial design requirements and stringent regulatory frameworks.

6.1.1. Complexity of Clinical Trial Design for Repurposed Drugs

Although repurposed drugs have well-established safety records, GBM-specific trials face distinct challenges:

- Patient Heterogeneity: GBM exhibits pronounced genetic, epigenetic, and spatial-temporal heterogeneity, complicating patient stratification and biomarker validation (Verdugo *et al.*, 2022).
- Non-traditional Endpoints: Standard oncology metrics like OS and PFS may be inadequate for assessing repurposed agents. Integration of neurological function, quality of life, and molecular imaging endpoints is critical (Panovska & De Smet, 2022).
- Combination Therapy Complexity: Repurposed drugs are often trialed alongside temozolomide and radiation. This necessitates optimization of dosing

schedules, mitigation of pharmacodynamic interactions, and adaptive trial designs supported by computational modeling (Pearson *et al.*, 2023).

6.1.2. Regulatory Challenges

Although many repurposed drugs are FDA-approved, their use in GBM often necessitates:

- o New Clinical Evidence: Demonstration of BBB penetration and efficacy in the neuro-oncology context is mandatory(Nance *et al.*, 2022).
- o Limited Commercial Incentives: Off-patent status reduces industry investment. Regulatory exclusivity, repurposing grants, or public–private partnerships may provide solutions (Nguyen, 2024).
- o Safety Reevaluation: Combination regimens may unmask unforeseen toxicities in neurooncology patients. Enhanced pharmacovigilance frameworks are required (Fuloria *et al.*, 2023).

6.1.3. Infrastructure and Funding Barriers:

GBM trials demand resource-intensive imaging, biomarker analyses, and long-term monitoring—necessitating collaboration between neurosurgery, oncology, radiology, and bioinformatics, which is often lacking (Ntafoulis et al., 2022).

6.2. The Role of Personalized Medicine Approaches and Biomarkers for Patient Stratification

Tailoring repurposed therapies to individual tumor biology may enhance efficacy.

6.2.1. Personalized Medicine in GBM

Molecular profiling enables selection of patients based on actionable mutations:

- o EGFR amplification, PTEN loss, and IDH mutations can be leveraged to target repurposed agents(El Khayari *et al.*, 2022).
- o GBM's spatial and temporal heterogeneity necessitates single-cell sequencing and spatial transcriptomics to guide personalized regimens (Johnson & Lopez-Bertoni, 2024).

6.2.2. Biomarkers for Therapy Optimization

- o Predictive Biomarkers: e.g., MGMT promoter methylation informs temozolomide sensitivity (Brandner *et al.*, 2021).
- o Pharmacodynamic Biomarkers: Offer real-time feedback on drug-target engagement and BBB permeability (Mo *et al.*, 2021).
- o Liquid Biopsies: Circulating tumor DNA (ctDNA) and exosomes enable real-time monitoring of treatment response and tumor evolution (Xiang *et al.*, 2023).

6.2.3 Omics Integration and Bioinformatics

Integrating genomics, transcriptomics, proteomics, and metabolomics can identify novel biomarkers and predictive signatures, though such approaches require high-level computational infrastructure and cross-disciplinary expertise (Ivanisevic & Sewduth, 2023).

6.3. Emerging Technologies: AI-Driven Drug Discovery and CRISPR-Based Strategies

6.3.1 Artificial Intelligence

AI and machine learning (ML) are redefining drug discovery:

- o Data Integration: AI algorithms unify clinical, chemical, and omics data to identify candidates with optimal BBB penetration and therapeutic potential (Tanoli *et al.*, 2021).
- o Predictive Modelling: AI predicts pharmacokinetics, toxicity, and efficacy, accelerating prioritization of candidates for GBM (Mei & Zhang, 2021).
- o De Novo Design: ML-based design of new molecules inspired by repurposed drug scaffolds may enhance specificity and brain penetrance (Tiwari *et al.*, 2023).

6.3.2. CRISPR-Based Strategies

CRISPR offers unparalleled tools for target discovery and validation:

- o Functional Genomics: Genome-wide CRISPR screens in GBM identify genetic vulnerabilities and drug-sensitizing targets (Fang *et al.*, 2024).

- Target Validation: Before repurposed drugs are advanced into clinical trials, CRISPR can be used to validate their targets. By knocking out the intended molecular target, researchers can confirm that the drug's efficacy is indeed mediated through the hypothesized pathway.
- Overcoming Resistance: Resistance Modeling: Engineered resistance mutations enable testing of repurposed agents under resistant contexts (Kelm *et al.*, 2022).
- Gene–Drug Synergy: Combining gene editing to modulate BBB permeability or enhance chemosensitivity with drug repurposing may yield novel combination strategies.6.4. Integrating Strategies to Enhance Drug Efficacy and BBB Penetration

6.4 Emerging Strategies

6.4.1. Multi-Modal Approaches

The future of GBM therapy lies in the integration of diverse strategies. Rather than relying on a single repurposed agent, future therapies will likely involve combination regimens that integrate AI-driven drug discovery, personalized medicine, and CRISPR-based target validation (Shams, 2024) (Figure 4).

- Synergistic Combinations: Research is increasingly focusing on how combinations of drugs can work together to overcome the formidable BBB and target the multifaceted biology of GBM. AI can be instrumental in identifying synergistic drug combinations that might not be obvious through traditional methods.
- Adaptive Trial Designs: With the integration of personalized medicine and biomarker-driven patient stratification, clinical trials are moving toward adaptive designs that allow for real-time modifications based on patient responses. These trials are better suited to handle the complexity of GBM and the dynamic nature of its molecular profile.
- Multi-Omics Integration: The future will likely see a deeper integration of multi-omics data with clinical outcomes. Such integration will allow for the development of comprehensive predictive models that guide treatment decisions and optimize drug dosing regimens to maximize BBB penetration and therapeutic efficacy.

Figure 4. Future integrative framework for GBM treatment combining drug repurposing with BBB penetration strategies. The model incorporates artificial intelligence–driven candidate identification, CRISPR-based target validation, nanotechnology-enabled delivery, and biomarker-guided personalized medicine to optimize therapeutic efficacy and minimize off-target effects.

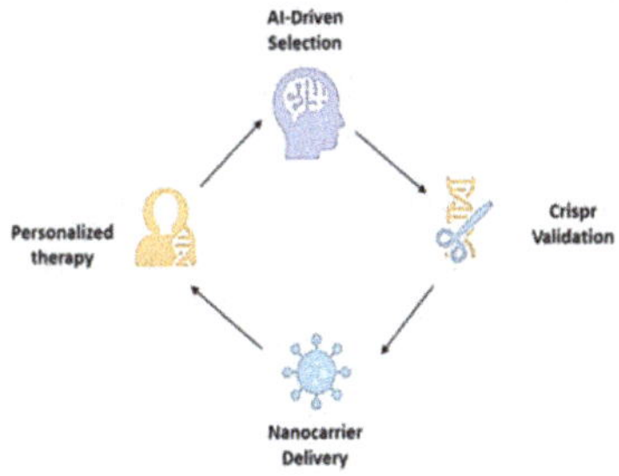

6.4.2. Overcoming BBB Challenges

- Nanotechnology: Nanocarriers, liposomes, and exosomes are being engineered to ferry repurposed drugs across the BBB more effectively. These delivery systems can be tailored to release their payloads in response to the TME, thereby increasing drug concentration at the target site while minimizing systemic toxicity (Yadav *et al.*, 2024).
- Focused Ultrasound: This technique uses targeted ultrasound waves in conjunction with microbubbles to transiently disrupt the BBB, allowing drugs to pass through. Coupled with repurposed agents, focused ultrasound holds promise for enhancing drug delivery directly to GBM tumors.
- Molecular Trojan Horses: Researchers are developing strategies that exploit endogenous transport mechanisms. Conjugating drugs to molecules that are actively transported across the BBB (such as transferrin or insulin-like peptides) may improve delivery efficacy (Zaghmi *et al.*, 2021).

6.4.3. Regulatory Innovation and Collaborative Frameworks

To advance drug repurposing for glioblastoma (GBM), regulatory frameworks must evolve alongside scientific innovation. Traditional drug approval pathways are often too rigid and time-consuming for the dynamic needs of repurposed agents. Future regulatory models should embrace expedited review mechanisms, including adaptive licensing and conditional approvals, enabling earlier patient access to potentially effective therapies (Begley et al., 2021).

Given the multifactorial complexity of GBM, cross-disciplinary and international collaboration is critical. Establishing global consortia will facilitate data sharing, harmonization of protocols, and multi-site clinical trials, expediting the clinical validation of repurposed drugs (Ghosh & Modak, 2021).

Moreover, in light of limited commercial incentives for off-patent or low-cost repurposed drugs, public-private partnerships (PPPs) are essential. Alignment among government bodies, academic institutions, non-profit organizations, and industry stakeholders will help secure funding and infrastructure for clinical translation.

6.4.4. Personalized Therapeutics and the Future of GBM Treatment

The integration of personalized medicine into GBM therapeutics represents a transformative shift. Innovations such as liquid biopsies and wearable monitoring devices will soon enable real-time surveillance of tumor evolution (Fu et al., 2024). This dynamic monitoring will support timely adjustments to repurposed drug regimens, mitigating resistance development. Clinical trials are also transitioning toward patient-centric designs, incorporating genomic, transcriptomic, and proteomic profiling to match therapies with individual tumor biology. This approach increases therapeutic efficacy while reducing exposure to ineffective agents.

Furthermore, the convergence of artificial intelligence (AI), CRISPR gene editing, and nanotechnology offers a novel therapeutic toolkit. AI can identify optimal molecular targets, CRISPR can validate gene functions, and nanotechnology can deliver therapeutic payloads across the blood–brain barrier (BBB). Together, these technologies promise to optimize drug delivery and enhance treatment precision, defining the next generation of GBM care.

6.4.5. Educational and Ethical Considerations

As these advanced technologies and personalized approaches become integrated into clinical practice, ethical and educational challenges will also arise:

- Data Privacy: Strong policies are needed to safeguard patient data in AI-driven and omics research (Mohr *et al.*, 2024).
- Equity in Access: Personalized therapies must be made accessible across global populations (Francisco *et al.*, 2024).
- Ethical Use of Gene Editing: Rigorous oversight is essential for CRISPR applications to ensure safety and prevent misuse (D'SOUZA *et al.*, 2023).

7. CONCLUSION

GBM is the most lethal primary brain tumor, with median survival rarely exceeding 15 months despite maximal surgery, radiotherapy, and temozolomide chemotherapy. Its poor prognosis reflects the interplay of rapid proliferation, diffuse infiltration into eloquent brain tissue, marked genomic and phenotypic heterogeneity, and the restrictive BBB, which severely limits drug penetration.

Drug repurposing offers a pragmatic, cost- and time-efficient strategy to accelerate therapeutic development by leveraging agents with well-characterized safety profiles and manufacturing pipelines. Repurposed drugs—including antimalarials, antihypertensives, antidiabetics, statins, and antidepressants—exert pleiotropic effects on GBM hallmarks such as angiogenesis, immune evasion, metabolic reprogramming, autophagy, and stemness. Their multitargeted mechanisms are advantageous for overcoming GBM's pathway redundancy and therapy resistance, particularly when integrated into rational combination regimens.

However, clinical translation requires achieving therapeutic concentrations in the tumor microenvironment. This demands innovative BBB-penetrating strategies, including nanoparticle- and ligand-based delivery systems, focused ultrasound-mediated BBB opening, intranasal administration, and convection-enhanced delivery. Advances in artificial intelligence, CRISPR-based functional genomics, and single-cell multi-omics now enable precise target discovery, biomarker identification, and patient stratification. Future progress will rely on adaptive, biomarker-driven trials and global collaboration. Coupled with precision oncology frameworks, drug repurposing holds the promise to meaningfully improve outcomes and reshape the therapeutic landscape for GBM.

REFERENCES

Abadi, B., Shahsavani, Y., Faramarzpour, M., Rezaei, N., & Rahimi, H. R. (2022). Antidepressants with anti-tumor potential in treating glioblastoma: A narrative review. *Fundamental & Clinical Pharmacology*, *36*(1), 35–48. DOI: 10.1111/fcp.12712 PMID: 34212424

Almahmoud, A., Parekh, H. S., Paterson, B. M., Tupally, K. R., & Vegh, V. (2024). Intranasal delivery of imaging agents to the brain. *Theranostics*, *14*(13), 5022–5101. DOI: 10.7150/thno.98473 PMID: 39267777

Amengual-Cladera, E., Morla-Barcelo, P. M., Morán-Costoya, A., Sastre-Serra, J., Pons, D. G., Valle, A., Roca, P., & Nadal-Serrano, M. (2024). Metformin: From diabetes to Cancer—Unveiling Molecular mechanisms and therapeutic strategies. *Biology (Basel)*, *13*(5), 302. DOI: 10.3390/biology13050302 PMID: 38785784

Angom, R. S., Nakka, N. M. R., & Bhattacharya, S. (2023). Advances in glioblastoma therapy: An update on current approaches. *Brain Sciences*, *13*(11), 1536. DOI: 10.3390/brainsci13111536 PMID: 38002496

Asija, S., Chatterjee, A., Yadav, S., Chekuri, G., Karulkar, A., Jaiswal, A. K., Goda, J. S., & Purwar, R. (2022). Combinatorial approaches to effective therapy in glioblastoma (GBM): Current status and what the future holds. *International Reviews of Immunology*, *41*(6), 582–605. DOI: 10.1080/08830185.2022.2101647 PMID: 35938932

Bae, W. H., Maraka, S., & Daher, A. (2024). Challenges and advances in glioblastoma targeted therapy: The promise of drug repurposing and biomarker exploration. *Frontiers in Oncology*, *14*, 1441460. DOI: 10.3389/fonc.2024.1441460 PMID: 39439947

Begley, C. G., Ashton, M., Baell, J., Bettess, M., Brown, M. P., Carter, B., Charman, W. N., Davis, C., Fisher, S., Frazer, I., Gautam, A., Jennings, M. P., Kearney, P., Keeffe, E., Kelly, D., Lopez, A. F., McGuckin, M., Parker, M. W., Rayner, C., & Sullivan, M. (2021). Drug repurposing: Misconceptions, challenges, and opportunities for academic researchers. *Science Translational Medicine*, *13*(612), eabd5524. DOI: 10.1126/scitranslmed.abd5524 PMID: 34550729

Benmameri, M. (2022) In silico exploration of membrane transport events: prediction of passive permeation coefficients and binding sites of human MRP4. Thesis, Université de Limoges.

Bianchimano, P., Britton, G. J., Wallach, D. S., Smith, E. M., Cox, L. M., Liu, S., Iwanowski, K., Weiner, H. L., Faith, J. J., Clemente, J. C., & Tankou, S. K. (2022). Mining the microbiota to identify gut commensals modulating neuroinflammation in a mouse model of multiple sclerosis. *Microbiome, 10*(1), 174. DOI: 10.1186/s40168-022-01364-2 PMID: 36253847

Borovcanin, M. M., Stojanovic, B., Dimitrijevic Stojanovic, M., Stojanovic, B. S., Lazovic, A., & Mitrovic, M. (2024). *Anticancer Properties of Antipsychotic Drugs. p.^pp*. Springer. DOI: 10.1007/16833_2024_394

Brandner, S., McAleenan, A., Kelly, C., Spiga, F., Cheng, H.-Y., Dawson, S., Schmidt, L., Faulkner, C. L., Wragg, C., Jefferies, S., Higgins, J. P. T., & Kurian, K. M. (2021). MGMT promoter methylation testing to predict overall survival in people with glioblastoma treated with temozolomide: A comprehensive meta-analysis based on a Cochrane Systematic Review. *Neuro-Oncology, 23*(9), 1457–1469. DOI: 10.1093/neuonc/noab105 PMID: 34467991

Chang, Y.-L., Chou, C.-H., Li, Y.-F., Huang, L.-C., Kao, Y., Hueng, D.-Y., & Tsai, C.-K. (2023). Antiproliferative and apoptotic effects of telmisartan in human glioma cells. *Cancer Cell International, 23*(1), 111. DOI: 10.1186/s12935-023-02963-1 PMID: 37291545

Chen, K.-T., Wei, K.-C., & Liu, H.-L. (2021). Focused ultrasound combined with microbubbles in central nervous system applications. *Pharmaceutics, 13*(7), 1084. DOI: 10.3390/pharmaceutics13071084 PMID: 34371774

Chen, L., Peng, J., Wang, Y., Jiang, H., Wang, W., Dai, J., Tang, M., Wei, Y., Kuang, H., & Xu, G. (2020). Fenofibrate-induced mitochondrial dysfunction and metabolic reprogramming reversal: The anti-tumor effects in gastric carcinoma cells mediated by the PPAR pathway. *American Journal of Translational Research, 12*, 428. PMID: 32194894

Chien, C.-H., Hsueh, W.-T., Chuang, J.-Y., & Chang, K.-Y. (2019). Role of autophagy in therapeutic resistance of glioblastoma. *Journal of Cancer Metastasis and Treatment, 5*(66). DOI: 10.20517/2394-4722.2019.016

Chiu, C.-F., Guerrero, J. J. G., Regalado, R. R. H., Zhou, J., Notarte, K. I., Lu, Y.-W., Encarnacion, P. C., Carles, C. D. D., Octavo, E. M., Limbaroc, D. C. I., Saengboonmee, C., & Huang, S.-Y. (2024). Insights into Metabolic Reprogramming in Tumor Evolution and Therapy. *Cancers (Basel), 16*(20), 3513. DOI: 10.3390/cancers16203513 PMID: 39456607

Correia, A., Monteiro, A., Silva, R., Moreira, J., Lobo, J. S., & Silva, A. (2022). Lipid nanoparticles strategies to modify pharmacokinetics of central nervous system targeting drugs: Crossing or circumventing the blood–brain barrier (BBB) to manage neurological disorders. *Advanced Drug Delivery Reviews, 189*, 114485. DOI: 10.1016/j.addr.2022.114485 PMID: 35970274

D'Souza, R., MathEw, M. & SuRapanEni, K.M. (2023). A Scoping Review on the Ethical Issues in the Use of CRISPR-Cas9 in the Creation of Human Disease Models. *Journal of Clinical and Diagnostic Research, 17(12).*

Delgado-Martín, B., & Medina, M. Á. (2020). Advances in the knowledge of the molecular biology of glioblastoma and its impact in patient diagnosis, stratification, and treatment. *Advancement of Science*, *7*(9), 1902971. DOI: 10.1002/advs.201902971 PMID: 32382477

Dixon, S., O'connor, A. T., Brooks-Noreiga, C., Clark, M. A., Levy, A., & Castejon, A. M. (2024). Role of renin angiotensin system inhibitors and metformin in Glioblastoma Therapy: A review. *Cancer Chemotherapy and Pharmacology*, *94*(1), 1–23. DOI: 10.1007/s00280-024-04686-0 PMID: 38914751

Du, W., Chen, H., Gróf, I., Lemaitre, L., Bocsik, A., Perdyan, A., Mieczkowski, J., Deli, M. A., Hortobágyi, T., Wan, Q., & Glebov, O. O. (2024). Antidepressant-induced membrane trafficking regulates blood-brain barrier permeability. *Molecular Psychiatry*, *29*(11), 3590–3598. DOI: 10.1038/s41380-024-02626-1 PMID: 38816584

Duarte, Y., Márquez-Miranda, V., Miossec, M. J., & González-Nilo, F. (2019). Integration of target discovery, drug discovery and drug delivery: A review on computational strategies. *Wiley Interdisciplinary Reviews. Nanomedicine and Nanobiotechnology*, *11*(4), e1554. DOI: 10.1002/wnan.1554 PMID: 30932351

El Khayari, A., Bouchmaa, N., Taib, B., Wei, Z., Zeng, A., & El Fatimy, R. (2022). Metabolic rewiring in glioblastoma cancer: EGFR, IDH and beyond. *Frontiers in Oncology*, *12*, 901951. DOI: 10.3389/fonc.2022.901951 PMID: 35912242

El Kheir, W., Marcos, B., Virgilio, N., Paquette, B., Faucheux, N., & Lauzon, M.-A. (2022). Drug delivery systems in the development of novel strategies for glioblastoma treatment. *Pharmaceutics*, *14*(6), 1189. DOI: 10.3390/pharmaceutics14061189 PMID: 35745762

Fang, Y., Li, X., & Tian, R. (2024). Unlocking glioblastoma vulnerabilities with CRISPR-based genetic screening. *International Journal of Molecular Sciences*, *25*(11), 5702. DOI: 10.3390/ijms25115702 PMID: 38891890

Ferreira, P. M. P., de Sousa, R. W. R., de Oliveira Ferreira, J. R., Militão, G. C. G., & Bezerra, D. P. (2021). Chloroquine and hydroxychloroquine in antitumor therapies based on autophagy-related mechanisms. *Pharmacological Research, 168*, 105582. DOI: 10.1016/j.phrs.2021.105582 PMID: 33775862

Fiorica, F., Tebano, U., Napoli, G., Franceschetto, A., Muraro, M., Giorgi, C., & Pinton, P. (2024). Metabolic-Modulating Effects of Radiation: Undetectable Yet Deadly—A Review on Radiotherapy. *Cancers (Basel), 17*(1), 54. DOI: 10.3390/cancers17010054 PMID: 39796683

Francisco, K. K. Y., Apuhin, A. E. C., Tan, M. J. T., Byers, M. C., Maravilla, N. M. A. T., Karim, H. A., & AlDahoul, N. (2024) Can Personalized Medicine Coexist with Health Equity? Examining the Cost Barrier and Ethical Implications. *arXiv preprint arXiv:241102307.*

Fu, S. W., Tang, C., Tan, X., & Srivastava, S. (2024). Liquid biopsy for early cancer detection: Technological revolutions and clinical dilemma. *Expert Review of Molecular Diagnostics, 24*(10), 937–955. DOI: 10.1080/14737159.2024.2408744 PMID: 39360748

Fuloria, N. K., Malviya, R., Verma, S., & Balusamy, B. (2023). *Big Data in Oncology: Impact, Challenges, and Risk Assessment.* CRC Press. DOI: 10.1201/9781003442639

Fusco, W., Lorenzo, M. B., Cintoni, M., Porcari, S., Rinninella, E., Kaitsas, F., Lener, E., Mele, M. C., Gasbarrini, A., Collado, M. C., Cammarota, G., & Ianiro, G. (2023). Short-chain fatty-acid-producing bacteria: Key components of the human gut microbiota. *Nutrients, 15*(9), 2211. DOI: 10.3390/nu15092211 PMID: 37432351

Gangwal, A., Ansari, A., Ahmad, I., Azad, A. K., & Sulaiman, W. M. A. W. (2024). Current strategies to address data scarcity in artificial intelligence-based drug discovery: A comprehensive review. *Computers in Biology and Medicine, 179*, 108734. DOI: 10.1016/j.compbiomed.2024.108734 PMID: 38964243

Ghosh, N., & Modak, S. (2021). What governance lesson does Mekong bear for Ganges–Brahmaputra–Meghna (GBM) basin? *Journal of Asian Economic Integration, 3*(2), 211–234. DOI: 10.1177/26316846211038421

Goenka, A., Tiek, D., Song, X., Huang, T., Hu, B., & Cheng, S.-Y. (2021). The many facets of therapy resistance and tumor recurrence in glioblastoma. *Cells, 10*(3), 484. DOI: 10.3390/cells10030484 PMID: 33668200

Gugu M (2023) Pivotal role of cyclooxygenase 2 (COX-2) in temozolomide-resistance of glioblastoma cell lines.

Gyimesi, G., & Hediger, M. A. (2023). Transporter-mediated drug delivery. *Molecules (Basel, Switzerland)*, *28*(3), 1151. DOI: 10.3390/molecules28031151 PMID: 36770817

Haqqani, A. S., Bélanger, K., & Stanimirovic, D. B. (2024). Receptor-mediated transcytosis for brain delivery of therapeutics: Receptor classes and criteria. *Frontiers in Drug Delivery*, *4*, 1360302. DOI: 10.3389/fddev.2024.1360302 PMID: 40836978

Harilal, S., Jose, J., Kumar, R., Unnikrishnan, M. K., Uddin, M. S., Mathew, G. E., Pratap, R., Marathakam, A., & Mathew, B. (2020). Revisiting the blood-brain barrier: A hard nut to crack in the transportation of drug molecules. *Brain Research Bulletin*, *160*, 121–140. DOI: 10.1016/j.brainresbull.2020.03.018 PMID: 32315731

Huang, D., Sun, L., Huang, L., & Chen, Y. (2021). Nanodrug delivery systems modulate tumor vessels to increase the enhanced permeability and retention effect. *Journal of Personalized Medicine*, *11*(2), 124. DOI: 10.3390/jpm11020124 PMID: 33672813

Iturrioz-Rodríguez, N., Sampron, N., & Matheu, A. (2023). Current advances in temozolomide encapsulation for the enhancement of glioblastoma treatment. *Theranostics*, *13*(9), 2734–2756. DOI: 10.7150/thno.82005 PMID: 37284445

Ivanisevic, T., & Sewduth, R. N. (2023). Multi-omics integration for the design of novel therapies and the identification of novel biomarkers. *Proteomes*, *11*(4), 34. DOI: 10.3390/proteomes11040034 PMID: 37873876

Javia, A., Bardoliwala, D., & Patel, M. (2021). *Ligands and Receptors for Targeted Delivery of Nanoparticles: Recent Updates and Challenges. Drug Delivery with Targeted Nanoparticles,p*. Jenny Stanford Publishing.

Johnson, A. L., & Lopez-Bertoni, H. (2024). Cellular diversity through space and time: Adding new dimensions to GBM therapeutic development. *Frontiers in Genetics*, *15*, 1356611. DOI: 10.3389/fgene.2024.1356611 PMID: 38774283

Kanderi, T., Munakomi, S., & Gupta, V. (2024) Glioblastoma multiforme. *StatPearls [Internet]*,p.^pp. StatPearls Publishing.

Karim, N. A., Ullah, A., Ahmad, I., Bahassi, E., Olowokure, O., Khaled, A., Davis, H., & Morris, J. C. (2022). A phase I trial to determine the safety and tolerability of autophagy inhibition using chloroquine or hydroxychloroquine in combination with carboplatin and gemcitabine in patients with advanced solid tumors. *Frontiers in Oncology*, *12*, 811411. DOI: 10.3389/fonc.2022.811411 PMID: 35574311

Kelm, J. M., Samarbakhsh, A., Pillai, A., VanderVere-Carozza, P. S., Aruri, H., Pandey, D. S., Pawelczak, K. S., Turchi, J. J., & Gavande, N. S. (2022). Recent advances in the development of non-PIKKs targeting small molecule inhibitors of DNA double-strand break repair. *Frontiers in Oncology, 12*, 850883. DOI: 10.3389/fonc.2022.850883 PMID: 35463312

Krajcer, A., Grzywna, E., & Lewandowska-Łańcucka, J. (2023). Strategies increasing the effectiveness of temozolomide at various levels of anti-GBL therapy. *Biomedicine and Pharmacotherapy, 165*, 115174. DOI: 10.1016/j.biopha.2023.115174 PMID: 37459661

Krishnamurthy, N., Grimshaw, A. A., Axson, S. A., Choe, S. H., & Miller, J. E. (2022). Drug repurposing: A systematic review on root causes, barriers and facilitators. *BMC Health Services Research, 22*(1), 970. DOI: 10.1186/s12913-022-08272-z PMID: 35906687

LaMoia, T. E., & Shulman, G. I. (2021). Cellular and molecular mechanisms of metformin action. *Endocrine Reviews, 42*(1), 77–96. DOI: 10.1210/endrev/bnaa023 PMID: 32897388

Lan, Z., Li, X., & Zhang, X. (2024). Glioblastoma: An update in pathology, molecular mechanisms and biomarkers. *International Journal of Molecular Sciences, 25*(5), 3040. DOI: 10.3390/ijms25053040 PMID: 38474286

Lee JH, Chapman DV & Saltzman WM (2023) Nanoparticle targeting with antibodies in the central nervous system. *BME frontiers* 4: 0012.

Mei, S., & Zhang, K. (2021). A machine learning framework for predicting drug–drug interactions. *Scientific Reports, 11*(1), 17619. DOI: 10.1038/s41598-021-97193-8 PMID: 34475500

Mo, F., Pellerino, A., Soffietti, R., & Rudà, R. (2021). Blood–brain barrier in brain tumors: Biology and clinical relevance. *International Journal of Molecular Sciences, 22*(23), 12654. DOI: 10.3390/ijms222312654 PMID: 34884457

Mohr, A. E., Ortega-Santos, C. P., Whisner, C. M., Klein-Seetharaman, J., & Jasbi, P. (2024). Navigating challenges and opportunities in multi-omics integration for personalized healthcare. *Biomedicines, 12*(7), 1496. DOI: 10.3390/biomedicines12071496 PMID: 39062068

Moreira, R., Nóbrega, C., de Almeida, L. P., & Mendonça, L. (2024). Brain-targeted drug delivery-nanovesicles directed to specific brain cells by brain-targeting ligands. *Journal of Nanobiotechnology, 22*(1), 260. DOI: 10.1186/s12951-024-02511-7 PMID: 38760847

Nance, E., Pun, S. H., Saigal, R., & Sellers, D. L. (2022). Drug delivery to the central nervous system. *Nature Reviews. Materials*, *7*(4), 314–331. DOI: 10.1038/s41578-021-00394-w PMID: 38464996

Neuss MN (2017) 2016 updated American Society of Clinical Oncology/Oncology Nursing Society chemotherapy administration safety standards, including standards for pediatric oncology. *Number 1/January 2017* 44: 31-43.

Nguyen, S. (2024) From Barriers to Solution Pathways: Drug Repurposing's Path Forward for Off-Patent Drugs. Thesis.

Niazi, S. K. (2023). Non-invasive drug delivery across the blood–brain barrier: A prospective analysis. *Pharmaceutics*, *15*(11), 2599. DOI: 10.3390/pharmaceutics15112599 PMID: 38004577

Noebauer-Huhmann, I. M., Weber, M.-A., Lalam, R. K., Trattnig, S., Bohndorf, K., Vanhoenacker, F., Tagliafico, A., van Rijswijk, C., Vilanova, J. C., & Afonso, P. D. (2015) Soft tissue tumors in adults: ESSR-approved guidelines for diagnostic imaging. Vol. 19 p.^pp. 475-482. Thieme Medical Publishers.

Ntafoulis, I., Koolen, S. L., Leenstra, S., & Lamfers, M. L. (2022). Drug repurposing, a fast-track approach to develop effective treatments for glioblastoma. *Cancers (Basel)*, *14*(15), 3705. DOI: 10.3390/cancers14153705 PMID: 35954371

Nwagwu, C. D., Immidisetti, A. V., Jiang, M. Y., Adeagbo, O., Adamson, D. C., & Carbonell, A.-M. (2021). Convection enhanced delivery in the setting of high-grade gliomas. *Pharmaceutics*, *13*(4), 561. DOI: 10.3390/pharmaceutics13040561 PMID: 33921157

Ortiz, R., Perazzoli, G., Cabeza, L., Jiménez-Luna, C., Luque, R., Prados, J., & Melguizo, C. (2021). Temozolomide: An updated overview of resistance mechanisms, nanotechnology advances and clinical applications. *Current Neuropharmacology*, *19*, 513–537. PMID: 32589560

Ou, A., Yung, W. A., & Majd, N. (2020). Molecular mechanisms of treatment resistance in glioblastoma. *International Journal of Molecular Sciences*, *22*(1), 351. DOI: 10.3390/ijms22010351 PMID: 33396284

Panovska, D., & De Smet, F. (2022). Functional precision oncology: The next frontier to improve glioblastoma outcome? *International Journal of Molecular Sciences*, *23*(15), 8637. DOI: 10.3390/ijms23158637 PMID: 35955765

Partridge, B., Eardley, A., Morales, B. E., Campelo, S. N., Lorenzo, M. F., Mehta, J. N., Kani, Y., Mora, J. K. G., Campbell, E.-O. Y., Arena, C. B., Platt, S., Mintz, A., Shinn, R. L., Rylander, C. G., Debinski, W., Davalos, R. V., & Rossmeisl, J. H. (2022). Advancements in drug delivery methods for the treatment of brain disease. *Frontiers in Veterinary Science*, *9*, 1039745. DOI: 10.3389/fvets.2022.1039745 PMID: 36330152

Patil, N, & Ranjan, A, Gaurav, Mukherjee D, Panda BK, Diksha, Komal, Narang RK & Singh A. (2024). Navigating Biosimilar Regulatory Pathways in Emerging Markets: Insights from Brics Nations. *Applied Drug Research, Clinical Trials and Regulatory Affairs*.

Pearson, R. A., Wicha, S. G., & Okour, M. (2023). Drug combination modeling: Methods and applications in drug development. *Journal of Clinical Pharmacology*, *63*(2), 151–165. DOI: 10.1002/jcph.2128 PMID: 36088583

Pęczek, P., Gajda, M., Rutkowski, K., Fudalej, M., Deptała, A., & Badowska-Kozakiewicz, A. M. (2023). Cancer-associated inflammation: Pathophysiology and clinical significance. *Journal of Cancer Research and Clinical Oncology*, *149*(6), 2657–2672. DOI: 10.1007/s00432-022-04399-y PMID: 36260158

Puris, E., Fricker, G., & Gynther, M. (2022). Targeting transporters for drug delivery to the brain: Can we do better? *Pharmaceutical Research*, *39*(7), 1415–1455. DOI: 10.1007/s11095-022-03241-x PMID: 35359241

Rechberger, J. S., Toll, S. A., Biswas, S., You, H. B., Chow, W. D., Kendall, N., Navalkele, P., & Khatua, S. (2025). Advances in the Repurposing and Blood–Brain Barrier Penetrance of Drugs in Pediatric Brain Tumors. *Cancers (Basel)*, *17*(3), 439. DOI: 10.3390/cancers17030439 PMID: 39941807

Ricco, N., & Kron, S. J. (2023). Statins in cancer prevention and therapy. *Cancers (Basel)*, *15*(15), 3948. DOI: 10.3390/cancers15153948 PMID: 37568764

Rodrigues, P., Bangali, H., Hammoud, A., Mustafa, Y. F., Al-Hetty, H. R. A. K., Alkhafaji, A. T., Deorari, M. M., Al-Taee, M. M., Zabibah, R. S., & Alsalamy, A. (2024). COX 2-inhibitors; a thorough and updated survey into combinational therapies in cancers. *Medical Oncology (Northwood, London, England)*, *41*(1), 41. DOI: 10.1007/s12032-023-02256-7 PMID: 38165473

Rudrapal M, Khairnar SJ & Jadhav AG (2020) Drug Repurposing (DR): An Emerging Approach in Drug. *Drug Repurposing: Hypothesis, Molecular Aspects and Therapeutic Applications* 3.

Salomonsson, S. E., & Clelland, C. D. (2024). Building CRISPR gene therapies for the central nervous system: A review. *JAMA Neurology*, *81*(3), 283–290. DOI: 10.1001/jamaneurol.2023.4983 PMID: 38285472

Saltarella, I., Altamura, C., Campanale, C., Laghetti, P., Vacca, A., Frassanito, M. A., & Desaphy, J.-F. (2023). Anti-angiogenic activity of drugs in multiple myeloma. *Cancers (Basel)*, *15*(7), 1990. DOI: 10.3390/cancers15071990 PMID: 37046651

Sanchez-Cano, F., Hernández-Kelly, L. C., & Ortega, A. (2021). The blood–brain barrier: Much more than a selective access to the brain. *Neurotoxicity Research*, *39*(6), 2154–2174. DOI: 10.1007/s12640-021-00431-0 PMID: 34677787

Schmitt, M., & Greten, F. R. (2021). The inflammatory pathogenesis of colorectal cancer. *Nature Reviews. Immunology*, *21*(10), 653–667. DOI: 10.1038/s41577-021-00534-x PMID: 33911231

Schwartz, N. C. (2021) Analysis of Hyperosmotic Changes in Tight Junctions Using Immunocytochemistry and Electric Cell-Substrate Impedance Sensing. Thesis, Tulane University.

Segarra, M., Aburto, M. R., & Acker-Palmer, A. (2021). Blood–brain barrier dynamics to maintain brain homeostasis. *Trends in Neurosciences*, *44*(5), 393–405. DOI: 10.1016/j.tins.2020.12.002 PMID: 33423792

Seker-Polat, F., Pinarbasi Degirmenci, N., Solaroglu, I., & Bagci-Onder, T. (2022). Tumor cell infiltration into the brain in glioblastoma: From mechanisms to clinical perspectives. *Cancers (Basel)*, *14*(2), 443. DOI: 10.3390/cancers14020443 PMID: 35053605

Shah, S., Mansour, H. M., Aguilar, T. M., & Lucke-Wold, B. (2024). Advances in anti-cancer drug development: Metformin as anti-angiogenic supplemental treatment for glioblastoma. *International Journal of Molecular Sciences*, *25*(11), 5694. DOI: 10.3390/ijms25115694 PMID: 38891882

Shams, A. (2024). Leveraging state-of-the-art ai algorithms in personalized oncology: From transcriptomics to treatment. *Diagnostics (Basel)*, *14*(19), 2174. DOI: 10.3390/diagnostics14192174 PMID: 39410578

Singh, G., Kumar, P., & Aran, K. R. (2025). Targeting EGFR and PI3K/mTOR pathways in glioblastoma: Innovative therapeutic approaches. *Medical Oncology (Northwood, London, England)*, *42*(4), 1–17. DOI: 10.1007/s12032-025-02652-1 PMID: 40064710

Tang, J., Karbhari, N., & Campian, J. L. (2025). Therapeutic Targets in Glioblastoma: Molecular Pathways, Emerging Strategies, and Future Directions. *Cells, 14*(7), 494. DOI: 10.3390/cells14070494 PMID: 40214448

Tanoli, Z., Vähä-Koskela, M., & Aittokallio, T. (2021). Artificial intelligence, machine learning, and drug repurposing in cancer. *Expert Opinion on Drug Discovery, 16*(9), 977–989. DOI: 10.1080/17460441.2021.1883585 PMID: 33543671

Teleanu, R. I., Preda, M. D., Niculescu, A.-G., Vladâcenco, O., Radu, C. I., Grumezescu, A. M., & Teleanu, D. M. (2022). Current strategies to enhance delivery of drugs across the blood–brain barrier. *Pharmaceutics, 14*(5), 987. DOI: 10.3390/pharmaceutics14050987 PMID: 35631573

Thenuwara, G., Curtin, J., & Tian, F. (2023). Advances in diagnostic tools and therapeutic approaches for gliomas: A comprehensive review. *Sensors (Basel), 23*(24), 9842. DOI: 10.3390/s23249842 PMID: 38139688

Tiwari, P. C., Pal, R., Chaudhary, M. J., & Nath, R. (2023). Artificial intelligence revolutionizing drug development: Exploring opportunities and challenges. *Drug Development Research, 84*(8), 1652–1663. DOI: 10.1002/ddr.22115 PMID: 37712494

Torrisi, F., Alberghina, C., D'Aprile, S., Pavone, A. M., Longhitano, L., Giallongo, S., Tibullo, D., Di Rosa, M., Zappalà, A., Cammarata, F. P., Russo, G., Ippolito, M., Cuttone, G., Li Volti, G., Vicario, N., & Parenti, R. (2022). The hallmarks of glioblastoma: Heterogeneity, intercellular crosstalk and molecular signature of invasiveness and progression. *Biomedicines, 10*(4), 806. DOI: 10.3390/biomedicines10040806 PMID: 35453557

Verdugo, E., Puerto, I., & Medina, M. Á. (2022). An update on the molecular biology of glioblastoma, with clinical implications and progress in its treatment. *Cancer Communications, 42*(11), 1083–1111. DOI: 10.1002/cac2.12361 PMID: 36129048

Wang, T., Liu, M., Peng, B., Song, X., Zhang, C., Sun, X., Niu, Q., Liu, J., Chen, S., & Chen, K. (2024) From Bench to Bedside: A Review of Clinical Trialsin Drug Discovery and Development. *arXiv preprint arXiv:241209378.*

Weth, F. R., Hoggarth, G. B., Weth, A. F., Paterson, E., White, M. P., Tan, S. T., Peng, L., & Gray, C. (2024). Unlocking hidden potential: Advancements, approaches, and obstacles in repurposing drugs for cancer therapy. *British Journal of Cancer, 130*(5), 703–715. DOI: 10.1038/s41416-023-02502-9 PMID: 38012383

Wu, J., Chu, Y., Jiang, Z., & Yu, Q. (2020). Losartan protects against intermittent hypoxia-induced peritubular capillary loss by modulating the renal renin–angiotensin system and angiogenesis factors. *Acta Biochimica et Biophysica Sinica*, *52*(1), 38–48. DOI: 10.1093/abbs/gmz136 PMID: 31836883

Xia, Y., Sun, M., Huang, H., & Jin, W.-L. (2024). Drug repurposing for cancer therapy. *Signal Transduction and Targeted Therapy*, *9*(1), 92. DOI: 10.1038/s41392-024-01808-1 PMID: 38637540

Xiang, Z., Xie, Q., & Yu, Z. (2023). Exosomal DNA: Role in reflecting tumor genetic heterogeneity, diagnosis, and disease monitoring. *Cancers (Basel)*, *16*(1), 57. DOI: 10.3390/cancers16010057 PMID: 38201485

Xiao, L., Li, X., Fang, C., Yu, J., & Chen, T. (2023). Neurotransmitters: Promising immune modulators in the tumor microenvironment. *Frontiers in Immunology*, *14*, 1118637. DOI: 10.3389/fimmu.2023.1118637 PMID: 37215113

Yadav, K., Vijayalakshmi, R., Sahu, K. K., Sure, P., Chahal, K., Yadav, R., Dubey, A., Jha, M., & Pradhan, M. (2024). Exosome-based macromolecular neurotherapeutic drug delivery approaches in overcoming the blood-brain barrier for treating brain disorders. *European Journal of Pharmaceutics and Biopharmaceutics*, *199*, 114298. DOI: 10.1016/j.ejpb.2024.114298 PMID: 38642716

Yalamarty, S. S. K., Filipczak, N., Li, X., Subhan, M. A., Parveen, F., Ataide, J. A., Rajmalani, B. A., & Torchilin, V. P. (2023). Mechanisms of resistance and current treatment options for glioblastoma multiforme (GBM). *Cancers (Basel)*, *15*(7), 2116. DOI: 10.3390/cancers15072116 PMID: 37046777

Yamaura, K., Nelson, A., Nishimura, H., Rutledge, J., Ravuri, S., Bahney, C., Philippon, M., & Huard, J. (2023). The effects of losartan or angiotensin II receptor antagonists on cartilage: A systematic review. *Osteoarthritis and Cartilage*, *31*(4), 435–446. DOI: 10.1016/j.joca.2022.11.014 PMID: 36586717

Zaghmi, A., Drouin-Ouellet, J., Brambilla, D., & Gauthier, M. (2021). Treating brain diseases using systemic parenterally administered protein therapeutics: Dysfunction of the brain barriers and potential strategies. *Biomaterials*, *269*, 120461. DOI: 10.1016/j.biomaterials.2020.120461 PMID: 33218788

Zhai, K., Siddiqui, M., Abdellatif, B., Liskova, A., Kubatka, P., & Büsselberg, D. (2021). Natural compounds in glioblastoma therapy: Preclinical insights, mechanistic pathways, and outlook. *Cancers (Basel)*, *13*(10), 2317. DOI: 10.3390/cancers13102317 PMID: 34065960

Zhou, G. (2024). Exploring Ester Prodrugs: A Comprehensive Review of Approaches, Applications, and Methods. *Pharmacology & Pharmacy*, *15*(8), 269–284. DOI: 10.4236/pp.2024.158016

Chapter 9
Novel Drug Delivery and Dosage Forms for Glioblastoma

Pindiprolu S. S. Sai Kiran
Aditya University, Surampalem, India

Dasari Nagasen
https://orcid.org/0000-0002-8305-7277
Aditya University, Surampalem, India

Andhavarapu Santosh Kumar
CDSCO, New Delhi, India

Shnati Amala
Krishna University College of Pharmaceutical Science and Research, India

ABSTRACT

Glioblastoma multiforme (GBM) is an aggressive, treatment-resistant brain tumor with poor prognosis. Current therapies, including surgery, radiotherapy, and temozolomide, are limited by the blood-brain barrier (BBB), tumor heterogeneity, and resistant glioma stem-like cells (GSCs). Novel drug delivery systems (NDDS)—including nanoparticles (liposomes, SLNs, dendrimers), cell-based carriers (exosomes, stem cells), and localized delivery (Gliadel® wafers, hydrogels)—aim to overcome these barriers. Intranasal administration and focused ultrasound (FUS) are under investigation for BBB bypass. Emerging theranostic platforms integrate targeting and imaging for precision therapy. Despite progress, translational chal-

DOI: 10.4018/979-8-3373-2695-5.ch009

lenges persist due to BBB variability, immune evasion, and scalability issues. A multidisciplinary approach incorporating nanotechnology, molecular oncology, and regulatory insight is essential for advancing GBM treatment.

1. INTRODUCTION

Glioblastoma multiforme (GBM) is the most aggressive and lethal primary brain tumor in adults, classified as a grade IV astrocytoma by the World Health Organization (WHO). Arising from glial cells, specifically astrocytes, GBM is characterized by rapid proliferation, diffuse infiltration, extensive angiogenesis, necrosis, and resistance to standard therapies. Despite decades of research, the median survival for patients with GBM remains dismally low, typically 12 to 15 months post-diagnosis, with a 5-year survival rate of less than 5%. This poor prognosis is largely attributed to the tumor's highly invasive nature, its ability to infiltrate surrounding brain tissues, and its unique tumor microenvironment.

Conventional therapies for GBM include maximal safe surgical resection followed by radiotherapy and chemotherapy, primarily with the alkylating agent temozolomide (TMZ). However, these strategies offer only modest improvements in survival. Surgical resection is often incomplete due to the tumor's diffuse boundaries and critical localization within functional brain regions. Furthermore, even with post-surgical therapies, recurrence is nearly universal, highlighting the limited efficacy of current approaches.

A major obstacle in the treatment of GBM is the presence of the blood-brain barrier (BBB), a tightly regulated endothelial membrane that selectively restricts the passage of substances from the bloodstream into the brain parenchyma. While the BBB is partially disrupted in glioblastoma due to neoangiogenesis and abnormal vasculature forming what is known as the blood-tumor barrier (BTB) this disruption is heterogeneous. As a result, many therapeutic agents fail to reach effective concentrations across all tumor regions. Even temozolomide, which is one of the few drugs capable of crossing the BBB, has shown limited efficacy due to intrinsic or acquired resistance, often driven by the expression of DNA repair enzymes such as O6-methylguanine-DNA methyltransferase (MGMT).

Moreover, GBM exhibits profound genetic and molecular heterogeneity, with subpopulations of therapy-resistant glioma stem-like cells (GSCs) that contribute to tumor recurrence and treatment failure. These GSCs can self-renew and differentiate, mirroring developmental pathways, and are often located in protective niches within the tumor microenvironment. Traditional chemotherapy and radiotherapy are largely ineffective against these cells, which necessitates alternative, more targeted therapeutic strategies.

In response to these challenges, the development of novel drug delivery systems and advanced dosage forms for GBM has gained significant momentum. These innovative approaches aim not only to improve drug penetration across the BBB but also to provide site-specific, sustained, and controlled release of therapeutic agents, reduce systemic toxicity, and target the tumor microenvironment and GSCs more effectively.

Nanotechnology-based platforms, such as liposomes, dendrimers, polymeric nanoparticles, and solid lipid nanoparticles, have shown promise in enhancing drug delivery to the brain. These nanocarriers can be engineered with surface modifications such as ligands, antibodies, or peptides that facilitate active targeting of tumor cells or endothelial receptors involved in BBB transport. Additionally, cell-based delivery systems, including mesenchymal stem cells and exosomes, are being investigated for their intrinsic ability to home to tumor sites, potentially serving as carriers for chemotherapeutics or gene therapies.

Non-invasive delivery routes such as intranasal administration have emerged as promising alternatives, bypassing the BBB via olfactory and trigeminal neural pathways. Likewise, localized delivery strategies, including implantable biodegradable wafers (e.g., Gliadel®) and injectable hydrogels, are being utilized to achieve high local drug concentrations while minimizing systemic exposure.

Furthermore, novel technologies such as focused ultrasound (FUS) combined with microbubbles offer transient and localized BBB disruption, enabling enhanced delivery of macromolecules or nanoparticles directly to the tumor site. Integration of such delivery platforms with advanced imaging and diagnostic tools is paving the way for personalized, image-guided therapy.

The complex biology of glioblastoma and the limitations of conventional treatment modalities necessitate a paradigm shift toward novel drug delivery systems. These innovations hold the potential to revolutionize the clinical management of GBM, offering new hope for improved therapeutic outcomes in a disease that has long been deemed incurable.

Glioblastoma accounts for approximately 15% of all primary brain tumors and 45–50% of malignant gliomas globally. Its incidence ranges from 3 to 5 cases per 100,000 people annually, with a slightly higher prevalence in males and individuals over 50 years of age. While rare in children, pediatric glioblastomas often exhibit different genetic signatures and clinical trajectories compared to adult-onset forms, requiring distinct therapeutic approaches.

The economic burden of GBM is substantial, involving not just direct medical costs such as surgery, hospitalization, and chemotherapy, but also long-term supportive care, palliative interventions, and indirect costs including loss of productivity. The average annual cost per patient can exceed $100,000 USD in developed nations, underscoring the critical need for more effective and affordable interventions.

Moreover, the quality of life for GBM patients is significantly impaired due to neurological deterioration, cognitive deficits, and the psychological toll of a terminal diagnosis. Functional impairments often require intensive caregiving and social support. Given the poor prognosis and the aggressive clinical course, early palliative care integration is now being recommended in treatment guidelines.

In this context, the emergence of novel drug delivery platforms offers a paradigm shift in glioblastoma management. These systems aim not only to extend survival but also to preserve neurological function and quality of life. The integration of precision medicine, nanotechnology, and localized delivery platforms reflects a multidisciplinary approach to tackle the multifactorial challenges posed by this deadly disease (Esemen et al., 2022).

2. PATHOPHYSIOLOGY AND BARRIERS IN GLIOBLASTOMA TREATMENT

Glioblastoma multiforme (GBM) presents a multifaceted pathophysiology rooted in intricate genetic mutations, signaling pathway dysregulation, and a uniquely hostile tumor microenvironment. Understanding these molecular and structural barriers is crucial for designing effective therapeutic strategies

2.1 Molecular Biology and Genetic Profile of GBM

GBM arises due to the accumulation of multiple genetic and epigenetic aberrations that drive uncontrolled cell proliferation, resistance to apoptosis, and invasive behavior. The Cancer Genome Atlas (TCGA) has classified GBM into four molecular subtypes: classical, proneural, neural, and mesenchymal each with distinct genomic alterations and clinical behaviors (Verhaak et al., 2010).

- Classical subtype frequently exhibits epidermal growth factor receptor (EGFR) amplification and chromosome 10 loss.
- Proneural subtype often shows IDH1 mutations and PDGFRA amplification.
- The mesenchymal subtype, which is more aggressive, is associated with NF1 mutations and a strong inflammatory profile (Lan et al., 2024).

One of the most clinically significant biomarkers is O6-methylguanine-DNA methyltransferase (MGMT), a DNA repair enzyme. Methylation of the MGMT promoter is associated with better responses to alkylating agents like temozolomide (TMZ) (Hegi et al., 2005).

Moreover, IDH1/2 mutations are commonly seen in secondary GBM and are associated with a better prognosis and slower disease progression. These mutations alter cellular metabolism, producing 2-hydroxyglutarate, which contributes to epigenetic reprogramming (Yan et al., 2009; Verdugo et al., 2022).

Another key hallmark of GBM is altered tumor metabolism. GBM cells often rely on aerobic glycolysis (known as the Warburg effect), wherein they preferentially convert glucose to lactate even in the presence of sufficient oxygen. This metabolic reprogramming supports rapid proliferation and resistance to apoptosis by generating biosynthetic precursors and maintaining redox balance. Enzymes such as hexokinase-2 (HK2), pyruvate kinase M2 (PKM2), and isocitrate dehydrogenase (IDH) are commonly dysregulated in this context, and are being explored as therapeutic targets.

Epigenetic modifications also contribute significantly to the tumor's progression and treatment resistance. These include DNA methylation, histone modifications (e.g., acetylation, methylation), and non-coding RNA-mediated gene silencing. Notably, mutations in genes encoding histone variants (e.g., H3F3A) are associated with poor prognosis in pediatric high-grade gliomas. Epigenetic plasticity further enables GBM cells to transition between subtypes, complicating treatment efforts.

Additionally, immune checkpoint molecules such as PD-1, PD-L1, and CTLA-4 are frequently overexpressed in the tumor microenvironment, allowing tumor cells to evade immune surveillance. This immune escape, combined with the immunosuppressive milieu of GBM, has limited the efficacy of immunotherapies that are successful in other cancers. Research is ongoing to improve the therapeutic response by combining checkpoint inhibitors with delivery systems that enhance local drug availability.

2.2 Role of the Blood-Brain Barrier (BBB) and Blood-Tumor Barrier (BTB)

A major impediment to effective chemotherapy in GBM is the blood-brain barrier (BBB) a dynamic, tightly-regulated barrier formed by endothelial cells connected by tight junctions, supported by astrocytes and pericytes. This barrier restricts nearly 98% of small-molecule drugs and nearly 100% of large-molecule drugs from entering the brain parenchyma (Pardridge, 2005).

In GBM, while the BBB is often disrupted due to neovascularization and inflammatory processes, this leads to the formation of a blood-tumor barrier (BTB), which is heterogeneously permeable. Some tumor regions exhibit a leaky vasculature allowing partial drug entry, whereas infiltrative edges remain shielded by an intact BBB, leading to inadequate drug distribution across the entire tumor (Pouyan et al., 2025)

Additionally, GBM upregulates efflux transporters like P-glycoprotein (P-gp) and breast cancer resistance protein (BCRP), which actively pump drugs out of the brain, reducing intracellular drug accumulation. This is a key mechanism for multi-drug resistance and necessitates the design of novel delivery systems that can bypass or modulate these transport mechanisms (Zhang et al., 2020)

2.3 Tumor Heterogeneity and Microenvironment

GBM is not a uniform mass of malignant cells; rather, it displays extensive intertumoral and intratumoral heterogeneity. Multiple subclones coexist within the same tumor, each with distinct genetic and phenotypic traits. This diversity is a major driver of therapeutic resistance and recurrence (Mansour et al., 2025)

A critical component of this heterogeneity is the presence of glioma stem-like cells (GSCs), a subpopulation with self-renewal capacity and resistance to chemotherapy and radiotherapy. GSCs reside in specialized niches such as hypoxic zones and perivascular regions, where they are protected from conventional therapies and sustain tumor regeneration (Xu et al., 2024)

The tumor microenvironment (TME) in GBM is immunosuppressive and hypoxic, promoting tumor growth and resistance. It includes tumor-associated macrophages (TAMs), microglia, myeloid-derived suppressor cells (MDSCs), and T-regulatory cells (Tregs), all contributing to immune evasion. GBM secretes factors like TGF-β and IL-10, which dampen anti-tumor immunity and support angiogenesis via VEGF upregulation (Quail & Joyce, 2017).

Moreover, the extracellular matrix (ECM) in GBM is rich in hyaluronic acid, tenascin-C, and proteoglycans, which not only facilitate invasion but also act as drug reservoirs or barriers, impeding drug diffusion. The dense ECM further supports mesenchymal transition, enhancing cellular motility and treatment resistance (Guo et al., 2023)

3. LIMITATIONS OF CONVENTIONAL DRUG DELIVERY IN GBM

Glioblastoma multiforme (GBM) presents formidable challenges to conventional drug delivery due to its aggressive biology, complex tumor microenvironment, and the presence of physiological barriers such as the blood-brain barrier (BBB). Despite advancements in surgical, chemotherapeutic, and radiotherapeutic approaches, current treatments remain palliative rather than curative. The failure of conventional drug delivery systems is primarily due to limitations in invasiveness, lack of tumor specificity, systemic toxicity, and poor pharmacokinetic profiles of existing anti-GBM drugs (Hart et al., 2013).

3.1 Invasive Techniques

The first line of GBM treatment is surgical resection, aimed at debulking the tumor and relieving intracranial pressure. However, the infiltrative nature of GBM prevents complete excision, as malignant cells often invade surrounding healthy brain tissue. This makes radical resection nearly impossible without compromising neurological function (Stupp et al., 2005; Tripathy et al., 2024).

To circumvent the limitations of systemic drug delivery, local delivery techniques like intracranial implants have been developed. One prominent example is the Gliadel® wafer, a biodegradable polymer impregnated with carmustine (BCNU) that is surgically implanted into the tumor resection cavity (Jezierzański et al., 2024). While this method provides localized drug release, it is highly invasive and limited to post-surgical use. Additionally, drug diffusion is often inadequate, particularly in targeting infiltrative tumor margins (Brem et al., 1995). These approaches also fail to address distant microinvasions that extend beyond the implant's effective range.

Moreover, convection-enhanced delivery (CED), which uses catheters to infuse drugs directly into brain parenchyma, poses risks including catheter misplacement, backflow, infection, and brain tissue damage. Its clinical translation remains limited due to variability in distribution and patient response (Vogelbaum & Aghi, 2015).

3.2 Systemic Toxicity and Non-Specificity

One of the most significant limitations of conventional systemic therapies is non-specific drug distribution, leading to systemic toxicity. For example, temozolomide (TMZ), the current standard chemotherapeutic agent, is administered orally and acts as a DNA alkylator. Although TMZ crosses the BBB, it lacks specificity for tumor cells, affecting rapidly dividing normal cells, particularly in the bone marrow and gastrointestinal tract, resulting in myelosuppression, nausea, and fatigue (Stupp et al., 2015).

Drugs like lomustine and procarbazine, also part of GBM regimens, have poor therapeutic indices and pose risks of hematologic toxicity, hepatotoxicity, and neurotoxicity. In pediatric GBM, these toxicities are especially concerning due to long-term developmental side effects (Ivy Brain Tumor Center, n.d.)

Additionally, off-target drug exposure can compromise the immune system and alter organ function, precluding high-dose regimens that might be more effective. Thus, systemic toxicity creates a therapeutic ceiling, where increasing doses to kill tumor cells becomes clinically unacceptable (Zhao et al., 2025).

Furthermore, the failure of numerous high-profile clinical trials underscores the limitations of conventional approaches. For example, the anti-angiogenic agent bevacizumab, though initially promising, failed to show a survival benefit in phase

III trials when added to standard chemoradiotherapy. Similarly, immune checkpoint inhibitors such as nivolumab, which have revolutionized treatment in melanoma and lung cancer, have shown limited efficacy in GBM, likely due to the tumor's immune-excluded phenotype and adaptive resistance mechanisms.

Patient compliance also emerges as a critical issue, especially in elderly individuals or those with poor performance status. The cumulative toxicities of temozolomide and radiation therapy often lead to treatment interruptions, dose reductions, or early discontinuation. These alterations not only reduce treatment efficacy but also complicate trial outcomes and survival statistics.

Additionally, GBM patients frequently suffer from comorbidities, steroid-induced complications, and treatment-related cognitive decline, all of which necessitate a careful balance between therapeutic intensity and quality of life. The risk of opportunistic infections due to prolonged corticosteroid use further complicates systemic therapy.

Taken together, these limitations make it clear that conventional drug delivery methods fall short in addressing the unique challenges posed by GBM. This has accelerated the development of novel delivery systems that promise better therapeutic targeting, improved tolerability, and enhanced patient outcomes.

3.3 Poor Pharmacokinetic Profiles of Anti-GBM Drugs

The pharmacokinetics of most anti-GBM agents are suboptimal for brain delivery. Effective treatment requires not just BBB penetration, but adequate concentration at the tumor site, sustained release, and retention within tumor cells all of which are limited in traditional formulations.

Temozolomide, though BBB-permeable, has a short plasma half-life (~1.8 hours) and is rapidly degraded into its active metabolite, MTIC (3-methyl-(triazen-1-yl) imidazole-4-carboxamide), which is itself unstable and exhibits poor tumor selectivity (23). Furthermore, many GBM patients express high levels of the MGMT repair enzyme, which reverses TMZ-induced DNA damage, leading to drug resistance and tumor recurrence.

Drugs such as paclitaxel, doxorubicin, and etoposide, though highly cytotoxic to GBM cells in vitro, are largely ineffective in vivo because of poor BBB permeability and P-glycoprotein (P-gp) mediated efflux. As a result, their plasma profiles do not correlate with intracranial tumor concentrations.

Moreover, conventional delivery fails to provide controlled or sustained release, leading to drug washout and subtherapeutic exposure. This intermittent exposure is insufficient to eliminate tumor cells, especially the glioma stem-like cells (GSCs), which require prolonged targeting (Stupp et al., 2017).

4. EMERGING DRUG DELIVERY SYSTEMS FOR GBM

Overcoming the limitations of conventional therapies in glioblastoma multiforme (GBM) has driven the exploration of advanced drug delivery platforms that can enhance brain targeting, reduce systemic toxicity, and cross physiological barriers such as the blood-brain barrier (BBB). Recent developments have brought forth a spectrum of promising strategies, including nanoparticle-based formulations, cell-mediated delivery, localized administration, and non-invasive BBB disruption techniques like focused ultrasound (FUS). These innovative approaches hold the potential to revolutionize the therapeutic landscape of GBM (Noorani & de la Rosa, 2023; Mokarram et al., 2025).

4.1 Nanoparticle-Based Delivery

Liposomes: Liposomes are spherical vesicles with phospholipid bilayers capable of encapsulating both hydrophilic and hydrophobic drugs. They offer biocompatibility, biodegradability, and surface modification potential. Liposomal doxorubicin (Doxil®), though primarily used in other cancers, has shown preclinical promise in GBM. Modified liposomes coated with transferrin or folic acid can actively target glioma cells by exploiting receptor-mediated endocytosis (Raju et al., 2023).

Solid Lipid Nanoparticles (SLNs): SLNs are composed of solid lipid cores stabilized by surfactants. They enhance the stability of encapsulated drugs, permit controlled release, and bypass the BBB via endocytosis or transporter-mediated mechanisms. SLNs loaded with temozolomide or curcumin have demonstrated improved brain delivery and prolonged circulation in animal models (Surender & Deepika, 2016).

Polymeric Nanoparticles: Biodegradable polymers like PLGA (poly(lactic-co-glycolic acid)) are widely used in nanoparticle systems for GBM. These particles can be tailored for sustained release and BBB permeability. For instance, PLGA nanoparticles loaded with paclitaxel and conjugated with glioma-homing peptides have enhanced accumulation in GBM xenografts (Kreuter, 2014).

Dendrimers: Dendrimers are highly branched, tree-like macromolecules with functionalizable surfaces. Their nanometric size and multivalency make them suitable for targeted delivery. PEGylated polyamidoamine (PAMAM) dendrimers have shown BBB penetration and selective delivery of siRNA and anticancer drugs to glioma cells (Aboody et al., 2013).

4.2 Cell-based Delivery Systems

Stem Cell-mediated Drug Delivery: Mesenchymal stem cells (MSCs) and neural stem cells (NSCs) have inherent tumor-homing abilities, allowing them to serve as drug carriers. Engineered stem cells can be loaded with nanoparticles or modified to express prodrug-converting enzymes. NSCs expressing cytosine deaminase, which converts 5-fluorocytosine to 5-fluorouracil, have shown tumor regression in GBM models (Narsinh et al., 2024).

Exosomes and Extracellular Vesicles (EVs): Exosomes are nano-sized vesicles secreted by cells that naturally carry RNA, proteins, and lipids. They can cross the BBB and target glioma cells through receptor-ligand interactions. Exosomes derived from dendritic cells or MSCs, engineered to carry miRNA or chemotherapeutics like doxorubicin, have exhibited tumor-suppressive effects in GBM preclinical studies (Yang et al., 2015).

In recent years, cell-based drug delivery systems have expanded to include genetically engineered mesenchymal stem cells (MSCs) and immune cell-derived exosomes. These systems can be loaded not only with chemotherapeutic agents but also with gene editing tools like CRISPR-Cas9, mRNA, and small interfering RNA (siRNA), enabling precise regulation of oncogenic pathways in GBM. For example, engineered MSCs expressing cytosine deaminase can convert the prodrug 5-fluorocytosine into the cytotoxic agent 5-fluorouracil directly within the tumor, reducing systemic toxicity.

Additionally, exosomes derived from tumor-educated immune cells (such as dendritic cells and T cells) have shown an inherent ability to target glioma cells via surface integrins and adhesion molecules. These exosomes can be engineered to carry multiple payloads, including miRNA cocktails, STAT3 inhibitors, and immunomodulators, to simultaneously suppress tumor growth and reprogram the tumor microenvironment.

A key advantage of exosomes over synthetic nanoparticles lies in their low immunogenicity, innate BBB-penetration ability, and potential to evade phagocytosis. Furthermore, they exhibit natural tropism toward inflamed or tumorigenic tissues due to their parental cell origin. Comparative studies have demonstrated that exosome-mediated delivery of doxorubicin or paclitaxel results in higher tumor accumulation and reduced systemic toxicity compared to conventional nanoparticles.

To maximize targeting specificity, hybrid systems combining exosomes with synthetic nanocarriers are being developed. These "biohybrid vesicles" leverage the targeting capabilities of exosomes with the customizable features of nanoparticles. For instance, exosome-coated polymeric nanoparticles have demonstrated improved stability, brain targeting, and intracellular uptake in orthotopic GBM models.

The scalability and standardization of cell-derived systems remain key translational challenges. However, advancements in biomanufacturing technologies such as microfluidic exosome isolation and cell bioreactor platforms are improving production yields and reproducibility, paving the way for clinical applications.

4.3 Intranasal and Intra-tumoral Delivery Mechanism and Advantages

Intranasal delivery offers a non-invasive pathway that bypasses the BBB via the olfactory and trigeminal nerves. This method enables rapid and direct brain targeting with reduced systemic exposure. Drugs like insulin, temozolomide, and even nanoparticles have been successfully delivered intranasally in GBM models, showing improved brain bioavailability (Illum, 2000).

Clinical Relevance: Although still largely experimental, intranasal delivery is gaining traction due to its safety and repeatability. Combined with nanoparticles or cell-derived vesicles, it offers a synergistic approach for enhanced drug targeting in glioma treatment (ter Linden et al., 2024).

4.4 Focused Ultrasound and BBB Disruption

Principles of Focused Ultrasound (FUS): FUS is a non-invasive method that uses acoustic waves to transiently open the BBB in targeted brain regions. When combined with circulating microbubbles, FUS can temporarily disrupt endothelial tight junctions, allowing drug passage into the brain parenchyma (Ahmed et al., 2023).

Microbubbles and Targeted Delivery: Microbubbles are gas-filled carriers that oscillate under ultrasound, creating mechanical forces that enhance vascular permeability. FUS combined with microbubbles has been used to deliver antibodies, chemotherapy agents, and nanoparticles across the BBB in preclinical GBM models. Clinical trials using FUS-BBB disruption (e.g., SonoCloud) in glioma patients have shown feasibility and safety as shown in Table 1 (Carpentier et al., 2016; Gong et al., 2025).

Table 1. Summary of emerging drug delivery systems for GBM

Delivery System	Key Features	Therapeutic Agents	Advantages	Reference
Liposomes	Phospholipid vesicles, modifiable surface	Doxorubicin, Paclitaxel	Biocompatible, can be functionalized for targeting	(Raju et al., 2023)
Solid Lipid Nanoparticles (SLNs)	Solid lipid matrix stabilized with surfactants	Temozolomide, Curcumin	Stable, controlled release, BBB penetration	(Surender & Deepika, 2016)
Polymeric Nanoparticles (PNPs)	Biodegradable polymers (e.g., PLGA)	Paclitaxel, TMZ, siRNA	Sustained release, modifiable for targeting	(Kreuter, 2014)
Dendrimers	Branched polymers, high drug loading	siRNA, Methotrexate	Nanoscale, multivalent targeting capability	(Westphal et al., 2003)
Hydrogels	Injectable, thermo-responsive scaffolds	TMZ, Anti-angiogenic agents	In situ gelation, localized sustained delivery	(Basso et al., 2018)
Microneedle Arrays	Minimally invasive polymeric patches	Chemotherapeutic agents	Localized release, minimal invasiveness	(Seetharam et al., 2020)
Focused Ultrasound (FUS)	Acoustic BBB disruption with microbubbles	Antibodies, nanoparticles	Non-invasive, site-specific BBB opening	(Carpentier et al., 2016)
Stem Cell-mediated Delivery	MSCs/NSCs with tumor-tropic properties	5-FC, Oncolytic viruses	Homing ability to tumor sites	(Aboody et al., 2013)
Exosomes	Endogenous vesicles from stem cells or immune cells	miRNA, Doxorubicin	Natural BBB crossing, low immunogenicity	(Yang et al., 2015)

5. ADVANCED DOSAGE FORMS IN GBM THERAPY

The treatment of glioblastoma multiforme (GBM) is severely constrained by the inability of many chemotherapeutic agents to reach the tumor site in effective concentrations due to the restrictive blood-brain barrier (BBB) and systemic toxicity. To address these limitations, advanced dosage forms have been developed to enable localized, sustained, and targeted drug delivery within the brain. Innovations such as injectable implants, thermoresponsive hydrogels, and minimally invasive microneedle systems are transforming GBM therapy (Roque et al., 2023).

5.1 Injectable Implants

Biodegradable Polymeric Wafers (e.g., Gliadel®): Gliadel® wafer is a landmark FDA-approved implantable system for GBM treatment. Composed of the biodegradable polymer polifeprosan 20 impregnated with carmustine (BCNU), each wafer delivers a sustained release of chemotherapy directly into the resection cavity post-surgery. This local administration bypasses the BBB, enabling high drug concentrations at the tumor site with minimal systemic exposure. Clinical trials have shown that Gliadel implantation increases median survival rates when used alongside radiotherapy and systemic chemotherapy (Westphal et al., 2003; Ghaznavi et al., 2024).

Reservoir-Based Systems: Reservoir-based implants involve a drug reservoir enclosed in a semi-permeable membrane or polymer matrix that regulates drug diffusion over time. These can be surgically implanted into or near the tumor bed, offering programmable and extended drug release profiles. For example, silicone-based reservoir implants loaded with temozolomide or paclitaxel have been explored for intracranial use in animal models, demonstrating enhanced local concentrations and tumor suppression (Weiser & Saltzman, 2014).

5.2 Hydrogels and Thermoresponsive Systems

Design and Function: Hydrogels are three-dimensional, hydrophilic polymeric networks capable of retaining large amounts of water or biological fluids. When loaded with drugs, they enable sustained and localized release upon implantation. Their physical properties, including porosity and degradation rate, can be tailored to suit various therapeutic needs (Liu et al., 2022).

Thermoresponsive Hydrogels: Thermoresponsive hydrogels, such as those composed of poly(N-isopropylacrylamide) (PNIPAAm) or poloxamers, remain in liquid form at room temperature but solidify into gels at body temperature. This property allows for injectable formulations that solidify in situ after administration, minimizing invasiveness (Lai et al., 2024).

An example is a PLGA–PEG–PLGA thermoresponsive hydrogel carrying temozolomide, which forms a depot in the tumor cavity and gradually releases the drug, achieving prolonged local exposure (46). Such systems have shown promising results in glioma-bearing rodent models, significantly enhancing drug retention and tumor regression (Gregory et al., 2020).

Hydrogels can also be co-loaded with multiple agents, including chemotherapeutics, siRNA, or immunomodulators, providing combinatorial therapy through a single injection.

5.3 Microneedle and Implantable Devices

Emerging Trends in Minimally Invasive Delivery: Microneedles, traditionally explored for dermal applications, are now being repurposed for intracranial drug delivery. These devices consist of tiny needles, often fabricated from biodegradable polymers or silicon, which can be loaded with chemotherapeutic agents and inserted with minimal tissue disruption (Shi et al., 2019).

Microneedle arrays implanted into brain parenchyma offer localized, controlled drug release with less invasiveness than traditional surgical implants. Recent developments have included hydrogel-forming microneedles that respond to pH or enzymatic triggers in the tumor microenvironment (Seetharam et al., 2020).

Miniaturized Implantable Pumps and Devices: Devices such as mini-pumps can provide programmable and long-term infusion of anticancer drugs directly into the tumor or surrounding tissues. For example, Alzet® osmotic pumps have been widely used in preclinical models for continuous infusion of temozolomide or doxorubicin in GBM. These devices are now being explored in smart implantable systems that can be wirelessly controlled or respond to external stimuli like magnetic fields or light (Wei et al., 2023; Qindeel et al., 2024).

6. TARGETING STRATEGIES IN GBM THERAPY

- Targeted drug delivery in glioblastoma multiforme (GBM) aims to improve therapeutic efficacy while minimizing off-target effects by directing therapeutic agents specifically to tumor tissues (Wang et al., 2016).

6.1 Passive Targeting: Enhanced Permeability and Retention (EPR) Effect

- **Basic Principle:** Passive targeting leverages the enhanced permeability and retention (EPR) effect, a phenomenon observed in solid tumors due to their leaky vasculature and poor lymphatic drainage. Nanocarriers such as liposomes, micelles, and nanoparticles accumulate preferentially in tumor tissues via the EPR effect when administered systemically (Di Filippo et al., 2023).
- **Challenges in GBM:** However, the application of the EPR effect in GBM is limited by the intact blood-brain barrier (BBB) in many regions of the tumor, especially in early-stage or infiltrative zones. Moreover, heterogeneity in BBB disruption and tumor vasculature among patients affects therapeutic outcomes (Sun et al., 2025).

Examples

- Doxil®, a PEGylated liposomal formulation of doxorubicin, exploits the EPR effect and has shown limited success in GBM, primarily due to suboptimal BBB penetration.
- Temozolomide-loaded PLGA nanoparticles have demonstrated passive accumulation in glioma models, but their efficiency depends heavily on tumor vasculature integrity (Kreuter, 2001).

6.2 Active Targeting: Ligand and Antibody-Mediated Delivery

Overview: Active targeting involves surface functionalization of drug carriers with ligands, antibodies, peptides, or aptamers that bind to overexpressed receptors on GBM cells or endothelial cells of the tumor vasculature, facilitating receptor-mediated endocytosis.

Key Receptors and Ligands

- **Transferrin receptors (TfR):** Widely expressed on GBM cells and the BBB. Nanoparticles conjugated with transferrin or anti-TfR antibodies have shown enhanced penetration and uptake (Qian et al., 2002).
- **Epidermal Growth Factor Receptor variant III (EGFRvIII):** A GBM-specific mutation. Antibody-functionalized nanoparticles targeting EGFRvIII can provide high tumor specificity.
- **Folate receptors and RGD peptides:** Used for targeting angiogenic endothelium in glioma.

Examples

- Lactoferrin-modified liposomes carrying paclitaxel showed higher cellular uptake in glioma cells and better brain penetration (Liu et al., 2011).
- Angiopep-2-functionalized polymersomes have demonstrated efficient BBB crossing and glioma targeting via low-density lipoprotein receptor-related protein 1 (LRP1) (Xin et al., 2011).
- Advantages and Limitations

Active targeting increases specificity and internalization but faces challenges such as receptor heterogeneity, receptor saturation, and immune recognition of ligands.

6.3 Multifunctional Platforms

Concept and Rationale: Multifunctional or "theranostic" platforms combine targeting, therapeutic delivery, and imaging in a single system (Nayak et al., 2024).

Examples

- Magnetic nanoparticles functionalized with both doxorubicin and targeting ligands (e.g., folic acid) enable MRI imaging alongside therapy.
- Gold nanoparticles conjugated with siRNA and peptides allow photothermal therapy and gene silencing specifically in glioma cells (Vines et al., 2019).
- pH-sensitive liposomes that release their payload in the acidic tumor microenvironment improve drug stability in circulation and enhance tumor targeting.

7. PRECLINICAL AND CLINICAL STATUS

Glioblastoma multiforme (GBM) is a highly aggressive brain tumor with poor prognosis and limited treatment options. In response, a wide range of novel drug delivery systems (NDDSs) are undergoing preclinical and clinical evaluations aimed at improving therapeutic efficacy, tumor specificity, and blood-brain barrier (BBB) penetration.

7.1 Formulations in the Preclinical Pipeline

Numerous nanotechnology-based and implantable systems have shown promise in preclinical GBM models:

- Polymeric nanoparticles (PNPs) loaded with doxorubicin or paclitaxel have been engineered to cross the BBB using ligands such as transferrin or angiopep-2 (Kreuter et al., 2003).
- Lipid-based nanoparticles, including solid lipid nanoparticles (SLNs) and nanostructured lipid carriers (NLCs), have been used to encapsulate TMZ, curcumin, and siRNA.
- Cell-based delivery systems, such as mesenchymal stem cells (MSCs) loaded with oncolytic viruses, offer tumor tropism, enabling site-specific drug release. Exosome-based delivery of miRNAs has also demonstrated anti-tumor activity in xenograft models.

- Hydrogel-based systems, incorporating anti-angiogenic agents, allow localized, post-surgical delivery of drugs directly into the resection cavity, reducing systemic exposure and increasing tumor control (Basso et al., 2018).

7.2 Clinical Trials Overview

Several novel GBM delivery platforms have entered clinical evaluation, focusing on nanoparticles, local delivery devices, and immunotherapies as shown in table 2:

- Gliadel® wafer, an FDA-approved carmustine-impregnated biodegradable polymer implant, remains one of the few clinically successful localized delivery systems. Implanted post-tumor resection, it releases drug directly at the site, bypassing the BBB.
- NanoTherm® therapy, which uses superparamagnetic iron oxide nanoparticles injected intratumorally and activated by alternating magnetic fields, has been tested in Europe (Grzegorzewski et al., 2025). This thermal ablation technique is combined with radiotherapy.
- Immunoliposomes targeting EGFRvIII, such as 2B3-101 (GlioLip) a glutathione pegylated liposomal doxorubicin has completed phase I/II trials, showing increased drug penetration across the BBB and tumor accumulation.
- Clinical trials involving focused ultrasound (FUS) to transiently disrupt the BBB, such as those using the Exablate system, have demonstrated increased drug delivery and safety in GBM patients (Carpentier et al., 2016).
- Stem cell therapies, including engineered neural stem cells delivering prodrugs like 5-FC, are under clinical evaluation for their ability to home to residual tumor cells and convert prodrugs to cytotoxic agents at the site of action.

Despite these advances, few systems have moved beyond Phase II trials, highlighting the gap between innovation and clinical adoption.

Despite numerous innovations, many experimental therapies have failed to translate into clinical success. For instance, the ACT IV trial evaluating the EGFRvIII-targeted vaccine rindopepimut was terminated due to lack of survival benefit, despite promising early-phase results. Such failures highlight the complex interplay of tumor heterogeneity, immune suppression, and adaptive resistance in GBM.

Similarly, checkpoint inhibitors like nivolumab have shown disappointing outcomes in randomized trials (e.g., CheckMate 143), which tested nivolumab against bevacizumab in recurrent GBM. While the safety profile was acceptable, overall survival was not significantly improved. This underscores the need for better patient stratification and combinatorial approaches, such as combining immunotherapy with localized or nanoparticle-based delivery platforms to overcome the immune-inert tumor microenvironment.

In contrast, CRISPR/Cas9-based genome-editing systems are entering early-stage investigation for glioblastoma. These platforms aim to disrupt oncogenes such as EGFRvIII, TERT, or PDGFRA with precision. Preclinical studies using lipid or exosome-mediated CRISPR delivery have demonstrated downregulation of these targets, leading to suppressed tumor growth and reduced stemness in glioma stem-like cells.

Moreover, RNA interference (RNAi) therapies are gaining attention. For instance, siRNA-loaded nanoparticles targeting STAT3, a key immunosuppressive transcription factor, have been shown to sensitize tumors to immunotherapy and inhibit GBM progression in vivo.

Clinical translation is beginning to benefit from more adaptive and umbrella trial designs, such as the GBM AGILE platform, which allows real-time modulation of therapeutic arms based on interim efficacy and biomarker analysis. This model increases trial efficiency and facilitates rapid evaluation of personalized delivery technologies.

7.3 Translational Challenges

Several barriers hamper the seamless translation of promising preclinical delivery systems to clinical practice:

- Blood-brain barrier (BBB) heterogeneity across GBM tumors reduces uniform drug delivery, necessitating personalized delivery strategies.
- Tumor heterogeneity, particularly in genetic and phenotypic profiles, complicates universal targeting approaches and may lead to drug resistance.
- Manufacturing complexity and scalability issues, especially for ligand-targeted or cell-based systems, often delay clinical transition due to stringent regulatory requirements.
- **Immunogenicity and toxicity:** Surface-modified or multifunctional nanocarriers may trigger immune responses or show off-target accumulation in organs like the liver and spleen.
- **Regulatory hurdles:** Regulatory approval requires comprehensive data on pharmacokinctics, biodistribution, and long-term safety, which are often lacking or inconsistent in early studies.
- **Cost and accessibility:** High manufacturing costs and lack of reimbursement pathways can restrict patient access, especially in low- and middle-income countries.

To address these challenges, a multidisciplinary approach involving materials science, pharmacology, oncology, and regulatory science is essential. Collaborative efforts and public-private partnerships are also needed to bridge the translational gap.

Table 2. Clinical trail overview

System/Strategy	Clinical Phase	Target	Mechanism/Approach	Outcome/ Status	Reference
Gliadel® wafer	Approved	Residual tumor post-surgery	Biodegradable carmustine wafer placed in resection cavity	Extended median survival with radiotherapy	(Westphal et al., 2003)
2B3-101 (GlioLip)	Phase I/II	BBB/ EGFRvIII	Glutathione-PEGylated liposomal doxorubicin	Improved BBB penetration and tumor accumulation	(Kreuter, 2001)
NanoTherm® Therapy	EU-approved (pilot)	Tumor core	Magnetic nanoparticles activated by AMF for hyperthermia	Early promise in combination with radiotherapy	(Grzegorzewski ry al., 2025)
FUS with Microbubbles	Phase I/II	BBB	Pulsed ultrasound induces transient BBB opening	Increased drug delivery; safe and reversible	(Carpentier et al., 2016)
NSC-mediated prodrug	Phase I	Tumor tissue	Neural stem cells expressing cytosine deaminase convert 5-FC to 5-FU	Tumor regression seen in preclinical studies	(Aboody et al., 2013)
Angiopep-2 nanoparticles	Preclinical/ early	LRP1 receptor on BBB	Enhanced uptake via receptor-mediated transcytosis	Promising BBB penetration and glioma targeting	(Xin et al., 2011)

7.4 Advanced Preclinical Models: BBB-on-a-Chip & Humanized Immunotherapy

BBB-on-a-Chip

Microfluidic BBB-on-a-chip models recreate human BBB architecture using endothelial cells, astrocytes, and pericytes, allowing real-time assessment of drug/ nanoparticle permeability with higher translational accuracy than animal models.

Humanized Immunotherapy Models

Humanized mice engrafted with human immune cells enable accurate testing of CAR-T and checkpoint inhibitors by mimicking human immune tumor interactions better than conventional xenografts.

8. REGULATORY AND ETHICAL CONSIDERATIONS

As the landscape of glioblastoma multiforme (GBM) therapy advances with innovative drug delivery systems, regulatory and ethical frameworks must evolve to ensure patient safety, product efficacy, and scientific integrity. These considerations are essential, especially given the high vulnerability of GBM patients, the complexity of brain-targeted delivery, and the experimental nature of many proposed therapies.

8.1 Safety and Biocompatibility

Safety and biocompatibility are core regulatory requirements for any novel drug delivery system. For GBM, these parameters are particularly stringent due to the proximity of therapeutic agents to sensitive central nervous system (CNS) structures.

- Biocompatibility involves ensuring that delivery systems, whether nanoparticles, hydrogels, or implants, do not provoke neuroinflammation, gliosis, or systemic toxicity. Materials like PLGA, chitosan, and PEGylated lipids are widely studied for their biocompatibility and FDA acceptance in CNS applications.
- Toxicological profiles must be rigorously assessed. For instance, surface-modified nanoparticles with cationic charges may cross the BBB effectively but can disrupt neuronal function and cause oxidative stress.
- Sterility, stability, and degradation products are also crucial for implants and injectable systems. Gliadel® wafers, for example, underwent extensive preclinical toxicological testing to validate the safety of their polyanhydride matrix before FDA approval in 1996.
- Immunogenicity remains a concern for cell-based systems (e.g., stem cells or exosomes) and viral vectors. Long-term immune surveillance studies are needed to avoid late-onset adverse events.

8.2 Regulatory Hurdles

The regulatory landscape for GBM therapies is evolving, but several challenges persist due to the innovative nature of these delivery systems:

- **Lack of standardized guidelines:** Most regulatory frameworks (FDA, EMA) are tailored for conventional small molecules or biologics. Nanoparticles, multifunctional systems, and hybrid materials often do not fit into existing categories.

- **Complexity of combination products:** Many NDDSs for GBM combine diagnostics and therapeutics ("theranostics") or involve multiple agents, making regulatory assessment multifactorial.
- **Pharmacokinetics (PK) and pharmacodynamics (PD)** for brain-targeting systems are hard to predict due to the dynamic nature of the BBB/BTB and tumor heterogeneity. Regulatory agencies require detailed PK/PD modeling, biodistribution studies, and in vivo tracking.
- **Translational gaps:** Many promising preclinical results are not reproducible in human models. For example, nanoparticle penetration and accumulation in murine GBM models often overestimate efficacy compared to human GBM due to anatomical and physiological differences.
- **Good Manufacturing Practices (GMP)** compliance for novel platforms like stem cell-derived exosomes or microfluidic-fabricated nanoparticles is still a developing area.
- The FDA's Breakthrough Therapy designation and Orphan Drug Act have been used to fast-track some GBM therapies (e.g., Toca 511, Optune), but many NDDSs fall short of the criteria, especially due to lack of Phase I human safety data.

8.3 Ethical Aspects in Neuro-Oncology Trials

Given the terminal nature of GBM, ethical considerations in clinical trials are paramount. These involve patient rights, trial design, informed consent, and equity of access:

- Informed consent must be thoroughly managed, especially for patients with impaired cognitive function due to tumor location. Proxy consent or legal representatives are sometimes involved, raising ethical dilemmas about autonomy and voluntariness.
- Risk-benefit analysis must be conservative. While patients and families may be eager for novel treatments, investigators must ensure interventions are justified by robust preclinical data. The ethical principle of *non-maleficence* guides against undue harm.
- Trial transparency and data sharing are ethical imperatives. Negative results from failed trials (e.g., of immune checkpoint inhibitors in GBM) must be published to avoid duplication and patient risk.
- Placebo-controlled trials in terminal GBM can be ethically challenging. Adaptive trial designs, such as Bayesian or platform trials (e.g., GBM AGILE), are increasingly favored as they offer real-time adjustments and reduce the number of patients exposed to ineffective treatments.

- Equitable access is critical. Advanced therapies, especially those requiring high-tech equipment (e.g., focused ultrasound or intratumoral pumps), may not be accessible in low-resource settings, raising concerns of global health disparity.

9. FUTURE PERSPECTIVES AND CHALLENGES

Glioblastoma multiforme (GBM) remains one of the most aggressive and treatment-resistant brain tumors despite decades of research. As novel drug delivery systems continue to evolve, the future of GBM therapy is increasingly leaning towards personalization, integration of diagnostics with therapy (theranostics), and computational tools like AI for optimizing treatment. These emerging directions offer promising avenues, yet also pose significant scientific, logistical, and ethical challenges.

9.1 Personalized Nanomedicine

Personalized medicine aims to tailor treatments based on an individual's molecular profile, tumor heterogeneity, and genetic landscape. This strategy holds immense promise for GBM, which exhibits considerable inter- and intra-patient variability.

- Nanomedicine enables this approach by designing delivery vehicles responsive to patient-specific tumor environments. For instance, nanoparticles can be surface-modified with ligands targeting overexpressed markers such as EGFRvIII, IL-13Rα2, or CD133, which are variably expressed in GBM subtypes.
- Genomic sequencing of patient tumors can guide the choice of drugs and carriers. For example, a patient with MGMT promoter methylation may benefit more from temozolomide-loaded nanocarriers, while EGFR-amplified GBM may be targeted using anti-EGFR antibody-functionalized systems.
- Advanced nanocarriers such as stimuli-responsive nanoparticles (responsive to pH, enzymes, or redox potential) offer precise spatial and temporal control, minimizing off-target effects. These carriers can be customized to match the microenvironmental cues of a specific tumor.
- Patient-derived glioblastoma stem cells (GSCs) are being used in preclinical studies to develop and screen personalized nanoparticle formulations. For instance, Mahmud et al. (2018) developed GSC-targeting liposomes modified with chlorotoxin, demonstrating improved tumor specificity in individualized models.

9.2 Integration with Diagnostics (Theranostics)

The concept of theranostics combines diagnostic imaging and therapeutic delivery in one platform. In GBM, this dual functionality is especially valuable for real-time monitoring of drug distribution and therapeutic response.

- Quantum dots, iron oxide nanoparticles, and gold nanoparticles are being explored for their imaging capabilities via MRI, CT, and photoacoustic techniques. When conjugated with drugs or siRNAs, they offer the potential for simultaneous tumor visualization and treatment.
- For example, Chan et al. (2022) designed a superparamagnetic iron oxide nanoparticle (SPION) system loaded with doxorubicin and decorated with transferrin ligands. The system facilitated both MRI tracking and targeted drug delivery to GBM cells.
- Theranostic implants are also being tested. Hydrogels embedded with imaging agents and chemotherapeutics allow for post-surgical implantation, sustained release, and tracking of therapeutic efficacy.

Theranostics may reduce treatment uncertainty and enable adaptive therapy, wherein dosage and drug combinations can be altered based on feedback from real-time imaging. However, toxicity of imaging agents, regulatory approval hurdles for combination devices, and integration with hospital imaging protocols remain substantial barriers.

9.3 AI and Computational Modeling in Drug Delivery Design

Artificial Intelligence (AI) and computational modeling are revolutionizing the design, prediction, and optimization of drug delivery systems for GBM.

- Machine learning (ML) algorithms can predict nanoparticle behavior in the brain, including BBB penetration, biodistribution, and cellular uptake, based on physicochemical properties like size, surface charge, and ligand density.
- In silico simulations are used to model drug release kinetics, diffusion through brain parenchyma, and interaction with tumor microenvironments. For example, computational fluid dynamics (CFD) has been employed to optimize convection-enhanced delivery (CED) parameters in GBM therapy.
- AI platforms such as DeepChem and BioSymphony are being explored for high-throughput screening of nanocarrier formulations and identifying optimal drug-ligand-carrier combinations with minimal experimental trials.

- Personalized predictive models using patient MRI data can guide the placement of implantable devices or predict the most effective delivery route (e.g., intranasal vs. intratumoral).

Limitations of AI integration include the need for high-quality, diverse datasets, interdisciplinary collaboration, and validation in clinical settings. Additionally, algorithmic bias and explainability (black-box models) present ethical concerns.

Future research may also integrate wearable biosensors and implantable telemetry devices to monitor intracranial drug concentrations, pH shifts, or enzymatic activity, enabling feedback-controlled drug release. Such closed-loop systems could enhance the precision of therapy, especially in high-risk or recurrent GBM cases.

10. CONCLUSION

Glioblastoma multiforme (GBM) continues to pose a significant clinical challenge due to its highly invasive nature, profound genetic heterogeneity, and poor prognosis despite aggressive multimodal therapy. Conventional approaches, including surgical resection, radiotherapy, and chemotherapy (primarily with temozolomide), are insufficient to eradicate infiltrative tumor cells and often fail due to resistance mechanisms and limited drug penetration across the blood-brain barrier (BBB). The emergence of innovative drug delivery systems and advanced dosage forms marks a transformative shift in GBM therapy, aiming to overcome these intrinsic limitations.

Over the past history, a multitude of nanoparticle-based carriers, such as liposomes, solid lipid nanoparticles, polymeric nanoparticles, and dendrimers, have been developed to enhance the targeted delivery of chemotherapeutic agents, siRNAs, and immunomodulators. These platforms can improve pharmacokinetics, reduce systemic toxicity, and facilitate penetration across the BBB through surface functionalization with ligands or stimuli-responsive materials. Liposomal formulations such as Doxil and experimental polymeric systems targeting receptors like EGFR, transferrin, or IL-13Rα2 exemplify this advancement.

Moreover, cell-based delivery systems, including exosomes and stem-cell-derived vesicles, offer biologically compatible carriers with intrinsic homing abilities to GBM tissue. Intranasal and intra-tumoral delivery methods have further enhanced localized and non-invasive administration. In parallel, technologies like focused ultrasound (FUS) in combination with microbubbles have demonstrated real-time, non-invasive BBB modulation, creating transient permeability windows that facilitate drug entry without damaging healthy brain tissue.

In terms of advanced dosage forms, biodegradable implants (e.g., Gliadel® wafers) and thermoresponsive hydrogels have enabled sustained, localized release of chemotherapeutics directly at the tumor resection site, bypassing systemic circulation. Microneedle patches and miniaturized implantable pumps represent the next generation of minimally invasive delivery devices, ensuring continuous dosing with programmable controls.

The integration of active and passive targeting strategies using ligands, antibodies, and enhanced permeability and retention (EPR) effects has significantly improved drug accumulation within tumor tissues. Multifunctional platforms, combining imaging and therapy (theranostics), have brought forward a personalized approach, enabling real-time monitoring and adaptive treatment.

Despite these advances, translating these innovations from bench to bedside remains a substantial hurdle. A relatively small number of nanomedicine formulations have entered clinical trials, and even fewer have achieved regulatory approval for GBM. Challenges include issues of scalability, reproducibility, long-term toxicity, immunogenicity, and patient-specific variability in tumor biology. Furthermore, the complex anatomy and immunoprivileged nature of the central nervous system (CNS) demand stringent safety evaluations and robust preclinical models.

Looking forward, the road to clinical implementation of these novel drug delivery systems will be shaped by several key factors:

1. Personalized nanomedicine approaches, guided by genomics and molecular profiling, will be vital in tailoring therapies to individual patients, enhancing efficacy and minimizing resistance.
2. Theranostic platforms will play an essential role in providing feedback on drug distribution, tumor response, and treatment adaptation, especially in aggressive and evolving tumors like GBM.
3. Artificial Intelligence (AI) and computational modeling will revolutionize drug design, dosage optimization, and delivery predictions, enabling accelerated discovery and development cycles.
4. Multidisciplinary collaboration among oncologists, neuroscientists, pharmaceutical scientists, bioengineers, and regulatory experts will be critical to overcoming translational bottlenecks.
5. Ethical considerations, particularly around experimental therapies in terminal patients and pediatric populations, must be addressed transparently with robust consent procedures and regulatory oversight.

REFERENCES

Aboody, K. S., Najbauer, J., Metz, M. Z., D'Apuzzo, M., Gutova, M., Annala, A. J., Synold, T. W., Couture, L. A., Blanchard, M. S., Moats, R. A., Garcia, E., Aramburo, S., Valenzuela, V. V., Frank, R. T., Barish, M. E., Brown, C. E., Kim, S. U., Badie, B., & Portnow, J. (2013). Neural stem cell-mediated enzyme/prodrug therapy for glioma: Preclinical studies. *Science Translational Medicine*, *5*(184), 184ra59. Advance online publication. DOI: 10.1126/scitranslmed.3005365 PMID: 23658244

Ahmed, M. H., Canney, M., Carpentier, A., & Idbaih, A. (2023). Overcoming the blood brain barrier in glioblastoma: Status and future perspective. *Revue Neurologique*, *179*(5), 430–436. DOI: 10.1016/j.neurol.2023.03.013 PMID: 37062676

Basso, J., Miranda, A., Nunes, S., Cova, T., Sousa, J., Vitorino, C., & Pais, A. (2018). Hydrogel-based drug delivery nanosystems for the treatment of brain tumors. *Gels (Basel, Switzerland)*, *4*(3), 62. Advance online publication. DOI: 10.3390/gels4030062 PMID: 30674838

Brem, H., Piantadosi, S., Burger, P. C., Walker, M., Selker, R., Vick, N. A., Black, K., Sisti, M., Brem, S., Mohr, G., Muller, P., Morawetz, R., & Schold, S. C. (1995). Placebo-controlled trial of safety and efficacy of intraoperative controlled delivery by biodegradable polymers of chemotherapy for recurrent gliomas. *Lancet*, *345*(8956), 1008–1012. DOI: 10.1016/S0140-6736(95)90755-6 PMID: 7723496

Carpentier, A., Canney, M., Vignot, A., Reina, V., Beccaria, K., Horodyckid, C., Karachi, C., Leclercq, D., Lafon, C., Chapelon, J.-Y., Capelle, L., Cornu, P., Sanson, M., Hoang-Xuan, K., Delattre, J.-Y., & Idbaih, A. (2016). Clinical trial of blood-brain barrier disruption by pulsed ultrasound. *Science Translational Medicine*, *8*(343), 343re2. Advance online publication. DOI: 10.1126/scitranslmed.aaf6086 PMID: 27306666

Chan, M.-H., Huang, W.-T., Satpathy, A., Su, T.-Y., Hsiao, M., & Liu, R.-S. (2022). Progress and viewpoints of multifunctional composite nanomaterials for glioblastoma theranostics. *Pharmaceutics*, *14*(2), 456. Advance online publication. DOI: 10.3390/pharmaceutics14020456 PMID: 35214188

Di Filippo, L. D., de Carvalho, S. G., Duarte, J. L., Luiz, M. T., Paes Dutra, J. A., de Paula, G. A., & Duarte, M. C. K. H. (2023). A receptor-mediated landscape of druggable and targeted nanomaterials for gliomas. *Materials Today. Bio*, *20*, 100671. Advance online publication. DOI: 10.1016/j.mtbio.2023.100671 PMID: 37273792

Esemen, Y., Awan, M., Parwez, R., Baig, A., Rahman, S., Masala, I., Poyiadji, N., & Han, X. (2022). Molecular pathogenesis of glioblastoma in adults and future perspectives: A systematic review. *International Journal of Molecular Sciences*, *23*(5), 2607. Advance online publication. DOI: 10.3390/ijms23052607 PMID: 35269752

Ghaznavi, H., Afzalipour, R., Khoei, S., Sargazi, S., Shirvalilou, S., & Sheervalilou, R. (2024). New insights into targeted therapy of glioblastoma using smart nanoparticles. *Cancer Cell International*, *24*(1), 160. Advance online publication. DOI: 10.1186/s12935-024-03331-3 PMID: 38715021

Gong, Z., Zhou, D., Wu, D., Han, Y., Yu, H., Shen, H., Feng, W., Hou, L., Chen, Y., & Xu, T. (2025). Challenges and material innovations in drug delivery to central nervous system tumors. *Biomaterials*, *319*, 123180. Advance online publication. DOI: 10.1016/j.biomaterials.2025.123180 PMID: 39985979

Gregory, J. V., Kadiyala, P., Doherty, R., Cadena, M., Habeel, S., Ruoslahti, E., Lowenstein, P. R., Castro, M. G., & Lahann, J. (2020). Systemic brain tumor delivery of synthetic protein nanoparticles for glioblastoma therapy. *Nature Communications*, *11*(1), 5687. Advance online publication. DOI: 10.1038/s41467-020-19225-7 PMID: 33173024

Grzegorzewski, J., Michalak, M., Wołoszczuk, M., Bulicz, M., & Majchrzak-Celińska, A. (2025). Nanotherapy of glioblastoma—Where hope grows. *International Journal of Molecular Sciences*, *26*(5), 1814. Advance online publication. DOI: 10.3390/ijms26051814 PMID: 40076445

Guo, X., Gu, L., Li, Y., Zheng, Z., Chen, W., Wang, Y., & Zhang, J. (2023). Histological and molecular glioblastoma, IDH-wildtype: A real-world landscape using the 2021 WHO classification of central nervous system tumors. *Frontiers in Oncology*, *13*, 1200815. Advance online publication. DOI: 10.3389/fonc.2023.1200815 PMID: 37483487

Hart, M. G., Garside, R., Rogers, G., Stein, K., & Grant, R. (2013). Temozolomide for high grade glioma. *Cochrane Database of Systematic Reviews*, *4*(9), CD007415. Advance online publication. DOI: 10.1002/14651858.CD007415.pub2 PMID: 23633341

Hegi, M. E., Diserens, A.-C., Gorlia, T., Hamou, M.-F., de Tribolet, N., Weller, M., Kros, J. M., Hainfellner, J. A., Mason, W., Mariani, L., Bromberg, J. E. C., Hau, P., Mirimanoff, R. O., Cairncross, J. G., Janzer, R. C., & Stupp, R. (2005). MGMT gene silencing and benefit from temozolomide in glioblastoma. *The New England Journal of Medicine*, *352*(10), 997–1003. DOI: 10.1056/NEJMoa043331 PMID: 15758010

Illum, L. (2000). Transport of drugs from the nasal cavity to the central nervous system. *European Journal of Pharmaceutical Sciences, 11*(1), 1–18. DOI: 10.1016/S0928-0987(00)00087-7 PMID: 10913748

Ivy Brain Tumor Center. (n.d.). *Glioblastoma current standard of care*. Retrieved May 21, 2025, from https://www.ivybraintumorcenter.org/the-challenge/current-standard-of-care/

Jezierzański, M., Nafalska, N., Stopyra, M., Furgoł, T., Miciak, M., Kabut, J., & Szczylik, C. (2024). Temozolomide (TMZ) in the treatment of glioblastoma multiforme—A literature review and clinical outcomes. *Current Oncology (Toronto, Ont.), 31*(7), 3994–4002. DOI: 10.3390/curroncol31070296 PMID: 39057168

Kreuter, J. (2001). Nanoparticulate systems for brain delivery of drugs. *Advanced Drug Delivery Reviews, 47*(1), 65–81. DOI: 10.1016/S0169-409X(00)00122-8 PMID: 11251246

Kreuter, J. (2014). Drug delivery to the central nervous system by polymeric nanoparticles: What do we know? *Advanced Drug Delivery Reviews, 71*, 2–14. DOI: 10.1016/j.addr.2013.08.008 PMID: 23981489

Kreuter, J., Ramge, P., Petrov, V., Hamm, S., Gelperina, S. E., Engelhardt, B., Alyautdin, R., von Briesen, H., & Begley, D. J. (2003). Direct evidence that polysorbate-80-coated poly(butylcyanoacrylate) nanoparticles deliver drugs to the CNS via specific mechanisms requiring prior binding of drug to the nanoparticles. *Pharmaceutical Research, 20*(3), 409–416. DOI: 10.1023/A:1022604120952 PMID: 12669961

Lai, G., Wu, H., Yang, K., Hu, K., Zhou, Y., Chen, X., Fu, F., Li, J., Xie, G., Wang, H. F., Lv, Z., & Wu, X. (2024). Progress of nanoparticle drug delivery system for the treatment of glioma. *Frontiers in Bioengineering and Biotechnology, 12*, 1403511. Advance online publication. DOI: 10.3389/fbioe.2024.1403511 PMID: 38919382

Lan, Z., Li, X., & Zhang, X. (2024). Glioblastoma: An update in pathology, molecular mechanisms and biomarkers. *International Journal of Molecular Sciences, 25*(5), 3040. Advance online publication. DOI: 10.3390/ijms25053040 PMID: 38474286

Liu, Z., Ji, X., He, D., Zhang, R., Liu, Q., & Xin, T. (2022). Nanoscale drug delivery systems in glioblastoma. *Nanoscale Research Letters, 17*(1), 27. Advance online publication. DOI: 10.1186/s11671-022-03668-6 PMID: 35171358

Mahmud, H., Kasai, T., Khayrani, A. C., Asakura, M., Oo, A. K. K., Du, J., Seno, M., & Yagi, K. (2018). Targeting glioblastoma cells expressing CD44 with liposomes encapsulating doxorubicin and displaying chlorotoxin-IgG Fc fusion protein. *International Journal of Molecular Sciences*, *19*(3), 659. Advance online publication. DOI: 10.3390/ijms19030659 PMID: 29495404

Mansour, M. A., Kamer-Eldawla, A. M., Malaeb, R. W., Aboelhassan, R., Nabawi, D. H., Aziz, M. M., & Choudhry, H. (2025). Unlocking the code: The role of molecular and genetic profiling in revolutionizing glioblastoma treatment. *Cancer Treatment and Research Communications*, *43*, 100881. Advance online publication. DOI: 10.1016/j.ctarc.2025.100881 PMID: 39985914

Mokarram, N., Case, A., Hossainy, N. N., Lyon, J. G., MacDonald, T. J., & Bellamkonda, R. V. (2025). Device-assisted strategies for drug delivery across the blood-brain barrier to treat glioblastoma. *Communications Materials*, *6*(1), 1–22. DOI: 10.1038/s43246-024-00721-y PMID: 39790893

Narsinh, K. H., Perez, E., Haddad, A. F., Young, J. S., Savastano, L., Villanueva-Meyer, J. E., & Aghi, M. K. (2024). Strategies to improve drug delivery across the blood–brain barrier for glioblastoma. *Current Neurology and Neuroscience Reports*, *24*(5), 123–139. DOI: 10.1007/s11910-024-01338-x PMID: 38578405

Nayak, A., Warrier, N. M., Raman, R., Prabhu, V., & Kumar, P. (2024). Targeted delivery of nanomedicines to glioblastoma: Overcoming the clinical barrier. *Journal of Drug Delivery Science and Technology*, *99*, 105980. Advance online publication. DOI: 10.1016/j.jddst.2024.105980

Noorani, I., & de la Rosa, J. (2023). Breaking barriers for glioblastoma with a path to enhanced drug delivery. *Nature Communications*, *14*(1), 5909. Advance online publication. DOI: 10.1038/s41467-023-41694-9 PMID: 37737212

Pardridge, W. M. (2005). The blood-brain barrier: Bottleneck in brain drug development. *NeuroRx : the Journal of the American Society for Experimental NeuroTherapeutics*, *2*(1), 3–14. DOI: 10.1602/neurorx.2.1.3 PMID: 15717053

Pouyan, A., Ghorbanlo, M., Eslami, M., Jahanshahi, M., Ziaei, E., Salami, A., & Farhadi, M. (2025). Glioblastoma multiforme: Insights into pathogenesis, key signaling pathways, and therapeutic strategies. *Molecular Cancer*, *24*(1), 58. Advance online publication. DOI: 10.1186/s12943-025-02267-0 PMID: 40011944

Qian, Z. M., Li, H., Sun, H., & Ho, K. (2002). Targeted drug delivery via the transferrin receptor-mediated endocytosis pathway. *Pharmacological Reviews*, *54*(4), 561–587. DOI: 10.1124/pr.54.4.561 PMID: 12429868

Qindeel, M., Irfan, M., Ullah, S., Fathi-karkan, S., Kharaba, Z., Rahdar, A., & Bilal, M. (2024). Nanotechnology in glioblastoma therapy: Advances in drug delivery systems and diagnostic approaches. *Journal of Drug Delivery Science and Technology*, *102*, 106322. Advance online publication. DOI: 10.1016/j.jddst.2024.106322

Quail, D. F., & Joyce, J. A. (2017). The microenvironmental landscape of brain tumors. *Cancer Cell*, *31*(3), 326–341. DOI: 10.1016/j.ccell.2017.02.009 PMID: 28292436

Raju, R., Abuwatfa, W. H., Pitt, W. G., & Husseini, G. A. (2023). Liposomes for the treatment of brain cancer—A review. *Pharmaceuticals (Basel, Switzerland)*, *16*(8), 1056. Advance online publication. DOI: 10.3390/ph16081056 PMID: 37630971

Roque, D., Cruz, N., Ferreira, H. A., Reis, C. P., Matela, N., Herculano-Carvalho, M., Cascão, R., & Faria, C. C. (2023). Nanoparticle-based treatment in glioblastoma. *Journal of Personalized Medicine*, *13*(9), 1328. Advance online publication. DOI: 10.3390/jpm13091328 PMID: 37763096

Seetharam, A. A., Choudhry, H., Bakhrebah, M. A., Abdulaal, W. H., Gupta, M. S., Rizvi, S. M. D., Alam, Q., & Gupta, R. (2020). Microneedles drug delivery systems for treatment of cancer: A recent update. *Pharmaceutics*, *12*(11), 1101. Advance online publication. DOI: 10.3390/pharmaceutics12111101 PMID: 33212921

Shi, D., Mi, G., Shen, Y., & Webster, T. J. (2019). Glioma-targeted dual functionalized thermosensitive Ferri-liposomes for drug delivery through an in vitro blood-brain barrier. *Nanoscale*, *11*(32), 15057–15071. DOI: 10.1039/C9NR03931G PMID: 31369016

Stupp, R., Mason, W. P., van den Bent, M. J., Weller, M., Fisher, B., Taphoorn, M. J. B., Belanger, K., Brandes, A. A., Marosi, C., Bogdahn, U., Curschmann, J., Janzer, R. C., Ludwin, S. K., Gorlia, T., Allgeier, A., Lacombe, D., Cairncross, J. G., Eisenhauer, E., & Mirimanoff, R. O. (2005). Radiotherapy plus concomitant and adjuvant temozolomide for glioblastoma. *The New England Journal of Medicine*, *352*(10), 987–996. DOI: 10.1056/NEJMoa043330 PMID: 15758009

Stupp, R., Taillibert, S., Kanner, A., Read, W., Steinberg, D. M., Lhermitte, B., Toms, S., Idbaih, A., Ahluwalia, M. S., Fink, K. L., Di Meco, F., Lieberman, F., Zhu, J.-J., Stragliotto, G., Tran, D. D., Brem, S., Hottinger, A. F., Kirson, E. D., & Ram, Z. (2017). Effect of tumor-treating fields plus maintenance temozolomide vs maintenance temozolomide alone on survival in patients with glioblastoma: A randomized clinical trial. *Journal of the American Medical Association*, *318*(23), 2306–2316. DOI: 10.1001/jama.2017.18718 PMID: 29260225

Stupp, R., Taillibert, S., Kanner, A. A., Kesari, S., Steinberg, D. M., Toms, S. A., Taylor, L. P., Lieberman, F., Silvani, A., Fink, K. L., Barnett, G. H., Zhu, J.-J., Henson, J. W., Engelhard, H. H., Chen, T. C., Tran, D. D., Sroubek, J., Tran, N. D., Hottinger, A. F., & Ram, Z. (2015). Maintenance therapy with tumor-treating fields plus temozolomide vs temozolomide alone for glioblastoma: A randomized clinical trial. *Journal of the American Medical Association*, *314*(23), 2535–2543. DOI: 10.1001/jama.2015.16669 PMID: 26670971

Sun, B., Li, R., Ji, N., Liu, H., Wang, H., Chen, C., Bai, L., Su, J., & Chen, J. (2025). Brain-targeting drug delivery systems: The state of the art in treatment of glioblastoma. *Materials Today. Bio*, *30*, 101443. Advance online publication. DOI: 10.1016/j.mtbio.2025.101443 PMID: 39866779

Surender, V., & Deepika, M. (2016). *Solid lipid nanoparticles: A comprehensive review*. LAP LAMBERT Academic Publishing.

ter Linden, E., Abels, E. R., van Solinge, T. S., Neefjes, J., & Broekman, M. L. D. (2024). Overcoming barriers in glioblastoma—Advances in drug delivery strategies. *Cells*, *13*(12), 998. Advance online publication. DOI: 10.3390/cells13120998 PMID: 38920629

Tripathy, D. K., Panda, L. P., Biswal, S., & Barhwal, K. (2024). Insights into the glioblastoma tumor microenvironment: Current and emerging therapeutic approaches. *Frontiers in Pharmacology*, *15*, 1355242. Advance online publication. DOI: 10.3389/fphar.2024.1355242 PMID: 38523646

Verdugo, E., Puerto, I., & Medina, M. Á. (2022). An update on the molecular biology of glioblastoma, with clinical implications and progress in its treatment. *Cancer Communications*, *42*(11), 1083–1111. DOI: 10.1002/cac2.12361 PMID: 36129048

Verhaak, R. G. W., Hoadley, K. A., Purdom, E., Wang, V., Qi, Y., Wilkerson, M. D., Miller, C. R., Ding, L., Golub, T., Mesirov, J. P., Alexe, G., Lawrence, M., O'Kelly, M., Tamayo, P., Weir, B. A., Gabriel, S., Winckler, W., Gupta, S., Jakkula, L., & Hayes, D. N.Cancer Genome Atlas Research Network. (2010). Integrated genomic analysis identifies clinically relevant subtypes of glioblastoma characterized by abnormalities in PDGFRA, IDH1, EGFR, and NF1. *Cancer Cell*, *17*(1), 98–110. DOI: 10.1016/j.ccr.2009.12.020 PMID: 20129251

Vines, J. B., Yoon, J.-H., Ryu, N.-E., Lim, D.-J., & Park, H. (2019). Gold nanoparticles for photothermal cancer therapy. *Frontiers in Chemistry*, *7*, 167. Advance online publication. DOI: 10.3389/fchem.2019.00167 PMID: 31024882

Vogelbaum, M. A., & Aghi, M. K. (2015). Convection-enhanced delivery for the treatment of glioblastoma. *Neuro-Oncology*, *17*(Suppl. 2), ii3–ii8. DOI: 10.1093/neuonc/nou354 PMID: 25746090

Wang, S., Meng, Y., Li, C., Qian, M., & Huang, R. (2016). Receptor-mediated drug delivery systems targeting to glioma. *Nanomaterials (Basel, Switzerland)*, *6*(1), 3. Advance online publication. DOI: 10.3390/nano6010003 PMID: 28344260

Wei, D., Zhang, N., Qu, S., Wang, H., & Li, J. (2023). Advances in nanotechnology for the treatment of GBM. *Frontiers in Neuroscience*, *17*, 1180943. Advance online publication. DOI: 10.3389/fnins.2023.1180943 PMID: 37214394

Weiser, J. R., & Saltzman, W. M. (2014). Controlled release for local delivery of drugs: Barriers and models. *Journal of Controlled Release*, *190*, 664–673. DOI: 10.1016/j.jconrel.2014.04.048 PMID: 24801251

Westphal, M., Hilt, D. C., Bortey, E., Delavault, P., Olivares, R., Warnke, P. C., Whittle, I. R., Jääskeläinen, J., & Ram, Z. (2003). A phase 3 trial of local chemotherapy with biodegradable carmustine (BCNU) wafers (Gliadel wafers) in patients with primary malignant glioma. *Neuro-Oncology*, *5*(2), 79–88. DOI: 10.1093/neuonc/5.2.79 PMID: 12672279

Xin, H., Jiang, X., Gu, J., Sha, X., Chen, L., Law, K., Chen, Y., Wang, X., Jiang, Y., & Fang, X. (2011). Angiopep-conjugated poly(ethylene glycol)-co-poly(ε-caprolactone) nanoparticles as dual-targeting drug delivery system for brain glioma. *Biomaterials*, *32*(18), 4293–4305. DOI: 10.1016/j.biomaterials.2011.02.044 PMID: 21427009

Xu, C., Hou, P., Li, X., Xiao, M., Zhang, Z., Li, Z., & Liu, Y. (2024). Comprehensive understanding of glioblastoma molecular phenotypes: Classification, characteristics, and transition. *Cancer Biology & Medicine*, 1–19. Advance online publication. DOI: 10.20892/j.issn.2095-3941.2023.0510 PMID: 38712813

Yan, H., Parsons, D. W., Jin, G., McLendon, R., Rasheed, B. A., Yuan, W., Kos, I., Batinic-Haberle, I., Jones, S., Riggins, G. J., Friedman, H., Friedman, A., Reardon, D., Herndon, J., Kinzler, K. W., Velculescu, V. E., Vogelstein, B., & Bigner, D. D. (2009). IDH1 and IDH2 mutations in gliomas. *The New England Journal of Medicine*, *360*(8), 765–773. DOI: 10.1056/NEJMoa0808710 PMID: 19228619

Yang, T., Martin, P., Fogarty, B., Brown, A., Schurman, K., Phipps, R., Yin, Y., Spence, A., & Bellamkonda, R. V. (2015). Exosome delivered anticancer drugs across the blood-brain barrier for brain cancer therapy in Danio rerio. *Pharmaceutical Research*, *32*(6), 2003–2014. DOI: 10.1007/s11095-014-1593-y PMID: 25609010

Zhang, P., Xia, Q., Liu, L., Li, S., & Dong, L. (2020). Current opinion on molecular characterization for GBM classification in guiding clinical diagnosis, prognosis, and therapy. *Frontiers in Molecular Biosciences*, *7*, 562798. Advance online publication. DOI: 10.3389/fmolb.2020.562798 PMID: 33102518

. Zhao, W., Zhang, Z., Xie, M., Ding, F., Zheng, X., & Sun, S. (2025). Exploring tumor-associated macrophages in glioblastoma: From diversity to therapy. *npj Precision Oncology, 9*(1), Article 1–18. https://doi.org/DOI: 10.1038/s41698-025-00678-4

Chapter 10
Nanomaterial-Based Strategies for Overcoming the Blood–Brain Barrier in Glioblastoma Therapy

Aida Loshaj Shala
https://orcid.org/0000-0003-2640-4356
University of Prishtina, Kosovo

Toskë Kryeziu
https://orcid.org/0000-0002-5591-2520
University of Prishtina, Kosovo

Dafina Fondaj
https://orcid.org/0009-0008-2279-8822
University of Bari, Italy

Nunzio Denora
University of Bari, Italy

Mimoza Basholli Salihu
University of Prishtina, Kosovo

ABSTRACT

Glioblastoma (GBM) is among the most aggressive and therapy-resistant brain tumors, due to its invasive growth, heterogeneity, and limited response to standard treatments. This chapter reviews GBM pathology, including molecular features,

DOI: 10.4018/979-8-3373-2695-5.ch010

glioma-initiating cells, hypoxia, and challenges posed by the blood–brain barrier (BBB). It explores nanotechnology-based strategies—liposomes, micelles, dendrimers, solid lipid, and biomimetic nanoparticles—focused on targeting, uptake, drug release, and BBB penetration. Preclinical studies show improved biodistribution and tumor accumulation. Clinical trials with liposomal doxorubicin and irinotecan show modest outcomes, underscoring a gap in clinical translation. The chapter highlights the need for improved delivery systems and personalized approaches. Nanotechnology offers promising potential for advancing GBM therapy.

1. INTRODUCTION

1.1. Epidemiology and Prognosis

According to the National Brain Tumour Society, there are over 120 different types of brain tumors (Society, 2025). Astrocytomas, or the star-shaped glial cell tumours of astrocytes, are the most frequent of them. World Health Organization (WHO) classifies astrocytomas into four grades depending on cellular atypia, mitotic activity, and vascular proliferation. Grade 1 astrocytomas are typically indolent and benign, whereas grade 4 astrocytomas are very malignant. Glioblastoma multiforme (GBM), the most infiltrative and malignant, is classified as the highest grade. It is associated with poor prognosis: one-year survival following diagnosis is approximately 40 %, it falls to 17 % at two years, and less than 10 % at five years (Tan et al., 2020).

1.2. Current Treatment and Limitations

Treatment for glioblastoma is usually individualized, taking into consideration the characteristics of the tumour and the patient's response to various treatments. The primary approaches are surgery, radiotherapy, and chemotherapy, known as the Stupp protocol, which combines maximal safe surgical resection with radiotherapy and the chemotherapeutic agent temozolomide (TMZ).

TMZ, the only FDA-approved therapy for newly diagnosed GBM. Apart from this standard treatment, GBM is still challenging to treat due to the tumor's tendency to recur, its molecular heterogeneity, and low blood–brain barrier (BBB) permeability, which limits drug delivery. (Jia et al., 2023)

Second-line treatment in the cases of tumour progression includes bevacizumab and lomustine, a monoclonal antibody targeting vascular endothelial growth factor (VEGF), through the mechanism of blocking tumour angiogenesis. In addition, the second FDA-approved option for treatment of both newly diagnosed and recurrent

GBM is tumour-treating fields (TTF), an external, non-invasive modality which applies alternating electric fields to block cancer cell division, offering a complementary option to usual treatments (Guo et al., 2022).

While conventional treatments remain essential in managing glioblastoma, they often come with side effects that can significantly impact patients' quality of life.

1.3. Therapeutic Resistance Mechanisms in Glioblastoma

Even though advancements in the treatment have been made, glioblastoma usually manages to survive. The most challenging part of managing this form of cancer is that it becomes therapy resistant. There are a number of biological mechanisms that reduce treatment effectiveness, which may range from chemotherapy to radiation. Figure 1 illustrates the key mechanisms responsible for glioma cell survival and contribute to therapeutic resistance, while the following sections provide a detailed overview of these factors.

Figure 1. Overview of mechanisms contributing to glioma cell survival and therapeutic resistance. Abbreviations: GICs, glioma-initiating cells; MMR, mismatch repair; BBB, blood–brain barrier; HIF-1, hypoxia-inducible factor 1; ABC, ATP-binding cassette transporters.

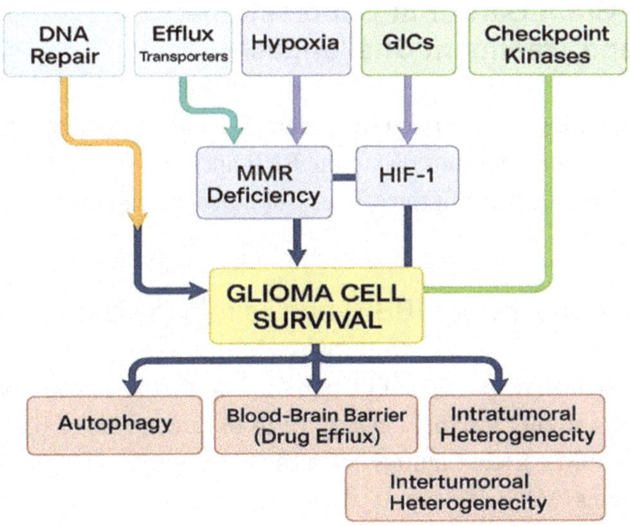

1.3.1. Mechanisms of Therapeutic Resistance in Glioblastoma

Glioblastoma resists therapy through several mechanisms:

- **DNA repair enzymes:** Temozolomide (TMZ) induces DNA damage, but many tumors express high levels of MGMT, which repairs this damage and drives resistance in most recurrent cases (Z. Yang et al., 2019).
- **Backup repair systems:** Even when MGMT is absent, defects in mismatch repair (MMR) allow tumor cells to tolerate TMZ-induced DNA lesions, sustaining growth (Erasimus et al., 2016).
- **Glioma-initiating cells (GICs):** These stem-like cells drive relapse and are highly resistant, partly due to overexpression of drug efflux pumps that expel chemotherapy agents (Dirkse et al., 2019)
- **Hypoxia and autophagy:** Low oxygen in the tumor microenvironment promotes survival pathways. Autophagy, a recycling process, helps cancer cells resist stress, but inhibition (e.g., chloroquine) may improve chemotherapy outcomes (Monteiro et al., 2017).

2. TREATMENT CHALLENGES

2.1. Blood–Brain Barrier in Glioblastoma: Structure and Treatment Challenges

A major limitation in effective GBM therapy is the restricted delivery of drugs to tumor and infiltrative regions due to the BBB and BBTB. This section addresses important challenges that limit the efficacy of current treatments for GBM (Jiawei Li et al., 2023).

2.1.1. Blood-Brain Barrier (BBB) and its role in glioblastoma therapy.

Though its selective permeability plays a major role in the control of CNS homeostasis, it presents the main challenge to the treatment of brain tumors like glioblastoma (GBM). Efflux pumps, such as P-glycoprotein (P-gp) and multidrug resistance proteins (MDRPs), export chemotherapy drugs out of the brain, reducing drug retention and significantly impairing the effectiveness of therapy (Minniti et al., 2005; Shala et al., 2023).

2.1.2. Blood–Brain Tumor Barrier (BBTB)

Closely associated with the BBB is the concept of the blood–brain tumor barrier (BBTB). Whereas the BBB defines the physiological barrier in healthy brain tissue, the BBTB is the disrupted barrier at the tumor edge. The BBTB, although more permeable in certain GBM areas, still prevents many therapeutic agents from reaching to tumor cells (Arvanitis et al., 2021).

2.2. Tissue Penetration and Tumor Heterogeneity

After crossing the BBB, drugs must diffuse through dense brain tissue where infiltrative GBM cells reside, often resulting in suboptimal concentrations. This challenge is intensified by the tumor's marked intertumoral and intratumoral heterogeneity, with genetically diverse subpopulations, cancer stem-like cells, and variable microenvironmental conditions affecting treatment response. These combined barriers highlight the need for advanced delivery systems, such as nanocarriers, which can improve tissue penetration and better address the biological diversity of GBM (Tzeng & Green, 2013).

3. NANOTECHNOLOGY IN GBM THERAPY

Glioblastoma multiforme presents a recalcitrant therapeutic challenge, largely because of the obstacle of providing effective therapy across the brain's protective barriers. Such a setting underlines the need for novel delivery systems, especially those capable of delivering into tumor cells without affecting normal tissue. Nanocarrier systems present a promising solution with the capacity to deliver site-specifically anticancer therapeutics, minimizing off-target toxicity, and evade biological barriers. Due to their nanoscale size and favorable surface features, such systems can transport therapeutic molecules across the BBB and accumulate in the tumor microenvironment (Laquintana et al., 2009).

For brain-targeted delivery, the success of nanocarriers depends significantly on molecular interactions between the surface-bound ligand and the overexpressed receptors in the target area of the disease. As shown by numerous studies, the optimal particle size is generally 100–300 nm, which improves penetration and retention in cerebral tissues. (H. Li et al., 2021).

The increased effectiveness of nanoparticle-based treatments often relies on their capacity to stabilize drugs, prevent premature degradation, enhance solubility and bioavailability.

Several classes of nanocarriers are under investigation for their potential to cross the BBB and enhance drug delivery across GBM. Some of these are lipid nanoparticles, polymeric nanoparticles, dendrimers, cyclodextrin complexes, magnetic nanoparticles, gold nanoparticles, quantum dots, and carbon nanotubes (Arduino et al., 2020). Figure 2 illustrates the main types of nanoparticle-based delivery systems currently investigated for glioblastoma treatment.

Figure 2. Schematic representation of nanodelivery systems that facilitate blood–brain barrier (BBB) penetration and enable target-specific drug action in glioma cells.

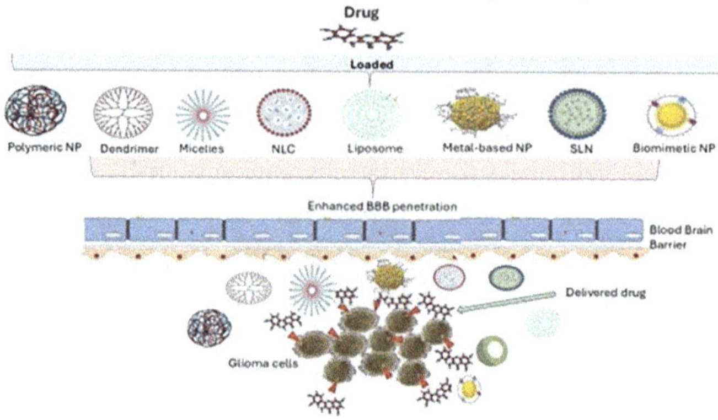

4. TRANSPORT MECHANISMS OF NANOCARRIERS ACROSS THE BLOOD–BRAIN BARRIER

Novel advances in nanomedicine have introduced nanocarriers, i.e., liposomes, micelles, polymeric nanoparticles, and biomimetic nanoparticles as promising tools for crossing the BBB (Ishihara et al., 2008).

Nanotechnology offers novel ways by which the BBB's restricted features can be bypassed or even modulated. Designed nanoparticles may be engineered to encapsulate or bind therapeutic molecules while facilitating transport across the BBB, further minimizing invasiveness and thus improving safety and patient compliance (Mittal et al., 2022).

By accurately adjusting the physicochemical properties of nanoparticles, i.e., size, shape, surface charge, and functional groups, enhanced cell uptake and penetration across the BBB can be facilitated. One approach includes surface decoration of nanocarriers with targeting ligands that bind to specific receptors on BBB endothelial cells (Asimakidou et al., 2024).

Apart from that, cationic nanoparticles can utilize electrostatic interactions between themselves and the negatively charged surface of endothelial cells to acquire adsorptive-mediated transcytosis (AMT) (Ahlawat et al., 2020).

Nanocarriers can pass the BBB through several well-defined pathways, such as (Puris et al., 2022):

- Paracellular transport across tight junctions (restricted in most drugs)
- Passive transcellular diffusion (predominantly for lipophilic small molecules)
- Carrier-mediated transport (CMT) for essential nutrients
- Receptor-mediated transcytosis (RMT), facilitated through receptor-ligand interactions
- Adsorptive-mediated transcytosis (AMT) due to surface charge interactions
- Cell-mediated transport, where immune or stem cells transport nanoparticles across the barrier

All these mechanisms provide a multi-faceted approach for designing the next-generation drug delivery systems that can overcome the biological barriers to successful GBM therapy.

5. NANOCARRIER-BASED THERAPEUTIC STRATEGIES IN GLIOBLASTOMA

5.1. Polymeric Nanoparticles

Polymeric nanoparticles are submicron-sized drug carriers constructed from biodegradable and biocompatible polymers and have been widely studied due to their potential in targeted anticancer therapy, particularly for the treatment of glioblastoma.

They can encapsulate drugs within their matrix or adsorb on their surface, allowing versatility in drug delivery design. The preferred polymers for brain application are poly(lactic acid) (PLA), poly(ε-caprolactone) (PCL), poly(butyl cyanoacrylate) (PBCA), poly(glycolic acid) (PGA), poly(lactic-co-glycolic acid) (PLGA), and poly(amino acids) because they degrade to lactic and glycolic acid—metabolites which are physiologically excreted through the Krebs cycle as carbon dioxide and water (S. Liu et al., 2024).

These nanosystems exhibit several advantages, including controlled drug release, active drug stability against enzymatic hydrolysis, structural stability, and surface susceptibility to functionalization.

Anticancer agents as paclitaxel (PTX), which acts by interrupting microtubule dynamics, and etoposide (ETP)—a topoisomerase II inhibitor, are hampered by low solubility, poor BBB permeability, and high systemic toxicity. To overcome these limitations, Maleki et al. in 2019 designed dual-drug-loaded mPEG-PLGA nanoparticles. Formulated through nanoprecipitation, the nanoparticles had diameters less than 150 nm and exhibited excellent drug encapsulation efficiencies (92.5% for PTX and 86.2% for ETP). The system facilitated controlled release of the drug for six days, thereby enhancing the therapeutic potential (Maleki et al., 2019).

Similarly, PTX-loaded PLGA nanoparticles (~216 nm) were evaluated for brain-targeted delivery via both intranasal and intravenous routes (Abdel-haq et al., 2023).

Bevacizumab, a VEGF-targeting monoclonal antibody approved for the treatment of recurrent GBM, faces challenges in BBB permeation, thus requiring a higher systemic dose that can lead to off-target risk effects. This challenge has been addressed by Sousa et al., in 2019 through the preparation of bevacizumab-loaded PLGA nanoparticles for intranasal administration in animal studies, which showed increased anti-angiogenic activity (Sousa et al., 2019).

Polymer nanoparticles have also shown promising results in gene delivery. Poly(β-amino ester) (PBAE) nanoparticles encapsulating non-viral DNA targeted BTICs—the subpopulation believed responsible for tumor relapse and drug resistance. With BTIC-derived oncospheres from patient-derived samples, researchers have been able to attain up to 76% transfection efficiency while maintaining cell viability. These nanoparticles preferentially targeted BTICs over neural progenitor cells and remained effective after extended storage at –20 °C (Guerrero-Cázares et al., 2014).

Recently, polymeric nanoparticles have also been used in photothermal therapy (PTT), a less invasive treatment based on near-infrared (NIR) light-induced hyperthermia (Bastiancich et al., 2021). One example is diketopyrrolopyrrole (DPP), a photostable NIR-absorbing molecule. Li et al. prepared DPP-loaded polymeric nanoparticles from a conjugated polymer (PBDPP) functionalized with DSPE-PEG. These particles showed high photothermal conversion and strong anti-glioma effects in vitro and in vivo, reflecting their promise as a dual-modal theranostic platform for GBM therapy (S. Li et al., 2019).

Besides therapy, polymeric nanoparticles are also explored as diagnostic tools. Bernal et al. in their study synthesized magnetite-based polymeric nanoparticles (PMNPs) for convection-enhanced delivery (CED) of temozolomide (TMZ) with imaging capability through magnetic resonance. While drug delivery was limited, the results showed that future modification through targeting ligands could significantly enhance therapeutic outcomes. More importantly, this work addresses the promise of polymeric NPs as not just drug carriers, but also image-guided therapy platforms for glioma treatment (Bernal et al., 2014).

5.2. Dendrimers

Dendrimers are synthetic, tree-like branched polymers with a defined and uniform architecture, consisting of a central core, repetitive internal layers (generations), and multiple terminal functional groups. Their unique structure allows precise control over size, surface functionality, and molecular weight, making them attractive candidates for drug delivery, imaging, and theranostic applications in glioma therapy.

These macromolecules may be designed to release hydrophobic and hydrophilic drugs either by encapsulation within their cavities or through surface conjugation. In glioblastoma, dendrimers have been used as carriers to deliver traditional chemotherapeutic agents like doxorubicin, cisplatin, rapamycin, and temozolomide. These nanocarriers help in solubilization, stabilization of the drug against degradation, extended circulation, and drug retention within the tumor (A. K. Sharma et al., 2018).

In addition to small-molecule drugs, dendrimers demonstrated strong potential as vehicles for gene delivery. Their capacity for nucleic acid compacting and protecting, including siRNA, plasmid DNA, and microRNA, has made them effective non-viral vectors for gene delivery. PAMAM dendrimers loaded with plasmids carrying tumor-suppressing genes such as interferon-beta or microRNA-7, have been reported to have high transfection efficiency and specific gene silencing in glioma models with less tumor growth and improved survival (Gaballu et al., 2017).

Dendrimers have also been explored for imaging applications. Their geometric structure may be precisely defined, allowing their conjugation with contrast agents. Therefore, they are suitable for MRI, PET, and optical imaging (Longmire et al., 2014).

Another recent application of dendrimer technology for glioma treatment is targeting the tumor microenvironment, particularly tumor-associated macrophages (TAMs). These immune cells, normally hijacked by glioma to support tumor growth and inhibit the immune response, are selectively targetable by ligand-functionalized dendrimers. It has been reported that glucose-grafted PAMAM dendrimers increase uptake by TAMs and microglia, leading to increased drug concentration within tumor tissue and improved therapeutic efficacy (R. Sharma et al., 2021).

Although very versatile and promising, dendrimer-based glioma therapy is at the preclinical stage. Issues of optimal generation size achievement, surface modification optimization, ensuring reproducible synthesis, and long-term safety determination need to be resolved before clinical translation is feasible.

5.3. Micelles

Polymeric micelles are spherical nanoscale aggregates produced by amphiphilic block copolymer self-assembly in aqueous media. They have the core–shell structure of having a hydrophobic core and hydrophilic shell, and they are particularly suitable for encapsulation and delivery of diverse therapeutic agents such as small-molecule drugs, nucleic acids, proteins, and monoclonal antibodies (Prencipe et al., 2021).

Micelles can be functionalized to enhance the sensitivity and specificity of drug release towards targets. The most common targeting mechanism utilized in glioblastoma treatment is the utilization of overexpressed integrins αvβ3 and αvβ5 on glioblastoma endothelial cells. One such ligand that has been used to target micelles towards GBM vasculature and cancer cells is cyclic Arg-Gly-Asp (cRGD) peptide (Quader et al., 2017).

To address the particular challenge of the glioblastoma microenvironment, various stimulus-responsive micellar designs have been developed. These designs are intended to provide controlled drug release upon the application of internal or external stimuli (Jiao et al., 2019).

Targeting strategies have also been explored, taking advantage of the dual expression of certain receptors on the BBB and glioblastoma cells, presenting the potential for synchronized transport through the BBB and accumulation within the tumor (Do et al., 2016).

Together, these advancements highlight the versatility and potential of micellar systems for overcoming the physiological and pharmacological barriers to glioblastoma treatment. Polymeric micelles are being established as valuable tools for site-specific, responsive, and effective drug delivery to brain tumors and multi-scale targeting.

5.4. Lipid Nanoparticles

Lipid-based nanocarriers, including liposomes, solid lipid nanoparticles (SLNs), and nanostructured lipid carriers (NLCs), have shown considerable potential in oncology. Their major advantages include high biocompatibility and biodegradability, the ability to deliver both hydrophilic and lipophilic drugs, controlled release of drugs, and sustained drug release. Moreover, their formulation methods are easily scalable for clinical translation (Blasi et al., 2011).

To enhance therapeutic effects and to limit off-target ones, lipid nanoparticles can be targeted using ligands. In GBM, lipid nanocarriers are made to cross the BBB by employing ligands that utilize endogenous transport mechanisms, thereby facilitating targeted delivery of the drug into the brain tumor microenvironment (Tosi et al., 2016).

5.4.1. Lipid Nanoparticles: SLNs and NLCs in Drug Delivery

Solid lipid nanoparticles (SLNs) are colloidal carriers made up of physiological lipids that remain a solid state at body temperature. With particle sizes ranging between 50 and 1000 nanometers, SLNs provide numerous advantages such as high physical and chemical stability and good biocompatibility (Sommonte et al., 2024).

To overcome these limitations, the NLCs were designed by blending the solid lipids with a proportion of liquid lipids, which disrupts the crystalline structure, creating the amorphous matrix capable of accommodating greater drug payloads and limiting expulsion of drugs during storage.

Qu et al. compared the efficacy of temozolomide (TMZ)-loaded polymeric nanoparticles (PNPs), SLNs, and NLCs in the therapy of GBM. All three nanoparticle systems had diameters ranging from 90 to 125 nm, with efficiencies of drug entrapment >80%. In vivo studies on mice implanted with U87 tumors showed that TMZ-NLCs have yielded the highest tumor regression, with inhibition levels of 85%, while TMZ-SLNs had 59%, TMZ-PNPs 45%, and free TMZ 27%. These results have highlighted NLCs as the most promising formulation for effective GBM treatment (Qu et al., 2016).

Later on, Kadari et al. formulated docetaxel-loaded SLNs functionalized with angiopep-2 to enhance brain delivery. In vivo studies in mice bearing GL261 glioma cells demonstrated that docetaxel-SLNs improved drug bioavailability without evident toxicity or notable weight fluctuations (Kadari et al., 2018). While recently, Wang et al. employed SLNs to deliver a TMZ-resistant GBM prodrug, CAT3. When administered, the SLN formulation facilitated effective bioconversion of the prodrug to its active state in vivo, leading to the possibility of SLNs potential to enhance prodrug efficacy against resistant gliomas (H. Wang et al., 2020).

While in animal models, efficacy of targeted delivery systems has been evaluated using extensive research in NLCs for glioblastoma therapy. Song et al. investigated TMZ-loaded NLCs that were functionalized with the arginine-glycine-aspartic acid (RGD) peptide, known for its affinity to integrins highly expressed on glioblastoma cells and tumor-associated endothelium. When injected into BALB/c nude mice with U87MG-derived tumors, these RGD-modified NLCs led to more than 80% decline in tumor volume, which was a threefold improvement compared to traditional TMZ treatment (Song et al., 2016).

5.4.2. Liposomes

Among the suitable nanocarrier systems for brain tumors, liposomes present one of the most promising options. These nanoscale vesicles consist of one or more phospholipid bilayers surrounding an aqueous core, allowing them to encapsulate water-soluble and lipid-soluble therapeutic agents (Fondaj et al., 2023)

What makes liposomes unique in glioma therapy is their versatility. Besides the fact, they can deliver a wide variety of drug molecules, they also protect them from enzymatic hydrolysis and enable sustained delivery at the site of action. Their surfaces can be modified with a wide array of ligands, such as transferin, folic acid, RGD peptides, or even dual-targeting moieties that bind specifically to receptors overexpressed on the BBB or glioma cells. These modifications enhance the ability of liposomes to pass through BBB and increase the concentration within the tumor tissue, which presents a significant limitation in traditional glioma chemotherapy (Arduino et al., 2024).

The process by which liposomes pass through the BBB may be active and passive transport. Cationic liposomes, for instance, electrostatically interact with negatively charged endothelial cells of the BBB, facilitating their internalization through non-specific endocytosis. Furthermore, receptor-mediated endocytosis has been widely used by incorporating a ligand that interacts with a specific BBB transporter into liposomes, resulting in more targeted and efficient delivery (Agrawal et al., 2017).

Promising outcomes have been reported in preclinical research studies on liposomal formulations designed specifically for the treatment of glioma. One of these is a transferrin-conjugated liposome doubly loaded with cabazitaxel and elemene, which showed strong tumor-targeting in glioma-bearing mice, resulting in significant survival improvements (Jie Li et al., 2021).

Benefits of the targeted delivery were also demonstrated in the experiment of functionalized liposomes with cyclic RGD peptide, improving drug permeation across the BBB and enhancing drug uptake by glioma cells for drugs such as procaine (D. Li et al., 2021). More sophisticated systems have incorporated mixtures of ligands or responsive elements into the liposome structure. For example, T7 and DA7R peptide-loaded double-modified liposomes were employed for co-delivery of doxorubicin and vincristine, achieving increased tumor cell killing activity compared to free drugs (Zhang et al., 2017). Redox and pH-sensitive liposomes have also been designed to release the payload selectively in the acidic and redox environment of the tumor to achieve higher drug concentration in the tumor site and decrease systemic toxicity (Pacheco-Torres et al., 2015).

Although they have numerous advantages, liposomal systems have some limitations. Rapid clearance by the mononuclear phagocyte system, decreased drug loading capacity, while disruption of receptor-mediated interactions at the BBB may limit their therapeutic potential. In order to address these limitations, researchers have explored the possibility of including synthetic phospholipids for formulation stability improvement, replacing natural cholesterol with safer analogs, and integrating "smart release" mechanisms that can be stimulated by tumor-specific triggers (Vieira & Gamarra, 2016).

Overall, liposomes have shown promising results in preclinical studies as a nanocarrier in glioma therapy. Their capacity to deliver various therapeutic agents, pass through the BBB, and selectively target tumor cells makes them a cornerstone of current nanomedicine research. Although further research on their optimization is needed for broader clinical application, recent studies suggest that liposomal systems could play a major role in future approaches for glioma treatment.

5.5. Metal-Based Nanoparticles

Among the novel approaches that have been explored for the treatment of glioblastoma, metal nanoparticles (NPs) have drawn significant attention due to their multimodal character and the possibility to overcome important therapeutic challenges. Biological and non-biological metallic nanoarchitectures such as gold (AuNPs), silver (AgNPs), iron oxide nanoparticles, and quantum dots are being studied for their capacity to cross the blood–brain barrier (BBB) and target sites of tumors (Amina & Guo, 2020).

Gold nanoparticles are among the most investigated due to their acceptable safety profile, favorable stability, and biocompatibility. Their size and shape can be controlled, while their diversity in configurations, such as nanospheres, rods, stars, and cubes, offers distinct pharmacokinetic profiles. In a very promising investigation, an intranasal formulation of gold nanoparticles containing the drug temozolomide (TMZ) and an anti-EphA3 functionalizing antibody (targeting ephrin type-A receptor 3) was used to bypass the BBB completely. The route of administration not only decreased systemic toxicity but also enhanced accumulation at the tumor site. The nanoparticles, which were under 50 nm in size, exhibited increased uptake in glioma cells and improved in vitro cytotoxicity, with an IC50 approximately 18 times lower than that of free TMZ. Additionally, the formulation decreased MGMT expression, the primary mediator of TMZ resistance, and improved survival in GBM animal models (L. Wang et al., 2021).

Silver nanomaterials are another group of metal nanomaterials that are investigated, predominantly for their chemical and biological properties. In glioma animal models, the effect of AgNPs was explored by investigating the impact of AgNPs combined with a single fraction of radiotherapy. This combination therapy resulted in an extended survival rate compared to monotherapies and controls. The groups that were treated with a combination of AgNPs and radiation showed over 500% increases in median survival, with cure rates exceeding 40%. What is important to note is that these results were achieved without causing significant toxicity, indicating a synergistic therapeutic effect (Haque et al., 2021).

Iron oxide nanoparticles studies are also advancing in oncology, mainly through their application in magnetic hyperthermia—a treatment method in which heat caused locally by an external alternating magnetic field kills tumor cells. The treatment is approved clinically within Europe as an adjuvant therapy for recurrent glioblastoma.

Although these metal nanoparticles provide unique benefits, such as controlled drug release and imaging capabilities, their safety profiles must be carefully considered. While numerous formulations have shown promising results in preclinical investigations and several have entered the clinical trials level, crucial challenges that need to be addressed are still present (Gawel et al., 2022).

5.6. Biomimetic Nanoparticles

Biomimetic nanoparticles represent a novel generation of nanotherapeutics that can mimic essential biological characteristics of cells to enhance drug targeting, delivery, and immune evasion for the treatment of glioblastoma (Arduino et al., 2024).

One of the most promising biomimetic nanotechnology approaches is M@HLPC, a hybrid nanoparticle with a lipid–polymer core coated with chlorin e6 and lactate oxidase and covered by glioblastoma cell membranes. This covering allows for the particles to cross the BBB and identify cancer cells. A patient-derived derivative (hM@HLPC), which contains patient tumor membrane, showed efficient tumor targeting and therapeutic activity in animal models (Lu et al., 2022).

Additional research has been made supporting this strategy based on biomimetic delivery platforms, including tumor-membrane-coated nanoparticles, RBC-mimetic particles designed to maintain circulation over weeks, and immune cell-derived carriers (e.g., macrophage or neutrophil membranes) that utilize inflammation-targeting mechanisms (Arduino et al., 2024; Sommonte et al., 2024).

The other promising approach is based on extracellular vesicles (EVs) and exosomes as endogenous nanocarriers. Targeted exosomes, usually surface-functionalized with targeting ligands such as Angiopep-2 or transferrin, have shown BBB penetration and delivery of siRNAs or chemotherapeutics into glioma cells (M. Wang et al., 2021).

Besides the promising results, biomimetic systems face several limitations. These include large-scale production, batch reproducibility, long-term safety, and regulatory frameworks needed for their further development in clinical development. Their multifunctionality, patient-specific optimization, and capacity to penetrate physiological barriers make them a powerful approach to next-generation glioblastoma nanomedicine (Y. Yang et al., 2023).

Table 1 provides a comparative overview of some of the most promising nanocarrier systems under investigation for glioblastoma therapy.

Table 1. Summary of nanocarrier systems investigated for glioblastoma therapy and their key outcomes.

Nanoparticles	Key Findings	References
Polymeric Nanoparticles	Enable controlled release, protect drugs from degradation, support gene delivery and imaging; shown to improve survival and drug targeting in preclinical models.	Maleki et al., 2019; Guerrero-Cázares et al., 2014; Abdel-haq et al., 2023; Li et al., 2019; Bernal et al., 2014
Dendrimers	Precisely engineered carriers for drugs and genes; demonstrated BBB crossing, tumor targeting, immune modulation, and dual imaging in glioma models.	Gaballu et al., 2017; Sharma et al., 2021
Micelles	Stimuli-responsive and ligand-targeted systems effective in drug delivery, dual therapy (PTT/PDT), and tumor-selective accumulation; used for overcoming drug resistance and BBB penetration.	Quader et al., 2017; Liu et al., 2020; Jiao et al., 2019;
Solid Lipid Nanoparticles (SLNs)	Provide high stability and biocompatibility; shown to improve brain delivery and therapeutic effect of drugs like docetaxel and RSV in GBM models.	Kadari et al., 2018; ; Wang et al., 2020
Nanostructured Lipid Carriers (NLCs)	Offer higher drug loading capacity and better in vivo tumor inhibition than SLNs and PNPs; suitable for functionalization and nasal delivery.	Qu et al., 2016; Song et al., 2016;
Liposomes	Versatile and biocompatible carriers, modifiable for targeted delivery (e.g., TfR, RGD); effective in reducing tumor size and enhancing BBB crossing in GBM models.	Gan et al., 2024; Li et al., 2021;
Gold Nanoparticles	Functionalized AuNPs enhance cytotoxicity, reduce chemoresistance, and extend survival; shown effective with intranasal delivery bypassing BBB.	Wang et al., 2021
Silver Nanoparticles	AgNPs combined with radiation significantly improved survival; shown to induce apoptosis and disrupt glioma cell cycle without major toxicity.	Haque et al., 2021
Iron Oxide Nanoparticles	Used in magnetic hyperthermia for GBM treatment; clinically approved in EU; shown to ablate tumor with minimal systemic toxicity.	Maier-Hauff et al., 2011; Martinkova et al., 2018
Biomimetic Nanoparticles	Membrane-coated or biologically inspired systems that enable homotypic targeting, immune evasion, and BBB penetration; demonstrated enhanced tumor accumulation and photodynamic effects in preclinical GBM models.	Zhao et al., 2022; Ahmed et al., 2025; Li et al., 2024; Wu et al., 2023

6. COMPARATIVE PERFORMANCE OF NANOCARRIER SYSTEMS

Although multiple classes of nanocarriers demonstrate encouraging preclinical activity, their performance varies substantially when comparing stability, BBB penetration mechanisms, tumor selectivity, and translational feasibility. Polymeric nanoparticles offer excellent versatility and controlled release profiles, but their performance is strongly dependent on polymer composition, degradation rate, and surface modification; they often require ligand functionalization to achieve adequate BBB transport (Maleki et al., 2019). Liposomes, in contrast, remain the most clinically validated platform because of their biocompatibility and scalable manufacturing, yet they face rapid clearance by the mononuclear phagocyte system and demonstrate limited penetration into infiltrative tumor borders unless decorated with BBB-targeting ligands such as transferrin or RGD peptides (Jie Li et al., 2021). Dendrimers provide unmatched structural precision and multivalent surface chemistry that enable high drug-loading and efficient siRNA/gene delivery, but their clinical translation is slowed by cytotoxicity concerns associated with cationic surface groups and the complexity of reproducible large-scale synthesis (Gaballu et al., 2017). Micelles excel in solubilizing hydrophobic therapeutics and allow stimulus-responsive release, but they may dissociate in circulation, reducing drug availability at the tumor site unless crosslinking strategies are employed (Quader et al., 2017). Lipid nanoparticles (SLNs and NLCs) demonstrate strong stability, compatibility with both hydrophilic and lipophilic drugs, and high payload capacity; however, crystallization phenomena in SLNs may expel drugs during storage, whereas NLCs offer better long-term stability but still face challenges in penetrating intact BBB regions (Qu et al., 2016). Metal-based nanoparticles, including gold and iron oxide systems, provide theranostic capabilities such as imaging and hyperthermia, yet concerns over biodegradability and long-term accumulation limit their acceptability for human use (L. Wang et al., 2021). Lastly, biomimetic nanoparticles coated with tumor-cell membranes or immune-cell membranes, offer superior immune evasion and homotypic targeting; however, their clinical translation is hindered by challenges in large-scale production, reproducibility, and regulatory standardization (Lu et al., 2022).

Taken together, no single nanocarrier system is universally superior; rather, each platform addresses different aspects of the delivery problem, highlighting the need for hybrid and multifunctional approaches capable of crossing the BBB, penetrating the tumor microenvironment, and overcoming the profound molecular heterogeneity of GBM.

7. CLINICAL TRANSLATION OF NANOFORMULATIONS FOR GLIOBLASTOMA: PROGRESS AND CHALLENGES

Besides the achieved progress in the development of nanoparticle drug delivery systems, clinical translation for GBM treatment remains limited. Among the several nanoformulations that have been explored, liposomal carriers, particularly PEGylated liposomes, are in the most advanced phase for clinical evaluation.

A number of Phase I and II trials have also evaluated PEGylated liposomal doxorubicin (PLD, commercially known as Caelyx) in recurrent high-grade glioma patients. Single-agent Caelyx has caused disease stabilization, without complete or partial response. Combination therapies with temozolomide (TMZ) were investigated but did not statistically provide significant benefits over TMZ alone, leading to termination in some cases. Other trials have investigated combinations with tamoxifen or other scheduling regimens, resulting in modest improvements in progression-free survival (PFS), but limited results in the overall survival rates (OS).

More recently, nanoliposomal irinotecan (nal-IRI) was tested in GBM, including combinations with TMZ. However, minimal therapeutic benefit was observed, and one trial was discontinued. A novel combination of liposomal curcumin and TMZ is currently under investigation, with trial completion anticipated in 2027.

These clinical trials indicate the potential and challenges of translating nanoparticle drug delivery systems into effective therapies. Liposomes are more advanced in clinical trials, but other nanoparticle platforms like chitosan, adeno-associated viruses (AAV), and neutrophil-based carriers are still in preclinical development. Translational progress has been limited by safety concerns, ineffective targeting, expensive production, and lack of consistency between animal models and human outcomes. However, developments with surface ligand and peptide modification may address these challenges and increase clinical relevance in the near future. A summary of nanoformulations that have entered clinical trials for glioblastoma therapy is presented in Table 2.

Table 2. Summary of clinical trials involving nanoformulations in GBM treatment.

Formulation	Clinical Phase	Key Notes	Trial Identifier
PEGylated liposomal doxorubicin (Caelyx)	Phase II	Showed disease stabilization in recurrent high-grade glioma (HGG), but no complete or partial responses.	(Fabel et al., 2001)
Caelyx + Temozolomide (TMZ)	Phase II	Some disease stabilization was observed; however, no statistically significant benefits over TMZ alone. The trial was terminated due to a low objective response rate.	(Chua et al., 2004)
PEG-DOX with or without Tamoxifen	Phase II	Some long-term progression-free survival in Grade III glioma; no significant improvement in overall survival	(Hau et al., 2004)
PEG-DOX + TMZ	Phase I/II	Compared with a control group (EORTC/NCI-C); Completed 2002–2009; well-tolerated, no OS/PFS benefit	(Beier et al., 2009)
Nanoliposomal irinotecan (nal-IRI)	Phase I	Tested alone and with TMZ. Minimal activity observed; one trial terminated during interim analysis.Completed 2008–2015; safe, but no clear efficacy signal	(Sun et al., 2025)
Liposomal curcumin + TMZ	Phase I/II (Ongoing)	This combination is currently recruiting participants and is expected to be completed in 2027.	(Holdhoff et al., 2025)
2B3-101 (glutathione-PEG DOX)	Phase I/IIa	Studied recurrent glioma and brain metastases	(Brendsma et al., 2014)
NKTR-102 (etirinotecan pegol)	Phase II	Investigated in high-grade glioma	(Nagpal et al., 2014)

8. CONCLUSIONS AND FUTURE PERSPECTIVES

Glioblastoma (GBM) remains one of the most challenging and lethal brain tumors with a high invasiveness, intense intratumoral heterogeneity, and resistance to conventional therapies. Despite the availability of surgical resection, radiotherapy, and chemotherapy, especially notably with temozolomide, long-term survival is still limited, with median survival being frequently below 15 months. These constraints have driven intensive research into new therapeutic strategies, among which nanotechnology-based treatments have shown very promising results.

Preclinical studies of nanomaterials such as liposomes, polymeric micelles, dendrimers, lipid nanoparticles, and biomimetic nanoparticles have shown strong potential in increasing drug solubility, prolonging systemic circulation half-lives, and achieving more targeted tumor targeting.

Transitioning into clinical research has revealed several challenges that need to be addressed. Only a limited number of nanoformulations, led by liposomal doxorubicin and liposomal irinotecan, have entered clinical trials for GBM. While generally well tolerated, these trials have yielded modest outcomes in terms of progression-free and overall survival results.

In conclusion, nanotechnology has yet to transform glioblastoma treatment; nevertheless, it has laid a strong platform for novel, targeted therapies that can overcome the limitations of current standard treatments. Ongoing investigation and clinical translation of nanomedicines driven by biological complexity and patient specificity will open new insights for GBM management.Top of FormBottom of Form

REFERENCES

Abdel-haq, M., Kumar, A., Mohand, F. A., Kravchenko-balasha, N., Rottenberg, Y., & Domb, A. J. (2023). Paclitaxel Delivery to the Brain for Glioblastoma Treatment. *International Journal of Pharmaceutical Sciences*, 1–14.

Agrawal, M., Ajazuddin, , Tripathi, D. K., Saraf, S., Saraf, S., Antimisiaris, S. G., Mourtas, S., Hammarlund-Udenaes, M., & Alexander, A. (2017). Recent advancements in liposomes targeting strategies to cross blood-brain barrier (BBB) for the treatment of Alzheimer's disease. *Journal of Controlled Release, 260*(April), 61–77. DOI: 10.1016/j.jconrel.2017.05.019 PMID: 28549949

Ahlawat, J., Barroso, G., Narayan, M., Alvarado, M., Armendariz, I., Bernal, J., Carabaza, X., Chavez, S., Cruz, P., Escalante, V., Estorga, S., Fernandez, D., Lozano, C., Marrufo, M., Ahmad, N., Negrete, S., Olvera, K., Parada, X., Portillo, B., & Viel, S. (2020). Nanocarriers as Potential Drug Delivery Candidates for Overcoming the Blood-Brain Barrier: Challenges and Possibilities. *ACS Omega, 5*(22), 12583–12595. DOI: 10.1021/acsomega.0c01592 PMID: 32548442

Amina, S. J., & Guo, B. (2020). A review on the synthesis and functionalization of gold nanoparticles as a drug delivery vehicle. *International Journal of Nanomedicine, 15*, 9823–9857. DOI: 10.2147/IJN.S279094 PMID: 33324054

Arduino, I., Depalo, N., Re, F., Dal Magro, R., Panniello, A., Margiotta, N., Fanizza, E., Lopalco, A., Laquintana, V., Cutrignelli, A., Lopedota, A. A., Franco, M., & Denora, N. (2020). PEGylated solid lipid nanoparticles for brain delivery of lipophilic kiteplatin Pt(IV) prodrugs: An in vitro study. *International Journal of Pharmaceutics, 583*(January), 119351. DOI: 10.1016/j.ijpharm.2020.119351 PMID: 32339634

Arduino, I., Di Fonte, R., Sommonte, F., Lopedota, A. A., Porcelli, L., Li, J., Serrati, S., Bártolo, R., Santos, H. A., Iacobazzi, R. M., Azzariti, A., & Denora, N. (2024). Fabrication of Biomimetic Hybrid Liposomes via Microfluidic Technology: Homotypic Targeting and Antitumor Efficacy Studies in Glioma Cells. *International Journal of Nanomedicine, 19*, 13217–13233. DOI: 10.2147/IJN.S489872 PMID: 39679250

Arduino, I., Di Fonte, R., Tiboni, M., Porcelli, L., Serratì, S., Fondaj, D., Rafaschieri, T., Cutrignelli, A., Guida, G., Casettari, L., Azzariti, A., Lopedota, A. A., Denora, N., & Iacobazzi, R. M. (2024). Microfluidic development and biological evaluation of targeted therapy-loaded biomimetic nano system to improve the metastatic melanoma treatment. *International Journal of Pharmaceutics, 650*(December 2023), 123697. DOI: 10.1016/j.ijpharm.2023.123697

Arvanitis, C. D., Ferraro, G. B., Jain, R. K., Laboratories, L. S., & General, M. (2021). The blood–brain barrier and blood–tumour barrier in brain tumours and metastases. *Nature Reviews. Cancer*, *20*(1), 26–41. DOI: 10.1038/s41568-019-0205-x PMID: 31601988

Asimakidou, E., Tan, J. K. S., Zeng, J., & Lo, C. H. (2024). Blood–Brain Barrier-Targeting Nanoparticles: Biomaterial Properties and Biomedical Applications in Translational Neuroscience. *Pharmaceuticals (Basel, Switzerland)*, *17*(5), 612. Advance online publication. DOI: 10.3390/ph17050612 PMID: 38794182

Bastiancich, C., Da Silva, A., & Estève, M. A. (2021). Photothermal Therapy for the Treatment of Glioblastoma: Potential and Preclinical Challenges. *Frontiers in Oncology*, *10*(January), 1–16. DOI: 10.3389/fonc.2020.610356 PMID: 33520720

Beier, C. P., Schmid, C., Gorlia, T., Kleinletzenberger, C., Beier, D., Grauer, O., Steinbrecher, A., Hirschmann, B., Brawanski, A., Dietmaier, C., Jauch-Worley, T., Kölbl, O., Pietsch, T., Proescholdt, M., Rümmele, P., Muigg, A., Stockhammer, G., Hegi, M., Bogdahn, U., & Hau, P. (2009). RNOP-09: Pegylated liposomal doxorubicine and prolonged temozolomide in addition to radiotherapy in newly diagnosed glioblastoma - A phase II study. *BMC Cancer*, *9*(1), 308. DOI: 10.1186/1471-2407-9-308 PMID: 19725960

Bernal, G. M., LaRiviere, M. J., Mansour, N., Pytel, P., Cahill, K. E., Voce, D. J., Kang, S., Spretz, R., Welp, U., Noriega, S. E., Nuñez, L., Larsen, G., Weichselbaum, R. R., & Yamini, B. (2014). Convection-enhanced delivery and in vivo imaging of polymeric nanoparticles for the treatment of malignant glioma. *Nanomedicine; Nanotechnology, Biology, and Medicine*, *10*(1), 149–157. DOI: 10.1016/j.nano.2013.07.003 PMID: 23891990

Blasi, P., Giovagnoli, S., Schoubben, A., Puglia, C., Bonina, F., Rossi, C., & Ricci, M. (2011). Lipid nanoparticles for brain targeting I. Formulation optimization. *International Journal of Pharmaceutics*, *419*(1–2), 287–295. DOI: 10.1016/j.ijpharm.2011.07.035 PMID: 21827844

Brendsma, D., Krtolica, A., Le Moan, N., Getz, J., Davis, T., Ng, S., Bedard, C., Davis, A., Leung, P., Serwer, L., Tanaka, K., Keating, T., Yan, F., Winger, J., & Cary, S. (2014). GLUTATHIONE PEGYLATED LIPOSOMAL DOXORUBICIN, IN PATIENTS WITH RECURRENT HIGH GRADE GLIOMAS AND BREAST CANCER BRAIN METASTASES. *Neuro-Oncology*, *16*(suppl 2), 2014. DOI: 10.1093/neuonc/nou174.191

Chua, S. L., Rosenthal, M. A., Wong, S. S., Ashley, D. M., Woods, A. M., Dowling, A., & Cher, L. M. (2004). Phase 2 study of temozolomide and Caelyx in patients with recurrent glioblastoma multiforme. *Neuro-Oncology*, *6*(1), 38–43. DOI: 10.1215/S1152851703000188 PMID: 14769139

Dirkse, A., Golebiewska, A., Buder, T., Nazarov, P. V., Muller, A., Poovathingal, S., Brons, N. H. C., Leite, S., Sauvageot, N., Sarkisjan, D., Seyfrid, M., Fritah, S., Stieber, D., Michelucci, A., Hertel, F., Herold-Mende, C., Azuaje, F., Skupin, A., Bjerkvig, R., & Niclou, S. P. (2019). Stem cell-associated heterogeneity in Glioblastoma results from intrinsic tumor plasticity shaped by the microenvironment. *Nature Communications*, *10*(1), 1–16. DOI: 10.1038/s41467-019-09853-z PMID: 30992437

Do, H. T., Bruelle, C., Pham, D. D., Jauhiainen, M., Eriksson, O., Korhonen, L. T., & Lindholm, D. (2016). Nerve growth factor (NGF) and pro-NGF increase low-density lipoprotein (LDL) receptors in neuronal cells partly by different mechanisms: Role of LDL in neurite outgrowth. *Journal of Neurochemistry*, *136*(2), 306–315. DOI: 10.1111/jnc.13397 PMID: 26484803

Erasimus, H., Gobin, M., Niclou, S., & Van Dyck, E. (2016). DNA repair mechanisms and their clinical impact in glioblastoma. *Mutation Research/Reviews in Mutation Research*, *769*, 19–35. DOI: 10.1016/j.mrrev.2016.05.005 PMID: 27543314

Fabel, K., Dietrich, J., Hau, P., Wismeth, C., Winner, B., Przywara, S., Steinbrecher, A., Ullrich, W., & Bogdahn, U. (2001). Long-term stabilization in patients with malignant glioma after treatment with liposomal doxorubicin. *Cancer*, *92*(7), 1936–1942. DOI: 10.1002/1097-0142(20011001)92:7<1936::AID-CNCR1712>3.0.CO;2-H PMID: 11745268

Fondaj, D., Arduino, I., Lopedota, A. A., Denora, N., & Iacobazzi, R. M. (2023). Exploring the Microfluidic Production of Biomimetic Hybrid Nanoparticles and Their Pharmaceutical Applications. *Pharmaceutics*, *15*(7), 1953. Advance online publication. DOI: 10.3390/pharmaceutics15071953 PMID: 37514139

Gaballu, F. A., Dehghan, G., Ghaffaria, M., Yekta, R., Abbaspour-Ravasjanid, S., Baradarana, B., Ezzati, J., Dolatabadie, N., & Hamblinf, M. R. (2017). PAMAM dendrimers as efficient drug and gene delivery nanosystems for cancer therapy. *Applied Materials Today*, *176*(3), 139–148. DOI: 10.1002/hep.30150.Ductular

Gan, Y., Yu, Y., Xu, H., & Piao, H. (2024). Liposomal Nanomaterials: A Rising Star in Glioma Treatment. *International Journal of Nanomedicine*, *19*(June), 6757–6776. DOI: 10.2147/IJN.S470478 PMID: 38983132

Gawel, A. M., Singh, R., & Debinski, W. (2022). Metal-Based Nanostructured Therapeutic Strategies for Glioblastoma Treatment—An Update. *Biomedicines*, *10*(7), 1–31. DOI: 10.3390/biomedicines10071598 PMID: 35884903

Guerrero-Cázares, H., Tzeng, S. Y., Young, N. P., Abutaleb, A. O., Quiñones-Hinojosa, A., & Green, J. J. (2014). Biodegradable polymeric nanoparticles show high efficacy and specificity at DNA delivery to human glioblastoma in vitro and in vivo. *ACS Nano*, *8*(5), 5141–5153. DOI: 10.1021/nn501197v PMID: 24766032

Guo, X., Yang, X., Wu, J., Yang, H., Li, Y., Li, J., Liu, Q., Wu, C., Xing, H., Liu, P., Wang, Y., Hu, C., & Ma, W. (2022). Tumor-Treating Fields in Glioblastomas: Past, Present, and Future. *Cancers (Basel)*, *14*(15), 3669. DOI: 10.3390/cancers14153669 PMID: 35954334

Haque, S., Norbert, C. C., Acharyya, R., Mukherjee, S., Kathirvel, M., & Patra, C. R. (2021). Biosynthesized silver nanoparticles for cancer therapy and in vivo bioimaging. *Cancers (Basel)*, *13*(23), 6114. Advance online publication. DOI: 10.3390/cancers13236114 PMID: 34885224

Hau, P., Fabel, K., Baumgart, U., Rümmele, P., Grauer, O., Bock, A., Dietmaier, C., Dietmaier, W., Dietrich, J., Dudel, C., Hübner, F., Jauch, T., Drechsel, E., Kleiter, I., Wismeth, C., Zellner, A., Brawanski, A., Steinbrecher, A., Marienhagen, J., & Bogdahn, U. (2004). Pegylated Liposomal Doxorubicin-Efficacy in Patients with Recurrent High-Grade Glioma. *Cancer*, *100*(6), 1199–1207. DOI: 10.1002/cncr.20073 PMID: 15022287

Holdhoff, M., Sahebjam, S., Huang, P., Kamson, D. O., Iacoboni, M., Dobson-brown, T., Schreck, K. C., Kleinberg, L., Redmond, K. J., Croog, V. J., Kut, C., Ozer, B., Grossman, S. A., Comas, M., Plehn, J., Fisher, J. D., & Sordillo, P. P. (2025). Liposomal curcumin and standard radiation and temozolomide for newly diagnosed high-grade gliomas : A phase 1 / 2 study. *Journal of Clinical Oncology*, *5768919*(16_suppl). Advance online publication. DOI: 10.1200/JCO.2025.43.16_suppl.TPS2095

Ishihara, H., Kubota, H., Lindberg, R. L. P., Leppert, D., Gloor, S. M., Errede, M., Virgintino, D., Fontana, A., Yonekawa, Y., & Frei, K. (2008). Endothelial cell barrier impairment induced by glioblastomas and transforming growth factor β2 involves matrix metalloproteinases and tight junction proteins. *Journal of Neuropathology and Experimental Neurology*, *67*(5), 435–448. DOI: 10.1097/NEN.0b013e31816fd622 PMID: 18431253

Jia, J. L., Alshamsan, B., & Ng, T. L. (2023). Temozolomide Chronotherapy in Glioma: A Systematic Review. *Current Oncology (Toronto, Ont.)*, *30*(2), 1893–1902. DOI: 10.3390/curroncol30020147 PMID: 36826108

Jiao, X., Yu, Y., Meng, J., He, M., Zhang, C. J., Geng, W., Ding, B., Wang, Z., & Ding, X. (2019). Dual-targeting and microenvironment-responsive micelles as a gene delivery system to improve the sensitivity of glioma to radiotherapy. *Acta Pharmaceutica Sinica. B, 9*(2), 381–396. DOI: 10.1016/j.apsb.2018.12.001 PMID: 30972284

Kadari, A., Pooja, D., Gora, R. H., Gudem, S., Kolapalli, V. R. M., Kulhari, H., & Sistla, R. (2018). Design of multifunctional peptide collaborated and docetaxel loaded lipid nanoparticles for antiglioma therapy. *European Journal of Pharmaceutics and Biopharmaceutics, 132*, 168–179. DOI: 10.1016/j.ejpb.2018.09.012 PMID: 30244167

Laquintana, V., Trapani, A., Denora, N., Wang, F., Gallo, J., & Trapani, G. (2009). New strategies to deliver anticancer drugs to brain tumors. *Expert Opinion on Drug Delivery, 6*(10), 1017–1032. DOI: 10.1517/17425240903167942 PMID: 19732031

Li, D., Gao, J., Yang, C., Li, B., Sun, J., Yu, M., Wang, Y., Wang, H., & Lu, Y. (2021). cRGDyK-modified procaine liposome inhibits the proliferation and motility of glioma cells via the ERK/p38MAPK pathway. *Experimental and Therapeutic Medicine, 22*(2), 1–11. DOI: 10.3892/etm.2021.10291 PMID: 34178132

Li, H., Li, M., Fu, J., Ao, H., Wang, W., & Wang, X. (2021). Enhancement of oral bioavailability of quercetin by metabolic inhibitory nanosuspensions compared to conventional nanosuspensions. *Drug Delivery, 28*(1), 1226–1236. DOI: 10.1080/10717544.2021.1927244 PMID: 34142631

Li, J., Feng, L., & Lu, Y. (2023). Glioblastoma multiforme: Diagnosis, treatment, and invasion. *Journal of Biomedical Research, 37*(1), 47–58. DOI: 10.7555/JBR.36.20220156 PMID: 36403983

Li, J., Zeng, H., You, Y., Wang, R., Tan, T., Wang, W., Yin, L., Zeng, Z., Zeng, Y., & Xie, T. (2021). Active targeting of orthotopic glioma using biomimetic liposomes co-loaded elemene and cabazitaxel modified by transferritin. *Journal of Nanobiotechnology, 19*(1), 1–19. DOI: 10.1186/s12951-021-01048-3 PMID: 34565383

Li, S., Deng, Q., Li, X., Huang, Y., Li, X., Liu, F., Wang, H., Qing, W., Liu, Z., & Lee, C. S. (2019). Bis-diketopyrrolopyrrole conjugated polymer nanoparticles as photothermic nanoagonist for specific and synergistic glioblastoma therapy. *Biomaterials, 216*(June), 119252. DOI: 10.1016/j.biomaterials.2019.119252 PMID: 31212086

Liu, S., Tan, B., Wang, F., & Yu, Y. (2024). Applications of polymeric nanoparticles in drug delivery for glioblastoma. *Frontiers in Pharmacology, 15*(January), 1–17. DOI: 10.3389/fphar.2024.1519479 PMID: 39834835

Longmire, M. R., Ogawa, M., Choyke, P. L., & Kobayashi, H. (2014). Dendrimers as high relaxivity MR contrast agents. *Wiley Interdisciplinary Reviews. Nanomedicine and Nanobiotechnology*, *123*(2), 40–43. DOI: 10.1002/wnan.1250 PMID: 24155241

Lu, G., Wang, X., Li, F., Wang, S., Zhao, J., Wang, J., Liu, J., Lyu, C., Ye, P., Tan, H., Li, W., Ma, G., & Wei, W. (2022). Engineered biomimetic nanoparticles achieve targeted delivery and efficient metabolism-based synergistic therapy against glioblastoma. *Nature Communications*, *13*(1), 4214. Advance online publication. DOI: 10.1038/s41467-022-31799-y PMID: 35864093

Maleki, H., Naghibzadeh, M., Amani, A., Adabi, M., & Khosravani, M. (2019). Preparation of Paclitaxel and Etoposide Co-loaded mPEG-PLGA Nanoparticles: An Investigation with Artificial Neural Network. *Journal of Pharmaceutical Innovation*, *16*(1), 11–25. DOI: 10.1007/s12247-019-09419-y

Minniti, G., De Sanctis, V., Muni, R., Filippone, F., Bozzao, A., Valeriani, M., Osti, M. F., De Paula, U., Lanzetta, G., Tombolini, V., & Maurizi Enrici, R. (2005). Radiotherapy plus concomitant and adjuvant temozolomide for glioblastoma in elderly patients. *The New England Journal of Medicine*, *88*(1), 97–103. DOI: 10.1007/s11060-008-9538-0 PMID: 18250965

Mittal, K. R., Pharasi, N., Sarna, B., Singh, M., Rachana, , Haider, S., Singh, S. K., Dua, K., Jha, S. K., Dey, A., Ojha, S., Mani, S., & Jha, N. K. (2022). Nanotechnology-based drug delivery for the treatment of CNS disorders. *Translational Neuroscience*, *13*(1), 527–546. DOI: 10.1515/tnsci-2022-0258 PMID: 36741545

Monteiro, A. R., Hill, R., Pilkington, G. J., & Madureira, P. A. (2017). The role of hypoxia in glioblastoma invasion. *Cells*, *6*(4), 45. Advance online publication. DOI: 10.3390/cells6040045 PMID: 29165393

Nagpal, S., Recht, C. K., Imtiaz, U., Bertrand, S., Thomas, R. P., Ajlan, A., Pena, J., Gershon, M., Kunz, P. L., Li, G., & Recht, L. D. (2014). Etirinotecan pegol (EP, NKTR-102) in the treatment of high-grade glioma (HGG): A phase 2 trial. *Journal of Clinical Oncology*, *32*(15, suppl), 2096–2096. DOI: 10.1200/jco.2014.32.15_suppl.2096

Pacheco-Torres, J., Mukherjee, N., Walko, M., López-Larrubia, P., Ballesteros, P., Cerdan, S., & Kocer, A. (2015). Image guided drug release from pH-sensitive Ion channel-functionalized stealth liposomes into an in vivo glioblastoma model. *Nanomedicine; Nanotechnology, Biology, and Medicine*, *11*(6), 1345–1354. DOI: 10.1016/j.nano.2015.03.014 PMID: 25888277

Prencipe, F., Diaferia, C., Rossi, F., Ronga, L., & Tesauro, D. (2021). Forward precision medicine: Micelles for active targeting driven by peptides. *Molecules (Basel, Switzerland)*, *26*(13), 4049. Advance online publication. DOI: 10.3390/molecules26134049 PMID: 34279392

Puris, E., Fricker, G., & Gynther, M. (2022). Targeting Transporters for Drug Delivery to the Brain: Can We Do Better? In *Pharmaceutical Research* (Vol. 39, Issue 7). Springer US. DOI: 10.1007/s11095-022-03241-x

Qu, J., Zhang, L., Chen, Z., Mao, G., Gao, Z., Lai, X., Zhu, X., & Zhu, J. (2016). Nanostructured lipid carriers, solid lipid nanoparticles, and polymeric nanoparticles: Which kind of drug delivery system is better for glioblastoma chemotherapy? *Drug Delivery*, *23*(9), 3408–3416. DOI: 10.1080/10717544.2016.1189465 PMID: 27181462

Quader, S., Liu, X., Chen, Y., Mi, P., Chida, T., Ishii, T., Miura, Y., Nishiyama, N., Cabral, H., & Kataoka, K. (2017). cRGD peptide-installed epirubicin-loaded polymeric micelles for effective targeted therapy against brain tumors. *Journal of Controlled Release*, *258*, 56–66. DOI: 10.1016/j.jconrel.2017.04.033 PMID: 28483513

Shala, A. L., Arduino, I., Salihu, M. B., & Denora, N. (2023). Quercetin and Its Nano-Formulations for Brain Tumor Therapy—Current Developments and Future Perspectives for Paediatric Studies. *Pharmaceutics*, *15*(3), 963. Advance online publication. DOI: 10.3390/pharmaceutics15030963 PMID: 36986827

Sharma, A. K., Gupta, L., Sahu, H., Qayum, A., Singh, S. K., Nakhate, K. T., Ajazuddin, , & Gupta, U. (2018). Chitosan Engineered PAMAM Dendrimers as Nanoconstructs for the Enhanced Anti-Cancer Potential and Improved In vivo Brain Pharmacokinetics of Temozolomide. *Pharmaceutical Research*, *35*(1), 9. Advance online publication. DOI: 10.1007/s11095-017-2324-y PMID: 29294212

Sharma, R., Liaw, K., Sharma, A., Jimenez, A., Chang, M., Salazar, S., Amlani, I., Kannan, S., & Kannan, R. M. (2021). Glycosylation of PAMAM dendrimers significantly improves tumor macrophage targeting and specificity in glioblastoma. *Journal of Controlled Release*, *337*, 179–192. DOI: 10.1016/j.jconrel.2021.07.018 PMID: 34274384

Society, N. B. T. (2025). *Brain Tumors Types*. https://braintumor.org/brain-tumors/about-brain-tumors/brain-tumor-types/

Sommonte, F., Arduino, I., Iacobazzi, R. M., Laera, L., Silvestri, T., Lopedota, A. A., Castegna, A., & Denora, N. (2024). Microfluidic development of brain-derived neurotrophic factor loaded solid lipid nanoparticles: An in vitro evaluation in the post-traumatic brain injury neuroinflammation model. *Journal of Drug Delivery Science and Technology*, *96*(April), 105699. DOI: 10.1016/j.jddst.2024.105699

Song, S., Mao, G., Du, J., & Zhu, X. (2016). Novel RGD containing, temozolomide-loading nanostructured lipid carriers for glioblastoma multiforme chemotherapy. *Drug Delivery*, *23*(4), 1404–1408. DOI: 10.3109/10717544.2015.1064186 PMID: 26203687

Sousa, F., Dhaliwal, H. K., Gattacceca, F., Sarmento, B., & Amiji, M. M. (2019). Enhanced anti-angiogenic effects of bevacizumab in glioblastoma treatment upon intranasal administration in polymeric nanoparticles. *Journal of Controlled Release*, *309*(July), 37–47. DOI: 10.1016/j.jconrel.2019.07.033 PMID: 31344424

Sun, B., Li, R., Ji, N., Liu, H., Wang, H., Chen, C., Bai, L., Su, J., & Chen, J. (2025). Brain-targeting drug delivery systems: The state of the art in treatment of glioblastoma. *Materials Today Bio, 30*(December 2024), 101443. DOI: 10.1016/j.mtbio.2025.101443

Tan, A. C., Ashley, D. M., López, G. Y., Malinzak, M., Friedman, H. S., & Khasraw, M. (2020). Management of glioblastoma: State of the art and future directions. *CA: a Cancer Journal for Clinicians*, *70*(4), 299–312. DOI: 10.3322/caac.21613 PMID: 32478924

Tosi, G., Musumeci, T., Ruozi, B., Carbone, C., Belletti, D., Pignatello, R., Vandelli, M. A., & Puglisi, G. (2016). The "fate" of polymeric and lipid nanoparticles for brain delivery and targeting: Strategies and mechanism of blood-brain barrier crossing and trafficking into the central nervous system. *Journal of Drug Delivery Science and Technology*, *32*, 66–76. DOI: 10.1016/j.jddst.2015.07.007

Tzeng, S. Y., & Green, J. J. (2013). Therapeutic nanomedicine for brain cancer. *Therapeutic Delivery*, *4*(6), 687–704. DOI: 10.4155/tde.13.38 PMID: 23738667

Vieira, D. B., & Gamarra, L. F. (2016). Getting into the brain: Liposome-based strategies for effective drug delivery across the blood–brain barrier. *International Journal of Nanomedicine*, *11*, 5381–5414. DOI: 10.2147/IJN.S117210 PMID: 27799765

Wang, H., Li, L., Ye, J., Wang, R., Wang, R., Hu, J., Wang, Y., Dong, W., Xia, X., Yang, Y., Gao, Y., Gao, L., & Liu, Y. (2020). Improving the oral bioavailability of an anti-glioma prodrug cat3 using novel solid lipid nanoparticles containing oleic acid-cat3 conjugates. *Pharmaceutics*, *12*(2), 126. Advance online publication. DOI: 10.3390/pharmaceutics12020126 PMID: 32028734

Wang, L., Tang, S., Yu, Y., Lv, Y., Wang, A., Yan, X., Li, N., Sha, C., Sun, K., & Li, Y. (2021). Intranasal Delivery of Temozolomide-Conjugated Gold Nanoparticles Functionalized with Anti-EphA3 for Glioblastoma Targeting. *Molecular Pharmaceutics*, *18*(3), 915–927. DOI: 10.1021/acs.molpharmaceut.0c00911 PMID: 33417456

Wang, M., Lv, C. Y., Li, S. A., Wang, J. K., Luo, W. Z., Zhao, P. C., Liu, X. Y., Wang, Z. M., Jiao, Y., Sun, H. W., Zhao, Y., & Zhang, P. (2021). Near infrared light fluorescence imaging-guided biomimetic nanoparticles of extracellular vesicles deliver indocyanine green and paclitaxel for hyperthermia combined with chemotherapy against glioma. *Journal of Nanobiotechnology*, *19*(1), 1–18. DOI: 10.1186/s12951-023-02253-y PMID: 34261493

Yang, S., Wallach, M., Krishna, A., Kurmasheva, R., & Sridhar, S. (2021). Recent developments in nanomedicine for pediatric cancer. *Journal of Clinical Medicine*, *10*(7), 1–22. DOI: 10.3390/jcm10071437 PMID: 33916177

Yang, Y., Cheng, N., Luo, Q., Shao, N., Ma, X., Chen, J., Luo, L., & Xiao, Z. (2023). How Nanotherapeutic Platforms Play a Key Role in Glioma? A Comprehensive Review of Literature. *International Journal of Nanomedicine*, *18*(June), 3663–3694. DOI: 10.2147/IJN.S414736 PMID: 37427368

Yang, Z., Wei, D., Dai, X., Stevens, M. F. G., Bradshaw, T. D., Luo, Y., & Zhang, J. (2019). C8-substituted imidazotetrazine analogs overcome temozolomide resistance by inducing DNA adducts and DNA damage. *Frontiers in Oncology*, *9*(JUN), 1–14. DOI: 10.3389/fonc.2019.00485 PMID: 31263673

Zhao, Y., Li, D., Zhao, J., Song, J., & Zhao, Y. (2016). The role of the low-density lipoprotein receptor-related protein 1 (LRP-1) in regulating blood-brain barrier integrity. *Reviews in the Neurosciences*, *27*(6), 623–634. DOI: 10.1515/revneuro-2015-0069 PMID: 27206317

KEY TERMS AND DEFINITIONS

Biomimetic Nanoparticles: Nanocarriers mimicking biological structures (cells, membranes, proteins) to improve targeting and therapeutic outcomes.

Blood–Brain Barrier (BBB): A selective barrier of endothelial cells and tight junctions that restricts passage of substances from blood to the brain.

Blood–Brain Tumor Barrier (BBTB): A modified BBB around gliomas; more permeable but still hinders drug delivery.

Dendrimers: Highly branched polymers that encapsulate or bind drugs and allow surface functionalization for targeting.

Glioblastoma Multiforme (GBM): The most aggressive form of primary brain tumor, with rapid growth, invasiveness, and resistance to treatment.

Liposomes: Phospholipid bilayer vesicles that encapsulate hydrophilic or hydrophobic drugs for targeted brain delivery.

Metal-based Nanoparticles: Nanoparticles containing metals such as gold, silver, or iron oxide, explored for drug delivery, imaging, and combined therapeutic and diagnostic applications (theranostics).

Micelles: Self-assembled nanoscale spheres formed by amphiphilic molecules, useful for solubilizing and delivering hydrophobic drugs.

Nanocarrier: Nanoscale drug delivery system designed to improve solubility, stability, targeting, and controlled release.

Nanostructured Lipid Carriers (NLCs): Blends of solid and liquid lipids with higher drug loading and stability than SLNs.

Polymeric Nanoparticles: Biodegradable polymer-based systems for sustained and controlled drug delivery.

Receptor-Mediated Transcytosis (RMT): Transport of nanoparticles across the BBB via binding to specific endothelial receptors.

Solid Lipid Nanoparticles (SLNs): Lipid-based carriers solid at body temperature, stabilizing drugs and enabling controlled release.

Compilation of References

Abadi, B., Shahsavani, Y., Faramarzpour, M., Rezaei, N., & Rahimi, H. R. (2022). Antidepressants with anti-tumor potential in treating glioblastoma: A narrative review. *Fundamental & Clinical Pharmacology*, *36*(1), 35–48. DOI: 10.1111/fcp.12712 PMID: 34212424

Abbott, R. C., Iliopoulos, M., Watson, K. A., Arcucci, V., Go, M., Hughes-Parry, H. E., & Darcy, P. K. (2023). Human EGFRvIII chimeric antigen receptor T cells demonstrate favorable safety profile and curative responses in orthotopic glioblastoma. *Journal for Immunotherapy of Cancer*, *11*(3), e006444. Advance online publication. DOI: 10.1136/jitc-2022-006444 PMID: 36890859

Abdel-haq, M., Kumar, A., Mohand, F. A., Kravchenko-balasha, N., Rottenberg, Y., & Domb, A. J. (2023). Paclitaxel Delivery to the Brain for Glioblastoma Treatment. *International Journal of Pharmaceutical Sciences*, 1–14.

Aboody, K. S., Najbauer, J., Metz, M. Z., D'Apuzzo, M., Gutova, M., Annala, A. J., Synold, T. W., Couture, L. A., Blanchard, M. S., Moats, R. A., Garcia, E., Aramburo, S., Valenzuela, V. V., Frank, R. T., Barish, M. E., Brown, C. E., Kim, S. U., Badie, B., & Portnow, J. (2013). Neural stem cell-mediated enzyme/prodrug therapy for glioma: Preclinical studies. *Science Translational Medicine*, *5*(184), 184ra59. Advance online publication. DOI: 10.1126/scitranslmed.3005365 PMID: 23658244

Acharekar, A., Bachal, K., Shirke, P., Thorat, R., Banerjee, A., Gardi, N., & Dutt, S. (2023). Substrate stiffness regulates the recurrent glioblastoma cell morphology and aggressiveness. *Journal of Neuro-Oncology*, *115*, 107–127. DOI: 10.1007/s11060-023-04412-1 PMID: 36563706

Acharya, M. M., Martirosian, V., Chmielewski, N. N., Hanna, N., Tran, K. K., Liao, A. C., Christie, L. A., Parihar, V. K., & Limoli, C. L. (2015). Stem cell transplantation reverses chemotherapy-induced cognitive dysfunction. *Cancer Research*, *75*(4), 676–686. DOI: 10.1158/0008-5472.CAN-14-2237 PMID: 25687405

Adair, J. E., Beard, B. C., Trobridge, G. D., Neff, T., Rockhill, J. K., Silbergeld, D. L., Mrugala, M. M., & Kiem, H. P. (2012). Extended survival of glioblastoma patients after chemoprotective HSC gene therapy. *Science Translational Medicine*, *4*(133). Advance online publication. DOI: 10.1126/scitranslmed.3003425 PMID: 22572881

Adair, J. E., Johnston, S. K., Mrugala, M. M., Beard, B. C., Guyman, L. A., Baldock, A. L., Bridge, C. A., Hawkins-Daarud, A., Gori, J. L., Born, D. E., Gonzalez-Cuyar, L. F., Silbergeld, D. L., Rockne, R. C., Storer, B. E., Rockhill, J. K., Swanson, K. R., & Kiem, H. P. (2014). Gene therapy enhances chemotherapy tolerance and efficacy in glioblastoma patients. *The Journal of Clinical Investigation*, *124*(9), 4082–4092. DOI: 10.1172/JCI76739 PMID: 25105369

Agemy, L., Friedmann-Morvinski, D., Kotamraju, V. R., Roth, L., Sugahara, K. N., Girard, O. M., Mattrey, R. F., Verma, I. M., & Ruoslahti, E. (2011). Targeted nanoparticle enhanced proapoptotic peptide as potential therapy for glioblastoma. *Proceedings of the National Academy of Sciences of the United States of America*, *108*(42), 17450–17455. DOI: 10.1073/pnas.1114518108 PMID: 21969599

Aggarwal, R., Italiano, A., Domchek, S., Goodman, O., Postel-Vinay, S., Garcia-Donas, J., & Shore, N. (2024). Abstract CT222: Efficacy and safety of ceralasertib in the PLANETTE study in patients (pts) with ATM-altered advanced solid tumors (ASTs) or metastatic castration-resistant prostate cancer (mCRPC). *Cancer Research*, *84*(7, Supplement), CT222–CT222. DOI: 10.1158/1538-7445.AM2024-CT222

Aghi, M., & Chiocca, E. A. (2006). Gene therapy for glioblastoma. *Neurosurgical Focus*, *20*(4), E18. Advance online publication. DOI: 10.3171/foc.2006.20.4.9 PMID: 16709023

Agnihotri, S., Gajadhar, A. S., Ternamian, C., Gorlia, T., Diefes, K. L., Mischel, P. S., & Carlson, B. L. (2012). Alkylpurine–DNA–N-glycosylase confers resistance to Temozolomide in xenograft models of glioblastoma multiforme and is associated with poor survival in patients. *The Journal of Clinical Investigation*, *122*(1), 253–266. DOI: 10.1172/JCI59334 PMID: 22156195

Agosti, E., Zeppieri, M., De Maria, L., Tedeschi, C., Fontanella, M. M., Panciani, P. P., Ius, T., & Skrap, M. (2023). Glioblastoma immunotherapy: A systematic review of the present strategies and prospects for advancements. *International Journal of Molecular Sciences*, *24*(20), 15037. Advance online publication. DOI: 10.3390/ijms242015037 PMID: 37894718

Agrawal, M., Ajazuddin, , Tripathi, D. K., Saraf, S., Saraf, S., Antimisiaris, S. G., Mourtas, S., Hammarlund-Udenaes, M., & Alexander, A. (2017). Recent advancements in liposomes targeting strategies to cross blood-brain barrier (BBB) for the treatment of Alzheimer's disease. *Journal of Controlled Release*, *260*(April), 61–77. DOI: 10.1016/j.jconrel.2017.05.019 PMID: 28549949

Ahlawat, J., Barroso, G., Narayan, M., Alvarado, M., Armendariz, I., Bernal, J., Carabaza, X., Chavez, S., Cruz, P., Escalante, V., Estorga, S., Fernandez, D., Lozano, C., Marrufo, M., Ahmad, N., Negrete, S., Olvera, K., Parada, X., Portillo, B., & Viel, S. (2020). Nanocarriers as Potential Drug Delivery Candidates for Overcoming the Blood-Brain Barrier: Challenges and Possibilities. *ACS Omega*, *5*(22), 12583–12595. DOI: 10.1021/acsomega.0c01592 PMID: 32548442

Ahmed, M. H., Canney, M., Carpentier, A., & Idbaih, A. (2023). Overcoming the blood brain barrier in glioblastoma: Status and future perspective. *Revue Neurologique*, *179*(5), 430–436. DOI: 10.1016/j.neurol.2023.03.013 PMID: 37062676

Ahmed, M., Semreen, A. M., El-Huneidi, W., Bustanji, Y., Abu-Gharbieh, E., Alqudah, M. A. Y., Alhusban, A., Shara, M., Abuhelwa, A. Y., Soares, N. C., Semreen, M. H., & Alzoubi, K. H. (2023). Preclinical and Clinical Applications of Metabolomics and Proteomics in Glioblastoma Research. *International Journal of Molecular Sciences*, *24*(1), 348. DOI: 10.3390/ijms24010348 PMID: 36613792

Ahmed, T. J. (2023). Biomaterial-based in vitro 3D modeling of glioblastoma multiforme. *Current Pharmacology Reports*, *1*(03), 177–194. DOI: 10.1007/s40495-023-00334-5 PMID: 38327839

Ahuja, S., Gupta, P., Ajay, G., & Ghorai, A. (2025). *Hypoxia-Induced DNA Damage Response and Genomic Instability Dictate Cancer Treatment Response Hypoxia and Tumor Microenvironment: Implications for Cancer Therapy*. Springer.

Aime, S., & Caravan, P. (2009). Biodistribution of gadolinium-based contrast agents, including gadolinium deposition. *Journal of Magnetic Resonance Imaging*, *30*(6), 1259–1267. DOI: 10.1002/jmri.21969 PMID: 19938038

Aiyappa-Maudsley, R., Chalmers, A. J., & Parsons, J. L. (2022). Factors affecting the radiation response in glioblastoma. *Neuro-Oncology Advances*, *4*(1), vdac156. Advance online publication. DOI: 10.1093/noajnl/vdac156 PMID: 36325371

Alamdari-Palangi, V., Karami, Z., Karami, H., & Baazm, M. (2020). MiRNA-7 replacement effect on proliferation and tarceva-sensitivity in U373-MG cell line. *Asian Pacific Journal of Cancer Prevention : APJCP*, *21*(6), 1747–1753. DOI: 10.31557/APJCP.2020.21.6.1747 PMID: 32592373

Aldape, K., Zadeh, G., Mansouri, S., Reifenberger, G., & von Deimling, A. (2015). Glioblastoma: Pathology, molecular mechanisms and markers. *Acta Neuropathologica, 17*(1), 98–110. DOI: 10.1007/s00401-015-1432-1 PMID: 25943888

Aldoghachi, A. F., Aldoghachi, A. F., Breyne, K., Ling, K. H., & Cheah, P. S. (2022). Recent advances in the therapeutic strategies of glioblastoma multiforme. *Neuroscience, 491*, 240–270. DOI: 10.1016/j.neuroscience.2022.03.030 PMID: 35395355

Alifieris, C., & Trafalis, D. T. (2015). Glioblastoma multiforme: Pathogenesis and treatment. *Pharmacology & Therapeutics, 152*, 63–82. DOI: 10.1016/j.pharmthera.2015.05.005 PMID: 25944528

Almahmoud, A., Parekh, H. S., Paterson, B. M., Tupally, K. R., & Vegh, V. (2024). Intranasal delivery of imaging agents to the brain. *Theranostics, 14*(13), 5022–5101. DOI: 10.7150/thno.98473 PMID: 39267777

Alomari, S., Zhang, I., Hernandez, A., Kraft, C. Y., Raj, D., Kedda, J., & Chitneni, S. K. (2021). Drug repurposing for glioblastoma and current advances in drug delivery—A comprehensive review of the literature. *Biomolecules, 11*(12), 1870. Advance online publication. DOI: 10.3390/biom11121870 PMID: 34944514

Amengual-Cladera, E., Morla-Barcelo, P. M., Morán-Costoya, A., Sastre-Serra, J., Pons, D. G., Valle, A., Roca, P., & Nadal-Serrano, M. (2024). Metformin: From diabetes to Cancer—Unveiling Molecular mechanisms and therapeutic strategies. *Biology (Basel), 13*(5), 302. DOI: 10.3390/biology13050302 PMID: 38785784

Amina, S. J., & Guo, B. (2020). A review on the synthesis and functionalization of gold nanoparticles as a drug delivery vehicle. *International Journal of Nanomedicine, 15*, 9823–9857. DOI: 10.2147/IJN.S279094 PMID: 33324054

Amodio, V., Vitiello, P., Bardelli, A., & Germano, G. (2024). DNA repair-dependent immunogenic liabilities in colorectal cancer: Opportunities from errors. *British Journal of Cancer, 131*(10), 1576–1590. DOI: 10.1038/s41416-024-02848-8 PMID: 39271762

Anand, J., Chiou, L., Sciandra, C., Zhang, X., Hong, J., Wu, D., Zhou, P., & Vaziri, C. (2023). Roles of trans-lesion synthesis (TLS) DNA polymerases in tumorigenesis and cancer therapy. *NAR Cancer, 5*(1), zcad005. DOI: 10.1093/narcan/zcad005 PMID: 36755961

Angom, R. S., Nakka, N. M. R., & Bhattacharya, S. (2023). Advances in glioblastoma therapy: An update on current approaches. *Brain Sciences, 13*(11), 1536. DOI: 10.3390/brainsci13111536 PMID: 38002496

Anido, J., Sáez-Borderías, A., Gonzàlez-Juncà, A., Rodón, L., Folch, G., Carmona, M. A., Prieto-Sánchez, R. M., Barba, I., Martínez-Sáez, E., Prudkin, L., Cuartas, I., Raventós, C., Martínez-Ricarte, F., Poca, M. A., García-Dorado, D., Lahn, M. M., Yingling, J. M., Rodón, J., Sahuquillo, J., & Seoane, J. (2010). TGF-β Receptor Inhibitors Target the CD44(high)/Id1(high) Glioma-Initiating Cell Population in Human Glioblastoma. *Cancer Cell, 18*(6), 655–668. DOI: 10.1016/j.ccr.2010.10.023 PMID: 21156287

Annovazzi, L., Mellai, M., & Schiffer, D. (2017). Chemotherapeutic drugs: DNA damage and repair in glioblastoma. *Cancers (Basel), 9*(6), 57. DOI: 10.3390/cancers9060057 PMID: 28587121

Aragon-Sanabria, V.. (2022). Ultrasmall Nanoparticle Delivery of Doxorubicin Improves Therapeutic Index for High-Grade Glioma. *Molecular Cancer Therapeutics, 21*(5), 789–798. DOI: 10.1158/1535-7163.MCT-21-0720 PMID: 35499557

Arce, C., Rodríguez-Rovira, I., De Rycke, K., Durán, K., Campuzano, V., Fabregat, I., Jiménez-Altayó, F., Berraondo, P., & Egea, G. (2021). Anti-TGFβ (transforming growth factor β) therapy with betaglycan-derived P144 peptide gene delivery prevents the formation of aortic aneurysm in a mouse model of Marfan syndrome. *Arteriosclerosis, Thrombosis, and Vascular Biology, 41*(9), e440–e452. DOI: 10.1161/ATVBAHA.121.316496 PMID: 34162229

Arduino, I., Di Fonte, R., Tiboni, M., Porcelli, L., Serratì, S., Fondaj, D., Rafaschieri, T., Cutrignelli, A., Guida, G., Casettari, L., Azzariti, A., Lopedota, A. A., Denora, N., & Iacobazzi, R. M. (2024). Microfluidic development and biological evaluation of targeted therapy-loaded biomimetic nano system to improve the metastatic melanoma treatment. *International Journal of Pharmaceutics, 650*(December 2023), 123697. DOI: 10.1016/j.ijpharm.2023.123697

Arduino, I., Depalo, N., Re, F., Dal Magro, R., Panniello, A., Margiotta, N., Fanizza, E., Lopalco, A., Laquintana, V., Cutrignelli, A., Lopedota, A. A., Franco, M., & Denora, N. (2020). PEGylated solid lipid nanoparticles for brain delivery of lipophilic kiteplatin Pt(IV) prodrugs: An in vitro study. *International Journal of Pharmaceutics, 583*(January), 119351. DOI: 10.1016/j.ijpharm.2020.119351 PMID: 32339634

Arduino, I., Di Fonte, R., Sommonte, F., Lopedota, A. A., Porcelli, L., Li, J., Serrati, S., Bártolo, R., Santos, H. A., Iacobazzi, R. M., Azzariti, A., & Denora, N. (2024). Fabrication of Biomimetic Hybrid Liposomes via Microfluidic Technology: Homotypic Targeting and Antitumor Efficacy Studies in Glioma Cells. *International Journal of Nanomedicine, 19*, 13217–13233. DOI: 10.2147/IJN.S489872 PMID: 39679250

Arvanitis, C. D., Ferraro, G. B., Jain, R. K., Laboratories, L. S., & General, M. (2021). The blood–brain barrier and blood–tumour barrier in brain tumours and metastases. *Nature Reviews. Cancer*, *20*(1), 26–41. DOI: 10.1038/s41568-019-0205-x PMID: 31601988

Asija, S., Chatterjee, A., Yadav, S., Chekuri, G., Karulkar, A., Jaiswal, A. K., Goda, J. S., & Purwar, R. (2022). Combinatorial approaches to effective therapy in glioblastoma (GBM): Current status and what the future holds. *International Reviews of Immunology*, *41*(6), 582–605. DOI: 10.1080/08830185.2022.2101647 PMID: 35938932

Asimakidou, E., Tan, J. K. S., Zeng, J., & Lo, C. H. (2024). Blood–Brain Barrier-Targeting Nanoparticles: Biomaterial Properties and Biomedical Applications in Translational Neuroscience. *Pharmaceuticals (Basel, Switzerland)*, *17*(5), 612. Advance online publication. DOI: 10.3390/ph17050612 PMID: 38794182

Atkinson, A. P.. (2018). Aptamers in Glioblastoma Research: Potential for Targeted Therapy. *Cancer Letters*, *414*, 82–90. DOI: 10.1016/j.canlet.2017.11.017

Attique, I., Haider, Z., Khan, M., Hassan, S., Soliman, M. M., Ibrahim, W. N., & Anjum, S. (2025). Reactive Oxygen Species: From Tumorigenesis to Therapeutic Strategies in Cancer. *Cancer Medicine*, *14*(10), e70947. DOI: 10.1002/cam4.70947 PMID: 40377005

Azam, M. Z. (2021). Glioblastoma pathogenesis and diagnosis.

Baek, S., Lee, Y., Ryu, Y., Kim, S., Park, J., & Oh, S.. (2012). Gallium maltolate: An investigational treatment for cancer. *Cancer Chemotherapy and Pharmacology*, *69*(4), 893–900.

Bae, W. H., Maraka, S., & Daher, A. (2024). Challenges and advances in glioblastoma targeted therapy: The promise of drug repurposing and biomarker exploration. *Frontiers in Oncology*, *14*, 1441460. Advance online publication. DOI: 10.3389/fonc.2024.1441460 PMID: 39439947

Bagó, J. R., Alfonso-Pecchio, A., Okolie, O., Dumitru, R., Rinkenbaugh, A., Baldwin, A. S., Miller, C. R., Magness, S. T., & Hingtgen, S. D. (2016). Therapeutically engineered induced neural stem cells are tumour-homing and inhibit progression of glioblastoma. *Nature Communications*, *7*(1), 10593. Advance online publication. DOI: 10.1038/ncomms10593 PMID: 26830441

Bagó, J. R., Sheets, K. T., & Hingtgen, S. D. (2015). Neural stem cell therapy for cancer. *Methods (San Diego, Calif.)*, *99*, 37–43. DOI: 10.1016/j.ymeth.2015.08.013 PMID: 26314280

Bakhtiyari-Ramezani, M., Nohekhan, M., Akbari, M. E., Abbasvandi, F., Bayat, M., Akbari, A., & Rezaie, N. (2024). Comparative assessment of direct and indirect cold atmospheric plasma effects, based on helium and argon, on human glioblastoma: An in vitro and in vivo study. *Scientific Reports*, *14*(1), 3578. Advance online publication. DOI: 10.1038/s41598-024-54070-4 PMID: 38347045

Bao, P., Gu, H. Y., Jiang, Y. C., Wang, J. W., Wu, M., Yu, A., Wang, X., & Zhang, X. (2024). In situ sprayed exosome-cross-linked gel as artificial lymph nodes for postoperative glioblastoma immunotherapy. *ACS Nano*, *18*(20), 13266–13276. DOI: 10.1021/acsnano.4c02425 PMID: 38709874

Bao, S., Wu, Q., McLendon, R. E., Hao, Y., Shi, Q., Hjelmeland, A. B., Dewhirst, M. W., Bigner, D. D., & Rich, J. N. (2006). Glioma stem cells promote radioresistance by preferential activation of the DNA damage response. *Nature*, *444*(7120), 756–760. DOI: 10.1038/nature05236 PMID: 17051156

Barron, T., Yalçın, B., Mochizuki, A., Cantor, E., Shamardani, K., Tlais, D., & Monje, M. (2023). CNSC-01. GABAergic neuron-to-glioma synapses in diffuse midline gliomas. *Neuro-Oncology*, *25*(Supplement_1), i11. DOI: 10.1093/neuonc/noad073.044

Barzegar-Fallah, A., Gandhi, K., Rizwan, S. B., Slatter, T. L., & Reynolds, J. N. (2022). Harnessing ultrasound for targeting drug delivery to the brain and breaching the blood–brain tumour barrier. *Pharmaceutics*, *14*(10), 2231. Advance online publication. DOI: 10.3390/pharmaceutics14102231 PMID: 36297666

Basso, J., Miranda, A., Nunes, S., Cova, T., Sousa, J., Vitorino, C., & Pais, A. (2018). Hydrogel-based drug delivery nanosystems for the treatment of brain tumors. *Gels (Basel, Switzerland)*, *4*(3), 62. Advance online publication. DOI: 10.3390/gels4030062 PMID: 30674838

Bastiancich, C., Da Silva, A., & Estève, M. A. (2021). Photothermal Therapy for the Treatment of Glioblastoma: Potential and Preclinical Challenges. *Frontiers in Oncology*, *10*(January), 1–16. DOI: 10.3389/fonc.2020.610356 PMID: 33520720

Bausart, M., Préat, V., & Malfanti, A. (2022). Immunotherapy for glioblastoma: The promise of combination strategies. *Journal of Experimental & Clinical Cancer Research : CR*, *41*(1), 35. Advance online publication. DOI: 10.1186/s13046-022-02251-2 PMID: 35078492

Bayat, H., Pourgholami, M. H., Rahmani, S., Pournajaf, S., & Mowla, S. J. (2023). Synthetic miR-21 decoy circularized by tRNA splicing mechanism inhibited tumorigenesis in glioblastoma in vitro and in vivo models. *Molecular Therapy. Nucleic Acids*, *32*, 432–444. DOI: 10.1016/j.omtn.2023.04.001 PMID: 37181451

Becker, A. P., Sells, B. E., Jaharul Haque, S., & Chakravarti, A. (2021). Tumor Heterogeneity in Glioblastomas: From Light Microscopy to Molecular Pathology. *Cancers (Basel)*, *13*(4), 1–25. DOI: 10.3390/cancers13040761 PMID: 33673104

Begagić, E., Pugonja, R., Bečulić, H., Čeliković, A., Tandir Lihić, L., Kadić Vukas, S., & Dorić, M. (2023). Molecular targeted therapies in glioblastoma multiforme: A systematic overview of global trends and findings. *Brain Sciences*, *13*(11), 1602. Advance online publication. DOI: 10.3390/brainsci13111602 PMID: 38002561

Begley, C. G., Ashton, M., Baell, J., Bettess, M., Brown, M. P., Carter, B., Charman, W. N., Davis, C., Fisher, S., Frazer, I., Gautam, A., Jennings, M. P., Kearney, P., Keeffe, E., Kelly, D., Lopez, A. F., McGuckin, M., Parker, M. W., Rayner, C., & Sullivan, M. (2021). Drug repurposing: Misconceptions, challenges, and opportunities for academic researchers. *Science Translational Medicine*, *13*(612), eabd5524. DOI: 10.1126/scitranslmed.abd5524 PMID: 34550729

Behrooz, A. B., Latifi-Navid, H., Nezhadi, A., Świat, M., Los, M., Jamalpoor, Z., & Seif, F. (2023). Molecular mechanisms of microRNAs in glioblastoma pathogenesis. *Biochimica et Biophysica Acta (BBA) –. Revisiones en Cáncer*, *1870*(6), 119482. Advance online publication. DOI: 10.1016/j.bbcan.2023.188948

Beier, C. P., Schmid, C., Gorlia, T., Kleinletzenberger, C., Beier, D., Grauer, O., Steinbrecher, A., Hirschmann, B., Brawanski, A., Dietmaier, C., Jauch-Worley, T., Kölbl, O., Pietsch, T., Proescholdt, M., Rümmele, P., Muigg, A., Stockhammer, G., Hegi, M., Bogdahn, U., & Hau, P. (2009). RNOP-09: Pegylated liposomal doxorubicine and prolonged temozolomide in addition to radiotherapy in newly diagnosed glioblastoma - A phase II study. *BMC Cancer*, *9*(1), 308. DOI: 10.1186/1471-2407-9-308 PMID: 19725960

Benmameri, M. (2022) In silico exploration of membrane transport events: prediction of passive permeation coefficients and binding sites of human MRP4. Thesis, Université de Limoges.

Bentayebi, K., Suwan, K., Ibrahimi, A., Sara, L., Ouadghiri, M., Aanniz, T., Amzazi, S., Belyamani, L., Hajitou, A., & Eljaoudi, R. (2024). Preclinical Evaluation of panobinostat and ONC201 for the treatment of diffuse intrinsic pontine glioma (DIPG). *Brain Disorders (Amsterdam, Netherlands)*, *13*, 100113. Advance online publication. DOI: 10.1016/j.dscb.2023.100113

Bernal, G. M., LaRiviere, M. J., Mansour, N., Pytel, P., Cahill, K. E., Voce, D. J., Kang, S., Spretz, R., Welp, U., Noriega, S. E., Nuñez, L., Larsen, G., Weichselbaum, R. R., & Yamini, B. (2014). Convection-enhanced delivery and in vivo imaging of polymeric nanoparticles for the treatment of malignant glioma. *Nanomedicine; Nanotechnology, Biology, and Medicine*, *10*(1), 149–157. DOI: 10.1016/j.nano.2013.07.003 PMID: 23891990

Bhargava, R., Sandhu, M., Muk, S., Lee, G., Vaidehi, N., & Stark, J. M. (2018). C-NHEJ without indels is robust and requires synergistic function of distinct XLF domains. *Nature Communications*, *9*(1), 2484. DOI: 10.1038/s41467-018-04867-5 PMID: 29950655

Bialasek, M., Sun, M., Marszalek, I., Taciak, B., Weller, M., Rygiel, T., & Król, M. (2025). Abstract A037: Macrophage-ferritin-drug conjugates: A novel approach to overcome glioblastoma drug resistance and induce long-term tumor immunity. *Cancer Immunology Research*, *13*(2, Supplement), A037. DOI: 10.1158/2326-6074.IO2025-A037

Bianchimano, P., Britton, G. J., Wallach, D. S., Smith, E. M., Cox, L. M., Liu, S., Iwanowski, K., Weiner, H. L., Faith, J. J., Clemente, J. C., & Tankou, S. K. (2022). Mining the microbiota to identify gut commensals modulating neuroinflammation in a mouse model of multiple sclerosis. *Microbiome*, *10*(1), 174. DOI: 10.1186/s40168-022-01364-2 PMID: 36253847

Birzu, C., French, P., Caccese, M., Cerretti, G., Idbaih, A., Zagonel, V., & Lombardi, G. (2021). Recurrent glioblastoma: From molecular landscape to new treatment perspectives. *Cancers (Basel)*, *13*(1), 47. Advance online publication. DOI: 10.3390/cancers13010047 PMID: 33375286

Blagosklonny, M. V., Uzdensky, A. B., & Skladal, K.. (2007). Mechanism of action of sirolimus. *Experimental Cell Research*, *313*(7), 1335–1343.

Blanco, E., Shen, H., & Ferrari, M. (2015). Principles of nanoparticle design for overcoming biological barriers to drug delivery. *Nature Biotechnology*, *33*(9), 941–951. DOI: 10.1038/nbt.3330 PMID: 26348965

Blanding, W. M., & Gibney, B. C. (2023). Commentary: Neoadjuvant immunotherapy: A brave new world. *The Journal of Thoracic and Cardiovascular Surgery*, *166*(2), 356. DOI: 10.1016/j.jtcvs.2022.12.019 PMID: 36774207

Blasi, P., Giovagnoli, S., Schoubben, A., Puglia, C., Bonina, F., Rossi, C., & Ricci, M. (2011). Lipid nanoparticles for brain targeting I. Formulation optimization. *International Journal of Pharmaceutics*, *419*(1–2), 287–295. DOI: 10.1016/j.ijpharm.2011.07.035 PMID: 21827844

Bleeker, F. E., Molenaar, R. J., & Leenstra, S. (2012). Recent advances in the molecular understanding of glioblastoma. *Journal of Neuro-Oncology, 108*(1), 11–27. DOI: 10.1007/s11060-011-0793-0 PMID: 22270850

Blitz, S. E., Kappel, A. D., Gessler, F. A., Klinger, N. V., Arnaout, O., Lu, Y., Peruzzi, P. P., Smith, T. R., Chiocca, E. A., Friedman, G. K., & Bernstock, J. D. (2022). Tumor-associated macrophages/microglia in glioblastoma oncolytic virotherapy: A double-edged sword. *International Journal of Molecular Sciences, 23*(3), 1808. Advance online publication. DOI: 10.3390/ijms23031808 PMID: 35163730

Bobyk, L., Edouard, M., Deman, P., Vautrin, M., Pernet-Gallay, K., Delaroche, J., Adam, J. F., Estève, F., Ravanat, J. L., & Elleaume, H. (2013). Photoactivation of gold nanoparticles for glioma treatment. *Nanomedicine; Nanotechnology, Biology, and Medicine, 9*(7), 1089–1097. DOI: 10.1016/j.nano.2013.04.007 PMID: 23643529

Bohn, A., Braley, A., Rodriguez de la Vega, P., Zevallos, J. C., & Barengo, N. C. (2018, June 21). The association between race and survival in glioblastoma patients in the US: A retrospective cohort study. *PLoS One, 13*(6), e0198581. DOI: 10.1371/journal.pone.0198581 PMID: 29927955

Bona, N. P., Pedra, N. S., Spohr, L., da Silva dos Santos, F., Saraiva, J. T., Carvalho, F. B., & Stefanello, F. M. (2024). Antitumoral activity of Cecropia pachystachya leaves extract in vitro and in vivo model of rat glioma: Brain and blood effects. *Metabolic Brain Disease, 39*(10), 8234–8252. DOI: 10.1007/s11011-024-01392-6 PMID: 38483655

Bondy, M. L., Scheurer, M. E., Malmer, B., Barnholtz-Sloan, J. S., Davis, F. G., Il'yasova, D., Kruchko, C., McCarthy, B. J., Rajaraman, P., Schwartzbaum, J. A., Sadetzki, S., Schlehofer, B., Tihan, T., Wiemels, J. L., Wrensch, M., & Buffler, P. A. (2008). Brain tumor epidemiology: Consensus from the Brain Tumor EpidemiologyConsortium. *Cancer, 113*(S7), 1953–1968. DOI: 10.1002/cncr.23741 PMID: 18798534

Bonm, A., & Kesari, S. (2021). DNA damage response in glioblastoma: Mechanism for treatment resistance and emerging therapeutic strategies. *Cancer Journal (Sudbury, Mass.), 27*(5), 379–385. DOI: 10.1097/PPO.0000000000000540 PMID: 34570452

Bora, A., Pal, R., Mandi, C. S., & Dutta, S. (2024). DNA abasic sites act as rational therapeutic targets to synergize temozolomide response in both MMR-proficient and deficient cancer. *NAR Cancer, 6*(3), zcae034. DOI: 10.1093/narcan/zcae034 PMID: 39055333

Borovcanin, M. M., Stojanovic, B., Dimitrijevic Stojanovic, M., Stojanovic, B. S., Lazovic, A., & Mitrovic, M. (2024). *Anticancer Properties of Antipsychotic Drugs. p.^pp.* Springer. DOI: 10.1007/16833_2024_394

Bose, P., Dai, Y., & Grant, S. (2014). Histone deacetylase inhibitor (HDACI) mechanisms of action: Emerging insights. *Pharmacology & Therapeutics*, *143*(3), 323–336. DOI: 10.1016/j.pharmthera.2014.04.004 PMID: 24769080

Bostian, A. C., & Eoff, R. L. (2016). Aberrant kynurenine signaling modulates DNA replication stress factors and promotes genomic instability in gliomas. *Chemical Research in Toxicology*, *29*(9), 1369–1380. DOI: 10.1021/acs.chemrestox.6b00255 PMID: 27482758

Bovenkamp, D., Sentosa, R., Rank, E., Erkkilä, M. T., Placzek, F., Püls, J., Ntziachristos, V., & Rühm, A. (2018). Combination of high-resolution optical coherence tomography and Raman spectroscopy for improved staging and grading in bladder cancer. *Applied Sciences (Basel, Switzerland)*, *8*(12), 2371. Advance online publication. DOI: 10.3390/app8122371

Brada, M., Judson, I., Beale, P., Moore, S., Reidenberg, P., Statkevich, P., Dugan, M., Batra, V., & Cutler, D. (1999). Phase I dose-escalation and pharmacokinetic study of temozolomide (SCH 52365) for refractory or relapsing malignancies. *British Journal of Cancer*, *81*(6), 1022–1030. DOI: 10.1038/sj.bjc.6690802 PMID: 10576660

Brandner, S., McAleenan, A., Kelly, C., Spiga, F., Cheng, H.-Y., Dawson, S., Schmidt, L., Faulkner, C. L., Wragg, C., Jefferies, S., Higgins, J. P. T., & Kurian, K. M. (2021). MGMT promoter methylation testing to predict overall survival in people with glioblastoma treated with temozolomide: A comprehensive meta-analysis based on a Cochrane Systematic Review. *Neuro-Oncology*, *23*(9), 1457–1469. DOI: 10.1093/neuonc/noab105 PMID: 34467991

Brar, H. K., Jose, J., Wu, Z., & Sharma, M. (2022). Tyrosine kinase inhibitors for glioblastoma multiforme: Challenges and opportunities for drug delivery. *Pharmaceutics*, *15*(1), 59. DOI: 10.3390/pharmaceutics15010059 PMID: 36678688

Brat, D. J., Prayson, R. A., Ryken, T. C., & Olson, J. J. (2008). Diagnosis of malignant glioma: Role of neuropathology. *Journal of Neuro-Oncology*, *89*(3), 287–311. DOI: 10.1007/s11060-008-9618-1 PMID: 18712282

Brem, H., Piantadosi, S., Burger, P. C., Walker, M., Selker, R., Vick, N. A., Black, K., Sisti, M., Brem, S., Mohr, G., Muller, P., Morawetz, R., & Schold, S. C. (1995). Placebo-controlled trial of safety and efficacy of intraoperative controlled delivery by biodegradable polymers of chemotherapy for recurrent gliomas. *Lancet*, *345*(8956), 1008–1012. DOI: 10.1016/S0140-6736(95)90755-6 PMID: 7723496

Brendsma, D., Krtolica, A., Le Moan, N., Getz, J., Davis, T., Ng, S., Bedard, C., Davis, A., Leung, P., Serwer, L., Tanaka, K., Keating, T., Yan, F., Winger, J., & Cary, S. (2014). GLUTATHIONE PEGYLATED LIPOSOMAL DOXORUBICIN, IN PATIENTS WITH RECURRENT HIGH GRADE GLIOMAS AND BREAST CANCER BRAIN METASTASES. *Neuro-Oncology*, *16*(suppl 2), 2014. DOI: 10.1093/neuonc/nou174.191

Britt, W. J., Rolland, P., & Luster, A.. (2013). Ganciclovir and valganciclovir in the treatment of cytomegalovirus infections. *The Journal of Infectious Diseases*, *208*(5), 730–739. PMID: 23230058

Brown, T. J., Brennan, M. C., Li, M., Church, E. W., Brandmeir, N. J., Rakszawski, K. L., Patel, A. S., Sharma, S., Rizk, E., Florman, J. E., Feletti, A., & Glantz, M. J. (2016). Association of the extent of resection with survival in glioblastoma: A systematic review and meta-analysis. *JAMA Oncology*, *2*(11), 1460–1469. DOI: 10.1001/jamaoncol.2016.1373 PMID: 27310651

Brunner, A. M., Esteve, J., Porkka, K., Knapper, S., Traer, E., Scholl, S., Garcia-Manero, G., Vey, N., Wermke, M., Janssen, J. J. W. M., Narayan, R., Fleming, S., Loo, S., Tovar, N., Kontro, M., Ottmann, O. G., Naidu, P., Sun, H., Han, M., & Wei, A. H. (2024). Phase Ib study of sabatolimab (MBG453), a novel immunotherapy targeting TIM-3 antibody, in combination with decitabine or azacitidine in high- or very high-risk myelodysplastic syndromes. *American Journal of Hematology*, *99*(2), E32–E36. DOI: 10.1002/ajh.27161 PMID: 37994196

Bu, L., Lu, J., Zhang, J., & Wu, J. (2021). Intraoperative cognitive mapping tasks for direct electrical stimulation in clinical and neuroscientific contexts. *Frontiers in Human Neuroscience*, *15*, 612891. Advance online publication. DOI: 10.3389/fnhum.2021.612891 PMID: 33762913

Burström, G., Amini, M., El-Hajj, V. G., Arfan, A., Gharios, M., Buwaider, A., & Edström, E. (2024). Optical methods for brain tumor detection: A systematic review. *Journal of Clinical Medicine*, *13*(9), 2676. Advance online publication. DOI: 10.3390/jcm13092676 PMID: 38731204

Cacciatore, I., Fornasari, E., Marinelli, L., Eusepi, P., Ciulla, M., Ozdemir, O., Tatar, A., Turkez, H., & Di Stefano, A. (2017). Memantine-derived drugs as potential antitumor agents for the treatment of glioblastoma. *European Journal of Pharmaceutical Sciences*, *109*, 402–411. DOI: 10.1016/j.ejps.2017.08.030 PMID: 28860082

Calixto, G. M., Bernegossi, J., De Freitas, L. M., Fontana, C. R., & Chorilli, M. (2016). Nanotechnology-based drug delivery systems for photodynamic therapy of cancer: A review. *Molecules (Basel, Switzerland), 21*(3), 342. Advance online publication. DOI: 10.3390/molecules21030342 PMID: 26978341

Cao, T. Q., Wainwright, D. A., Lee-Chang, C., Miska, J., Sonabend, A. M., Heimberger, A. B., & Lukas, R. V. (2022). Next steps for immunotherapy in glioblastoma. *Cancers (Basel), 14*(16), 4023. Advance online publication. DOI: 10.3390/cancers14164023 PMID: 36011015

Carpentier, A., Canney, M., Vignot, A., Reina, V., Beccaria, K., Horodyckid, C., Karachi, C., Leclercq, D., Lafon, C., Chapelon, J.-Y., Capelle, L., Cornu, P., Sanson, M., Hoang-Xuan, K., Delattre, J.-Y., & Idbaih, A. (2016). Clinical trial of blood-brain barrier disruption by pulsed ultrasound. *Science Translational Medicine, 8*(343), 343re2. Advance online publication. DOI: 10.1126/scitranslmed.aaf6086 PMID: 27306666

Carson, K. A., Grossman, S. A., Fisher, J. D., & Shaw, E. G. (2007). Prognostic factors for survival in adult patients with recurrent glioma enrolled on New Approaches to Brain Tumor Therapy "NABTT" CNS Consortium Phase I and II clinical trials. *Journal of Clinical Oncology, 25*(18), 2601–2606. DOI: 10.1200/JCO.2006.08.1661 PMID: 17577040

Castro, M. P., Sipos, B., Biskup, S., & Kahn, N. (2023). Network-targeting combination therapy of leptomeningeal glioblastoma using multiple synthetic lethal strategies: A case report. *Frontiers in Oncology, 13*, 1210224. Advance online publication. DOI: 10.3389/fonc.2023.1210224 PMID: 38023264

Catania, G., Rodella, G., Vanvarenberg, K., Préat, V., & Malfanti, A. (2023). Combination of hyaluronic acid conjugates with immunogenic cell death inducer and CpG for glioblastoma local chemo-immunotherapy elicits an immune response and induces long-term survival. *Biomaterials, 294*, 122006. Advance online publication. DOI: 10.1016/j.biomaterials.2023.122006 PMID: 36701998

Chaichana, K. L., Garzon-Muvdi, T., Parker, S., Weingart, J. D., Olivi, A., Bennett, R., Brem, H., & Quinones-Hinojosa, A. (2011). Supratentorial glioblastoma multiforme: The role of surgical resection versus biopsy among older patients. *Annals of Surgical Oncology, 18*(1), 239–245. DOI: 10.1245/s10434-010-1242-6 PMID: 20697823

Chakkittukandiyil, A., Chakraborty, S., Kothandan, R., Rymbai, E., Muthu, S. K., Vasu, S., & Sajeev, A. (2024). Side effects based network construction and drug repositioning of ropinirole as a potential molecule for Alzheimer's disease: An in-silico, in-vitro, and in-vivo study. *Journal of Biomolecular Structure & Dynamics*, *42*(20), 10785–10799. DOI: 10.1080/07391102.2023.2258968 PMID: 37723871

Chamberlain, M. C. (2011). Treatment of glioblastoma with bevacizumab: Has a new standard therapy been defined? *CNS Drugs*, *25*(1), 1–4. DOI: 10.2165/11587880-000000000-00000 PMID: 21936584

Chang, Y.-L., Chou, C.-H., Li, Y.-F., Huang, L.-C., Kao, Y., Hueng, D.-Y., & Tsai, C.-K. (2023). Antiproliferative and apoptotic effects of telmisartan in human glioma cells. *Cancer Cell International*, *23*(1), 111. DOI: 10.1186/s12935-023-02963-1 PMID: 37291545

Chan, M.-H., Huang, W.-T., Satpathy, A., Su, T.-Y., Hsiao, M., & Liu, R.-S. (2022). Progress and viewpoints of multifunctional composite nanomaterials for glioblastoma theranostics. *Pharmaceutics*, *14*(2), 456. Advance online publication. DOI: 10.3390/pharmaceutics14020456 PMID: 35214188

Chari, A., Palumbo, A., & Sezer, O.. (2019). Selinexor in patients with relapsed or refractory multiple myeloma. *The New England Journal of Medicine*, *380*(23), 2219–2232. PMID: 31800987

Chatzikonstantinou, G., Ulrich, P., Archavlis, E., Zamboglou, N., Strouthos, I., Zoga, E., Baltas, D., & Tselis, N. (2019). Interstitial high-dose-rate brachytherapy in the primary treatment of inoperable glioblastoma multiforme. *Journal of Contemporary Brachytherapy*, *11*(3), 215–220. DOI: 10.5114/jcb.2019.85722 PMID: 31435428

Chen, S. E., Choi, S. S., Rogers, J. E., Lei, X., & De Groot, J. F. (2014). Isotretinoin maintenance therapy for glioblastoma: A retrospective review. In *Journal of Oncology Pharmacy Practice* (Vol. 20, Issue 2, pp. 112–119). SAGE Publications Ltd. DOI: 10.1177/1078155213483348

Cheng, L., Huang, Z., Zhou, W., & Wu, Q. (2021). Glioblastoma stem cells: Molecular characteristics and targeted therapies. *Frontiers in Oncology*, *11*, 638279. DOI: 10.3389/fonc.2021.638279

Cheng, X., Lou, S., Huang, S., Chen, H., & Liu, J. (2017). Primary spinal cord glioblastoma multiforme: A retrospective study of patients at a single institution. *World Neurosurgery*, *106*, 113–119. DOI: 10.1016/j.wneu.2017.03.120 PMID: 28377242

Cheng, Y., Morshed, R. A., Auffinger, B., Tobias, A. L., & Lesniak, M. S. (2014). Nanomedicine for brain tumor treatment: Overcoming the blood-brain barrier and drug resistance. *Frontiers in Pharmacology*, *5*, 105. DOI: 10.3389/fphar.2014.00105

Chen, J., Larsson, L., Swarbrick, A., & Lundeberg, J. (2024). Spatial landscapes of cancers: Insights and opportunities. *Nature Reviews. Clinical Oncology*, *21*(9), 660–674. DOI: 10.1038/s41571-024-00926-7 PMID: 39043872

Chen, K.-T., Wei, K.-C., & Liu, H.-L. (2021). Focused ultrasound combined with microbubbles in central nervous system applications. *Pharmaceutics*, *13*(7), 1084. DOI: 10.3390/pharmaceutics13071084 PMID: 34371774

Chen, L., Peng, J., Wang, Y., Jiang, H., Wang, W., Dai, J., Tang, M., Wei, Y., Kuang, H., & Xu, G. (2020). Fenofibrate-induced mitochondrial dysfunction and metabolic reprogramming reversal: The anti-tumor effects in gastric carcinoma cells mediated by the PPAR pathway. *American Journal of Translational Research*, *12*, 428. PMID: 32194894

Chen, S., Qiu, Q., Wang, D., She, D., Yin, B., Chai, M., Gu, G., & Chen, J. (2022). Long acting carmustine loaded natural extracellular matrix hydrogel for inhibition of glioblastoma recurrence after tumor resection. *Frontiers of Chemical Science and Engineering*, *16*(4), 536–545. DOI: 10.1007/s11705-021-2067-5

Chen, S., Qiu, Q., Wang, D., She, D., Yin, B., Gu, G., & Chen, J. (2022). Dual-sensitive drug-loaded hydrogel system for local inhibition of post-surgical glioma recurrence. *Journal of Controlled Release*, *349*, 565–579. DOI: 10.1016/j.jconrel.2022.07.011 PMID: 35835399

Chen, W.. (2021). Nanoparticle-Mediated Gene Editing: Progress and Challenges. *Trends in Biotechnology*, *39*(5), 456–469. DOI: 10.1016/j.tibtech.2020.12.002 PMID: 33036785

Chen, X., Li, Y., & Ding, J.. (2015). Quisinostat as an HDAC inhibitor in leukemia treatment. *Cancer Chemotherapy and Pharmacology*, *75*(2), 405–413.

Chen, X., Ma, X., Liu, X., Li, X., Jiang, S., & Zhang, Q. (2022). Origin, activation, and targeted therapy of glioma-associated macrophages. *Frontiers in Immunology*, *13*, 974702. Advance online publication. DOI: 10.3389/fimmu.2022.974702 PMID: 36275720

Chen, X., Wang, J., Liu, S., Han, Q., Zhang, H., & Wu, J. (2025). Research landscape of glioma and inflammation over the past two decades. *Frontiers in Immunology*, *16*, 1605346. Advance online publication. DOI: 10.3389/fimmu.2025.1605346 PMID: 40881678

Chiariello, M., Inzalaco, G., Barone, V., & Gherardini, L. (2023). Overcoming challenges in glioblastoma treatment: Targeting infiltrating cancer cells and harnessing the tumor microenvironment. *Frontiers in Cellular Neuroscience*, *17*, 1327621. Advance online publication. DOI: 10.3389/fncel.2023.1327621 PMID: 38188666

Chien, C.-H., Hsueh, W.-T., Chuang, J.-Y., & Chang, K.-Y. (2019). Role of autophagy in therapeutic resistance of glioblastoma. *Journal of Cancer Metastasis and Treatment*, *5*(66). DOI: 10.20517/2394-4722.2019.016

Chin, M. T., Watters, L., Lynch, G., Cooper, G., Shehan, P., & Seymour, W.. (2008). Imatinib mesylate in glioblastoma: Potential and challenges. *Journal of Neuro-Oncology*, *87*(2), 243–251.

Chiu, C.-F., Guerrero, J. J. G., Regalado, R. R. H., Zhou, J., Notarte, K. I., Lu, Y.-W., Encarnacion, P. C., Carles, C. D. D., Octavo, E. M., Limbaroc, D. C. I., Saengboonmee, C., & Huang, S.-Y. (2024). Insights into Metabolic Reprogramming in Tumor Evolution and Therapy. *Cancers (Basel)*, *16*(20), 3513. DOI: 10.3390/cancers16203513 PMID: 39456607

Choi, B. D., Yu, X., Castano, A. P., Darr, H., Henderson, D. B., Bouffard, A. A., & Maus, M. V. (2019). CRISPR-Cas9 disruption of PD-1 enhances activity of universal EGFRvIII CAR T cells in a preclinical model of human glioblastoma. *Journal for Immunotherapy of Cancer*, *7*(1), 304. Advance online publication. DOI: 10.1186/s40425-019-0806-7 PMID: 31727131

Choueiri, T. K., Motzer, R. J., & Barata, P. C.. (2021). Belzutifan for renal cell carcinoma. *The New England Journal of Medicine*, *384*(9), 907–918. PMID: 33657295

Chua, S. L., Rosenthal, M. A., Wong, S. S., Ashley, D. M., Woods, A. M., Dowling, A., & Cher, L. M. (2004). Phase 2 study of temozolomide and Caelyx in patients with recurrent glioblastoma multiforme. *Neuro-Oncology*, *6*(1), 38–43. DOI: 10.1215/S1152851703000188 PMID: 14769139

Chu, C., Jablonska, A., Gao, Y., Lan, X., Lesniak, W. G., Liang, Y., & Zhang, Y. (2022). Hyperosmolar blood-brain barrier opening using intra-arterial injection of hyperosmotic mannitol in mice under real-time MRI guidance. *Nature Protocols*, *17*(1), 76–94. DOI: 10.1038/s41596-021-00634-x PMID: 34903870

Chung, O. W., Yao, S., Yang, F., Wang, L., Cerda-Smith, C., Hutchinson, H. M., . . . Zou, L. (2025). BRCA1-A and LIG4 complexes mediate ecDNA biogenesis and cancer drug resistance. bioRxiv, 2025.2002. 2018.638901.

Ciechomska, I. A., Jayaprakash, C., Maleszewska, M., & Kaminska, B. (2020). Histone modifying enzymes and chromatin modifiers in glioma pathobiology and therapy responses. *Glioma Signaling*, 259-279.

Clarke, H. J., Chambers, J. E., Liniker, E., & Marciniak, S. J. (2014). Endoplasmic reticulum stress in malignancy. *Cancer Cell, 25*(5), 563–573. DOI: 10.1016/j.ccr.2014.03.015 PMID: 24823636

Clarke, J., Butowski, N., & Chang, S. (2010). Recent advances in therapy for glioblastoma. *Archives of Neurology, 67*(3), 279–283. DOI: 10.1001/archneurol.2010.5 PMID: 20212224

Clay, N. E., Whittenberg, J. J., Leong, J., Kumar, V., Chen, J., Choi, I., & Lee, K.-B. (2017). Chemical and mechanical modulation of polymeric micelle assembly. *Nanoscale, 9*(16), 5194–5204. DOI: 10.1039/C6NR08414A PMID: 28397883

Cloughesy, T. F., Landolfi, J., Vogelbaum, M. A., Ostertag, D., Elder, J. B., Bloomfield, S., Carter, B., Chen, C. C., Kalkanis, S. N., Kesari, S., Lai, A., Lee, I. Y., Liau, L. M., Mikkelsen, T., Nghiemphu, P., Piccioni, D., Accomando, W., Diago, O. R., Hogan, D. J., & Walbert, T. (2018). Durable complete responses in some recurrent high-grade glioma patients treated with Toca 511 + Toca FC. *Neuro-Oncology, 20*(10), 1383–1392. DOI: 10.1093/neuonc/noy075 PMID: 29762717

Correia, A., Monteiro, A., Silva, R., Moreira, J., Lobo, J. S., & Silva, A. (2022). Lipid nanoparticles strategies to modify pharmacokinetics of central nervous system targeting drugs: Crossing or circumventing the blood–brain barrier (BBB) to manage neurological disorders. *Advanced Drug Delivery Reviews, 189*, 114485. DOI: 10.1016/j.addr.2022.114485 PMID: 35970274

Cote, D. J., Balak, N., Brennum, J., Holsgrove, D. T., Kitchen, N., Kolenda, H., & Russell, S. M. (2017). Ethical difficulties in the innovative surgical treatment of patients with recurrent glioblastoma multiforme. *Journal of Neurosurgery, 126*(6), 2045–2050. DOI: 10.3171/2016.11.JNS162488 PMID: 28430037

Cramer, S. W., & Chen, C. C. (2020). Photodynamic therapy for the treatment of glioblastoma. *Frontiers in Surgery, 6*, 81. Advance online publication. DOI: 10.3389/fsurg.2019.00081 PMID: 32039232

Cruz Da Silva, E., Mercier, M. C., Etienne-Selloum, N., Dontenwill, M., & Choulier, L. (2021). A systematic review of glioblastoma-targeted therapies in phases II, III, IV clinical trials. *Cancers (Basel), 13*(8), 1795. Advance online publication. DOI: 10.3390/cancers13081795 PMID: 33918704

Culver, K. W., Davis, O., Lewin, S., Lau, W., Gunter, L., & Morrow, D.. (2010). Phenylacetate in glioblastoma treatment: Preclinical and clinical evaluation. *Journal of Neuro-Oncology*, *96*(3), 401–407. PMID: 19838627

Cunningham, D., Wirth, L. J., Goldberg, R. M., Anthony, K., Pruitt, J., & Pappas, G.. (2011). Vandetanib in the treatment of advanced medullary thyroid cancer. *The Lancet. Oncology*, *12*(1), 111–118.

Curran, W. J.Jr, Scott, C. B., Horton, J., Nelson, J. S., Weinstein, A. S., Fischbach, A. J., Chang, C. H., Rotman, M., Asbell, S. O., Krisch, R. E., & Nelson, D. F. (1993). Recursive partitioning analysis of prognostic factors in three Radiation Therapy Oncology Group malignant glioma trials. *Journal of the National Cancer Institute*, *85*(9), 704–710. DOI: 10.1093/jnci/85.9.704 PMID: 8478956

D'Amico, R. S., Aghi, M. K., Vogelbaum, M. A., & Bruce, J. N. (2021). Convection-enhanced drug delivery for glioblastoma: A review. *Journal of Neuro-Oncology*, *151*(3), 415–427. DOI: 10.1007/s11060-020-03408-9 PMID: 33611708

d'Angelo, M., Castelli, V., Benedetti, E., Antonosante, A., Catanesi, M., Dominguez-Benot, R., & Cimini, A. (2019). Theranostic nanomedicine for malignant gliomas. *Frontiers in Bioengineering and Biotechnology*, *7*, 325. Advance online publication. DOI: 10.3389/fbioe.2019.00325 PMID: 31799246

D'Souza, R., MathEw, M. & SuRapanEni, K.M. (2023). A Scoping Review on the Ethical Issues in the Use of CRISPR-Cas9 in the Creation of Human Disease Models. *Journal of Clinical and Diagnostic Research, 17(12).*

Dalma, S. (2020). Cancer Cell Specific Induction of Endoplasmic Reticulum Stress by Small Molecular Found in the Serum.

Damiati, S., Kompella, U. B., Damiati, S. A., & Kodzius, R. (2018). Microfluidic devices for drug delivery systems and drug screening. *Genes*, *9*(2), 103. Advance online publication. DOI: 10.3390/genes9020103 PMID: 29462948

Davis, M. E. (2016). Glioblastoma: Overview of disease and treatment. *Clinical Journal of Oncology Nursing*, *20*(5, Suppl.), S2–S8. DOI: 10.1188/16.CJON.S1.2-8 PMID: 27668386

De Lima, B. P., Ferraz, L. S., Devalle, S., & Borges, H. L. (2025). Liquid biopsy-derived tumor biomarkers for clinical applications in glioblastoma. *Biomolecules*, *15*(5), 658. Advance online publication. DOI: 10.3390/biom15050658 PMID: 40427551

Degl'Innocenti, A., Di Leo, N., & Ciofani, G. (2020). Genetic hallmarks and heterogeneity of glioblastoma in the single-cell omics era. *Advanced Therapeutics*, *3*(1), 1900152. Advance online publication. DOI: 10.1002/adtp.201900152 PMID: 31942443

Del Bene, M., Osti, D., Faletti, S., Beznoussenko, G. V., DiMeco, F., & Pelicci, G. (2022). Extracellular vesicles: The key for precision medicine in glioblastoma. *Neuro-Oncology*, *24*(2), 184–196. DOI: 10.1093/neuonc/noab229 PMID: 34581817

Delgado-Martín, B., & Medina, M. Á. (2020). Advances in the knowledge of the molecular biology of glioblastoma and its impact in patient diagnosis, stratification, and treatment. *Advancement of Science*, *7*(9), 1902971. DOI: 10.1002/advs.201902971 PMID: 32382477

Della Cuna, G. R., & Paoletti, P. (1976). BCNU and CCNU chemotherapy of tumours of the central nervous system. In Hellmann, K., & Connors, T. A. (Eds.), *Chemotherapy: Cancer chemotherapy II* (pp. 541–549). Springer., DOI: 10.1007/978-1-4613-4352-3_85

Denicolaï, E., Baeza-Kallee, N., Tchoghandjian, A., Carré, M., Colin, C., Jiglaire, C. J., Mercurio, S., Beclin, C., & Figarella-Branger, D. (2014). Proscillaridin A is cytotoxic for glioblastoma cell lines and controls tumor xenograft growth in vivo. *Oncotarget*, *5*(21), 10934–10948. DOI: 10.18632/oncotarget.2541 PMID: 25400117

Di Filippo, L. D., de Carvalho, S. G., Duarte, J. L., Luiz, M. T., Paes Dutra, J. A., de Paula, G. A., & Duarte, M. C. K. H. (2023). A receptor-mediated landscape of druggable and targeted nanomaterials for gliomas. *Materials Today. Bio*, *20*, 100671. Advance online publication. DOI: 10.1016/j.mtbio.2023.100671 PMID: 37273792

Dias, A. P., da Silva Santos, S., da Silva, J. V., Parise-Filho, R., Ferreira, E. I., El Seoud, O., & Giarolla, J. (2020). Dendrimers in the context of nanomedicine. *International Journal of Pharmaceutics*, *573*, 118814. Advance online publication. DOI: 10.1016/j.ijpharm.2019.118814 PMID: 31759101

Dimou, J., Beland, B., & Kelly, J. (2020). Supramaximal resection: A systematic review of its safety, efficacy and feasibility in glioblastoma. *Journal of Clinical Neuroscience*, *72*, 328–334. DOI: 10.1016/j.jocn.2019.12.021 PMID: 31864830

Dirkse, A., Golebiewska, A., Buder, T., Nazarov, P. V., Muller, A., Poovathingal, S., Brons, N. H. C., Leite, S., Sauvageot, N., Sarkisjan, D., Seyfrid, M., Fritah, S., Stieber, D., Michelucci, A., Hertel, F., Herold-Mende, C., Azuaje, F., Skupin, A., Bjerkvig, R., & Niclou, S. P. (2019). Stem cell-associated heterogeneity in Glioblastoma results from intrinsic tumor plasticity shaped by the microenvironment. *Nature Communications*, *10*(1), 1–16. DOI: 10.1038/s41467-019-09853-z PMID: 30992437

Dixon, S., O'connor, A. T., Brooks-Noreiga, C., Clark, M. A., Levy, A., & Castejon, A. M. (2024). Role of renin angiotensin system inhibitors and metformin in Glioblastoma Therapy: A review. *Cancer Chemotherapy and Pharmacology*, *94*(1), 1–23. DOI: 10.1007/s00280-024-04686-0 PMID: 38914751

Do, H. T., Bruelle, C., Pham, D. D., Jauhiainen, M., Eriksson, O., Korhonen, L. T., & Lindholm, D. (2016). Nerve growth factor (NGF) and pro-NGF increase low-density lipoprotein (LDL) receptors in neuronal cells partly by different mechanisms: Role of LDL in neurite outgrowth. *Journal of Neurochemistry*, *136*(2), 306–315. DOI: 10.1111/jnc.13397 PMID: 26484803

Dong, X. (2018). Current strategies for brain drug delivery. *Theranostics*, *8*(6), 1481–1493. DOI: 10.7150/thno.21254 PMID: 29556336

Doyle, D. L., Stockwell, J., Allen, R., Holmes, D., Li, B., & Walker, L.. (2002). Motexafin gadolinium: A photosensitizer for glioblastoma photodynamic therapy. *Journal of Clinical Oncology*, *20*(15), 3916–3922.

Drew, Y., Kim, J.-W., Penson, R. T., O'Malley, D. M., Parkinson, C., Roxburgh, P., & Ferguson, M. (2024). Olaparib plus durvalumab, with or without bevacizumab, as treatment in PARP inhibitor-naïve platinum-sensitive relapsed ovarian cancer: A phase II multicohort study. *Clinical Cancer Research*, *30*(1), 50–62. DOI: 10.1158/1078-0432.CCR-23-2249 PMID: 37939124

Drew, Y., Zenke, F. T., & Curtin, N. J. (2025). DNA damage response inhibitors in cancer therapy: Lessons from the past, current status and future implications. *Nature Reviews. Drug Discovery*, *24*(1), 19–39. DOI: 10.1038/s41573-024-01060-w PMID: 39533099

Drzewiecka, M., Jaśniak, D., Barszczewska-Pietraszek, G., Czarny, P., Kobrzycka, A., Wieczorek, M., Radek, M., Szemraj, J., Skorski, T., & Śliwiński, T. (2023). Class I HDAC Inhibition Leads to a Downregulation of FANCD2 and RAD51, and the Eradication of Glioblastoma Cells. *Journal of Personalized Medicine*, *13*(9), 1315. DOI: 10.3390/jpm13091315 PMID: 37763083

Duan, M., Cao, R., Yang, Y., Chen, X., Liu, L., Ren, B., Wang, L., & Goh, B.-C. (2024). Blood–brain barrier conquest in glioblastoma nanomedicine: Strategies, clinical advances, and emerging challenges. *Cancers (Basel)*, *16*(19), 3300. DOI: 10.3390/cancers16193300 PMID: 39409919

Duarte, Y., Márquez-Miranda, V., Miossec, M. J., & González-Nilo, F. (2019). Integration of target discovery, drug discovery and drug delivery: A review on computational strategies. *Wiley Interdisciplinary Reviews. Nanomedicine and Nanobiotechnology*, *11*(4), e1554. DOI: 10.1002/wnan.1554 PMID: 30932351

Durant, S. T., Zheng, L., Wang, Y., Chen, K., Zhang, L., Zhang, T., . . . Fok, J. H. (2018). The brain-penetrant clinical ATM inhibitor AZD1390 radiosensitizes and improves survival of preclinical brain tumor models. *Science advances, 4*(6), eaat1719.

Du, W., Chen, H., Gróf, I., Lemaitre, L., Bocsik, A., Perdyan, A., Mieczkowski, J., Deli, M. A., Hortobágyi, T., Wan, Q., & Glebov, O. O. (2024). Antidepressant-induced membrane trafficking regulates blood-brain barrier permeability. *Molecular Psychiatry, 29*(11), 3590–3598. DOI: 10.1038/s41380-024-02626-1 PMID: 38816584

Eckert, T., Walton, C., Bell, M., Small, C., Rowland, N. C., Rivers, C., & Mehta, A. (2025). The basis for targeting the tumor macrophage compartment in glioblastoma immunotherapy. *Cancers (Basel), 17*(10), 1631. Advance online publication. DOI: 10.3390/cancers17101631 PMID: 40427130

El Khayari, A., Bouchmaa, N., Taib, B., Wei, Z., Zeng, A., & El Fatimy, R. (2022). Metabolic rewiring in glioblastoma cancer: EGFR, IDH and beyond. *Frontiers in Oncology, 12*, 901951. DOI: 10.3389/fonc.2022.901951 PMID: 35912242

El Kheir, W., Marcos, B., Virgilio, N., Paquette, B., Faucheux, N., & Lauzon, M.-A. (2022). Drug delivery systems in the development of novel strategies for glioblastoma treatment. *Pharmaceutics, 14*(6), 1189. DOI: 10.3390/pharmaceutics14061189 PMID: 35745762

Elashwah, A., Alsuhaibani, A., Alzahrani, A., Azzam, A. Z., Moftah, B., Breakeit, M., Alharbi, A., & Alshaikh, A. (2023). The use of intraoperative radiation therapy (IORT) in multimodality management of cancer patients: A single institution experience. *Journal of Gastrointestinal Cancer, 54*(2), 433–441. DOI: 10.1007/s12029-021-00786-9 PMID: 35290599

Eljamel, M. S., Goodman, C., & Moseley, H. (2008). ALA and Photofrin® Fluorescence-guided resection and repetitive PDT in glioblastoma multiforme: A single centre Phase III randomised controlled trial. *Lasers in Medical Science, 23*(4), 361–367. DOI: 10.1007/s10103-007-0494-2 PMID: 17926079

Ellis, H. (2009). Harvey Cushing: A founding father of neurosurgery. *British Journal of Hospital Medicine, 70*(10), 600. DOI: 10.12968/hmed.2009.70.10.44633 PMID: 19966711

Ellor, S. V., Pagano-Young, T. A., & Avgeropoulos, N. G. (2014). Glioblastoma: Background, standard treatment paradigms, and supportive care considerations. *The Journal of Law, Medicine & Ethics, 42*(2), 171–182. DOI: 10.1111/jlme.12133 PMID: 25040381

Elshaer, S. S., Abulsoud, A. I., Fathi, D., Abdelmaksoud, N. M., Zaki, M. B., El-Mahdy, H. A., & Doghish, A. S. (2023). miRNAs role in glioblastoma pathogenesis and targeted therapy: Signaling pathways interplay. *Pathology, Research and Practice, 246*, 154511. Advance online publication. DOI: 10.1016/j.prp.2023.154511 PMID: 37178618

Engels, E. A.. (2005). Cancer risk in people infected with human immunodeficiency virus in the United States. *International Journal of Cancer, 113*(5), 829–835. DOI: 10.1002/ijc.23487 PMID: 15499619

Erasimus, H., Gobin, M., Niclou, S., & Van Dyck, E. (2016). DNA repair mechanisms and their clinical impact in glioblastoma. *Mutation Research/Reviews in Mutation Research, 769*, 19–35. DOI: 10.1016/j.mrrev.2016.05.005 PMID: 27543314

Esemen, Y., Awan, M., Parwez, R., Baig, A., Rahman, S., Masala, I., Franchini, S., & Giakoumettis, D. (2022). Molecular pathogenesis of glioblastoma in adults and future perspectives: A systematic review. *International Journal of Molecular Sciences, 23*(5), 2607. DOI: 10.3390/ijms23052607 PMID: 35269752

Eyler, C. E., & Rich, J. N. (2008). Survival of the fittest: Cancer stem cells in therapeutic resistance and angiogenesis. *Journal of Clinical Oncology, 26*(17), 2839–2845. DOI: 10.1200/JCO.2007.15.1829 PMID: 18539962

Fabel, K., Dietrich, J., Hau, P., Wismeth, C., Winner, B., Przywara, S., Steinbrecher, A., Ullrich, W., & Bogdahn, U. (2001). Long-term stabilization in patients with malignant glioma after treatment with liposomal doxorubicin. *Cancer, 92*(7), 1936–1942. DOI: 10.1002/1097-0142(20011001)92:7<1936::AID-CNCR1712>3.0.CO;2-H PMID: 11745268

Fahrer, J., & Christmann, M. (2023). DNA alkylation damage by nitrosamines and relevant DNA repair pathways. *International Journal of Molecular Sciences, 24*(5), 4684. DOI: 10.3390/ijms24054684 PMID: 36902118

Fang, Y., Li, X., & Tian, R. (2024). Unlocking glioblastoma vulnerabilities with CRISPR-based genetic screening. *International Journal of Molecular Sciences, 25*(11), 5702. DOI: 10.3390/ijms25115702 PMID: 38891890

Fan, R., Chen, C., Mu, M., Chuan, D., Liu, H., Hou, H., Zhang, X., & Wang, J. (2023). Engineering MMP-2 activated nanoparticles carrying B7-H3 bispecific antibodies for ferroptosis-enhanced glioblastoma immunotherapy. *ACS Nano, 17*(10), 9126–9139. DOI: 10.1021/acsnano.2c12217 PMID: 37097811

Fan, Y., Nguyen, D. T., Akay, Y., Xu, F., & Akay, M. (2016). Engineering a Brain Cancer Chip for High-throughput Drug Screening. *Scientific Reports*, *6*(1), 25062. Advance online publication. DOI: 10.1038/srep25062 PMID: 27151082

Farahani, S., Hejazi, M., Tabassum, M., Ieva, A. D., Mahdavifar, N., & Liu, S. (2024). Diagnostic performance of deep learning for predicting gliomas' IDH and 1p/19q status in MRI: A systematic review and meta-analysis. arXiv. Retrieved May 17, 2025, from https://arxiv.org/abs/2411.02426

Fayaz, A., Aziz, T., & Qadir, M.. (2016). Levetiracetam in glioblastoma: A potential neuroprotective agent. *Journal of Neuro-Oncology*, *128*(2), 205–212.

Feldman, L. (2024). Hypoxia within the glioblastoma tumor microenvironment: A master saboteur of novel treatments. *Frontiers in Immunology*, *15*, 1384249. Advance online publication. DOI: 10.3389/fimmu.2024.1384249 PMID: 38994360

Ferrara, N., & Kerbel, R. S. (2018). Angiogenesis in Glioblastoma. *The New England Journal of Medicine*, *373*(17), 1657–1665. DOI: 10.1056/NEJMra1614713 PMID: 30354954

Ferreira, P. M. P., de Sousa, R. W. R., de Oliveira Ferreira, J. R., Militão, G. C. G., & Bezerra, D. P. (2021). Chloroquine and hydroxychloroquine in antitumor therapies based on autophagy-related mechanisms. *Pharmacological Research*, *168*, 105582. DOI: 10.1016/j.phrs.2021.105582 PMID: 33775862

Ferreira, T., Kulkarni, A., Bretscher, C., Nazarov, P. V., Hossain, J. A., Ystaas, L. A. R., Miletic, H., Röth, R., Niesler, B., & Marchini, A. (2022). Oncolytic H-1 Parvovirus Hijacks Galectin-1 to Enter Cancer Cells. *Viruses*, *14*(5), 1018. DOI: 10.3390/v14051018 PMID: 35632759

Fiedler, T., Strauss, M., Hering, S., Redanz, U., William, D., Rosche, Y., & Podbielski, A. (2015). Arginine deprivation by arginine deiminase of Streptococcus pyogenes controls primary glioblastoma growth in vitro and in vivo. *Cancer Biology & Therapy*, *16*(7), 1047–1055. DOI: 10.1080/15384047.2015.1026478 PMID: 25774632

Filipczak, N., Yalamarty, S. S. K., Li, X., Parveen, F., & Torchilin, V. (2021). Developments in treatment methodologies using dendrimers for infectious diseases. *Molecules (Basel, Switzerland)*, *26*(11), 3304. Advance online publication. DOI: 10.3390/molecules26113304 PMID: 34072765

Fiorica, F., Tebano, U., Napoli, G., Franceschetto, A., Muraro, M., Giorgi, C., & Pinton, P. (2024). Metabolic-Modulating Effects of Radiation: Undetectable Yet Deadly—A Review on Radiotherapy. *Cancers (Basel)*, *17*(1), 54. DOI: 10.3390/cancers17010054 PMID: 39796683

Fondaj, D., Arduino, I., Lopedota, A. A., Denora, N., & Iacobazzi, R. M. (2023). Exploring the Microfluidic Production of Biomimetic Hybrid Nanoparticles and Their Pharmaceutical Applications. *Pharmaceutics, 15*(7), 1953. Advance online publication. DOI: 10.3390/pharmaceutics15071953 PMID: 37514139

Francisco, K. K. Y., Apuhin, A. E. C., Tan, M. J. T., Byers, M. C., Maravilla, N. M. A. T., Karim, H. A., & AlDahoul, N. (2024) Can Personalized Medicine Coexist with Health Equity? Examining the Cost Barrier and Ethical Implications. *arXiv preprint arXiv:241102307.*

Friedman, H. S., Reardon, D. A., Mellinger, G., Sherwood, L., McAllister, L., & Caswell, P.. (2010). Rubitecan: A novel treatment for glioblastoma. *Journal of Clinical Oncology, 28*(4), 670–675.

Friedmann-Morvinski, D. (2014). Glioblastoma heterogeneity and cancer cell plasticity. *Critical Reviews in Oncogenesis, 19*(5), 327–336. DOI: 10.1615/CritRevOncog.2014011777 PMID: 25404148

Fuentes-Fayos, A. C., García-García, M. E., Pérez-Gómez, J. M., Montero-Hidalgo, A. J., Martín-Colom, J., Doval-Rosa, C., & Luque, R. M. (2023). Metformin and simvastatin exert additive antitumour effects in glioblastoma via senescence-state: Clinical and translational evidence. *EBioMedicine, 90*, 104519. Advance online publication. DOI: 10.1016/j.ebiom.2023.104484 PMID: 36907105

Fukuta, T., Shaha, S., da Silva-Candal, A., Zhao, Z., & Mitragotri, S. (2025). Cell therapies against brain tumors: Clinical development and emerging prospects. *Bioengineering & Translational Medicine, 10*(5), 70018. DOI: 10.1002/btm2.70018 PMID: 41030289

Fuloria, N. K., Malviya, R., Verma, S., & Balusamy, B. (2023). *Big Data in Oncology: Impact, Challenges, and Risk Assessment*. CRC Press. DOI: 10.1201/9781003442639

Funakoshi, Y., Hata, N., Kuga, D., Hatae, R., Sangatsuda, Y., Fujioka, Y., Takigawa, K., Mizoguchi, M., & Iihara, K. (2020). Update on chemotherapeutic approaches and management of bevacizumab usage for glioblastoma. *Pharmaceuticals (Basel, Switzerland), 13*(12), 470. Advance online publication. DOI: 10.3390/ph13120470 PMID: 33339404

Fu, S. W., Tang, C., Tan, X., & Srivastava, S. (2024). Liquid biopsy for early cancer detection: Technological revolutions and clinical dilemma. *Expert Review of Molecular Diagnostics, 24*(10), 937–955. DOI: 10.1080/14737159.2024.2408744 PMID: 39360748

Fusco, W., Lorenzo, M. B., Cintoni, M., Porcari, S., Rinninella, E., Kaitsas, F., Lener, E., Mele, M. C., Gasbarrini, A., Collado, M. C., Cammarota, G., & Ianiro, G. (2023). Short-chain fatty-acid-producing bacteria: Key components of the human gut microbiota. *Nutrients*, *15*(9), 2211. DOI: 10.3390/nu15092211 PMID: 37432351

Gaballu, F. A., Dehghan, G., Ghaffaria, M., Yekta, R., Abbaspour-Ravasjanid, S., Baradarana, B., Ezzati, J., Dolatabadie, N., & Hamblinf, M. R. (2017). PAMAM dendrimers as efficient drug and gene delivery nanosystems for cancer therapy. *Applied Materials Today*, *176*(3), 139–148. DOI: 10.1002/hep.30150.Ductular

Gallo, M., Coutinho, F. J., Vanner, R. J., Gayden, T., Mack, S. C., Murison, A., Remke, M., Li, R., Takayama, N., Desai, K., Lee, L., Lan, X., Park, N. I., Barsyte-Lovejoy, D., Smil, D., Sturm, D., Kushida, M. M., Head, R., Cusimano, M. D., & Dirks, P. B. (2015). MLL5 orchestrates a cancer self-renewal state by repressing the histone variant H3.3 and globally reorganizing chromatin. *Cancer Cell*, *28*(5), 715–729. DOI: 10.1016/j.ccell.2015.10.005 PMID: 26626085

Gangwal, A., Ansari, A., Ahmad, I., Azad, A. K., & Sulaiman, W. M. A. W. (2024). Current strategies to address data scarcity in artificial intelligence-based drug discovery: A comprehensive review. *Computers in Biology and Medicine*, *179*, 108734. DOI: 10.1016/j.compbiomed.2024.108734 PMID: 38964243

Gan, Y., Yu, Y., Xu, H., & Piao, H. (2024). Liposomal Nanomaterials: A Rising Star in Glioma Treatment. *International Journal of Nanomedicine*, *19*(June), 6757–6776. DOI: 10.2147/IJN.S470478 PMID: 38983132

Gawel, A. M., Singh, R., & Debinski, W. (2022). Metal-Based Nanostructured Therapeutic Strategies for Glioblastoma Treatment—An Update. *Biomedicines*, *10*(7), 1–31. DOI: 10.3390/biomedicines10071598 PMID: 35884903

Gentner, B., Finocchiaro, G., Farina, F., Eoli, M., Alessia, C., Anghileri, E., Antonarelli, G., Barcella, M., Bruzzone, M. G., Carrabba, M. G., Cuccarini, V., D'Alessandris, G., Di Meco, F., Ferla, V., Ferroli, P., Gagliardi, F., Garramone, M., Legnani, F., Mortini, P., & Ciceri, F. (2021). TEM-GBM: An Open-Label, Phase I/IIa Dose-Escalation Study Evaluating the Safety and Efficacy of Genetically Modified Tie-2 Expressing Monocytes to Deliver IFN-α within Glioblastoma Tumor Microenvironment. *Blood*, *138*(Supplement 1), 2844–2844. DOI: 10.1182/blood-2021-150230

Ge, Y.-F., Sun, J., Jin, C.-J., Cao, B.-Q., Jiang, Z.-F., & Shao, J.-F. (2013). AntagomiR-27a targets FOXO3a in glioblastoma and suppresses U87 cell growth in vitro and in vivo. *Asian Pacific Journal of Cancer Prevention : APJCP*, *14*(2), 963–968. DOI: 10.7314/APJCP.2013.14.2.963 PMID: 23621269

Ghaznavi, H., Afzalipour, R., Khoei, S., Sargazi, S., Shirvalilou, S., & Sheervalilou, R. (2024). New insights into targeted therapy of glioblastoma using smart nanoparticles. *Cancer Cell International*, *24*(1), 160. Advance online publication. DOI: 10.1186/s12935-024-03331-3 PMID: 38715021

Gherardini, L., Vetri Buratti, V., Maturi, M., Inzalaco, G., Locatelli, E., Sambri, L., & Comes Franchini, M. (2023). Loco-regional treatment with temozolomide-loaded thermogels prevents glioblastoma recurrences in orthotopic human xenograft models. *Communications Biology*, *6*(1), 4630. Advance online publication. DOI: 10.1038/s42003-023-04630-5 PMID: 36944737

Ghosh, B., & Biswas, S. (2021). Polymeric micelles in cancer therapy: State of the art. *Journal of Controlled Release*, *332*, 127–147. DOI: 10.1016/j.jconrel.2021.02.016 PMID: 33609621

Ghosh, N., & Modak, S. (2021). What governance lesson does Mekong bear for Ganges–Brahmaputra–Meghna (GBM) basin? *Journal of Asian Economic Integration*, *3*(2), 211–234. DOI: 10.1177/26316846211038421

Gibson, V. P., Tahiri, H., Yang, C., Phan, Q. T., Banquy, X., & Hardy, P. J. (2023). Hyaluronan decorated layer-by-layer assembled lipid nanoparticles for miR-181a delivery in glioblastoma treatment. *International Journal of Pharmaceutics*, *302*, 122341. Advance online publication. DOI: 10.1016/j.ijpharm.2023.122341 PMID: 37778056

Giese, A., Bjerkvig, R., Berens, M. E., & Westphal, M. (2003). Cost of migration: Invasion of malignant gliomas and implications for treatment. *Journal of Clinical Oncology*, *21*(8), 1624–1636. DOI: 10.1200/JCO.2003.05.063 PMID: 12697889

Ginat, D. T. (2022). 1,3-Bis(2-chloroethyl)-1-nitrosourea (BCNU; carmustine) polymer wafer (Gliadel). In Ginat, D. T., Small, J. E., & Schaefer, P. W. (Eds.), *Neuroimaging pharmacopoeia* (pp. 141–148). Springer., DOI: 10.1007/978-3-031-08774-5_18

Giordano, R. J.. (2019). Integrin-targeted therapies for glioblastoma: New directions and challenges. *Molecular Cancer Therapeutics*, *18*(9), 1424–1432. DOI: 10.1158/1535-7163.MCT-18-0736

Giordano, R. J., Cardó-Vila, M., Lahdenranta, J., Pasqualini, R., & Arap, W. (2001). From combinatorial peptide selection to drug prototype [Review]. *Nature Reviews. Drug Discovery*, *1*(1), 68–76. DOI: 10.1038/35095083

Glaser, T., Han, I., Wu, L., & Zeng, X. (2017). Targeted nanotechnology in glioblastoma multiforme. *Frontiers in Pharmacology, 8*(MAR), 238646. DOI: 10.3389/FPHAR.2017.00166/PD PMID: 28408882

Goenka, A., Tiek, D., Song, X., Huang, T., Hu, B., & Cheng, S.-Y. (2021). The many facets of therapy resistance and tumor recurrence in glioblastoma. *Cells, 10*(3), 484. DOI: 10.3390/cells10030484 PMID: 33668200

Gong, Z., Zhou, D., Wu, D., Han, Y., Yu, H., Shen, H., Feng, W., Hou, L., Chen, Y., & Xu, T. (2025). Challenges and material innovations in drug delivery to central nervous system tumors. *Biomaterials, 319*, 123180. Advance online publication. DOI: 10.1016/j.biomaterials.2025.123180 PMID: 39985979

Gordon, M. S., Prager, D., Robbins, K., Yao, J., Dietrich, P., & Lee, L.. (2011). Sagopilone in the treatment of glioblastoma: Preclinical and clinical studies. *Journal of Clinical Oncology, 29*(14), 1842–1848.

Gostimskaya, I. (2022). CRISPR–Cas9: A history of its discovery and ethical considerations of its use in genome editing. *Biochemistry (Moscow), 87*(8), 777–788. DOI: 10.1134/S0006297922080090 PMID: 36171658

Gousias, K., Theocharous, T., & Simon, M. (2022). Mechanisms of cell cycle arrest and apoptosis in glioblastoma. *Biomedicines, 10*(3), 564. DOI: 10.3390/biomedicines10030564 PMID: 35327366

Gozdz, A. (2023). Proteasome inhibitors against glioblastoma—Overview of molecular mechanisms of cytotoxicity, progress in clinical trials, and perspective for use in personalized medicine. *Current Oncology (Toronto, Ont.), 30*(11), 9676–9688. DOI: 10.3390/curroncol30110702 PMID: 37999122

Gregory, J. V., Kadiyala, P., Doherty, R., Cadena, M., Habeel, S., Ruoslahti, E., Lowenstein, P. R., Castro, M. G., & Lahann, J. (2020). Systemic brain tumor delivery of synthetic protein nanoparticles for glioblastoma therapy. *Nature Communications, 11*(1), 5687. Advance online publication. DOI: 10.1038/s41467-020-19225-7 PMID: 33173024

Grochans, S., Cybulska, A. M., Simińska, D., Korbecki, J., Kojder, K., Chlubek, D., & Baranowska-Bosiacka, I. (2022). Epidemiology of Glioblastoma Multiforme-Literature Review. *Cancers (Basel), 14*(10), 2412. Advance online publication. DOI: 10.3390/cancers14102412 PMID: 35626018

Groth, P., Ausländer, S., Majumder, M. M., Schultz, N., Johansson, F., Petermann, E., & Helleday, T. (2010). Methylated DNA causes a physical block to replication forks independently of damage signaling, O6-methylguanine or DNA single-strand breaks and results in DNA damage. *Journal of Molecular Biology*, *402*(1), 70–82. DOI: 10.1016/j.jmb.2010.07.010 PMID: 20643142

Gruden, Š., & Poklar Ulrih, N. (2021). Diverse mechanisms of antimicrobial activities of lactoferrins, lactoferricins, and other lactoferrin-derived peptides. *International Journal of Molecular Sciences*, *22*(20), 11264. Advance online publication. DOI: 10.3390/ijms222011264 PMID: 34681923

Grzegorzewski, J., Michalak, M., Wołoszczuk, M., Bulicz, M., & Majchrzak-Celińska, A. (2025). Nanotherapy of glioblastoma—Where hope grows. *International Journal of Molecular Sciences*, *26*(5), 1814. Advance online publication. DOI: 10.3390/ijms26051814 PMID: 40076445

Guerrero-Cázares, H., Tzeng, S. Y., Young, N. P., Abutaleb, A. O., Quiñones-Hinojosa, A., & Green, J. J. (2014). Biodegradable polymeric nanoparticles show high efficacy and specificity at DNA delivery to human glioblastoma in vitro and in vivo. *ACS Nano*, *8*(5), 5141–5153. DOI: 10.1021/nn501197v PMID: 24766032

Gugu M (2023) Pivotal role of cyclooxygenase 2 (COX-2) in temozolomide-resistance of glioblastoma cell lines.

Guo, Q. L., Dai, X. L., Yin, M. Y., Cheng, H. W., Qian, H. S., Wang, H., Chen, D. W., & Zhang, X. (2022). Nanosensitizers for sonodynamic therapy for glioblastoma multiforme: Current progress and future perspectives. *Military Medical Research*, *9*(1), 26. Advance online publication. DOI: 10.1186/s40779-022-00386-z PMID: 35676737

Guo, X., Gu, L., Li, Y., Zheng, Z., Chen, W., Wang, Y., & Zhang, J. (2023). Histological and molecular glioblastoma, IDH-wildtype: A real-world landscape using the 2021 WHO classification of central nervous system tumors. *Frontiers in Oncology*, *13*, 1200815. Advance online publication. DOI: 10.3389/fonc.2023.1200815 PMID: 37483487

Guo, X., Yang, X., Wu, J., Yang, H., Li, Y., Li, J., Liu, Q., Wu, C., Xing, H., Liu, P., Wang, Y., Hu, C., & Ma, W. (2022). Tumor-Treating Fields in Glioblastomas: Past, Present, and Future. *Cancers (Basel)*, *14*(15), 3669. DOI: 10.3390/cancers14153669 PMID: 35954334

Gupta, S., Kumar, A., Patel, R., & Kumar, V. (2021). Genetically modified crop regulations: Scope and opportunity using the CRISPR-Cas9 genome editing approach. *Molecular Biology Reports*, *48*(5), 4851–4863. DOI: 10.1007/s11033-021-06477-9 PMID: 34114124

Gyimesi, G., & Hediger, M. A. (2023). Transporter-mediated drug delivery. *Molecules (Basel, Switzerland)*, *28*(3), 1151. DOI: 10.3390/molecules28031151 PMID: 36770817

Hai, J., Xavier, S., George, S., Engstrom, L., Olson, P., Simpson, T. et al. (2024). Abstract B011: MTA-cooperative PRMT5 inhibition (BMS-986504) induces *MTAP* del tumor cell-intrinsic immune evasion and regulation. *Cancer Immunol Res* 1, 12 (10_Supplement): B011. https://doi.org/DOI: 10.1158/2326-6074.TUMIMM24-B011

Hailozian, C., Luftig, J., Liang, A., Outhay, M., Ullal, M., Anderson, E. S., Kalmin, M., Shoptaw, S., Greenwald, M. K., & Herring, A. A. (2022). Synergistic effect of ketamine and buprenorphine observed in the treatment of buprenorphine precipitated opioid withdrawal in a patient with fentanyl use. *Journal of Addiction Medicine*, *16*(4), 483–487. Advance online publication. DOI: 10.1097/ADM.0000000000000929 PMID: 34789683

Hamad, A., Yusubalieva, G. M., Baklaushev, V. P., Chumakov, P. M., & Lipatova, A. V. (2023). Recent developments in glioblastoma therapy: Oncolytic viruses and emerging future strategies. *Viruses*, *15*(2), 547. Advance online publication. DOI: 10.3390/v15020547 PMID: 36851761

Hambardzumyan, D., Gutmann, D. H., & Kettenmann, H. (2016). The role of microglia and macrophages in glioma maintenance and progression. *Nature Neuroscience*, *19*(1), 20–27. DOI: 10.1038/nn.4185 PMID: 26713745

Hamilton, A. J., Seid, J., Verdecchia, K., & Chuba, P. (2018). Abscopal Effect after Radiosurgery for Solitary Brain Metastasis from Non-small Cell Lung Cancer. *Cureus*, *10*(12). Advance online publication. DOI: 10.7759/cureus.3777 PMID: 30854265

Han, S., Liu, Y., Cai, S. J., Qian, M., Ding, J., Larion, M., Gilbert, M. R., & Yang, C. (2020). IDH mutation in glioma: Molecular mechanisms and potential therapeutic targets. *British Journal of Cancer*, *122*(11), 1580–1589. DOI: 10.1038/s41416-020-0814-x PMID: 32291392

Hao, X., Bahia, R. K., Cseh, O., Bozek, D. A., Blake, S., Rinnenthal, J., & McDermott, D. F. (2023). BI-907828, a novel potent MDM2 inhibitor, inhibits glioblastoma brain tumor stem cells in vitro and prolongs survival in orthotopic xenograft mouse models. *Neuro-Oncology*, *25*(5), 913–926. DOI: 10.1093/neuonc/noac271 PMID: 36521007

Haqqani, A. S., Bélanger, K., & Stanimirovic, D. B. (2024). Receptor-mediated transcytosis for brain delivery of therapeutics: Receptor classes and criteria. *Frontiers in Drug Delivery*, *4*, 1360302. DOI: 10.3389/fddev.2024.1360302 PMID: 40836978

Haque, S., Norbert, C. C., Acharyya, R., Mukherjee, S., Kathirvel, M., & Patra, C. R. (2021). Biosynthesized silver nanoparticles for cancer therapy and in vivo bioimaging. *Cancers (Basel)*, *13*(23), 6114. Advance online publication. DOI: 10.3390/cancers13236114 PMID: 34885224

Hardaker, E. L., Sanseviero, E., Karmokar, A., Taylor, D., Milo, M., Michaloglou, C., & Solanki, A. (2024). The ATR inhibitor ceralasertib potentiates cancer checkpoint immunotherapy by regulating the tumor microenvironment. *Nature Communications*, *15*(1), 1700. DOI: 10.1038/s41467-024-45996-4 PMID: 38402224

Harilal, S., Jose, J., Kumar, R., Unnikrishnan, M. K., Uddin, M. S., Mathew, G. E., Pratap, R., Marathakam, A., & Mathew, B. (2020). Revisiting the blood-brain barrier: A hard nut to crack in the transportation of drug molecules. *Brain Research Bulletin*, *160*, 121–140. DOI: 10.1016/j.brainresbull.2020.03.018 PMID: 32315731

Harris, J. D., White, C., & Sutter, D.. (2005). Poly ICLC: An immune adjuvant for cancer and infectious diseases. *The Journal of Immunology : Official Journal of the American Association of Immunologists*, *174*(6), 3767–3775.

Hart, M. G., Garside, R., Rogers, G., Stein, K., & Grant, R. (2013). Temozolomide for high grade glioma. *Cochrane Database of Systematic Reviews*, *4*(9), CD007415. Advance online publication. DOI: 10.1002/14651858.CD007415.pub2 PMID: 23633341

Hasegawa, K., Saga, R., & Hosokawa, Y. (2023). Radiotherapeutic review: Acquisition of radioresistance and cancer stem cell properties via irradiation. *Radiation Environment and Medicine*, *12*(1), 25–36.

Haslam, A., & Prasad, V. (2019). Estimation of the percentage of US patients with cancer who are eligible for and respond to checkpoint inhibitor immunotherapy drugs. *JAMA Network Open*, *2*(5), e192535. Advance online publication. DOI: 10.1001/jamanetworkopen.2019.2535 PMID: 31050774

Hassanzadeganroudsari, M., Soltani, M., Heydarinasab, A., Apostolopoulos, V., Akbarzadehkhiyavi, A., Nurgali, K., & Mantzorou, M. (2020). Targeted nano-drug delivery system for glioblastoma therapy: In vitro and in vivo study. *Journal of Drug Delivery Science and Technology*, *60*, 102039. Advance online publication. DOI: 10.1016/j.jddst.2020.102039

Hau, P., Fabel, K., Baumgart, U., Rümmele, P., Grauer, O., Bock, A., Dietmaier, C., Dietmaier, W., Dietrich, J., Dudel, C., Hübner, F., Jauch, T., Drechsel, E., Kleiter, I., Wismeth, C., Zellner, A., Brawanski, A., Steinbrecher, A., Marienhagen, J., & Bogdahn, U. (2004). Pegylated Liposomal Doxorubicin-Efficacy in Patients with Recurrent High-Grade Glioma. *Cancer*, *100*(6), 1199–1207. DOI: 10.1002/cncr.20073 PMID: 15022287

Hayashi, C., Ueda, R., & Tasaki, A. (1997). *Ultra-fine particles: Exploratory science and technology*. Noyes Publications.

Hazafa, A., Mumtaz, M., Farooq, M. F., Bilal, S., Chaudhry, S. N., Firdous, M., Naeem, M., Ullah, M. O., Yameen, M., Mukhtiar, M. S., & Zafar, F. (2020). CRISPR/Cas9: A powerful genome editing technique for the treatment of cancer cells with present challenges and future directions. *Life Sciences*, *263*, 118525. Advance online publication. DOI: 10.1016/j.lfs.2020.118525 PMID: 33031826

Hegi, M. E., Diserens, A.-C., Gorlia, T., Hamou, M.-F., de Tribolet, N., Weller, M., Kros, J. M., Hainfellner, J. A., Mason, W., Mariani, L., Bromberg, J. E. C., Hau, P., Mirimanoff, R. O., Cairncross, J. G., Janzer, R. C., & Stupp, R. (2005). MGMT gene silencing and benefit from temozolomide in glioblastoma. *The New England Journal of Medicine*, *352*(10), 997–1003. DOI: 10.1056/NEJMoa043331 PMID: 15758010

Helson, L. (2018). Radiation-induced Demyelination and Remyelination in the Central Nervous System: A Literature Review. *Anticancer Research*, *38*(9), 4999–5002. DOI: 10.21873/anticanres.12818 PMID: 30194143

Henssen, D., Meijer, F., Verburg, F. A., & Smits, M. (2023). Challenges and opportunities for advanced neuroimaging of glioblastoma. *The British Journal of Radiology*, *96*(1141), 20211232. Advance online publication. DOI: 10.1259/bjr.20211232 PMID: 36062962

Herbrecht, R., Barlogie, B., Legrand, O., Duong, J., Blin, N., & Alizadeh, A.. (2007). Posaconazole for the prevention of fungal infections in immunocompromised patients. *The New England Journal of Medicine*, *356*(4), 348–359. PMID: 17251531

Her, S., Jaffray, D. A., & Allen, C. (2017). Gold nanoparticles for applications in cancer radiotherapy: Mechanisms and recent advancements. *Advanced Drug Delivery Reviews*, *109*, 84–101. DOI: 10.1016/j.addr.2015.12.012 PMID: 26712711

He, S., Cen, B., Liao, L., Wang, Z., Qin, Y., Wu, Z., & Zhang, Z. (2017). A tumor-targeting cRGD-EGFR siRNA conjugate and its anti-tumor effect on glioblastoma in vitro and in vivo. *Drug Delivery*, *24*(1), 471–481. DOI: 10.1080/10717544.2016.1267821 PMID: 28181832

He, Y.. (2020). Nanoparticles for Efficient Gene Delivery in Cancer Therapy. *Frontiers in Pharmacology*, *11*, 585917. DOI: 10.3389/fphar.2020.585917

Holdhoff, M., Sahebjam, S., Huang, P., Kamson, D. O., Iacoboni, M., Dobson-brown, T., Schreck, K. C., Kleinberg, L., Redmond, K. J., Croog, V. J., Kut, C., Ozer, B., Grossman, S. A., Comas, M., Plehn, J., Fisher, J. D., & Sordillo, P. P. (2025). Liposomal curcumin and standard radiation and temozolomide for newly diagnosed high-grade gliomas : A phase 1 / 2 study. *Journal of Clinical Oncology*, *5768919*(16_suppl). Advance online publication. DOI: 10.1200/JCO.2025.43.16_suppl.TPS2095

Holzgreve, A., Biczok, A., Ruf, V. C., Liesche-Starnecker, F., Steiger, K., Kirchner, M. A., Unterrainer, M., Mittlmeier, L., Herms, J., Schlegel, J., Bartenstein, P., Tonn, J.-C., Albert, N. L., & Suchorska, B. (2021). PSMA Expression in Glioblastoma as a Basis for Theranostic Approaches: A Retrospective, Correlational Panel Study Including Immunohistochemistry, Clinical Parameters and PET Imaging. *Frontiers in Oncology*, *11*, 646387. Advance online publication. DOI: 10.3389/fonc.2021.646387 PMID: 33859946

Hoosemans, L., Vooijs, M., & Hoeben, A. (2024). Opportunities and challenges of small molecule inhibitors in glioblastoma treatment: Lessons learned from clinical trials. *Cancers (Basel)*, *16*(17), 3021. Advance online publication. DOI: 10.3390/cancers16173021 PMID: 39272879

Horta, M., Soares, P., Leite Pereira, C., & Lima, R. T. (2025). Emerging approaches in glioblastoma treatment: Modulating the extracellular matrix through nanotechnology. *Pharmaceutics*, *17*(2), 142. Advance online publication. DOI: 10.3390/pharmaceutics17020142 PMID: 40006509

Houweling, M., Abdul, U., Brahm, C., Lagerweij, T., Heukelom, S., Koken, P., & Verheul, H. M. W. (2023). Radio-sensitizing effect of MEK inhibition in glioblastoma in vitro and in vivo. *Journal of Neuro-Oncology*, *149*(1), 297–305. DOI: 10.1007/s11060-023-04362-8 PMID: 36451044

Houweling, M., Giczewska, A., Abdul, K., Nieuwenhuis, N., Küçükosmanoglu, A., Pastuszak, K., & French, P. J. (2023). Screening of predicted synergistic multi-target therapies in glioblastoma identifies new treatment strategies. *Neuro-Oncology Advances*, *5*(1), vdad073. Advance online publication. DOI: 10.1093/noajnl/vdad073 PMID: 37455945

Huang, D., Sun, L., Huang, L., & Chen, Y. (2021). Nanodrug delivery systems modulate tumor vessels to increase the enhanced permeability and retention effect. *Journal of Personalized Medicine*, *11*(2), 124. DOI: 10.3390/jpm11020124 PMID: 33672813

Huang, R.. (2021). Platelet-derived growth factor receptor signaling in Glioblastoma and its therapeutic targeting. *Journal of Neuro-Oncology*, *153*(2), 231–245. DOI: 10.1007/s11060-021-03753-7 PMID: 33206309

Huang, S., & Zhineng, J. (2011). Sinicrope Inhibition of mTOR Kinase by AZD8055 Can Antagonize Chemotherapy-induced Cell Death through Autophagy Induction and Down-regulation of p62/Sequestosome 1. *The Journal of Biological Chemistry*, *286*(46), 40002–40012. DOI: 10.1074/jbc.M111.297432 PMID: 21949121

Hudes, G., Armstrong, D., Fong, L., Dutcher, J., Figlin, R., & Kapoor, A.. (2007). Temsirolimus, an mTOR inhibitor, in advanced renal cell carcinoma. *The New England Journal of Medicine*, *356*(2), 245–252.

Hu, H., Mu, Q., Bao, Z., Chen, Y., Liu, Y., Chen, J., Wang, K., Wang, Z., Nam, Y., Jiang, B., Sa, J. K., Cho, H.-J., Her, N.-G., Zhang, C., Zhao, Z., Zhang, Y., Zeng, F., Wu, F., Kang, X., & Jiang, T. (2018). Mutational landscape of secondary glioblastoma guides MET-targeted trial in brain tumor. *Cell*, *175*(6), 1665–1678. DOI: 10.1016/j.cell.2018.09.038 PMID: 30343896

Hu, M., Ge, X., Chen, X., Mao, W., Qian, X., & Yuan, W. E. (2020). Micro/nanorobot: A promising targeted drug delivery system. *Pharmaceutics*, *12*(7), 665. Advance online publication. DOI: 10.3390/pharmaceutics12070665 PMID: 32679772

Hunt, W. A., Barnett, B., & O'Hara, M.. (2010). The role of disulfiram in the treatment of alcoholism. *The American Journal of Psychiatry*, *167*(5), 581–589.

Hu, Z., Ott, P. A., & Wu, C. J. (2018). Towards personalized, tumour-specific, therapeutic vaccines for cancer. *Nature Reviews. Immunology*, *18*(3), 168–182. DOI: 10.1038/nri.2017.131 PMID: 29226910

Ibrahim, R. S., Ibrahim, S. S., El-Naas, A., Koklesová, L., Kubatka, P., & Büsselberg, D. (2023). Could metformin and resveratrol support glioblastoma treatment? A mechanistic view at the cellular level. *Cancers (Basel)*, *15*(13), 3368. Advance online publication. DOI: 10.3390/cancers15133368 PMID: 37444478

Illum, L. (2000). Transport of drugs from the nasal cavity to the central nervous system. *European Journal of Pharmaceutical Sciences*, *11*(1), 1–18. DOI: 10.1016/S0928-0987(00)00087-7 PMID: 10913748

Incekara, F., Smits, M., Van der Voort, S. R., Dubbink, H. J., Atmodimedjo, P. N., Kros, J. M., Vincent, A. J. P. E., & van den Bent, M. (2020). The association between the extent of glioblastoma resection and survival in light of MGMT promoter methylation in 326 patients with newly diagnosed IDH-wildtype glioblastoma. *Frontiers in Oncology*, *10*, 1087. DOI: 10.3389/fonc.2020.01087 PMID: 32766140

Ip, K. L., Thomas, M. A., Behar, K. L., de Graaf, R. A., & De Feyter, H. M. (2023). Mapping of exogenous choline uptake and metabolism in rat glioblastoma using deuterium metabolic imaging (DMI). *Frontiers in Cellular Neuroscience, 17*, 1130816. Advance online publication. DOI: 10.3389/fncel.2023.1130816 PMID: 37187610

Ishihara, H., Kubota, H., Lindberg, R. L. P., Leppert, D., Gloor, S. M., Errede, M., Virgintino, D., Fontana, A., Yonekawa, Y., & Frei, K. (2008). Endothelial cell barrier impairment induced by glioblastomas and transforming growth factor β2 involves matrix metalloproteinases and tight junction proteins. *Journal of Neuropathology and Experimental Neurology, 67*(5), 435–448. DOI: 10.1097/NEN.0b013e31816fd622 PMID: 18431253

Iturrioz-Rodríguez, N., Sampron, N., & Matheu, A. (2023). Current advances in temozolomide encapsulation for the enhancement of glioblastoma treatment. *Theranostics, 13*(9), 2734–2756. DOI: 10.7150/thno.82005 PMID: 37284445

Ivanisevic, T., & Sewduth, R. N. (2023). Multi-omics integration for the design of novel therapies and the identification of novel biomarkers. *Proteomes, 11*(4), 34. DOI: 10.3390/proteomes11040034 PMID: 37873876

Ivy Brain Tumor Center. (n.d.). *Glioblastoma current standard of care*. Retrieved May 21, 2025, from https://www.ivybraintumorcenter.org/the-challenge/current-standard-of-care/

Iwanami, A., Gini, B., Zanca, C., Matsutani, T., Assuncao, A., Nael, A., Dang, J., Yang, H., Zhu, S., Kohyama, J., Kitabayashi, I., Cavenee, W. K., Cloughesy, T. F., Furnari, F. B., Nakamura, M., Toyam, Y., Okano, H., & Mischel, P. S. (2013). PML mediates glioblastoma resistance to mammalian target of rapamycin (mTOR)-targeted therapies. *Proceedings of the National Academy of Sciences of the United States of America, 110*(11), 4339–4344. DOI: 10.1073/pnas.1217602110 PMID: 23440206

Jackson, C. M., Choi, J., & Lim, M. (2019). Mechanisms of immunotherapy resistance: Lessons from glioblastoma. *Nature Immunology, 20*(9), 1100–1109. DOI: 10.1038/s41590-019-0433-y PMID: 31358997

Jackson, C. M., Lim, M., & Drake, C. G. (2014). Immunotherapy for brain cancer: Recent progress and future promise. *Clinical Cancer Research, 20*(14), 3651–3659. DOI: 10.1158/1078-0432.CCR-13-2057 PMID: 24771646

Jacot, W., Thezenas, S., Senal, R., Viglianti, C., Laberenne, A.-C., Lopez-Crapez, E., Bibeau, F., Bleuse, J.-P., Romieu, G., & Lamy, P.-J. (2013). BRCA1 promoter hypermethylation, 53BP1 protein expression and PARP-1 activity as biomarkers of DNA repair deficit in breast cancer. *BMC Cancer, 13*(1), 1–11. DOI: 10.1186/1471-2407-13-523 PMID: 24191908

Jain, K. K. (2018). A critical overview of targeted therapies for glioblastoma. *Frontiers in Oncology*, *8*(OCT), 418128. DOI: 10.3389/fonc.2018.00419 PMID: 30374421

Jaiswal, S., & Tyagi, A. (2022). Biocompatible Nanoparticles for Cancer Therapy: A Review. *Journal of Nanomedicine Research*, *10*(2), 55–64. DOI: 10.18231/j.jnanomed.2022.21

Jakola, A. S., Sagberg, L. M., Gulati, S., & Solheim, O. (2020). Advancements in predicting outcomes in patients with glioma: A surgical perspective. *Expert Review of Anticancer Therapy*, *20*(3), 167–177. DOI: 10.1080/14737140.2020.1735367 PMID: 32114857

Jang, H. J., Song, M. G., Park, C. R., Youn, H., Lee, Y.-S., Cheon, G. J., & Choi, S. H. (2023). Imaging of indocyanine green-human serum albumin (ICG-HSA) complex in secreted protein acidic and rich in cysteine (SPARC)-expressing glioblastoma. *European Journal of Nuclear Medicine and Molecular Imaging*, *51*(1), 850–861. DOI: 10.1007/s00259-023-06491-0 PMID: 36614294

Jatyan, R., Sahel, D. K., Singh, P., Sakhuja, R., Mittal, A., & Chitkara, D. (2023). Temozolomide-fatty acid conjugates for glioblastoma multiforme: In vitro and in vivo evaluation. *Journal of Controlled Release*, *359*, 161–174. DOI: 10.1016/j.jconrel.2023.05.012 PMID: 37182806

Javia, A., Bardoliwala, D., & Patel, M. (2021). *Ligands and Receptors for Targeted Delivery of Nanoparticles: Recent Updates and Challenges. Drug Delivery with Targeted Nanoparticles,p*. Jenny Stanford Publishing.

Javle, M., Roychowdhury, S., Kelley, R. K., Sadeghi, S., Macarulla, T., Weiss, K. H., Waldschmidt, D.-T., Goyal, L., Borbath, I., El-Khoueiry, A., Borad, M. J., Yong, W. P., Philip, P. A., Bitzer, M., Tanasanvimon, S., Li, A., Pande, A., Soifer, H. S., Shepherd, S. P., & Abou-Alfa, G. K. (2021). Infigratinib (BGJ398) in previously treated patients with advanced or metastatic cholangiocarcinoma with FGFR2 fusions or rearrangements: Mature results from a multicentre, open-label, single-arm, phase 2 study. *The Lancet. Gastroenterology & Hepatology*, *6*(10), 803–815. DOI: 10.1016/S2468-1253(21)00196-5 PMID: 34358484

Jensen, S. S., Petterson, S. A., Halle, B., Aaberg-Jessen, C., & Kristensen, B. W. (2017). Effects of the lysosomal destabilizing drug siramesine on glioblastoma in vitro and in vivo. *BMC Cancer*, *17*(1), 178. Advance online publication. DOI: 10.1186/s12885-017-3162-3 PMID: 28270132

Jezierzański, M., Nafalska, N., Stopyra, M., Furgoł, T., Miciak, M., Kabut, J., & Szczylik, C. (2024). Temozolomide (TMZ) in the treatment of glioblastoma multiforme—A literature review and clinical outcomes. *Current Oncology (Toronto, Ont.)*, *31*(7), 3994–4002. DOI: 10.3390/curroncol31070296 PMID: 39057168

Jhu, M. Y., Ellison, E. E., & Sinha, N. R. (2023). CRISPR gene editing to improve crop resistance to parasitic plants. *Frontiers in Genome Editing*, *5*, 1289416. Advance online publication. DOI: 10.3389/fgeed.2023.1289416 PMID: 37965302

Jia, J. L., Alshamsan, B., & Ng, T. L. (2023). Temozolomide Chronotherapy in Glioma: A Systematic Review. *Current Oncology (Toronto, Ont.)*, *30*(2), 1893–1902. DOI: 10.3390/curroncol30020147 PMID: 36826108

Jiao, X., Yu, Y., Meng, J., He, M., Zhang, C. J., Geng, W., Ding, B., Wang, Z., & Ding, X. (2019). Dual-targeting and microenvironment-responsive micelles as a gene delivery system to improve the sensitivity of glioma to radiotherapy. *Acta Pharmaceutica Sinica. B*, *9*(2), 381–396. DOI: 10.1016/j.apsb.2018.12.001 PMID: 30972284

Jia, X., Wang, L., Feng, X., Liu, W., Wang, X., Li, F., & Liu, Y. (2023). Cell membrane-coated oncolytic adenovirus for targeted treatment of glioblastoma. *ACS Nano*, *17*(23), 11120–11128. DOI: 10.1021/acsnano.3c07123 PMID: 38032110

Jnaidi, R., Almeida, A. J., & Gonçalves, L. M. (2020). Solid lipid nanoparticles and nanostructured lipid carriers as smart drug delivery systems in the treatment of glioblastoma multiforme. *Pharmaceutics*, *12*(9), 860. Advance online publication. DOI: 10.3390/pharmaceutics12090860 PMID: 32927610

Johnson, A. L., & Lopez-Bertoni, H. (2024). Cellular diversity through space and time: Adding new dimensions to GBM therapeutic development. *Frontiers in Genetics*, *15*, 1356611. DOI: 10.3389/fgene.2024.1356611 PMID: 38774283

Johnson, D. R., Fogh, S. E., Giannini, C., Kaufmann, T. J., Raghunathan, A., Theodosopoulos, P. V., & Jenkins, R. B. (2015). Case-based review: Newly diagnosed glioblastoma. *Neuro-Oncology Practice*, *2*(3), 106–121. DOI: 10.1093/nop/npv020 PMID: 31386093

Johnson, D. R., & O'Neill, B. P. (2012). Glioblastoma survival in the United States before and during the temozolomide era. *Journal of Neuro-Oncology*, *107*(2), 359–364. DOI: 10.1007/s11060-011-0749-4 PMID: 22045118

Jovčevska, I. (2020). Next generation sequencing and machine learning technologies are painting the epigenetic portrait of glioblastoma. *Frontiers in Oncology*, *10*, 798. Advance online publication. DOI: 10.3389/fonc.2020.00798 PMID: 32500035

Jung, H. (2022). Contributing factors for mutagenic DNA lesion bypass by DNA polymerase eta (polη). *DNA*, *2*(4), 205–220. DOI: 10.3390/dna2040015

Kadari, A., Pooja, D., Gora, R. H., Gudem, S., Kolapalli, V. R. M., Kulhari, H., & Sistla, R. (2018). Design of multifunctional peptide collaborated and docetaxel loaded lipid nanoparticles for antiglioma therapy. *European Journal of Pharmaceutics and Biopharmaceutics*, *132*, 168–179. DOI: 10.1016/j.ejpb.2018.09.012 PMID: 30244167

Kamran, N., Kadiyala, P., Saxena, M., Candolfi, M., Li, Y., Moreno-Ayala, M. A., Raja, N., Shah, D., Lowenstein, P. R., & Castro, M. G. (2017). Immunosuppressive Myeloid Cells' Blockade in the Glioma Microenvironment Enhances the Efficacy of Immune-Stimulatory Gene Therapy. *Molecular Therapy : the Journal of the American Society of Gene Therapy*, *25*(1), 232–248. DOI: 10.1016/j.ymthe.2016.10.003 PMID: 28129117

Kanderi, T., Munakomi, S., & Gupta, V. (2024) Glioblastoma multiforme. *StatPearls [Internet]*, p.^pp. StatPearls Publishing.

Karim, N. A., Ullah, A., Ahmad, I., Bahassi, E., Olowokure, O., Khaled, A., Davis, H., & Morris, J. C. (2022). A phase I trial to determine the safety and tolerability of autophagy inhibition using chloroquine or hydroxychloroquine in combination with carboplatin and gemcitabine in patients with advanced solid tumors. *Frontiers in Oncology*, *12*, 811411. DOI: 10.3389/fonc.2022.811411 PMID: 35574311

Karim, R., Palazzo, C., Evrard, B., & Piel, G. (2016). Nanocarriers for the treatment of glioblastoma multiforme: Current state-of-the-art. *Journal of Controlled Release*, *227*, 23–37. DOI: 10.1016/j.jconrel.2016.02.026 PMID: 26892752

Karschnia, P., Vogelbaum, M. A., van den Bent, M., Cahill, D. P., Bello, L., Narita, Y., Berger, M. S., Weller, M., & Tonn, J. C. (2021). Evidence-based recommendations on categories for extent of resection in diffuse glioma. *European Journal of Cancer*, *149*, 23–33. DOI: 10.1016/j.ejca.2021.03.002 PMID: 33819718

Kaufman, S. A., Badowski, M., Jones, D., Williams, S., Greenfield, S., & Dickson, M.. (2017). Cisplatin in glioblastoma: Clinical outcomes and future directions. *Oncology*, *92*(4), 162–170.

Kelkar, S. S., & Reineke, T. M. (2011). Theranostics: Combining imaging and therapy. *Bioconjugate Chemistry*, *22*(10), 1879–1903. DOI: 10.1021/bc200151q PMID: 21830812

Kelm, J. M., Samarbakhsh, A., Pillai, A., VanderVere-Carozza, P. S., Aruri, H., Pandey, D. S., Pawelczak, K. S., Turchi, J. J., & Gavande, N. S. (2022). Recent advances in the development of non-PIKKs targeting small molecule inhibitors of DNA double-strand break repair. *Frontiers in Oncology*, *12*, 850883. DOI: 10.3389/fonc.2022.850883 PMID: 35463312

Khagi, S., Kotecha, R., Gatson, N. T. N., Jeyapalan, S., Abdullah, H. I., Avgeropoulos, N. G., & Mehta, M. P. (2024). Recent advances in Tumor Treating Fields (TTFields) therapy for glioblastoma. *The Oncologist*, *30*(2), oyae227. Advance online publication. DOI: 10.1093/oncolo/oyae227 PMID: 39401002

Khan, I. N., Navaid, S., Waqar, W., Hussein, D., Ullah, N., Khan, M. U. A., & Amin, A. (2024). Chitosan-based polymeric nanoparticles as an efficient gene delivery system to cross blood brain barrier: In vitro and in vivo evaluations. *International Journal of Polymeric Materials*, *73*(2), 169–180. DOI: 10.1080/00914037.2023.2275588 PMID: 38399386

Kickingereder, P., Isensee, F., Tursunova, I., Petersen, J., Neuberger, U., Bonekamp, D., Brugnara, G., Schell, M., Kessler, T., Foltyn, M., Harting, I., Sahm, F., Prager, M., Nowosielski, M., Wick, A., Nolden, M., Radbruch, A., Debus, J., Schlemmer, H.-P., & Maier-Hein, K. H. (2019). Automated quantitative tumour response assessment of MRI in neuro-oncology with artificial neural networks: A multicentre, retrospective study. *The Lancet. Oncology*, *20*(5), 728–740. DOI: 10.1016/S1470-2045(19)30098-1 PMID: 30952559

Kim, K.. (2020). Intranasal delivery of cancer-targeting doxorubicin-loaded PLGA nanoparticles arrests glioblastoma growth. *Journal of Drug Targeting*, *28*(7-8), 617–626. DOI: 10.1080/1061186X.2020.1775736 PMID: 31852284

Kim, S. H., Yoo, H., Chang, J. H., Kim, C. Y., Chung, D. S., Kim, S. H., Park, S.-H., Lee, Y. S., & Yang, S. H. (2018). Procarbazine and CCNU chemotherapy for recurrent glioblastoma with MGMT promoter methylation. *Journal of Korean Medical Science*, *33*(24), e167. Advance online publication. DOI: 10.3346/jkms.2018.33.e167 PMID: 29892208

Kim, S., Jing, K., Shin, S., Jeong, S., Han, S.-H., Oh, H., & Lim, K. (2018). ω3-polyunsaturated fatty acids induce cell death through apoptosis and autophagy in glioblastoma cells: In vitro and in vivo. *Oncology Reports*, *39*(1), 239–246. DOI: 10.3892/or.2017.6107 PMID: 29192322

Klein, E., Hau, A.-C., Oudin, A., Golebiewska, A., & Niclou, S. P. (2020). Glioblastoma organoids: Pre-clinical applications and challenges in the context of immunotherapy. *Frontiers in Oncology, 10*, 604121. Advance online publication. DOI: 10.3389/fonc.2020.604121 PMID: 33364198

Koes, N., Taisto, M., Tschida, B. R., Carlson, D. F., Aftabizadeh, M., Thirimanne, H. N., & Largaespada, D. A. (2025). Abstract 6511: Immunocompetent large animal model of mesenchymal glioblastoma achieved through somatic gene editing technology. *Cancer Research, 85*(8, Supplement_1), 6511. DOI: 10.1158/1538-7445.AM2025-6511

Kostka, K., Sokolova, V., El-Taibany, A., Kruse, B., Porada, D., Wolff, N., Prymak, O., Seeds, M. C., Epple, M., & Atala, A. J. (2024). The Application of Ultrasmall Gold Nanoparticles (2 nm) Functionalized with Doxorubicin in Three-Dimensional Normal and Glioblastoma Organoid Models of the Blood–Brain Barrier. *Molecules (Basel, Switzerland), 29*(11), 2469. DOI: 10.3390/molecules29112469 PMID: 38893345

Krajcer, A., Grzywna, E., & Lewandowska-Łańcucka, J. (2023). Strategies increasing the effectiveness of temozolomide at various levels of anti-GBL therapy. *Biomedicine and Pharmacotherapy, 165*, 115174. DOI: 10.1016/j.biopha.2023.115174 PMID: 37459661

Krawczynski, K., Godlewski, J., & Bronisz, A. (2020). Oxidative stress—Part of the solution or part of the problem in the hypoxic environment of a brain tumor. *Antioxidants, 9*(8), 747. DOI: 10.3390/antiox9080747 PMID: 32823815

Kretowski, R., Kusaczuk, M., Naumowicz, M., Kotyńska, J., Szynaka, B., &Cechowska-Pasko, M. (2017). The Effects of Silica Nanoparticles on Apoptosis and Autophagy of Glioblastoma Cell Lines. *Nanomaterials 2017, Vol. 7, Page 230, 7*(8), 230. .DOI: 10.3390/nano7080230

Kreuter, J. (2001). Nanoparticulate systems for brain delivery of drugs. *Advanced Drug Delivery Reviews, 47*(1), 65–81. DOI: 10.1016/S0169-409X(00)00122-8 PMID: 11251246

Kreuter, J. (2014). Drug delivery to the central nervous system by polymeric nanoparticles: What do we know? *Advanced Drug Delivery Reviews, 71*, 2–14. DOI: 10.1016/j.addr.2013.08.008 PMID: 23981489

Kreuter, J., Ramge, P., Petrov, V., Hamm, S., Gelperina, S. E., Engelhardt, B., Alyautdin, R., von Briesen, H., & Begley, D. J. (2003). Direct evidence that polysorbate-80-coated poly(butylcyanoacrylate) nanoparticles deliver drugs to the CNS via specific mechanisms requiring prior binding of drug to the nanoparticles. *Pharmaceutical Research, 20*(3), 409–416. DOI: 10.1023/A:1022604120952 PMID: 12669961

Krishnamurthy, N., Grimshaw, A. A., Axson, S. A., Choe, S. H., & Miller, J. E. (2022). Drug repurposing: A systematic review on root causes, barriers and facilitators. *BMC Health Services Research, 22*(1), 970. DOI: 10.1186/s12913-022-08272-z PMID: 35906687

Kubben, P. L., Scholtes, F., Schijns, O. E., ter Laak-Poort, M. P., Teernstra, O. P., Kessels, A. G., van Overbeeke, J. J., Martin, D. H., & Van Santbrink, H. (2014). Intraoperative magnetic resonance imaging versus standard neuronavigation for the neurosurgical treatment of glioblastoma: A randomized controlled trial. *Surgical Neurology International, 5*(1), 70. DOI: 10.4103/2152-7806.132572 PMID: 24991473

Kucinska, M., Pospieszna, J., Tang, J., Lisiak, N., Toton, E., Rubis, B., Murias, M., & Hofmann, J. (2024). The combination therapy using tyrosine kinase receptors inhibitors and repurposed drugs to target patient-derived glioblastoma stem cells. *Biomedicine and Pharmacotherapy, 176*, 116892. Advance online publication. DOI: 10.1016/j.biopha.2024.116892 PMID: 38876048

Kumari, S., Gupta, R., Ambasta, R. K., & Kumar, P. (2023). Multiple therapeutic approaches of glioblastoma multiforme: From terminal to therapy. *Biochimica et Biophysica Acta (BBA) –. Revisiones en Cáncer, 1878*(4), 188913. Advance online publication. DOI: 10.1016/j.bbcan.2023.188913 PMID: 37182666

Kwiatkowska-Miernik, A., Mruk, B., Sklinda, K., Zaczyński, A., & Walecki, J. (2023). Radiomics in the diagnosis of glioblastoma. *Polish Journal of Radiology / Polish Medical Society of Radiology, 88*, e461–e466. DOI: 10.5114/pjr.2023.132168 PMID: 38020501

Laba, A. E., & Ziólkowski, P. (2021). Trends in glioblastoma treatment research: An analysis of clinical trials and literature. *Neurologia i Neurochirurgia Polska, 55*(3), 269–280. DOI: 10.5603/PJNNS.a2021.0024 PMID: 33710606

Lai, G., Wu, H., Yang, K., Hu, K., Zhou, Y., Chen, X., Fu, F., Li, J., Xie, G., Wang, H. F., Lv, Z., & Wu, X. (2024). Progress of nanoparticle drug delivery system for the treatment of glioma. *Frontiers in Bioengineering and Biotechnology, 12*, 1403511. Advance online publication. DOI: 10.3389/fbioe.2024.1403511 PMID: 38919382

Lal, S., & Mukherjee, J. (2016). Oncolytic viral therapy of glioblastoma: Will this soon become a reality. *Chemotherapy (Los Angeles, Calif.)*, *5*(2), e131. Advance online publication. DOI: 10.4172/2167-7700.1000e131

LaMoia, T. E., & Shulman, G. I. (2021). Cellular and molecular mechanisms of metformin action. *Endocrine Reviews*, *42*(1), 77–96. DOI: 10.1210/endrev/bnaa023 PMID: 32897388

Lansangan, C., Khoobchandani, M., Jain, R., Rudensky, S., Perry, C. C., & Patil, R. (2024). Designing gold nanoparticles for precise glioma treatment: Challenges and alternatives. *Materials (Basel)*, *17*(5), 1153. Advance online publication. DOI: 10.3390/ma17051153 PMID: 38473623

Lan, Z., Li, X., & Zhang, X. (2024). Glioblastoma: An update in pathology, molecular mechanisms and biomarkers. *International Journal of Molecular Sciences*, *25*(5), 3040. DOI: 10.3390/ijms25053040 PMID: 38474286

Lanza, C., Carriero, S., Buijs, E. F. M., Mortellaro, S., Pizzi, C., Sciacqua, L. V., & Venturini, M. (2023). Robotics in interventional radiology: Review of current and future applications. *Technology in Cancer Research & Treatment*, *22*, 15330338231152084. DOI: 10.1177/15330338231152084 PMID: 37113061

Laquintana, V., Trapani, A., Denora, N., Wang, F., Gallo, J., & Trapani, G. (2009). New strategies to deliver anticancer drugs to brain tumors. *Expert Opinion on Drug Delivery*, *6*(10), 1017–1032. DOI: 10.1517/17425240903167942 PMID: 19732031

Lathia, J. D., Mack, S. C., Mulkearns-Hubert, E. E., Valentim, C. L., & Rich, J. N. (2015). Cancer stem cells in glioblastoma. *Genes & Development*, *29*(12), 1203–1217. DOI: 10.1101/gad.261982.115 PMID: 26109046

Ledermann, J., & Luvero, D. (2015). Update on anti-angiogenic agents and PARP inhibitors: Is the combination a potential or a reality? *Cancer Breaking News*, *3*(2), 20–29.

Lee Bredlau, A., Dixit, S., Chen, C., & Broome, A.-M. (2017). Nanotechnology applications for diffuse intrinsic pontine glioma. *Current Neuropharmacology*, *15*(1), 104–115. DOI: 10.2174/1570159X14666160223121002 PMID: 26903150

Lee JH, Chapman DV & Saltzman WM (2023) Nanoparticle targeting with antibodies in the central nervous system. *BME frontiers* 4: 0012.

Lee, J. K., Wang, J., Sa, J. K., Ladewig, E., Lee, H. O., Lee, I. H., Kang, H. J., Rosenbloom, D. S., Camara, P. G., Liu, Z., Van Nieuwenhuizen, P., Jung, S. W., Choi, S. W., Kim, J., Chen, A., Kim, K. T., Shin, S., Seo, Y. J., Oh, J. M., & Nam, D. H. (2017). Spatiotemporal genomic architecture informs precision oncology in glioblastoma. *Nature Genetics*, *49*(4), 594–599. DOI: 10.1038/ng.3806 PMID: 28263318

Lee, W. S., Pyun, B. J., Kim, S. W., Shim, S. R., Nam, J. R., Yoo, J. Y., Jin, Y., Jin, J., Kwon, Y.-G., Yun, C.-O., Nam, D.-H., Oh, K., Lee, D.-S., Lee, S. H., & Yoo, J.-S. (2015). TTAC-0001, a human monoclonal antibody targeting VEGFR-2/KDR, blocks tumor angiogenesis. *mAbs*, *7*(5), 957–968. DOI: 10.1080/19420862.2015.1045168 PMID: 25942475

Leroy, H. A., Vermandel, M., Lejeune, J. P., Mordon, S., & Reyns, N. (2015). Fluorescence guided resection and glioblastoma in 2015: A review. *Lasers in Surgery and Medicine*, *47*(5), 441–451. DOI: 10.1002/lsm.22359 PMID: 25946082

Levin, V. A. (2010). Role of bevacizumab therapy in the management of glioblastoma. *Cancer Management and Research*, *2*, 97–104. DOI: 10.2147/CMAR.S6103 PMID: 21188100

Liau, C. T., Wei, K. C., Tseng, C. K., & Jung, S. M. (2005). Combination chemotherapy with carmustine and cisplatin followed by procarbazine, lomustine, and vincristine for adult high-grade astrocytoma. *Chang Gung Medical Journal*, *28*(1), 16–23. PMID: 15804144

Li, B., Zheng, Y., & Yang, L. (2019). The oncogenic potential of SUV39H2: A comprehensive and perspective view. *Journal of Cancer*, *10*(3), 721–729. DOI: 10.7150/jca.28254 PMID: 30719171

Li, D., Gao, J., Yang, C., Li, B., Sun, J., Yu, M., Wang, Y., Wang, H., & Lu, Y. (2021). cRGDyK-modified procaine liposome inhibits the proliferation and motility of glioma cells via the ERK/p38MAPK pathway. *Experimental and Therapeutic Medicine*, *22*(2), 1–11. DOI: 10.3892/etm.2021.10291 PMID: 34178132

Li, G., Wang, D., Zhai, Y., Pan, C., Zhang, J., Wang, C., & Chen, X. (2024). Glycometabolic reprogramming-induced XRCC1 lactylation confers therapeutic resistance in ALDH1A3-overexpressing glioblastoma. *Cell Metabolism*, *36*(8), 1696–1710.e10. DOI: 10.1016/j.cmet.2024.07.011 PMID: 39111285

Liguori, G. L. (2024). Challenges and promise for glioblastoma treatment through extracellular vesicle inquiry. *Cells*, *13*(4), 336. Advance online publication. DOI: 10.3390/cells13040336 PMID: 38391949

Li, H.. (2022). Targeted Nanoparticles for the Delivery of CRISPR-Cas9 Systems in Gene Editing. *Nature Communications*, *13*(1), 1827. DOI: 10.1038/s41467-022-29472-7 PMID: 35383166

Li, H., Li, M., Fu, J., Ao, H., Wang, W., & Wang, X. (2021). Enhancement of oral bioavailability of quercetin by metabolic inhibitory nanosuspensions compared to conventional nanosuspensions. *Drug Delivery*, *28*(1), 1226–1236. DOI: 10.1080/10717544.2021.1927244 PMID: 34142631

Li, J., Feng, L., & Lu, Y. (2023). Glioblastoma multiforme: Diagnosis, treatment, and invasion. *Journal of Biomedical Research*, *37*(1), 47–58. DOI: 10.7555/JBR.36.20220156 PMID: 36403983

Li, J., Zeng, H., You, Y., Wang, R., Tan, T., Wang, W., Yin, L., Zeng, Z., Zeng, Y., & Xie, T. (2021). Active targeting of orthotopic glioma using biomimetic liposomes co-loaded elemene and cabazitaxel modified by transferritin. *Journal of Nanobiotechnology*, *19*(1), 1–19. DOI: 10.1186/s12951-021-01048-3 PMID: 34565383

Li, L.. (2022). Recent Advances in Nanoparticle-Based Delivery Systems for Gene Therapy in Glioblastoma. *Nanotechnology Reviews*, *11*(1), 84–96. DOI: 10.1515/ntrev-2022-0079

Lim, M., Xia, Y., Bettegowda, C., & Weller, M. (2018). Current state of immunotherapy for glioblastoma. *Nature Reviews. Clinical Oncology*, *15*(7), 422–442. DOI: 10.1038/s41571-018-0003-5 PMID: 29643471

Lin, H., Liu, C., Hu, A., Zhang, D., Yang, H., & Mao, Y. (2024). Understanding the immunosuppressive microenvironment of glioma: Mechanistic insights and clinical perspectives. *Journal of Hematology & Oncology*, *17*(1), 31. Advance online publication. DOI: 10.1186/s13045-024-01544-7 PMID: 38720342

Linkous, , A., & Yazlovitskaya, E. (2011). Angiogenesis in glioblastoma multiforme: Navigating the maze. *Anti-cancer Agents in Medicinal Chemistry*, *11*(8), 712–718. DOI: 10.2174/187152011797378643 PMID: 21707499

Li, P.-J., Lai, S.-Z., Jin, T., Ying, H.-J., Chen, Y.-M., Zhang, P., & Cai, Q. (2023). Radiotherapy opens the blood–brain barrier and synergizes with anlotinib in treating glioblastoma. *Pharmacological Research*, *183*, 109633. Advance online publication. DOI: 10.1016/j.phrs.2023.106633 PMID: 36963438

Lipková, J., Menze, B., Wiestler, B., Koumoutsakos, P., & Lowengrub, J. S. (2022). Modelling glioma progression, mass effect and intracranial pressure in patient anatomy. *Journal of the Royal Society, Interface*, *19*(188), 20210922. Advance online publication. DOI: 10.1098/rsif.2021.0922 PMID: 35317645

Li, Q., Zhang, Z., Wu, X., Zhao, Y., & Liu, Y. (2025). Cascade-responsive nanoparticles for efficient CRISPR/Cas9-based glioblastoma gene therapy. *ACS Applied Materials & Interfaces, 17*(3), 4480–4489. DOI: 10.1021/acsami.4c15671 PMID: 39797776

Li, S., Deng, Q., Li, X., Huang, Y., Li, X., Liu, F., Wang, H., Qing, W., Liu, Z., & Lee, C. S. (2019). Bis-diketopyrrolopyrrole conjugated polymer nanoparticles as photothermic nanoagonist for specific and synergistic glioblastoma therapy. *Biomaterials, 216*(June), 119252. DOI: 10.1016/j.biomaterials.2019.119252 PMID: 31212086

Liu, Y., Cui, Z., Li, L., You, J., Feng, X., Wang, J., & Zhang, Y. (2025). Glioma multimodal MRI analysis system for tumor layered diagnosis via multi-task semi-supervised learning. arXiv. Retrieved May 17, 2025, from https://arxiv.org/abs/2501.17758

Liu, D., Dai, X., Zhang, W., Zhu, X., Zha, Z., Qian, H., & Cheng, H. (2023). Liquid exfoliation of ultrasmall zirconium carbide nanodots as a noninflammatory photothermal agent in the treatment of glioma. *Advanced Materials, 35*(2), 2210917. Advance online publication. DOI: 10.1002/adma.202210917 PMID: 36470160

Liu, G., & Sun, Y. (2025). Harnessing nanoparticles for Alzheimer's disease: Innovations in drug delivery and pathology-specific treatments. *Journal of Alzheimer's Disease, 107*(4), 1374–1399. DOI: 10.1177/13872877251374149 PMID: 40899976

Liu, G., Yuan, X., Zeng, Z., Tunici, P., Ng, H., Abdulkadir, I. R., Lu, L., Irvin, D., Black, K. L., & Yu, J. S. (2006). Analysis of gene expression and chemoresistance of CD133+ cancer stem cells in glioblastoma. *Molecular Cancer, 5*(1), 67. Advance online publication. DOI: 10.1186/1476-4598-5-67 PMID: 17140455

Liu, H.. (2021). CD133 as a marker for glioblastoma stem cells: Implications for drug resistance. *Stem Cell Research & Therapy, 12*(1), 107. DOI: 10.1186/s13287-021-02307-1 PMID: 33541421

Liu, J., Majd, N., Zou, C., Mirchia, K., Pak, J., Foster, K., & Pan, S. (2024). OS07. 1. A INTEGRATIVE SINGLE NUCLEI, SPATIAL, AND FUNCTIONAL GENOMIC ANALYSES REVEAL DNA-PK DRIVES GLIOBLASTOMA RADIORESISTANCE THROUGH TUMOR CELLS AND THE MYELOID MICROENVIRONMENT. *Neuro-Oncology, 26*(Supplement_5), v22–v23. DOI: 10.1093/neuonc/noae144.065

Liu, L., Liao, X., Wu, H., Li, Y., Zhu, Y., & Chen, Q. (2020). Mitophagy and its contribution to metabolic and aging-associated disorders. *Antioxidants & Redox Signaling, 32*(12), 906–927. DOI: 10.1089/ars.2019.8013 PMID: 31969001

Liu, M., Ji, Z., Jain, V., Smith, V. L., Hocke, E., Patel, A. P., McLendon, R. E., Ashley, D. M., Gregory, S. G., & López, G. Y. (2024). Spatial transcriptomics reveals segregation of tumor cell states in glioblastoma and marked immunosuppression within the perinecrotic niche. *Acta Neuropathologica Communications*, *12*(1), 64. DOI: 10.1186/s40478-024-01769-0 PMID: 38650010

Liu, S., Tan, B., Wang, F., & Yu, Y. (2024). Applications of polymeric nanoparticles in drug delivery for glioblastoma. *Frontiers in Pharmacology*, *15*(January), 1–17. DOI: 10.3389/fphar.2024.1519479 PMID: 39834835

Liu, S., Zhang, S. M., Ju, R. J., Xiao, Y., Wang, X., Song, X. L., Liu, Y., & Li, X. T. (2017). Antitumor efficacy of Lf modified daunorubicin plus honokiol liposomes in treatment of brain glioma. *European Journal of Pharmaceutical Sciences*, *106*, 185–197. DOI: 10.1016/j.ejps.2017.06.002 PMID: 28583810

Liu, X.. (2023). Functionalized Nanoparticles for Targeted Delivery in CRISPR/Cas9-Based Gene Editing. *Nanomedicine; Nanotechnology, Biology, and Medicine*, *27*, 42–52. DOI: 10.1016/j.nano.2022.102484

Liu, X., Zhao, Z., Dai, W., Liao, K., Sun, Q., Chen, D., & Liu, Z. (2023). The development of immunotherapy for the treatment of recurrent glioblastoma. *Cancers (Basel)*, *15*(17), 4308. Advance online publication. DOI: 10.3390/cancers15174308 PMID: 37686584

Liu, Y., Hu, D., Gao, D., Gong, P., Zheng, H., Sun, M., & Cai, L. (2023). Engineered apoptotic bodies hitchhiking across the blood-brain barrier achieved a combined photothermal-chemotherapeutic effect against glioma. *Advancement of Science*, *10*(9), 2206296. Advance online publication. DOI: 10.7150/thno.80632 PMID: 37284458

Liu, Z., Ji, X., He, D., Zhang, R., Liu, Q., & Xin, T. (2022). Nanoscale drug delivery systems in glioblastoma. *Nanoscale Research Letters*, *17*(1), 27. Advance online publication. DOI: 10.1186/s11671-022-03668-6 PMID: 35171358

Li, W., & Xu, X. (2023). Advances in mitophagy and mitochondrial apoptosis pathway-related drugs in glioblastoma treatment. *Frontiers in Pharmacology*, *14*, 1211719. DOI: 10.3389/fphar.2023.1211719 PMID: 37456742

Li, X., Li, M., Huang, M., Lin, Q., Fang, Q., Liu, J., Chen, X., Liu, L., Zhan, X., Shan, H., Lu, D., Li, Q., Li, Z., & Zhu, X. (2022). The multi-molecular mechanisms of tumor-targeted drug resistance in precision medicine. *Biomedicine and Pharmacotherapy*, *150*, 113064. Advance online publication. DOI: 10.1016/j.biopha.2022.113064 PMID: 35658234

Longmire, M. R., Ogawa, M., Choyke, P. L., & Kobayashi, H. (2014). Dendrimers as high relaxivity MR contrast agents. *Wiley Interdisciplinary Reviews. Nanomedicine and Nanobiotechnology*, *123*(2), 40–43. DOI: 10.1002/wnan.1250 PMID: 24155241

Lopes, J., Ferreira-Gonçalves, T., Ascensão, L., Viana, A. S., Carvalho, L., Catarino, J., & Reis, C. P. (2023). Safety of gold nanoparticles: From in vitro to in vivo testing array checklist. *Nanomaterials (Basel, Switzerland)*, *13*(4), 1120. Advance online publication. DOI: 10.3390/nano13041120 PMID: 37111608

Louis, D. N., Perry, A., Reifenberger, G., von Deimling, A., Figarella-Branger, D., Cavenee, W. K., Ohgaki, H., Wiestler, O. D., Kleihues, P., & Ellison, D. W. (2016). The 2016 World Health Organization Classification of Tumors of the Central Nervous System. *Acta Neuropathologica*, *131*(6), 803–820. DOI: 10.1007/s00401-016-1545-1 PMID: 27157931

Louis, D. N., Perry, A., Wesseling, P., Brat, D. J., Cree, I. A., Figarella-Branger, D., Hawkins, C., Ng, H. K., Pfister, S. M., Reifenberger, G., Soffietti, R., Von Deimling, A., & Ellison, D. W. (2021). The 2021 WHO Classification of Tumors of the Central Nervous System: A summary. *Neuro-Oncology*, *23*(8), 1231–1251. DOI: 10.1093/neuonc/noab106 PMID: 34185076

Louveau, A., Smirnov, I., Keyes, T. J., Eccles, J. D., Rouhani, S. J., Peske, J. D., Derecki, N. C., Castle, D., Mandell, J. W., Lee, K. S., Harris, T. H., & Kipnis, J. (2015). Structural and functional features of central nervous system lymphatic vessels. *Nature*, *523*(7560), 337–341. DOI: 10.1038/nature14432 PMID: 26030524

Lozinski, M., Bowden, N. A., Graves, M. C., Fay, M., & Tooney, P. A. (2021). DNA damage repair in glioblastoma: Current perspectives on its role in tumor progression, treatment resistance and PIKKing potential therapeutic targets. *Cellular Oncology (Dordrecht)*, *44*(5), 961–981. DOI: 10.1007/s13402-021-00613-0 PMID: 34057732

Lu, G., Wang, X., Li, F., Wang, S., Zhao, J., Wang, J., Liu, J., Lyu, C., Ye, P., Tan, H., Li, W., Ma, G., & Wei, W. (2022). Engineered biomimetic nanoparticles achieve targeted delivery and efficient metabolism-based synergistic therapy against glioblastoma. *Nature Communications*, *13*(1), 4214. Advance online publication. DOI: 10.1038/s41467-022-31799-y PMID: 35864093

Lu, R., Wu, C., Guo, L., Liu, Y., Mo, W., Wang, H., Ding, Y., Wong, E. T., & Yu, M. (2012). The role of brevican in glioma: Promoting tumor cell motility in vitro and in vivo. *BMC Cancer*, *12*(1), 607. Advance online publication. DOI: 10.1186/1471-2407-12-607 PMID: 23253190

Lu, V. M., Jue, T. R., McDonald, K. L., & Rovin, R. A. (2018). The survival effect of repeat surgery at glioblastoma recurrence and its trend: A systematic review and meta-analysis. *World Neurosurgery*, *115*, 453–459. DOI: 10.1016/j.wneu.2018.04.016 PMID: 29654958

Lyakhovich, A., Graifer, D., Stefanovie, B., & Krejci, L. (2016). Mitochondrial dysfunction in DDR-related cancer predisposition syndromes. *Biochimica et Biophysica Acta (BBA)-. Revisiones en Cáncer*, *1865*(2), 184–189. PMID: 26926806

Ly, P., Brunner, S. F., Shoshani, O., Kim, D. H., Lan, W., Pyntikova, T., & Campbell, P. J. (2019). Chromosome segregation errors generate a diverse spectrum of simple and complex genomic rearrangements. *Nature Genetics*, *51*(4), 705–715. DOI: 10.1038/s41588-019-0360-8 PMID: 30833795

Maeda, H., Wu, J., Sawa, T., Matsumura, Y., & Hori, K. (2000). Tumor vascular permeability and the EPR effect in macromolecular therapeutics. A review. *Journal of Controlled Release*, *65*(1–2), 271–284. DOI: 10.1016/S0168-3659(99)00248-5 PMID: 10699287

Magee, D. E., Hird, A. E., Klaassen, Z., Sridhar, S. S., Nam, R. K., Wallis, C. J. D., & Kulkarni, G. S. (2020). Adverse event profile for immunotherapy agents compared with chemotherapy in solid organ tumors: A systematic review and meta-analysis of randomized clinical trials. *Annals of Oncology : Official Journal of the European Society for Medical Oncology*, *31*(1), 50–60. DOI: 10.1016/j.annonc.2019.10.008 PMID: 31912796

Mahmoudi, K., Bouras, A., Bozec, D., Ivkov, R., & Hadjipanayis, C. (2018). Magnetic hyperthermia therapy for the treatment of glioblastoma: a review of the therapy's history, efficacy and application in humans. *International Journal of Hyperthermia : The Official Journal of European Society for Hyperthermic Oncology. International Journal of Hyperthermia*, *34*(8), 1316–1328. DOI: 10.1080/02656736.2018.1430867 PMID: 29353516

Mahmoudi, M.. (2011). Superparamagnetic iron oxide nanoparticles for biomedical applications: Opportunities and challenges. *Chemical Reviews*, *111*(2), 253–280. DOI: 10.1021/cr1001832 PMID: 21077606

Mahmud, H., Kasai, T., Khayrani, A. C., Asakura, M., Oo, A. K. K., Du, J., Seno, M., & Yagi, K. (2018). Targeting glioblastoma cells expressing CD44 with liposomes encapsulating doxorubicin and displaying chlorotoxin-IgG Fc fusion protein. *International Journal of Molecular Sciences*, *19*(3), 659. Advance online publication. DOI: 10.3390/ijms19030659 PMID: 29495404

Maity, S., Bhuyan, T., Jewell, C., Kawakita, S., Sharma, S., Nguyen, H. T., & Kim, Y. J. (2025). Recent developments in glioblastoma-on-a-chip for advanced drug screening applications. *Small*, *21*(1), e2405511. Advance online publication. DOI: 10.1002/smll.202405511 PMID: 39535474

Majc, B., Novak, M., Kopitar-Jerala, N., Jewett, A., & Breznik, B. (2021). Immunotherapy of glioblastoma: Current strategies and challenges in tumor model development. *Cells*, *10*(2), 265. Advance online publication. DOI: 10.3390/cells10020265 PMID: 33572835

Majumder, B., Nataraj, N. B., Maitreyi, L., & Datta, S. (2024). Mismatch repair-proficient tumor footprints in the sands of immune desert: Mechanistic constraints and precision platforms. *Frontiers in Immunology*, *15*, 1414376. DOI: 10.3389/fimmu.2024.1414376 PMID: 39100682

Maksoud, S. (2022). The DNA double-strand break repair in glioma: Molecular players and therapeutic strategies. *Molecular Neurobiology*, *59*(9), 5326–5365. DOI: 10.1007/s12035-022-02915-2 PMID: 35696013

Maleki, H., Naghibzadeh, M., Amani, A., Adabi, M., & Khosravani, M. (2019). Preparation of Paclitaxel and Etoposide Co-loaded mPEG-PLGA Nanoparticles: An Investigation with Artificial Neural Network. *Journal of Pharmaceutical Innovation*, *16*(1), 11–25. DOI: 10.1007/s12247-019-09419-y

Malhotra, P., & Rahman, R. (2024). Tumour heterogeneity and disease infiltration as paradigms of glioblastoma treatment resistance. *Onco*, *4*(4), 349–358. DOI: 10.3390/onco4040024

Malone, E. R., Oliva, M., Sabatini, P. J. B., Stockley, T. L., & Siu, L. L. (2020). Molecular profiling for precision cancer therapies. *Genome Medicine*, *12*(1), 8. Advance online publication. DOI: 10.1186/s13073-019-0703-1 PMID: 31937368

Mancera-Andrade, E. I., Parsaeimehr, A., Arevalo-Gallegos, A., Ascencio-Favela, G., & Parra-Saldivar, R. (2018). Microfluidics technology for drug delivery: A review. *Frontiers in Bioscience (Elite Edition)*, *10*(1), 74–91. DOI: 10.2741/e809 PMID: 28930605

Manek, E., & Petroianu, G. A. (2021). Brain delivery of antidotes by polymeric nanoparticles. *Journal of Applied Toxicology*, *41*(1), 20–32. DOI: 10.1002/jat.4029 PMID: 32666582

Mansour, M. A., Kamer-Eldawla, A. M., Malaeb, R. W., Aboelhassan, R., Nabawi, D. H., Aziz, M. M., & Choudhry, H. (2025). Unlocking the code: The role of molecular and genetic profiling in revolutionizing glioblastoma treatment. *Cancer Treatment and Research Communications*, *43*, 100881. Advance online publication. DOI: 10.1016/j.ctarc.2025.100881 PMID: 39985914

Markov, A. V., Moralev, A. D., & Odarenko, K. V. (2025). Sesquiterpene lactones as promising anti-glioblastoma drug candidates exerting complex effects on glioblastoma cell viability and proneural–mesenchymal transition. *Biomedicines*, *13*(1), 133. Advance online publication. DOI: 10.3390/biomedicines13010133 PMID: 39857717

Marniemi, J., & Parkki, M. G. (1975). Radiochemical assay of glutathione S-epoxide transferase and its enhancement by phenobarbital in rat liver in vivo. *Biochemical Pharmacology*, *24*(17), 1569–1572. DOI: 10.1016/0006-2952(75)90080-5 PMID: 9

Martuscello, R. T., Vedam-Mai, V., McCarthy, D. J., Schmoll, M. E., Jundi, M. A., Louviere, C. D., & Deleyrolle, L. P. (2016). A supplemented high-fat low-carbohydrate diet for the treatment of glioblastoma. *Clinical Cancer Research*, *22*(10), 2482–2495. DOI: 10.1158/1078-0432.CCR-15-0916 PMID: 26631612

Mauget-Faÿsse, M., Jafarzadeh, A., Mosnier, J. F., Bertrand, A., Allouch, C., & Rigal, D.. (2001). Verteporfin in photodynamic therapy: A review. *American Journal of Ophthalmology*, *132*(5), 757–765. PMID: 11704038

Mazzoleni, A., Awuah, W. A., Sanker, V., Bharadwaj, H. R., Aderinto, N., Tan, J. K., & Atallah, O. (2024). Chromosomal instability: A key driver in glioma pathogenesis and progression. *European Journal of Medical Research*, *29*(1), 451. DOI: 10.1186/s40001-024-02043-8 PMID: 39227895

McCague, C., Ramlee, S., Reinius, M., Selby, I., Hulse, D., Piyatissa, P., & Davies, R. (2023). Introduction to radiomics for a clinical audience. *Clinical Radiology*, *78*(2), 83–98. DOI: 10.1016/j.crad.2022.08.149 PMID: 36639175

McGranahan, T., Therkelsen, K. E., Ahmad, S., & Nagpal, S. (2019). Current State of Immunotherapy for Treatment of Glioblastoma. *Current Treatment Options in Oncology*, *20*(3), 24. Advance online publication. DOI: 10.1007/s11864-019-0619-4 PMID: 30790064

McMahon, S. A.. (2019). Monoclonal antibodies in glioblastoma treatment: Targeting EGFR and VEGF. *Journal of Clinical Oncology*, *37*(3), 234–240. DOI: 10.1200/JCO.18.01556

Mehta, M., Wen, P., Nishikawa, R., Reardon, D., & Peters, K. (2017). Critical review of the addition of tumor treating fields (TTFields) to the existing standard of care for newly diagnosed glioblastoma patients. *Critical Reviews in Oncology/ Hematology*, *111*, 60–65. DOI: 10.1016/j.critrevonc.2017.01.005 PMID: 28259296

Mei, S., & Zhang, K. (2021). A machine learning framework for predicting drug–drug interactions. *Scientific Reports*, *11*(1), 17619. DOI: 10.1038/s41598-021-97193-8 PMID: 34475500

Mendiratta, K., Singh, S., & Chattopadhyay, P. (2024). SKIPNet: Spatial attention skip connections for enhanced brain tumor classification. arXiv. Retrieved May 17, 2025, from https://arxiv.org/abs/2412.07736v1

Meng, W., Palmer, J. D., Siedow, M., Haque, S. J., & Chakravarti, A. (2022). Overcoming radiation resistance in gliomas by targeting metabolism and DNA repair pathways. *International Journal of Molecular Sciences*, *23*(4), 2246. DOI: 10.3390/ ijms23042246 PMID: 35216362

Mercier, B. D., Tizpa, E., Philip, E. J., Feng, Q., Huang, Z., Thomas, R. M., Pal, S. K., Dorff, T. B., & Li, Y. R. (2022). Dietary interventions in cancer treatment and response: A comprehensive review. *Cancers (Basel)*, *14*(20), 5149. DOI: 10.3390/ cancers14205149 PMID: 36291933

Merenzon, M. A., Arias, E. H., Bhatia, S., Shah, A. H., Higgins, D. M., Villaverde, M., & Eichberg, D. G. (2023). Nitric oxide synthase inhibitors as potential therapeutic agents for gliomas: A systematic review. *Nitric Oxide*, *138–139*, 10–16. DOI: 10.1016/j.niox.2023.06.002 PMID: 37279819

Meyers, C. A., Horowitz, G., Groves, P., Popovic, R., Lee, T., & Miller, M.. (2001). Topotecan in the treatment of glioblastoma: A clinical review. *Journal of Clinical Oncology*, *19*(6), 2227–2233.

Meyers, J. D., Cheng, Y., Broome, A.-M., Agnes, R. S., Schluchter, M. D., Margevicius, S., Wang, X., Kenney, M. E., Burda, C., & Basilion, J. P. (2015). Peptide-targeted gold nanoparticles for photodynamic therapy of brain cancer. *Particle & Particle Systems Characterization*, *32*(4), 448–457. DOI: 10.1002/ppsc.201400119 PMID: 25999665

Mikic, N., Gentilal, N., Cao, F., Lok, E., Wong, E. T., Ballo, M., & Kesari, S. (2024). Tumor-treating fields dosimetry in glioblastoma: Insights into treatment planning, optimization, and dose–response relationships. *Neuro-Oncology Advances*, *6*(1), vdae032. Advance online publication. DOI: 10.1093/noajnl/vdae032 PMID: 38560348

Millán-Zambrano, G., Burton, A., Bannister, A. J., & Schneider, R. (2022). Histone posttranslational modifications—Cause and consequence of genome function. *Nature Reviews. Genetics, 23*(9), 563–580. DOI: 10.1038/s41576-022-00468-7 PMID: 35338361

Mineo, J. F., Bordron, A., Baroncini, M., Ramirez, C., Maurage, C. A., Blond, S., & Dam-Hieu, P. (2007). Prognosis factors of survival time in patients with glioblastoma multiforme: A multivariate analysis of 340 patients. *Acta Neurochirurgica, 149*(3), 245–253. DOI: 10.1007/s00701-006-1092-y PMID: 17273889

Minniti, G., De Sanctis, V., Muni, R., Filippone, F., Bozzao, A., Valeriani, M., Osti, M. F., De Paula, U., Lanzetta, G., Tombolini, V., & Maurizi Enrici, R. (2005). Radiotherapy plus concomitant and adjuvant temozolomide for glioblastoma in elderly patients. *The New England Journal of Medicine, 88*(1), 97–103. DOI: 10.1007/s11060-008-9538-0 PMID: 18250965

Mittal, K. R., Pharasi, N., Sarna, B., Singh, M., Rachana, , Haider, S., Singh, S. K., Dua, K., Jha, S. K., Dey, A., Ojha, S., Mani, S., & Jha, N. K. (2022). Nanotechnology-based drug delivery for the treatment of CNS disorders. *Translational Neuroscience, 13*(1), 527–546. DOI: 10.1515/tnsci-2022-0258 PMID: 36741545

Miyai, M., Tomita, H., Soeda, A., Yano, H., Iwama, T., & Hara, A. (2017). Current trends in mouse models of glioblastoma. *Journal of Neuro-Oncology, 135*(3), 423–432. DOI: 10.1007/s11060-017-2626-2 PMID: 29052807

Mo, F., Pellerino, A., Soffietti, R., & Rudà, R. (2021). Blood–brain barrier in brain tumors: Biology and clinical relevance. *International Journal of Molecular Sciences, 22*(23), 12654. DOI: 10.3390/ijms222312654 PMID: 34884457

Mohammed, S., Dinesan, M., & Ajayakumar, T. (2022). Survival and quality of life analysis in glioblastoma multiforme with adjuvant chemoradiotherapy: A retrospective study. *Reports of Practical Oncology and Radiotherapy : Journal of Greatpoland Cancer Center in Poznan and Polish Society of Radiation Oncology, 27*(6), 1026–1036. DOI: 10.5603/RPOR.a2022.0113 PMID: 36632307

Mohan, A., Nair, S. V., & Lakshmanan, V.-K. (2018). Polymeric nanomicelles for cancer theragnostics. *International Journal of Polymeric Materials, 67*(2), 119–130. DOI: 10.1080/00914037.2017.1309540

Mohr, A. E., Ortega-Santos, C. P., Whisner, C. M., Klein-Seetharaman, J., & Jasbi, P. (2024). Navigating challenges and opportunities in multi-omics integration for personalized healthcare. *Biomedicines, 12*(7), 1496. DOI: 10.3390/biomedicines12071496 PMID: 39062068

Mokarram, N., Case, A., Hossainy, N. N., Lyon, J. G., MacDonald, T. J., & Bellamkonda, R. V. (2025). Device-assisted strategies for drug delivery across the blood-brain barrier to treat glioblastoma. *Communications Materials*, *6*(1), 1–22. DOI: 10.1038/s43246-024-00721-y PMID: 39790893

Molinaro, A. M., Hervey-Jumper, S., Morshed, R. A., Young, J., Han, S. J., Chunduru, P., Zhang, Y., Phillips, J. J., Shai, A., Lafontaine, M., Crane, J., Chandra, A., Flanigan, P., Jahangiri, A., Cioffi, G., Ostrom, Q., Anderson, J. E., Badve, C., Barnholtz-Sloan, J., & Berger, M. S. (2020). Association of maximal extent of resection of contrast-enhanced and non–contrast-enhanced tumor with survival within molecular subgroups of patients with newly diagnosed glioblastoma. *JAMA Oncology*, *6*(4), 495–503. DOI: 10.1001/jamaoncol.2019.6143 PMID: 32027343

Monteiro, A. R., Hill, R., Pilkington, G. J., & Madureira, P. A. (2017). The role of hypoxia in glioblastoma invasion. *Cells*, *6*(4), 45. Advance online publication. DOI: 10.3390/cells6040045 PMID: 29165393

Moreira, R., Nóbrega, C., de Almeida, L. P., & Mendonça, L. (2024). Brain-targeted drug delivery-nanovesicles directed to specific brain cells by brain-targeting ligands. *Journal of Nanobiotechnology*, *22*(1), 260. DOI: 10.1186/s12951-024-02511-7 PMID: 38760847

Mura, S., Nicolas, J., & Couvreur, P. (2013). Stimuli-responsive nanocarriers for drug delivery. *Nature Materials*, *12*(11), 991–1003. DOI: 10.1038/nmat3776 PMID: 24150417

Musielak, E., & Krajka-Kuźniak, V. (2025). Lipidic and inorganic nanoparticles for targeted glioblastoma multiforme therapy: Advances and strategies. *Micro*, *5*(1), 2. Advance online publication. DOI: 10.3390/micro5010002

Nafe, R., & Hattingen, E. (2023). Cellular components of the tumor environment in gliomas—What do we know today? *Biomedicines*, *12*(1), 14. DOI: 10.3390/biomedicines12010014 PMID: 38275375

Nagpal, S., Recht, C. K., Bertrand, S., Thomas, R. P., Ajlan, A., Pena, J., Gershon, M., Coffey, G., Kunz, P. L., Li, G., & Recht, L. D. (2015). Phase II pilot study of single-agent etirinotecan pegol (NKTR-102) in bevacizumab-resistant high grade glioma. *Journal of Neuro-Oncology*, *123*(2), 277–282. DOI: 10.1007/s11060-015-1795-0 PMID: 25935109

Nagpal, S., Recht, C. K., Imtiaz, U., Bertrand, S., Thomas, R. P., Ajlan, A., Pena, J., Gershon, M., Kunz, P. L., Li, G., & Recht, L. D. (2014). Etirinotecan pegol (EP, NKTR-102) in the treatment of high-grade glioma (HGG): A phase 2 trial. *Journal of Clinical Oncology*, *32*(15, suppl), 2096–2096. DOI: 10.1200/jco.2014.32.15_suppl.2096

Nahar Metu, C. L., Sutihar, S. K., Sohel, M., Zohora, F., Hasan, A., Miah, M. T., Rani Kar, T., Hossain, M. A., & Rahman, M. H. (2023). Unraveling the signaling mechanism behind astrocytoma and possible therapeutics strategies: A comprehensive review. *Cancer Reports*, *6*(10), e1889. DOI: 10.1002/cnr2.1889 PMID: 37675821

Nakabayashi, H., & Shimizu, K. (2012). Involvement of Akt/NF-κB pathway in antitumor effects of parthenolide on glioblastoma cells in vitro and in vivo. *BMC Cancer*, *12*(1), 453. Advance online publication. DOI: 10.1186/1471-2407-12-453 PMID: 23039130

Namba, H., Kawaji, H., & Yamasaki, T. (2015). Use of genetically engineered stem cells for glioma therapy. *Oncology Letters*, *11*(1), 9–15. DOI: 10.3892/ol.2015.3860 PMID: 26870161

Nance, E., Pun, S. H., Saigal, R., & Sellers, D. L. (2022). Drug delivery to the central nervous system. *Nature Reviews. Materials*, *7*(4), 314–331. DOI: 10.1038/s41578-021-00394-w PMID: 38464996

Nangare, S., Chandankar, S., & Patil, P. (2023). Design of carbon and graphene quantum dots based nanotheranostics applications for glioblastoma management: Recent advanced and future prospects. *Journal of Drug Delivery Science and Technology*, *89*, 105060. Advance online publication. DOI: 10.1016/j.jddst.2023.105060

Narsinh, K. H., Perez, E., Haddad, A. F., Young, J. S., Savastano, L., Villanueva-Meyer, J. E., & Aghi, M. K. (2024). Strategies to improve drug delivery across the blood–brain barrier for glioblastoma. *Current Neurology and Neuroscience Reports*, *24*(5), 123–139. DOI: 10.1007/s11910-024-01338-x PMID: 38578405

Nayak, A., Warrier, N. M., Raman, R., Prabhu, V., & Kumar, P. (2024). Targeted delivery of nanomedicines to glioblastoma: Overcoming the clinical barrier. *Journal of Drug Delivery Science and Technology*, *99*, 105980. Advance online publication. DOI: 10.1016/j.jddst.2024.105980

Neuss MN (2017) 2016 updated American Society of Clinical Oncology/Oncology Nursing Society chemotherapy administration safety standards, including standards for pediatric oncology. *Number 1/January 2017* 44: 31-43.

Neuwelt, E. A., Várallyay, C. G., Manninger, S., Solymosi, D., Haluska, M., Hunt, M. A., Nesbit, G., Stevens, A., Jerosch-Herold, M., Jacobs, J. M., & Hoffman, J. M. (2007). The potential of ferumoxytol nanoparticle magnetic resonance imaging, perfusion, and angiography in central nervous system malignancy: A pilot study. *Neurosurgery*, *60*(4), 601–612. DOI: 10.1227/01.NEU.0000255350.71700.37 PMID: 17415196

Ng, A. T., Steve, T., Jamouss, K. T., Arham, A., Kawtharani, S., & Assi, H. I. (2024). The challenges and clinical landscape of glioblastoma immunotherapy. *CNS Oncology*, *13*(1), 2415878. Advance online publication. DOI: 10.1080/20450907.2024.2415878 PMID: 39469854

Ngoi, N. Y., Peng, G., & Yap, T. A. (2022). A tale of two checkpoints: ATR inhibition and PD-(L) 1 blockade. *Annual Review of Medicine*, *73*(1), 231–250. DOI: 10.1146/annurev-med-042320-025136 PMID: 34644155

Nguyen, S. (2024) From Barriers to Solution Pathways: Drug Repurposing's Path Forward for Off-Patent Drugs. Thesis.

Nguyen, T. K., Sahgal, A., Detsky, J., Soliman, H., Myrehaug, S., Tseng, C. L., Husain, Z. A., Carty, A., Das, S., Yang, V., Lee, Y., Sarfehnia, A., Chugh, B. P., Yeboah, C., & Ruschin, M. (2019). Single-Fraction Stereotactic Radiosurgery Versus Hippocampal-Avoidance Whole Brain Radiation Therapy for Patients With 10 to 30 Brain Metastases: A Dosimetric Analysis. *International Journal of Radiation Oncology, Biology, Physics*, *105*(2), 394–399. DOI: 10.1016/j.ijrobp.2019.06.2543 PMID: 31283978

Niazi, S. K. (2023). Non-invasive drug delivery across the blood–brain barrier: A prospective analysis. *Pharmaceutics*, *15*(11), 2599. DOI: 10.3390/pharmaceutics15112599 PMID: 38004577

Niculescu, A.-G., Chircov, C., Bîrcă, A. C., & Grumezescu, A. M. (2021). Fabrication and applications of microfluidic devices: A review. *International Journal of Molecular Sciences*, *22*(4), 2011. Advance online publication. DOI: 10.3390/ijms22042011 PMID: 33670545

Nikam, D., & Jain, A. (2023). Advances in the discovery of DHPMs as Eg5 inhibitors for the management of breast cancer and glioblastoma: A review. *Results in Chemistry*, *5*, 100718. Advance online publication. DOI: 10.1016/j.rechem.2022.100718

Nishiyama, N., Matsumura, Y., & Kataoka, K. (2016). Development of polymeric micelles for targeting intractable cancers. *Cancer Science*, *107*(7), 867–874. DOI: 10.1111/cas.12960 PMID: 27116635

Noebauer-Huhmann, I. M., Weber, M.-A., Lalam, R. K., Trattnig, S., Bohndorf, K., Vanhoenacker, F., Tagliafico, A., van Rijswijk, C., Vilanova, J. C., & Afonso, P. D. (2015) Soft tissue tumors in adults: ESSR-approved guidelines for diagnostic imaging. Vol. 19 p.^pp. 475-482. Thieme Medical Publishers.

Nogueira, L., Ruiz-Ontañon, P., Vazquez-Barquero, A., Lafarga, M., Berciano, M., Aldaz, B., & Fernández-Luna, J. L. (2011). Blockade of the NFκB pathway drives differentiating glioblastoma-initiating cells into senescence both in vitro and in vivo. *Oncogene*, *30*(32), 3537–3548. DOI: 10.1038/onc.2011.74 PMID: 21423202

Noorani, I., & de la Rosa, J. (2023). Breaking barriers for glioblastoma with a path to enhanced drug delivery. *Nature Communications*, *14*(1), 5909. Advance online publication. DOI: 10.1038/s41467-023-41694-9 PMID: 37737212

Ntafoulis, I., Koolen, S. L., Leenstra, S., & Lamfers, M. L. (2022). Drug repurposing, a fast-track approach to develop effective treatments for glioblastoma. *Cancers (Basel)*, *14*(15), 3705. DOI: 10.3390/cancers14153705 PMID: 35954371

Nwagwu, C. D., Immidisetti, A. V., Jiang, M. Y., Adeagbo, O., Adamson, D. C., & Carbonell, A.-M. (2021). Convection enhanced delivery in the setting of high-grade gliomas. *Pharmaceutics*, *13*(4), 561. DOI: 10.3390/pharmaceutics13040561 PMID: 33921157

O'Hara, R., Tedone, E., Ludlow, A., Huang, E., Arosio, B., Mari, D., & Shay, J. W. (2019). Quantitative mitochondrial DNA copy number determination using droplet digital PCR with single-cell resolution. *Genome Research*, *29*(11), 1878–1888. DOI: 10.1101/gr.250480.119 PMID: 31548359

Obozina, A. S., Komedchikova, E. N., Kolesnikova, O. A., Iureva, A. M., Kovalenko, V. L., Zavalko, F. A., & Deyev, S. M. (2023). Genetically encoded self-assembling protein nanoparticles for the targeted delivery in vitro and in vivo. *Pharmaceutics*, *15*(1), 231. Advance online publication. DOI: 10.3390/pharmaceutics15010231 PMID: 36678860

Ohba, S., & Hirose, Y. (2016). Current and future drug treatments for glioblastomas. *Current Medicinal Chemistry*, *23*(38), 4309–4316. DOI: 10.2174/0929867323666161014132907 PMID: 27758718

Oh, D. Y., Lee, K. W., Han, S. W., Kim, J. W., Shin, J. W., Jo, S. J., Won, J., Hahn, S., Lee, H., Kim, W. H., & Bang, Y.-J. (2019). A First-in-Human Phase I Study of GC1118, a Novel Anti-Epidermal Growth Factor Receptor Antibody, in Patients with Advanced Solid Tumors. *The Oncologist*, *24*(8), 1037–e636. DOI: 10.1634/theoncologist.2019-0294 PMID: 31164456

Oh, G., Wang, A., Wang, L., Li, J., Werba, G., Weissinger, D., & Ackermann, A. (2023). POLQ inhibition elicits an immune response in homologous recombination–deficient pancreatic adenocarcinoma via cGAS/STING signaling. *The Journal of Clinical Investigation*, *133*(11), e165934. DOI: 10.1172/JCI165934 PMID: 36976649

Ohgaki, H., Dessen, P., Jourde, B., Horstmann, S., Nishikawa, T., Di Patre, P.-L., Burkhard, C., Schüler, D., Probst-Hensch, N. M., Maiorka, P. C., Baeza, N., Pisani, P., Yonekawa, Y., Yasargil, M. G., Lütolf, U. M., & Kleihues, P. (2004). Genetic pathways to glioblastoma: A population-based study. *Cancer Research*, *64*(19), 6892–6899. DOI: 10.1158/0008-5472.CAN-04-1337 PMID: 15466178

Oh, J. H.. (2020). Transferrin receptor-targeted nanoparticles for drug delivery in glioblastoma therapy. *International Journal of Nanomedicine*, *15*, 6439–6453. DOI: 10.2147/IJN.S268791

Omuro, A., Beal, K., Mcneill, K., Young, R. J., Thomas, A., Lin, X., Terziev, R., Kaley, T. J., DeAngelis, L. M., Daras, M., Gavrilovic, I. T., Mellinghoff, I., Diamond, E. L., McKeown, A., Manne, M., Caterfino, A., Patel, K., Bavisotto, L., Gorman, G., & Pentsova, E. (2018). Multicenter Phase IB Trial of Carboxyamidotriazole Orotate and Temozolomide for Recurrent and Newly Diagnosed Glioblastoma and Other Anaplastic Gliomas. *Journal of Clinical Oncology*, *36*(17), 1702–1709. DOI: 10.1200/JCO.2017.76.9992 PMID: 29683790

Onciul, R., Brehar, F.-M., Toader, C., Covache-Busuioc, R.-A., Glavan, L.-A., Bratu, B.-G., Costin, H. P., Dumitrascu, D.-I., Serban, M., & Ciurea, A. V. (2024). Deciphering glioblastoma: Fundamental and novel insights into the biology and therapeutic strategies of gliomas. *Current Issues in Molecular Biology*, *46*(3), 2402–2443. DOI: 10.3390/cimb46030153 PMID: 38534769

Oraiopoulou, M.-E., Tzamali, E., Psycharakis, S. E., Tzedakis, G., Makatounakis, T., Manolitsi, K., & Zacharakis, G. (2024). The temozolomide–doxorubicin paradox in glioblastoma in vitro–in silico preclinical drug-screening. *Cancers (Basel)*, *16*(1), 3759. Advance online publication. DOI: 10.3390/cancers16020375 PMID: 38355655

Ortiz, R., Perazzoli, G., Cabeza, L., Jiménez-Luna, C., Luque, R., Prados, J., & Melguizo, C. (2021). Temozolomide: An updated overview of resistance mechanisms, nanotechnology advances and clinical applications. *Current Neuropharmacology*, *19*(4), 513–537. DOI: 10.2174/1570159X19666201230133538 PMID: 32589560

Ostrom, Q. T., Patil, N., Cioffi, G., Waite, K., Kruchko, C., & Barnholtz-Sloan, J. S. (2020). CBTRUS statistical report: Primary brain and other central nervous system tumors diagnosed in the United States in 2013–2017. *Neuro-Oncology*, *22*(Suppl. 1), iv1–iv96. DOI: 10.1093/neuonc/noaa200 PMID: 33123732

Ou, A., Yung, W. K. A., & Majd, N. (2021). Molecular mechanisms of treatment resistance in glioblastoma. *International Journal of Molecular Sciences*, *22*(1), 351. Advance online publication. DOI: 10.3390/ijms22010351 PMID: 33396284

Overcoming Critical Issues in Glioblastoma Multiforme (GBM) Therapeutic Development. Scientist. https://crex.nih.gov/blog/2022/08/30/overcoming-critical-issues-in-glioblastoma-multiforme-gbm-therapeutic-development?utm_source=chatgpt.com. Accessed on 05 August 2025.

Ozair, A., Bhat, V., Alisch, R. S., Khosla, A. A., Kotecha, R. R., Odia, Y., McDermott, M. W., & Ahluwalia, M. S. (2023). DNA methylation and histone modification in low-grade gliomas: Current understanding and potential clinical targets. *Cancers (Basel)*, *15*(4), 1342. DOI: 10.3390/cancers15041342 PMID: 36831683

Ożarowski, M., Karpiński, T. M., Czerny, B., Kamiński, A., & Seremak-Mrozikiewicz, A. (2025). Plant alkaloids as promising anticancer compounds with blood–brain barrier penetration in the treatment of glioblastoma: In vitro and in vivo models. *Molecules (Basel, Switzerland)*, *30*(7), 1561. Advance online publication. DOI: 10.3390/molecules30071561 PMID: 40286187

Ozdemir-Kaynak, E., Qutub, A. A., & Yesil-Celiktas, O. (2018). Advances in glioblastoma multiforme treatment: New models for nanoparticle therapy. *Frontiers in Physiology*, *9*, 170. Advance online publication. DOI: 10.3389/fphys.2018.00170 PMID: 29615917

Pacheco-Torres, J., Mukherjee, N., Walko, M., López-Larrubia, P., Ballesteros, P., Cerdan, S., & Kocer, A. (2015). Image guided drug release from pH-sensitive Ion channel-functionalized stealth liposomes into an in vivo glioblastoma model. *Nanomedicine; Nanotechnology, Biology, and Medicine*, *11*(6), 1345–1354. DOI: 10.1016/j.nano.2015.03.014 PMID: 25888277

Panovska, D., & De Smet, F. (2022). Functional precision oncology: The next frontier to improve glioblastoma outcome? *International Journal of Molecular Sciences*, *23*(15), 8637. DOI: 10.3390/ijms23158637 PMID: 35955765

Pardridge, W. M. (2005). The blood-brain barrier: Bottleneck in brain drug development. *NeuroRx : the Journal of the American Society for Experimental NeuroTherapeutics*, *2*(1), 3–14. DOI: 10.1602/neurorx.2.1.3 PMID: 15717053

Pardridge, W. M. (2012). Drug transport across the blood–brain barrier. *Journal of Cerebral Blood Flow and Metabolism*, *32*(11), 1959–1972. DOI: 10.1038/jcbfm.2012.126 PMID: 22929442

Parker, N. R., Hudson, A. L., Khong, P., Parkinson, J. F., Dwight, T., Ikin, R. J., Zhu, Y., Chen, J., Wheeler, H. R., & Howell, V. M. (2016). Intratumoral heterogeneity identified at the epigenetic, genetic and transcriptional level in glioblastoma. *Scientific Reports*, *6*(1), 22477. Advance online publication. DOI: 10.1038/srep22477 PMID: 26940435

Park, J. I., Song, K. H., Jung, S. Y., Ahn, J., Hwang, S. G., Kim, J., Kim, E. H., & Kim, J. S. (2019). Tumor-treating fields induce RAW264.7 macrophage activation via NK-κB/MAPK signaling pathways. *Technology in Cancer Research & Treatment*, *18*, 1533033819868225. DOI: 10.1177/1533033819868225 PMID: 31401938

Partridge, B., Eardley, A., Morales, B. E., Campelo, S. N., Lorenzo, M. F., Mehta, J. N., Kani, Y., Mora, J. K. G., Campbell, E.-O. Y., Arena, C. B., Platt, S., Mintz, A., Shinn, R. L., Rylander, C. G., Debinski, W., Davalos, R. V., & Rossmeisl, J. H. (2022). Advancements in drug delivery methods for the treatment of brain disease. *Frontiers in Veterinary Science*, *9*, 1039745. DOI: 10.3389/fvets.2022.1039745 PMID: 36330152

Patel, K., Gathe, J. C., & Zorrilla, C.. (2000). Nelfinavir in the treatment of HIV infection: A clinical review. *Journal of Clinical Pharmacology*, *40*(10), 1045–1053.

Patel, R., Patel, D., Dani, U., & Kuperkar, K. (2025). Nanoparticle-driven drug delivery system for cardiovascular treatment. *Journal of Cardiology*. Advance online publication. DOI: 10.1016/j.jjcc.2025.06.004 PMID: 40518071

Patil, C. G., Pricola, K., Sarmiento, J. M., Garg, S. K., Bryant, A., & Black, K. L. (2017). Whole brain radiation therapy (WBRT) alone versus WBRT and radiosurgery for the treatment of brain metastases. *Cochrane Database of Systematic Reviews*, *9*(9). Advance online publication. DOI: 10.1002/14651858.CD006121.pub4 PMID: 28945270

Patil, C., Priyanka, R., Harshitha, B. M., Oshik, S., Yashwanth, S., Darshan, B. R., Patil, S., Prajwal, K. A., Naik, P., Goudanavar, P., & Mallamma, T. (2025). Advanced nanotheranostic approaches for targeted glioblastoma treatment: A synergistic fusion of CRISPR-Cas gene editing, AI-driven tumor profiling, and BBB-modulation. *Medical Oncology (Northwood, London, England)*, *42*(9), 229. Advance online publication. DOI: 10.1007/s12032-025-02944-6 PMID: 40773116

Patil, N, & Ranjan, A, Gaurav, Mukherjee D, Panda BK, Diksha, Komal, Narang RK & Singh A. (2024). Navigating Biosimilar Regulatory Pathways in Emerging Markets: Insights from Brics Nations. *Applied Drug Research, Clinical Trials and Regulatory Affairs*.

Paull, T. T. (2019). RNA–DNA hybrids and the convergence with DNA repair. *Critical Reviews in Biochemistry and Molecular Biology*, *54*(4), 371–384. DOI: 10.1080/10409238.2019.1670131 PMID: 31577154

Paul, S., Sinha, S., & Kundu, C. N. (2022). Targeting cancer stem cells in the tumor microenvironment: An emerging role of PARP inhibitors. *Pharmacological Research*, *184*, 106425. DOI: 10.1016/j.phrs.2022.106425 PMID: 36075511

Pearson, R. A., Wicha, S. G., & Okour, M. (2023). Drug combination modeling: Methods and applications in drug development. *Journal of Clinical Pharmacology*, *63*(2), 151–165. DOI: 10.1002/jcph.2128 PMID: 36088583

Pęczek, P., Gajda, M., Rutkowski, K., Fudalej, M., Deptała, A., & Badowska-Kozakiewicz, A. M. (2023). Cancer-associated inflammation: Pathophysiology and clinical significance. *Journal of Cancer Research and Clinical Oncology*, *149*(6), 2657–2672. DOI: 10.1007/s00432-022-04399-y PMID: 36260158

Pérez-López, A., Torres-Suárez, A. I., Martín-Sabroso, C., & Aparicio-Blanco, J. (2023). An overview of in vitro 3D models of the blood-brain barrier as a tool to predict the in vivo permeability of nanomedicines. *Advanced Drug Delivery Reviews*, *196*, 114816. Advance online publication. DOI: 10.1016/j.addr.2023.114816 PMID: 37003488

Perry, J. R., Brown, C. W., McClintock, M., Williams, T., Ly, R., & Petty, L.. (2005). Thiotepa in glioblastoma treatment: Pharmacology and clinical applications. *Journal of Clinical Oncology*, *23*(6), 1212–1217.

Perry, J., Zinman, L., Chambers, A., Spithoff, K., Lloyd, N., & Laperriere, N. (2006). The use of prophylactic anticonvulsants in patients with brain tumours—A systematic review. *Current Oncology (Toronto, Ont.)*, *13*(6), 222–229. DOI: 10.3747/co.v13i6.107 PMID: 22792022

Perryman, R., Renziehausen, A., Shaye, H., Kostagianni, A. D., Tsiailanis, A. D., Thorne, T., & Syed, N. (2022). Inhibition of the angiotensin II type 2 receptor AT2R is a novel therapeutic strategy for glioblastoma. *Proceedings of the National Academy of Sciences of the United States of America*, *119*(32), e2116289119. Advance online publication. DOI: 10.1073/pnas.2116289119 PMID: 35917342

Pessina, F., Navarria, P., Cozzi, L., Ascolese, A. M., Simonelli, M., Santoro, A., Clerici, E., Rossi, M., Scorsetti, M., & Bello, L. (2017). Maximize surgical resection beyond contrast-enhancing boundaries in newly diagnosed glioblastoma multiforme: Is it useful and safe? A single institution retrospective experience. *Journal of Neuro-Oncology*, *135*(1), 129–139. DOI: 10.1007/s11060-017-2559-9 PMID: 28689368

Petković, M., Henis, M., Heese, O., & Relógio, A. (2023). Chronotherapy in glioblastoma: State of the art and future perspectives. *EBioMedicine*, *89*, 104485. Advance online publication. DOI: 10.1016/j.ebiom.2023.104470 PMID: 36796229

Pichierri, A., Bradley, M., & Iyer, V. (2019). Intraoperative magnetic resonance imaging–guided glioma resections in awake or asleep settings and feasibility in the context of a public health system. *World Neurosurgery: X*, *3*, 100022. DOI: 10.1016/j.wnsx.2019.100022 PMID: 31225516

Pinheiro Lopes, B., O'Neill, L., Bourke, P., & Boehm, D. (2025). Enhanced cytotoxic effects of cold plasma deposition of topotecan: A novel approach for local cancer drug delivery to glioblastoma cells. *Cancers (Basel)*, *17*(2), 201. Advance online publication. DOI: 10.3390/cancers17020201 PMID: 39857983

Pourmasoumi, P., Banihashemian, S. A., Zamani, F., Rasouli-Nia, A., Mehrabani, D., & Karimi-Busheri, F. (2024). Nanoparticle-Based Approaches in the Diagnosis and Treatment of Brain Tumors. *Journal of Clinical Medicine*, *13*(23), 7449. DOI: 10.3390/jcm13237449 PMID: 39685907

Pouyan, A., Ghorbanlo, M., Eslami, M., Jahanshahi, M., Ziaei, E., Salami, A., & Farhadi, M. (2025). Glioblastoma multiforme: Insights into pathogenesis, key signaling pathways, and therapeutic strategies. *Molecular Cancer*, *24*(1), 58. Advance online publication. DOI: 10.1186/s12943-025-02267-0 PMID: 40011944

Prencipe, F., Diaferia, C., Rossi, F., Ronga, L., & Tesauro, D. (2021). Forward precision medicine: Micelles for active targeting driven by peptides. *Molecules (Basel, Switzerland)*, *26*(13), 4049. Advance online publication. DOI: 10.3390/molecules26134049 PMID: 34279392

Preusser, M., Lim, M., Hafler, D. A., Reardon, D. A., & Sampson, J. H. (2015). Prospects of immune checkpoint modulators in the treatment of glioblastoma. *Nature Reviews. Neurology*, *11*(9), 504–514. DOI: 10.1038/nrneurol.2015.139 PMID: 26260659

Puris, E., Fricker, G., & Gynther, M. (2022). Targeting transporters for drug delivery to the brain: Can we do better? *Pharmaceutical Research*, *39*(7), 1415–1455. DOI: 10.1007/s11095-022-03241-x PMID: 35359241

Qian, Z. M., Li, H., Sun, H., & Ho, K. (2002). Targeted drug delivery via the transferrin receptor-mediated endocytosis pathway. *Pharmacological Reviews*, *54*(4), 561–587. DOI: 10.1124/pr.54.4.561 PMID: 12429868

Qindeel, M., Irfan, M., Ullah, S., Fathi-karkan, S., Kharaba, Z., Rahdar, A., & Bilal, M. (2024). Nanotechnology in glioblastoma therapy: Advances in drug delivery systems and diagnostic approaches. *Journal of Drug Delivery Science and Technology, 102*, 106322. Advance online publication. DOI: 10.1016/j.jddst.2024.106322

Qin, H., Zhang, F., & Gao, S. (2024). Ketogenic Diet Therapy for Glioma: Combined Effects. *Current Cancer Therapy Reviews, 20*(2), 177–187. DOI: 10.2174/1573394719666230717160843

Qiu, J., Kong, L., Cao, X., Li, A., Wei, P., Wang, L., Mignani, S., Caminade, A. M., Majoral, J. P., & Shi, X. (2018). Enhanced Delivery of Therapeutic siRNA into Glioblastoma Cells Using Dendrimer-Entrapped Gold Nanoparticles Conjugated with β-Cyclodextrin. *Nanomaterials (Basel, Switzerland), 8*(3), 131. Advance online publication. DOI: 10.3390/nano8030131 PMID: 29495429

Quader, S., Liu, X., Chen, Y., Mi, P., Chida, T., Ishii, T., Miura, Y., Nishiyama, N., Cabral, H., & Kataoka, K. (2017). cRGD peptide-installed epirubicin-loaded polymeric micelles for effective targeted therapy against brain tumors. *Journal of Controlled Release, 258*, 56–66. DOI: 10.1016/j.jconrel.2017.04.033 PMID: 28483513

Quail, D. F., & Joyce, J. A. (2017). The microenvironmental landscape of brain tumors. *Cancer Cell, 31*(3), 326–341. DOI: 10.1016/j.ccell.2017.02.009 PMID: 28292436

Queirolo, P., Spagnolo, F., Ascierto, P. A., Simeone, E., Marchetti, P., Scoppola, A., Del Vecchio, M., Di Guardo, L., Maio, M., Di Giacomo, A. M., Antonuzzo, A., Cognetti, F., Ferraresi, V., Ridolfi, L., Guidoboni, M., Guida, M., Pigozzo, J., & Chiarion Sileni, V. (2014). Efficacy and safety of ipilimumab in patients with advanced melanoma and brain metastases. *Journal of Neuro-Oncology, 118*(1), 109–116. DOI: 10.1007/s11060-014-1400-y PMID: 24532241

Qu, J., Zhang, L., Chen, Z., Mao, G., Gao, Z., Lai, X., Zhu, X., & Zhu, J. (2016). Nanostructured lipid carriers, solid lipid nanoparticles, and polymeric nanoparticles: Which kind of drug delivery system is better for glioblastoma chemotherapy? *Drug Delivery, 23*(9), 3408–3416. DOI: 10.1080/10717544.2016.1189465 PMID: 27181462

Qureshi, S., Anjum, S., Hussain, M., Sheikh, A., Gupta, G., Almoyad, M. A., Wahab, S., & Kesharwani, P. (2024). A recent insight of applications of gold nanoparticles in glioblastoma multiforme therapy. *International Journal of Pharmaceutics, 660*, 124301. Advance online publication. DOI: 10.1016/j.ijpharm.2024.124301 PMID: 38851411

Rahban, M., Joushi, S., Bashiri, H., Saso, L., & Sheibani, V. (2024). Characterization of prevalent tyrosine kinase inhibitors and their challenges in glioblastoma treatment. *Frontiers in Chemistry, 11*, 1325214. Advance online publication. DOI: 10.3389/fchem.2023.1325214 PMID: 38264122

Rahman, M. A., & Ali, M. M. (2024). Recent treatment strategies and molecular pathways in resistance mechanisms of antiangiogenic therapies in glioblastoma. *Cancers (Basel), 16*(17), 2975. Advance online publication. DOI: 10.3390/cancers16172975 PMID: 39272834

Rahman, M. H., Rana, H. K., Peng, S., Hu, X., Chen, C., Quinn, J. M., & Moni, M. A. (2021). Bioinformatics and machine learning methodologies to identify the effects of central nervous system disorders on glioblastoma progression. *Briefings in Bioinformatics, 22*(5), bbaa365. Advance online publication. DOI: 10.1093/bib/bbaa365 PMID: 33406529

Rainer Wirtz, W. S., Albert, F. K., Schwaderer, M., Heuer, C., Staubert, A., Tronnier, V. M., Knauth, M., & Kunze, S. (2000). The benefit of neuronavigation for neurosurgery analyzed by its impact on glioblastoma surgery. *Neurological Research, 22*(4), 354–360. DOI: 10.1080/01616412.2000.11740684 PMID: 10874684

Rajan, R. G., Fernandez-Vega, V., Sperry, J., Nakashima, J., Do, L. H., Andrews, W., & Tran, N. L. (2023). In vitro and in vivo drug-response profiling using patient-derived high-grade glioma. *Cancers (Basel), 15*(13), 3289. Advance online publication. DOI: 10.3390/cancers15133289 PMID: 37444398

Rajendran, A. T., & Vadakkepushpakath, A. N. (2024). Targeting glioblastoma: Advances in precision drug delivery. *Journal of Young Pharmacists : JYP, 16*(4), 697–705. DOI: 10.5530/jyp.2024.16.89

Rajput, T. A. (2025). The role of microRNAs in glioblastoma: Gene therapy and diagnostic potentials. *Medical Science and Discovery, 12*(5), 154–162. DOI: 10.36472/msd.v12i5.1276

Raju, R., Abuwatfa, W. H., Pitt, W. G., & Husseini, G. A. (2023). Liposomes for the treatment of brain cancer—A review. *Pharmaceuticals (Basel, Switzerland), 16*(8), 1056. Advance online publication. DOI: 10.3390/ph16081056 PMID: 37630971

Ratliff, M., Kim, H., Qi, H., Kim, M., Ku, B., Azorin, D. D., Hausmann, D., Khajuria, R. K., Patel, A., Maier, E., Cousin, L., Ogier, A., Sahm, F., Etminan, N., Bunse, L., Winkler, F., El-Khoury, V., Platten, M., & Kwon, Y.-J. (2022). Patient-derived tumor organoids for guidance of personalized drug therapies in recurrent glioblastoma. *International Journal of Molecular Sciences, 23*(12), 6572. Advance online publication. DOI: 10.3390/ijms23126572 PMID: 35743016

Ravn-Boess, N., Roy, N., Hattori, T., Bready, D., Donaldson, H., Lawson, C., & Mischel, P. S. (2023). The expression profile and tumorigenic mechanisms of CD97 (ADGRE5) in glioblastoma render it a targetable vulnerability. *Cell Reports*, *42*(11), 113374. Advance online publication. DOI: 10.1016/j.celrep.2023.113374 PMID: 37938973

Reardon, D. A., & Wen, P. Y. (2015). Glioma in 2014: Unravelling tumour heterogeneity—Implications for therapy. *Nature Reviews. Clinical Oncology*, *12*(2), 69–70. DOI: 10.1038/nrclinonc.2014.223 PMID: 25560529

Rechberger, J. S., Toll, S. A., Biswas, S., You, H. B., Chow, W. D., Kendall, N., Navalkele, P., & Khatua, S. (2025). Advances in the Repurposing and Blood–Brain Barrier Penetrance of Drugs in Pediatric Brain Tumors. *Cancers (Basel)*, *17*(3), 439. DOI: 10.3390/cancers17030439 PMID: 39941807

Rehman, M., Madni, A., Shi, D., Ihsan, A., Tahir, N., Chang, K. R., Javed, I., & Webster, T. J. (2017). Enhanced blood brain barrier permeability and glioblastoma cell targeting via thermoresponsive lipid nanoparticles. *Nanoscale*, *9*(40), 15434–15440. DOI: 10.1039/C7NR05216B PMID: 28976512

Reina, C., Šabanović, B., Lazzari, C., Gregorc, V., & Heeschen, C. (2024). Unlocking the future of cancer diagnosis–promises and challenges of ctDNA-based liquid biopsies in non-small cell lung cancer. *Translational Research; the Journal of Laboratory and Clinical Medicine*, *272*, 41–53. DOI: 10.1016/j.trsl.2024.05.014 PMID: 38838851

Reithmeier, T., Graf, E., Piroth, T., Trippel, M., Pinsker, M. O., & Nikkhah, G. (2010). BCNU for recurrent glioblastoma multiforme: Efficacy, toxicity and prognostic factors. *BMC Cancer*, *10*(1), 30. Advance online publication. DOI: 10.1186/1471-2407-10-30 PMID: 20122270

Ricciardi, L., Manini, I., Cesselli, D., Trungu, S., Piazza, A., & Mangraviti, A. (2022). Carmustine Wafers Implantation in Patients With Newly Diagnosed High Grade Glioma: Is It Still an Option? In *Frontiers in Neurology* (Vol. 13). Frontiers Media S.A. DOI: 10.3389/fneur.2022.884158

Ricco, N., & Kron, S. J. (2023). Statins in cancer prevention and therapy. *Cancers (Basel)*, *15*(15), 3948. DOI: 10.3390/cancers15153948 PMID: 37568764

Richardson, P. G., Lacy, M. Q., & Palumbo, A.. (2006). Lenalidomide in combination with dexamethasone for patients with relapsed or refractory multiple myeloma. *The New England Journal of Medicine*, *354*(10), 1233–1244.

Riemenschneider, M. J., Jeuken, J. W. M., Wesseling, P., & Reifenberger, G. (2010). Molecular diagnostics of gliomas: State of the art. *Acta Neuropathologica*, *120*(5), 567–584. DOI: 10.1007/s00401-010-0736-4 PMID: 20714900

Robinson, S. D., Filippopoulou, C., Besta, S., Samuels, M., Betrán, A. L., Ajamieh, M. A., & Giamas, G. (2025). Spatial biology–unraveling complexity within the glioblastoma microenvironment. *Trends in Molecular Medicine*, *31*(9), 846–859. DOI: 10.1016/j.molmed.2025.01.014

Rodrigues, P., Bangali, H., Hammoud, A., Mustafa, Y. F., Al-Hetty, H. R. A. K., Alkhafaji, A. T., Deorari, M. M., Al-Taee, M. M., Zabibah, R. S., & Alsalamy, A. (2024). COX 2-inhibitors; a thorough and updated survey into combinational therapies in cancers. *Medical Oncology (Northwood, London, England)*, *41*(1), 41. DOI: 10.1007/s12032-023-02256-7 PMID: 38165473

Rodriguez-Berriguete, G., Ranzani, M., Prevo, R., Puliyadi, R., Machado, N., Bolland, H. R., & Cerutti, A. (2023). Small-molecule Polθ inhibitors provide safe and effective tumor radiosensitization in preclinical models. *Clinical Cancer Research*, *29*(8), 1631–1642. DOI: 10.1158/1078-0432.CCR-22-2977 PMID: 36689546

Rodríguez-Camacho, A., Flores-Vázquez, J. G., Moscardini-Martelli, J., Torres-Ríos, J. A., Olmos-Guzmán, A., Ortiz-Arce, C. S., Cid-Sánchez, R. B., Villafaña-Vázquez, V., & García-López, E. (2022). Glioblastoma treatment: State-of-the-art and future perspectives. *International Journal of Molecular Sciences*, *23*(13), 7207. Advance online publication. DOI: 10.3390/ijms23137207 PMID: 35806212

Rodriguez, S. M. B., Kamel, A., Ciubotaru, G. V., Onose, G., Sevastre, A.-S., Sfredel, V., & Mirea, A. (2023). An overview of EGFR mechanisms and their implications in targeted therapies for glioblastoma. *International Journal of Molecular Sciences*, *24*(13), 11110. Advance online publication. DOI: 10.3390/ijms241311110 PMID: 37446288

Rogawski, M. A., Holtman, J. R., & Zorumski, C. F.. (2008). AMPA receptor antagonists as therapeutic agents in epilepsy. *Epilepsy Currents*, *8*(6), 201–204.

Rong, L., Li, N., & Zhang, Z. (2022). Emerging therapies for glioblastoma: Current state and future directions. *Journal of Experimental & Clinical Cancer Research : CR*, *41*(1), 142. Advance online publication. DOI: 10.1186/s13046-022-02349-7 PMID: 35428347

Roque, D., Cruz, N., Ferreira, H. A., Reis, C. P., Matela, N., Herculano-Carvalho, M., Cascão, R., & Faria, C. C. (2023). Nanoparticle-based treatment in glioblastoma. *Journal of Personalized Medicine*, *13*(9), 1328. Advance online publication. DOI: 10.3390/jpm13091328 PMID: 37763096

Rosenblum, D., Joshi, N., Tao, W., Karp, J. M., & Peer, D. (2018). Progress and challenges towards targeted delivery of cancer therapeutics. *Nature Communications*, *9*(1), 1410. DOI: 10.1038/s41467-018-03705-y PMID: 29650952

Ruan, W., Jiao, M., Xu, S., Ismail, M., Xie, X., An, Y., Guo, H., Qian, R., Shi, B., & Zheng, M. (2022). Brain-targeted CRISPR/Cas9 nanomedicine for effective glioblastoma therapy. *Journal of Controlled Release*, *351*, 739–751. DOI: 10.1016/j.jconrel.2022.09.046 PMID: 36174804

Rubenich, D. S., de Souza, P. O., Omizzollo, N., Aubin, M. R., Basso, P. J., Silva, L. M., & Bonorino, C. (2023). Tumor-neutrophil crosstalk promotes in vitro and in vivo glioblastoma progression. *Frontiers in Immunology*, *14*, 1183465. Advance online publication. DOI: 10.3389/fimmu.2023.1183465 PMID: 37292196

Rucco, M., Falsetti, L., & Viticchi, G. (2020). Towards personalized diagnosis of glioblastoma in fluid-attenuated inversion recovery (FLAIR) by topological interpretable machine learning. arXiv. Retrieved May 17, 2025, from https://arxiv.org/abs/1912.08167

Rudrapal M, Khairnar SJ & Jadhav AG (2020) Drug Repurposing (DR): An Emerging Approach in Drug. *Drug Repurposing: Hypothesis, Molecular Aspects and Therapeutic Applications* 3.

Ryshkova, N. E., Oborotova, N. A., Shprakh, Z. S., Bagirova, V. L., Orlova, O. L., & Polozkova, A. P. (2000). Chemico-pharmacological investigation of a new medicinal form of 1,3-bis(2-chloroethyl)-1-nitrosourea. *Pharmaceutical Chemistry Journal*, *34*(9), 502–504. DOI: 10.1023/A:1005206728431

Sadelain, M., Rivière, I., & Riddell, S. (2017). Therapeutic T cell engineering. *Nature*, *545*(7655), 423–431. DOI: 10.1038/nature22395 PMID: 28541315

Sadetzki, S.. (2005). Radiation-induced meningioma: A descriptive study of 253 cases. *Journal of Neurosurgery*, *102*(2), 232–241. DOI: 10.3171/jns.2002.97.5.1078 PMID: 12450029

Sadowski, K., Jażdżewska, A., Kozłowski, J., Zacny, A., Lorenc, T., & Olejarz, W. (2024). Revolutionizing glioblastoma treatment: A comprehensive overview of modern therapeutic approaches. *International Journal of Molecular Sciences*, *25*(11), 5774. Advance online publication. DOI: 10.3390/ijms25115774 PMID: 38891962

Salomonsson, S. E., & Clelland, C. D. (2024). Building CRISPR gene therapies for the central nervous system: A review. *JAMA Neurology*, *81*(3), 283–290. DOI: 10.1001/jamaneurol.2023.4983 PMID: 38285472

Saltarella, I., Altamura, C., Campanale, C., Laghetti, P., Vacca, A., Frassanito, M. A., & Desaphy, J.-F. (2023). Anti-angiogenic activity of drugs in multiple myeloma. *Cancers (Basel), 15*(7), 1990. DOI: 10.3390/cancers15071990 PMID: 37046651

Salvato, I., & Marchini, A. (2024). Immunotherapeutic strategies for the treatment of glioblastoma: Current challenges and future perspectives. *Cancers (Basel), 16*(7), 1276. Advance online publication. DOI: 10.3390/cancers16071276 PMID: 38610954

Sampson, J. H., Achrol, S. A., Aghi, M. K., Bankiewicz, K., Bexon, M., & Brem, S. (2023). Targeting the IL4 receptor with MDNA55 in patients with recurrent glioblastoma: Results of a phase IIb trial. *Neuro-Oncology, 25*(6), 1085–1097. DOI: 10.1093/neuonc/noac285 PMID: 36640127

Sanai, N., Polley, M. Y., McDermott, M. W., Parsa, A. T., & Berger, M. S. (2011). An extent of resection threshold for newly diagnosed glioblastomas. *Journal of Neurosurgery, 115*(1), 3–8. DOI: 10.3171/2011.2.JNS10998 PMID: 21417701

Sanchez-Cano, F., Hernández-Kelly, L. C., & Ortega, A. (2021). The blood–brain barrier: Much more than a selective access to the brain. *Neurotoxicity Research, 39*(6), 2154–2174. DOI: 10.1007/s12640-021-00431-0 PMID: 34677787

Sancho, P., Barneda, D., & Heeschen, C. (2016). Hallmarks of cancer stem cell metabolism. *British Journal of Cancer, 114*(12), 1305–1312. DOI: 10.1038/bjc.2016.152 PMID: 27219018

Sandbhor, P., Goda, J., Mohanty, B., Gera, P., Yadav, S., Chekuri, G., & Moiyadi, A. (2023). Targeted nano-delivery of chemotherapy via intranasal route suppresses in vivo glioblastoma growth and prolongs survival in the intracranial mouse model. *PLoS One, 13*(2), 608–626. DOI: 10.1371/journal.pone.0287394 PMID: 36245060

Saxena, M., van der Burg, S. H., Melief, C. J. M., & Bhardwaj, N. (2021, June). (202*1). Therapeutic cancer* vaccines. *Nature Reviews. Cancer*, *21*(6), 360–378. DOI: 10.1038/s41568-021-00346-0 PMID: 33907315

Schiff, D., Lee, E. Q., Nayak, L., Norden, A. D., Reardon, D. A., & Wen, P. Y. (2015). Medical management of brain tumors and the sequelae of treatment. *Neuro-Oncology, 17*(4), 488–504. DOI: 10.1093/neuonc/nou304 PMID: 25358508

Schmitt, M., & Greten, F. R. (2021). The inflammatory pathogenesis of colorectal cancer. *Nature Reviews. Immunology, 21*(10), 653–667. DOI: 10.1038/s41577-021-00534-x PMID: 33911231

Schwartz, N. C. (2021) Analysis of Hyperosmotic Changes in Tight Junctions Using Immunocytochemistry and Electric Cell-Substrate Impedance Sensing. Thesis, Tulane University.

Schweiger, B., & Kievit, F. M. (2025). Glioblastoma induced blood-brain barrier dysfunction via a paracrine mechanism that increases claudin-1 expression. *Experimental Brain Research, 243*(3), 70. DOI: 10.1007/s00221-025-07018-7 PMID: 39960547

Seetharam, A. A., Choudhry, H., Bakhrebah, M. A., Abdulaal, W. H., Gupta, M. S., Rizvi, S. M. D., Alam, Q., & Gupta, R. (2020). Microneedles drug delivery systems for treatment of cancer: A recent update. *Pharmaceutics, 12*(11), 1101. Advance online publication. DOI: 10.3390/pharmaceutics12111101 PMID: 33212921

Segarra, M., Aburto, M. R., & Acker-Palmer, A. (2021). Blood–brain barrier dynamics to maintain brain homeostasis. *Trends in Neurosciences, 44*(5), 393–405. DOI: 10.1016/j.tins.2020.12.002 PMID: 33423792

Seker-Polat, F., Pinarbasi Degirmenci, N., Solaroglu, I., & Bagci-Onder, T. (2022). Tumor cell infiltration into the brain in glioblastoma: From mechanisms to clinical perspectives. *Cancers (Basel), 14*(2), 443. Advance online publication. DOI: 10.3390/cancers14020443 PMID: 35053605

Senders, J. T., Muskens, I. S., Schnoor, R., Karhade, A. V., Cote, D. J., Smith, T. R., & Broekman, M. L. (2017). Agents for fluorescence-guided glioma surgery: A systematic review of preclinical and clinical results. *Acta Neurochirurgica, 159*(1), 151–167. DOI: 10.1007/s00701-016-3028-5 PMID: 27878374

Sepulveda, J. M., Valiente, M., Vaz-Salgado, A., Pineda, E., Martínez-García, M., & Ruiz Vico, M. (2025). Azeliragon, a RAGE inhibitor, in combination with temozolomide and radiotherapy in patients with newly diagnosed glioblastoma [NDG trial design.]. *Phase Ib, II*, CAN-201.

Shah, S., Green, J., Graff, S. A., Li, Q., & Heiss, J. D. (2025). Gene Therapy for Glioblastoma Multiforme. *Viruses, 17*(1), 118. Advance online publication. DOI: 10.3390/v17010118 PMID: 39861907

Shah, S., Mansour, H. M., Aguilar, T. M., & Lucke-Wold, B. (2024). Advances in anti-cancer drug development: Metformin as anti-angiogenic supplemental treatment for glioblastoma. *International Journal of Molecular Sciences, 25*(11), 5694. DOI: 10.3390/ijms25115694 PMID: 38891882

Shala, A. L., Arduino, I., Salihu, M. B., & Denora, N. (2023). Quercetin and Its Nano-Formulations for Brain Tumor Therapy—Current Developments and Future Perspectives for Paediatric Studies. *Pharmaceutics, 15*(3), 963. Advance online publication. DOI: 10.3390/pharmaceutics15030963 PMID: 36986827

Shams, A. (2024). Leveraging state-of-the-art ai algorithms in personalized oncology: From transcriptomics to treatment. *Diagnostics (Basel)*, *14*(19), 2174. DOI: 10.3390/diagnostics14192174 PMID: 39410578

Shan, F. Y., Zhao, D., Tirado, C. A., Fonkem, E., Zhang, Y., Feng, D., Huang, J. H., Shan, F. Y., Zhao, D., Tirado, C. A., Fonkem, E., Zhang, Y., Feng, D., & Huang, J. H. (2022). *Glioblastomas: Molecular Diagnosis and Pathology*. Glioblastoma - Current Evidence., DOI: 10.5772/intechopen.105472

Shang, W., Zeng, C., Du, Y., Hui, H., Liang, X., Chi, C., Wang, K., Wang, Z., & Tian, J. (2017). Core–shell gold nanorod@metal–organic framework nanoprobes for multimodality diagnosis of glioma. *Advanced Materials*, *29*(3), 1604381. Advance online publication. DOI: 10.1002/adma.201604381 PMID: 27859713

Sharma, A. K., Gupta, L., Sahu, H., Qayum, A., Singh, S. K., Nakhate, K. T., Ajazuddin, , & Gupta, U. (2018). Chitosan Engineered PAMAM Dendrimers as Nanoconstructs for the Enhanced Anti-Cancer Potential and Improved In vivo Brain Pharmacokinetics of Temozolomide. *Pharmaceutical Research*, *35*(1), 9. Advance online publication. DOI: 10.1007/s11095-017-2324-y PMID: 29294212

Sharma, M.. (2023). Nanoparticle-based Delivery Systems for Gene Therapy. *Nanomedicine; Nanotechnology, Biology, and Medicine*, *34*(7), 356–371. DOI: 10.1016/j.nano.2023.102441

Sharma, R., Liaw, K., Sharma, A., Jimenez, A., Chang, M., Salazar, S., Amlani, I., Kannan, S., & Kannan, R. M. (2021). Glycosylation of PAMAM dendrimers significantly improves tumor macrophage targeting and specificity in glioblastoma. *Journal of Controlled Release*, *337*, 179–192. DOI: 10.1016/j.jconrel.2021.07.018 PMID: 34274384

Sharp, P. S., Stylianou, M., Arellano, L. M., Neves, J. C., Gravagnuolo, A. M., Dodd, A., & Stylianopoulos, T. (2023). Graphene oxide nanoscale platform enhances the anti-cancer properties of bortezomib in glioblastoma models. *Advanced Healthcare Materials*, *12*(3), 2201968. Advance online publication. DOI: 10.1002/adhm.202201968 PMID: 36300643

Shi, C., Qin, K., Lin, A., Jiang, A., Cheng, Q., Liu, Z., Zhang, J., & Luo, P. (2022). The role of DNA damage repair (DDR) system in response to immune checkpoint inhibitor (ICI) therapy. *Journal of Experimental & Clinical Cancer Research : CR*, *41*(1), 268. DOI: 10.1186/s13046-022-02469-0 PMID: 36071479

Shi, D., Mi, G., Shen, Y., & Webster, T. J. (2019). Glioma-targeted dual functionalized thermosensitive Ferri-liposomes for drug delivery through an in vitro blood-brain barrier. *Nanoscale, 11*(32), 15057–15071. DOI: 10.1039/C9NR03931G PMID: 31369016

Shikalov, A., Koman, I., & Kogan, N. M. (2024). Targeted glioma therapy—Clinical trials and future directions. *Pharmaceutics, 16*(1), 100. Advance online publication. DOI: 10.3390/pharmaceutics16010100 PMID: 38258110

Shin, K., Sung, H., Jung, J. H., & Kim, S. E. (2025). Abstract 1853: BIK-E715E, an integrin-targeting ligand-drug conjugate equipped with a novel drug delivery system, demonstrates enhanced antitumor efficacy in glioblastoma. *Cancer Research, 85*(8, Supplement_1), 1853. DOI: 10.1158/1538-7445.AM2025-1853

Shi, Y., He, X., Wang, H., Dai, J., Fang, J., He, Y., & Liu, Z. (2023). Construction of a novel blood brain barrier-glioma microfluidic chip model: Applications in the evaluation of permeability and anti-glioma activity of traditional Chinese medicine components. *Talanta, 253*, 123971. Advance online publication. DOI: 10.1016/j.talanta.2022.123971 PMID: 36201955

Sim, H.-W., Galanis, E., & Khasraw, M. (2022). PARP inhibitors in glioma: A review of therapeutic opportunities. *Cancers (Basel), 14*(4), 1003. DOI: 10.3390/cancers14041003 PMID: 35205750

Simhadri, S., Peterson, S., Patel, D. S., Huo, Y., Cai, H., Bowman-Colin, C., & Bhaumik, M. (2014). Male fertility defect associated with disrupted BRCA1-PALB2 interaction in mice. *The Journal of Biological Chemistry, 289*(35), 24617–24629. DOI: 10.1074/jbc.M114.566141 PMID: 25016020

Singh, G., Kumar, P., & Aran, K. R. (2025). Targeting EGFR and PI3K/mTOR pathways in glioblastoma: Innovative therapeutic approaches. *Medical Oncology (Northwood, London, England), 42*(4), 1–17. DOI: 10.1007/s12032-025-02652-1 PMID: 40064710

Singh, P., Tomar, R. S., & Rath, S. K. (2015). Anticancer potential of the histone deacetylase inhibitor-like effects of flavones, a subclass of polyphenolic compounds: A review. *Molecular Biology Reports, 42*(11), 1515–1531. DOI: 10.1007/s11033-015-3881-y PMID: 26033434

Singh, R. R., Mondal, I., Janjua, T., Popat, A., & Kulshreshtha, R. (2024). Engineered smart materials for RNA based molecular therapy to treat glioblastoma. *Bioactive Materials, 33*, 396–423. DOI: 10.1016/j.bioactmat.2023.11.007 PMID: 38059120

Singh, S., Dey, D., Barik, D., Mohapatra, I., Kim, S., Sharma, M., Prasad, S., Wang, P., Singh, A., & Singh, G. (2025). Glioblastoma at the crossroads: Current understanding and future therapeutic horizons. *Signal Transduction and Targeted Therapy*, *10*(1), 213. Advance online publication. DOI: 10.1038/s41392-025-02299-4 PMID: 40628732

Skaga, E., Skaga, I. Ø., Grieg, Z., Sandberg, C. J., Langmoen, I. A., & Vik-Mo, E. O. (2019). The efficacy of a coordinated pharmacological blockade in glioblastoma stem cells with nine repurposed drugs using the CUSP9 strategy. *Journal of Cancer Research and Clinical Oncology*, *145*(6), 1495–1507. DOI: 10.1007/s00432-019-02920-4 PMID: 31028540

Slika, H., Karimov, Z., Alimonti, P., Abou-Mrad, T., De Fazio, E., Alomari, S., & El Housheimi, K. (2023). Preclinical models and technologies in glioblastoma research: Evolution, current state, and future avenues. *International Journal of Molecular Sciences*, *24*(22), 16316. Advance online publication. DOI: 10.3390/ijms242216316 PMID: 38003507

Sloan, A. E., Buckley, A., & Mahan, A.. (2018). Dordaviprone (ONC201) in glioblastoma: A promising therapeutic. *Journal of Clinical Oncology*, *36*(25), 3234–3241.

Sloan, E. A., Hilz, S., Gupta, R., Cadwell, C., Ramani, B., Hofmann, J., Kline, C. N., Banerjee, A., Reddy, A., Oberheim Bush, N. A., Chang, S., Braunstein, S., Chang, E. F., Raffel, C., Gupta, N., Sun, P. P., Kim, J. Y. H., Moes, G., Alva, E., & Solomon, D. A. (2020). Gliomas arising in the setting of Li-Fraumeni syndrome stratify into two molecular subgroups with diver*gent clinicopathologic fea*tures. *Acta Neuropathologica*, *139*(5), 953–957. DOI: 10.1007/s00401-020-02144-8 PMID: 32157385

Smith, A. J., & Kumar, P. (2023). Advances in Nanoparticle-Based Drug Delivery for Gene Therapy. *International Journal of Nanomedicine*, *18*(1), 107–123. DOI: 10.2147/IJN.S359162

Smith, C. J., Perfetti, T. A., Chokshi, C., Venugopal, C., Ashford, J. W., & Singh, S. K. (2024). Risk factors for glioblastoma are shared by other brain tumor types. *Human and Experimental Toxicology*, *43*, 09603271241241796. Advance online publication. DOI: 10.1177/09603271241241796 PMID: 38520250

Smolen, J. S.. (2019). EGFRvIII: A truncated, constitutively active form of EGFR in glioblastoma. *Oncology Letters*, *18*(5), 5394–5403. DOI: 10.3892/ol.2019.10747

Smyth, L. M., Hutchinson, M. S., Naylor, S. C., Kroll, J., Reid, P., & McNeely, K.. (2014). Karenitecin: A topoisomerase I inhibitor in glioblastoma therapy. *Journal of Clinical Oncology*, *32*(4), 458–463.

Society, N. B. T. (2025). *Brain Tumors Types*. https://braintumor.org/brain-tumors/about-brain-tumors/brain-tumor-types/

Sommonte, F., Arduino, I., Iacobazzi, R. M., Laera, L., Silvestri, T., Lopedota, A. A., Castegna, A., & Denora, N. (2024). Microfluidic development of brain-derived neurotrophic factor loaded solid lipid nanoparticles: An in vitro evaluation in the post-traumatic brain injury neuroinflammation model. *Journal of Drug Delivery Science and Technology*, *96*(April), 105699. DOI: 10.1016/j.jddst.2024.105699

Song, H., & Lee, S. (2021). Advances in Nanoparticle-Mediated Gene Delivery. *Journal of Controlled Release*, *330*, 388–409. DOI: 10.1016/j.jconrel.2021.07.022

Song, S., Mao, G., Du, J., & Zhu, X. (2016). Novel RGD containing, temozolomide-loading nanostructured lipid carriers for glioblastoma multiforme chemotherapy. *Drug Delivery*, *23*(4), 1404–1408. DOI: 10.3109/10717544.2015.1064186 PMID: 26203687

Soni, V., Adhikari, M., Simonyan, H., Lin, L., Sherman, J. H., Young, C. N., & Keppel, T. R. (2021). In vitro and in vivo enhancement of temozolomide effect in human glioblastoma by non-invasive application of cold atmospheric plasma. *Cancers (Basel)*, *13*(17), 4485. Advance online publication. DOI: 10.3390/cancers13174485 PMID: 34503293

Son, M. J., Woolard, K., Nam, D. H., Lee, J., & Fine, H. A. (2009). SSEA-1 is an enrichment marker for tumor-initiating cells in human glioblastoma. *Cell Stem Cell*, *4*(5), 440–452. DOI: 10.1016/j.stem.2009.03.003 PMID: 19427293

Sousa, F., Dhaliwal, H. K., Gattacceca, F., Sarmento, B., & Amiji, M. M. (2019). Enhanced anti-angiogenic effects of bevacizumab in glioblastoma treatment upon intranasal administration in polymeric nanoparticles. *Journal of Controlled Release*, *309*(July), 37–47. DOI: 10.1016/j.jconrel.2019.07.033 PMID: 31344424

Sperring, C. P., Argenziano, M. G., Savage, W. M., Teasley, D. E., Upadhyayula, P. S., Winans, N. J., Canoll, P., & Bruce, J. N. (2023). Convection-enhanced delivery of immunomodulatory therapy for high-grade glioma. *Neuro-Oncology Advances*, *5*(1), vdad044. Advance online publication. DOI: 10.1093/noajnl/vdad044 PMID: 37215957

Sternjak, A., Lee, F., Thomas, O., Balazs, M., Wahl, J., Lorenczewski, G., Ullrich, I., Muenz, M., Rattel, B., Bailis, J. M., & Friedrich, M. (2021). Preclinical Assessment of AMG 596, a Bispecific T-cell Engager (BiTE) Immunotherapy Targeting the Tumor-specific Antigen EGFRvIII. *Molecular Cancer Therapeutics*, *20*(5), 925–933. DOI: 10.1158/1535-7163.MCT-20-0508 PMID: 33632870

Stichel, D., Ebrahimi, A., Reuss, D., Schrimpf, D., Ono, T., Shirahata, M., Reifenberger, G., Weller, M., Hänggi, D., Wick, W., Herold-Mende, C., Westphal, M., Brandner, S., Pfister, S. M., Capper, D., Sahm, F., & von Deimling, A. (2018). Distribution of EGFR amplification, combined chromosome 7 gain and chromosome 10 loss, and TERT promoter mutation in brain tumors and their potential for the reclassification of IDHwt astrocytoma to glioblastoma. *Acta Neuropathologica, 136*(5), 793–803. DOI: 10.1007/s00401-018-1905-0 PMID: 30187121

Strobel, H., Baisch, T., Fitzel, R., Schilberg, K., Siegelin, M. D., Karpel-Massler, G., Debatin, K.-M., & Westhoff, M.-A. (2019). Temozolomide and other alkylating agents in glioblastoma therapy. *Biomedicines, 7*(3), 69. DOI: 10.3390/biomedicines7030069 PMID: 31505812

Stupp, R., Hegi, M. E., Mason, W. P., van den Bent, M. J., Taphoorn, M. J. B., Janzer, R. C., Ludwin, S. K., Allgeier, A., Fisher, B., Belanger, K., Hau, P., Brandes, A. A., Gijtenbeek, J., Marosi, C., Vecht, C. J., Mokhtari, K., Wesseling, P., Villa, S., Eisenhauer, E., & Gorlia, T. (2009). Effects of radiotherapy with concomitant and adjuvant temozolomide versus radiotherapy alone on survival in glioblastoma in a randomised phase III study: 5-year analysis of the EORTC-NCIC trial. *The Lancet. Oncology, 10*(5), 459–466. DOI: 10.1016/S1470-2045(09)70025-7 PMID: 19269895

Stupp, R., Mason, W. P., van den Bent, M. J., Weller, M., Fisher, B., Taphoorn, M. J. B., Belanger, K., Brandes, A. A., Marosi, C., Bogdahn, U., Curschmann, J., Janzer, R. C., Ludwin, S. K., Gorlia, T., Allgeier, A., Lacombe, D., Cairncross, J. G., Eisenhauer, E., & Mirimanoff, R. O. (2005). Radiotherapy plus concomitant and adjuvant temozolomide for glioblastoma. *The New England Journal of Medicine, 352*(10), 987–996. DOI: 10.1056/NEJMoa043330 PMID: 15758009

Stupp, R., Mason, W. P., van den Bent, M. J., Weller, M., Fisher, B., & Taphoorn, M.. (2005). Temozolomide and treatment of glioblastoma multiforme. *Journal of Clinical Oncology, 23*(21), 5206–5212.

Stupp, R., Taillibert, S., Kanner, A. A., Kesari, S., Steinberg, D. M., Toms, S. A., Taylor, L. P., Lieberman, F., Silvani, A., Fink, K. L., Barnett, G. H., Zhu, J.-J., Henson, J. W., Engelhard, H. H., Chen, T. C., Tran, D. D., Sroubek, J., Tran, N. D., Hottinger, A. F., & Ram, Z. (2015). Maintenance therapy with tumor-treating fields plus temozolomide vs temozolomide alone for glioblastoma: A randomized clinical trial. *Journal of the American Medical Association, 314*(23), 2535–2543. DOI: 10.1001/jama.2015.16669 PMID: 26670971

Stupp, R., Taillibert, S., Kanner, A., Read, W., Steinberg, D. M., Lhermitte, B., Toms, S., Idbaih, A., Ahluwalia, M. S., Fink, K. L., Di Meco, F., Lieberman, F., Zhu, J.-J., Stragliotto, G., Tran, D. D., Brem, S., Hottinger, A. F., Kirson, E. D., & Ram, Z. (2017). Effect of tumor-treating fields plus maintenance temozolomide vs maintenance temozolomide alone on survival in patients with glioblastoma: A randomized clinical trial. *Journal of the American Medical Association*, *318*(23), 2306–2316. DOI: 10.1001/jama.2017.18718 PMID: 29260225

Stupp, R., & Weller, M. (2014). Questions regarding the optimal use of bevacizumab in glioblastoma: A moving target. *Neuro-Oncology*, *16*(6), 765–767. DOI: 10.1093/neuonc/nou092 PMID: 24826844

Suarez-Meade, P., Marenco-Hillembrand, L., Prevatt, C., Murguia-Fuentes, R., Mohamed, A., Alsaeed, T., Ghaith, A. K., Sabsevitz, D. S., Sherman, W. J., Quinones-Hinojosa, A., & Chaichana, K. L. (2020). Awake vs. asleep motor mapping for glioma resection: A systematic review and meta-analysis. *Acta Neurochirurgica*, *162*(7), 1709–1720. DOI: 10.1007/s00701-020-04357-y PMID: 32388682

Suchorska, B., Weller, M., Tabatabai, G., Senft, C., Hau, P., Sabel, M. C., Herrlinger, U., Ketter, R., Schlegel, U., Marosi, C., Reifenberger, G., Wick, W., Tonn, J. C., & Wirsching, H. G. (2016). Complete resection of contrast-enhancing tumor volume is associated with improved survival in recurrent glioblastoma—Results from the DIRECTOR trial. *Neuro-Oncology*, *18*(4), 549–556. DOI: 10.1093/neuonc/nov326 PMID: 26823503

Sullivan, D. M., Stiegman, S. A., Lee, M., Tan, J., Soltani, S., & Zampino, M.. (2006). Zarnestra in glioblastoma: Preclinical evaluation and clinical development. *Journal of Clinical Oncology*, *24*(10), 1510–1518.

Sun, B., Li, R., Ji, N., Liu, H., Wang, H., Chen, C., Bai, L., Su, J., & Chen, J. (2025). Brain-targeting drug delivery systems: The state of the art in treatment of glioblastoma. *Materials Today. Bio*, *30*, 101443. Advance online publication. DOI: 10.1016/j.mtbio.2025.101443 PMID: 39866779

Sun, L., Liu, H., Ye, Y., Lei, Y., Islam, R., Tan, S., & Fu, Y. (2023). Smart nanoparticles for cancer therapy. *Signal Transduction and Targeted Therapy*, *8*(1), 418. Advance online publication. DOI: 10.1038/s41392-023-01642-x PMID: 37919282

Sun, T., Krishnan, V., Pan, D. C., Filippov, S. K., Ravid, S., Sarode, A., & Yang, X. (2023). Ultrasound-mediated delivery of flexibility-tunable polymer drug conjugates for treating glioblastoma. *Bioengineering & Translational Medicine*, *8*(2), e10408. Advance online publication. DOI: 10.1002/btm2.10408 PMID: 36925708

Sun, Z.-Y., Wang, X.-N., Cheng, S.-Q., Su, X.-X., & Ou, T.-M. (2019). Developing novel G-quadruplex ligands: From interaction with nucleic acids to interfering with nucleic acid–protein interaction. *Molecules (Basel, Switzerland)*, *24*(3), 396. DOI: 10.3390/molecules24030396 PMID: 30678288

Surender, V., & Deepika, M. (2016). *Solid lipid nanoparticles: A comprehensive review*. LAP LAMBERT Academic Publishing.

Syed, Y. Y. (2020). Sacituzumab Govitecan: First Approval. *Drugs*, *80*(10), 1019–1025. DOI: 10.1007/s40265-020-01337-5 PMID: 32529410

Szklener, K., Mazurek, M., Wieteska, M., Wacławska, M., Bilski, M., & Mańdziuk, S. (2022). New directions in the therapy of glioblastoma. *Cancers (Basel)*, *14*(21), 5377. Advance online publication. DOI: 10.3390/cancers14215377 PMID: 36358795

Tamura, R., Tanaka, T., Miyake, K., Yoshida, K., & Sasaki, H. (2017). Bevacizumab for malignant gliomas: Current indications, mechanisms of action and resistance, and markers of response. *Brain Tumor Pathology*, *34*(2), 62–77. DOI: 10.1007/s10014-017-0284-x PMID: 28386777

Tan, A. C., Ashley, D. M., López, G. Y., Malinzak, M., Friedman, H. S., & Khasraw, M. (2020). Management of glioblastoma: State of the art and future directions. *CA: a Cancer Journal for Clinicians*, *70*(4), 299–312. DOI: 10.3322/caac.21613 PMID: 32478924

Tang, J., Karbhari, N., & Campian, J. L. (2025). Therapeutic Targets in Glioblastoma: Molecular Pathways, Emerging Strategies, and Future Directions. *Cells*, *14*(7), 494. DOI: 10.3390/cells14070494 PMID: 40214448

Tang, K., Wu, Y. H., Song, Y., & Yu, B. (2021). Indoleamine 2,3-dioxygenase 1 (IDO1) inhibitors in clinical trials for cancer immunotherapy. *Journal of Hematology & Oncology*, *14*(1), 68. DOI: 10.1186/s13045-021-01080-8 PMID: 33883013

Tang, M., Bolderson, E., O'Byrne, K. J., & Richard, D. J. (2021). Tumor hypoxia drives genomic instability. *Frontiers in Cell and Developmental Biology*, *9*, 626229. DOI: 10.3389/fcell.2021.626229 PMID: 33796526

Tang, T., Liang, H., Wei, W., Han, Y., Cao, L., Cong, Z., & Zhang, J. (2023). Aloperine targets lysosomes to inhibit late autophagy and induces cell death through apoptosis and paraptosis in glioblastoma. *Cell Death Discovery*, *9*(1), 42. Advance online publication. DOI: 10.1038/s41420-023-01333-6 PMID: 36732504

Tang, W., Fan, W., Lau, J., Deng, L., Shen, Z., & Chen, X. (2019). Emerging blood–brain-barrier-crossing nanotechnology for brain cancer theranostics. *Chemical Society Reviews*, *48*(11), 2967–3014. DOI: 10.1039/C8CS00805A PMID: 31089607

Tang, X., Zuo, C., Fang, P., Liu, G., Qiu, Y., Huang, Y., & Tang, R. (2021). Targeting Glioblastoma Stem Cells: A Review on Biomarkers, Signal Pathways and Targeted Therapy. *Frontiers in Oncology*, *11*, 701291. DOI: 10.3389/fonc.2021.701291 PMID: 34307170

Tanoli, Z., Vähä-Koskela, M., & Aittokallio, T. (2021). Artificial intelligence, machine learning, and drug repurposing in cancer. *Expert Opinion on Drug Discovery*, *16*(9), 977–989. DOI: 10.1080/17460441.2021.1883585 PMID: 33543671

Teleanu, R. I., Preda, M. D., Niculescu, A.-G., Vladâcenco, O., Radu, C. I., Grumezescu, A. M., & Teleanu, D. M. (2022). Current strategies to enhance delivery of drugs across the blood–brain barrier. *Pharmaceutics*, *14*(5), 987. DOI: 10.3390/pharmaceutics14050987 PMID: 35631573

ter Linden, E., Abels, E. R., van Solinge, T. S., Neefjes, J., & Broekman, M. L. D. (2024). Overcoming barriers in glioblastoma—Advances in drug delivery strategies. *Cells*, *13*(12), 998. Advance online publication. DOI: 10.3390/cells13120998 PMID: 38920629

Tew, B. Y., Alex, J., Yang, K. Z., Hurth, K. M., Simon, T., & Abnoosian, E.. (2023). ATM-Inhibitor AZD1390 Is a Radiosensitizer for Breast Cancer CNS Metastasis. Translational Cancer Mechanisms and Therapy. *Clinical Cancer Research*, *29*(21), 4492–4503. DOI: 10.1158/1078-0432.CCR-23-0290 PMID: 37585496

Thanh, H. D., Lee, S., Nguyen, T. T., Huu, T. N., Ahn, E. J., Cho, S. H., Kim, H. S., Moon, K.-S., & Jung, C. (2024). Temozolomide promotes matrix metalloproteinase 9 expression through p38 MAPK and JNK pathways in glioblastoma cells. *Scientific Reports*, *14*(1), 14341. Advance online publication. DOI: 10.1038/s41598-024-65398-2 PMID: 38906916

The 2024 Brain Tumor Segmentation (BraTS) Challenge: Glioma segmentation on post-treatment MRI. (n.d.). arXiv. Retrieved May 17, 2025, from https://arxiv.org/html/2405.18368

Thenuwara, G., Curtin, J., & Tian, F. (2023). Advances in diagnostic tools and therapeutic approaches for gliomas: A comprehensive review. *Sensors (Basel)*, *23*(24), 9842. Advance online publication. DOI: 10.3390/s23249842 PMID: 38139688

Thomas, S. S., & Lee, J. S. (2021). Lipid Nanoparticles for Gene Therapy: Innovations and Applications. *Molecular Therapy. Nucleic Acids*, *24*, 134–145. DOI: 10.1016/j.omtn.2021.06.023

Tian, H., Gao, Z., Li, H., Zhang, B., Wang, G., Zhang, Q., Pei, D. S., & Zheng, J. (2015). DNA damage response–a double-edged sword in cancer prevention and cancer therapy. *Cancer Letters, 358*(1), 8–16. DOI: 10.1016/j.canlet.2014.12.038 PMID: 25528631

Tiwari, P. C., Pal, R., Chaudhary, M. J., & Nath, R. (2023). Artificial intelligence revolutionizing drug development: Exploring opportunities and challenges. *Drug Development Research, 84*(8), 1652–1663. DOI: 10.1002/ddr.22115 PMID: 37712494

Tong, F., Zhao, J.-X., Fang, Z.-Y., Cui, X.-T., Su, D.-Y., Liu, X., & Zhang, J. (2023). MUC1 promotes glioblastoma progression and TMZ resistance by stabilizing EGFRvIII. *Pharmacological Research, 187*, 106606. Advance online publication. DOI: 10.1016/j.phrs.2022.106606 PMID: 36516884

Topalian, S. L., Drake, C. G., & Pardoll, D. M. (2015). Immune checkpoint blockade: A common denominator approach to cancer therapy. *Cancer Cell, 27*(4), 450–461. DOI: 10.1016/j.ccell.2015.03.001 PMID: 25858804

Torrisi, F., Alberghina, C., D'Aprile, S., Pavone, A. M., Longhitano, L., Giallongo, S., Tibullo, D., Di Rosa, M., Zappalà, A., Cammarata, F. P., Russo, G., Ippolito, M., Cuttone, G., Li Volti, G., Vicario, N., & Parenti, R. (2022). The hallmarks of glioblastoma: Heterogeneity, intercellular crosstalk and molecular signature of invasiveness and progression. *Biomedicines, 10*(4), 806. DOI: 10.3390/biomedicines10040806 PMID: 35453557

Tosi, G., Musumeci, T., Ruozi, B., Carbone, C., Belletti, D., Pignatello, R., Vandelli, M. A., & Puglisi, G. (2016). The "fate" of polymeric and lipid nanoparticles for brain delivery and targeting: Strategies and mechanism of blood-brain barrier crossing and trafficking into the central nervous system. *Journal of Drug Delivery Science and Technology, 32*, 66–76. DOI: 10.1016/j.jddst.2015.07.007

Tripathy, D. K., Panda, L. P., Biswal, S., & Barhwal, K. (2024). Insights into the glioblastoma tumor microenvironment: Current and emerging therapeutic approaches. *Frontiers in Pharmacology, 15*, 1355242. Advance online publication. DOI: 10.3389/fphar.2024.1355242 PMID: 38523646

Turcotte, E. L., Jones, B. A., Chhabra, N., Porter, A. B., Donev, K., Hu, L. S., & Bendok, B. R. (2023). Awake microsurgical resection of a motor cortex glioma with cortical and subcortical motor mapping, image guidance, and augmented reality: 2-dimensional operative video. *Operative Neurosurgery (Hagerstown, Md.), 24*(2), e122. DOI: 10.1227/ons.0000000000000525 PMID: 36637320

Tu, Z., Wang, C., Hu, Q., Tao, C., Fang, Z., Lin, L., & Zhang, J. (2023). Protein disulfide-isomerase A4 confers glioblastoma angiogenesis promotion capacity and resistance to anti-angiogenic therapy. *Journal of Experimental & Clinical Cancer Research : CR*, *42*(1), 77. Advance online publication. DOI: 10.1186/s13046-023-02640-1 PMID: 36997943

Tzeng, S. Y., & Green, J. J. (2013). Therapeutic nanomedicine for brain cancer. *Therapeutic Delivery*, *4*(6), 687–704. DOI: 10.4155/tde.13.38 PMID: 23738667

Urbanska, K., Sokolowska, J., Szmidt, M., & Sysa, P. (2014). Glioblastoma multiforme - an overview. *Contemporary Oncology = Współczesna Onkologia*, *18*(5), 307–312. DOI: 10.5114/wo.2014.40559 PMID: 25477751

Urzì, O., Gasparro, R., Costanzo, E., De Luca, A., Giavaresi, G., Fontana, S., & Alessandro, R. (2023). Three-dimensional cell cultures: The bridge between in vitro and in vivo models. *International Journal of Molecular Sciences*, *24*(15), 12046. Advance online publication. DOI: 10.3390/ijms241512046 PMID: 37569426

van den Bossche, W. B. L., Kleijn, A., Teunissen, C. E., Voerman, J. S. A., Teodosio, C., Noske, D. P., van den Bent, M. J., van den Bent, M. J., & van den Bent, M. J. (2018). Oncolytic virotherapy in glioblastoma patients induces a tumor macrophage phenotypic shift leading to an altered glioblastoma microenvironment. *Neuro-Oncology*, *20*(11), 1494–1504. DOI: 10.1093/neuonc/noy082 PMID: 29796615

van Linde, M. E., Brahm, C. G., de Witt Hamer, P. C., Reijneveld, J. C., Bruynzeel, A. M. E., Vandertop, W. P., van de Ven, P. M., Wagemakers, M., van der Hoeven, A. M., Enting, R. H., & Verheul, H. M. W. (2017). Treatment outcome of patients with recurrent glioblastoma multiforme: A retrospective multicenter analysis. *Journal of Neuro-Oncology*, *135*(1), 183–192. DOI: 10.1007/s11060-017-2564-z PMID: 28730289

Vaz-Salgado, M. A., Villamayor, M., Albarrán, V., Alía, V., Sotoca, P., Chamorro, J., & García-Barbero, J. (2023). Recurrent glioblastoma: A review of the treatment options. *Cancers (Basel)*, *15*(17), 4279. Advance online publication. DOI: 10.3390/cancers15174279 PMID: 37686553

Veneris, J. T., Matulonis, U. A., Liu, J. F., & Konstantinopoulos, P. A. (2020). Choosing wisely: Selecting PARP inhibitor combinations to promote anti-tumor immune responses beyond BRCA mutations. *Gynecologic Oncology*, *156*(2), 488–497. DOI: 10.1016/j.ygyno.2019.09.021 PMID: 31630846

Ventola, C. L. (2017). *Progress in nanomedicine*: Approved and investigational nanodrugs. *P&T : a Peer-Reviewed Journal for Formulary Management*, *42*(12), 742–755. https://pmc.ncbi.nlm.nih.gov/articles/PMC5720487/ PMID: 29234213

Verdugo, E., Puerto, I., & Medina, M. Á. (2022). An update on the molecular biology of glioblastoma, with clinical implications and progress in its treatment. *Cancer Communications*, *42*(11), 1083–1111. DOI: 10.1002/cac2.12361 PMID: 36129048

Verhaak, R. G. W., Hoadley, K. A., Purdom, E., Wang, V., Qi, Y., Wilkerson, M. D., Miller, C. R., Ding, L., Golub, T., Mesirov, J. P., Alexe, G., Lawrence, M., O'Kelly, M., Tamayo, P., Weir, B. A., Gabriel, S., Winckler, W., Gupta, S., Jakkula, L., & Hayes, D. N. (2010). Integrated genomic analysis identifies clinically relevant subtypes of glioblastoma characterized by abnormalities in PDGFRA, IDH1, EGFR, and NF1. *Cancer Cell*, *17*(1), 98–110. DOI: 10.1016/j.ccr.2009.12.020 PMID: 20129251

Vieira, D. B., & Gamarra, L. F. (2016). Getting into the brain: Liposome-based strategies for effective drug delivery across the blood–brain barrier. *International Journal of Nanomedicine*, *11*, 5381–5414. DOI: 10.2147/IJN.S117210 PMID: 27799765

Vilar, J. B., Christmann, M., & Tomicic, M. T. (2022). Alterations in molecular profiles affecting glioblastoma resistance to radiochemotherapy: Where does the good go? *Cancers (Basel)*, *14*(10), 2416. DOI: 10.3390/cancers14102416 PMID: 35626024

Vines, J. B., Yoon, J.-H., Ryu, N.-E., Lim, D.-J., & Park, H. (2019). Gold nanoparticles for photothermal cancer therapy. *Frontiers in Chemistry*, *7*, 167. Advance online publication. DOI: 10.3389/fchem.2019.00167 PMID: 31024882

Vogelbaum, M. A., & Aghi, M. K. (2015). Convection-enhanced delivery for the treatment of glioblastoma. *Neuro-Oncology*, *17*(Suppl. 2), ii3–ii8. DOI: 10.1093/neuonc/nou354 PMID: 25746090

Voloshin, T., Kaynan, N., Davidi, S., Porat, Y., Shteingauz, A., Schneiderman, R. S., Zeevi, E., Munster, M., Blumberg, G., & Giladi, M. (2020). Tumor-treating fields (TTFields) induce immunogenic cell death resulting in enhanced antitumor efficacy when combined with anti-PD-1 therapy. *Cancer Immunology, Immunotherapy : CII*, *69*(7), 1191–1204. DOI: 10.1007/s00262-020-02534-7 PMID: 32144446

Wang, T., Liu, M., Peng, B., Song, X., Zhang, C., Sun, X., Niu, Q., Liu, J., Chen, S., & Chen, K. (2024) From Bench to Bedside: A Review of Clinical Trialsin Drug Discovery and Development. *arXiv preprint arXiv:241209378.*

Wang, H., Li, L., Ye, J., Wang, R., Wang, R., Hu, J., Wang, Y., Dong, W., Xia, X., Yang, Y., Gao, Y., Gao, L., & Liu, Y. (2020). Improving the oral bioavailability of an anti-glioma prodrug cat3 using novel solid lipid nanoparticles containing oleic acid-cat3 conjugates. *Pharmaceutics*, *12*(2), 126. Advance online publication. DOI: 10.3390/pharmaceutics12020126 PMID: 32028734

Wang, L., Tang, S., Yu, Y., Lv, Y., Wang, A., Yan, X., Li, N., Sha, C., Sun, K., & Li, Y. (2021). Intranasal Delivery of Temozolomide-Conjugated Gold Nanoparticles Functionalized with Anti-EphA3 for Glioblastoma Targeting. *Molecular Pharmaceutics, 18*(3), 915–927. DOI: 10.1021/acs.molpharmaceut.0c00911 PMID: 33417456

Wang, M., Lv, C. Y., Li, S. A., Wang, J. K., Luo, W. Z., Zhao, P. C., Liu, X. Y., Wang, Z. M., Jiao, Y., Sun, H. W., Zhao, Y., & Zhang, P. (2021). Near infrared light fluorescence imaging-guided biomimetic nanoparticles of extracellular vesicles deliver indocyanine green and paclitaxel for hyperthermia combined with chemotherapy against glioma. *Journal of Nanobiotechnology, 19*(1), 1–18. DOI: 10.1186/s12951-023-02253-y PMID: 34261493

Wang, S. W., Gao, C., Zheng, Y. M., Yi, L., Lu, J. C., Huang, X. Y., & Li, B. (2022). Current applications and future perspective of CRISPR/Cas9 gene editing in cancer. *Molecular Cancer, 21*(1), 57. Advance online publication. DOI: 10.1186/s12943-022-01518-8 PMID: 35189910

Wang, S., Meng, Y., Li, C., Qian, M., & Huang, R. (2016). Receptor-mediated drug delivery systems targeting to glioma. *Nanomaterials (Basel, Switzerland), 6*(1), 3. Advance online publication. DOI: 10.3390/nano6010003 PMID: 28344260

Wang, S., Wei, W., Yuan, Y., Sun, B., Yang, D., Liu, N., & Zhang, J. (2023). Chimeric antigen receptor T cells targeting cell surface GRP78 efficiently kill glioblastoma and cancer stem cells. *Journal of Translational Medicine, 21*(1), 493. Advance online publication. DOI: 10.1186/s12967-023-04330-0 PMID: 37481592

Wang, Y.. (2021). Recent Progress in Nanoparticle-Mediated Delivery Systems for RNA-Based Therapeutics. *Journal of Controlled Release, 332*, 86–99. DOI: 10.1016/j.jconrel.2021.04.009

Wang, Y., Luo, R., Zhang, X., Xiang, H., Yang, B., Feng, J., Deng, M., Ran, P., Sujie, A., Zhang, F., Zhu, J., Tan, S., Xie, T., Chen, P., Yu, Z., Li, Y., Jiang, D., Zhang, X., Zhao, J. Y., & Ding, C. (2023). Proteogenomics of diffuse gliomas reveal molecular subtypes associated with specific therapeutic targets and immune-evasion mechanisms. *Nature Communications, 14*(1), 505. Advance online publication. DOI: 10.1038/s41467-023-36005-1 PMID: 36720864

Wang, Y., Luo, W., & Wang, Y. (2019). PARP-1 and its associated nucleases in DNA damage response. *DNA Repair, 81*, 102651. DOI: 10.1016/j.dnarep.2019.102651 PMID: 31302005

Wang, Y., Wang, Z., Hua, C., Xu, Y., Li, Y., & Zhao, G. (2022). Primary Malignant Brain Tumors following Systemic Malignancies: A Population-Based Analysis. *Neuroepidemiology, 56*(6), 452–459. DOI: 10.1159/000527437 PMID: 36244332

Wang, Z., Hu, P., Tang, F., Lian, H., Chen, X., Zhang, Y., He, X., Liu, Y., Wu, J., & Wang, Z. (2016). HDAC6 promotes cell proliferation and confers resistance to temozolomide in glioblastoma. *Cancer Letters*, *379*(1), 134–142. DOI: 10.1016/j.canlet.2016.06.001 PMID: 27267806

Wanigasekara, J., Carroll, L. J., Cullen, P. J., Tiwari, B., & Curtin, J. F. (2023). Three-dimensional (3D) in vitro cell culture protocols to enhance glioblastoma research. *PLoS One*, *18*(2), e0276248. Advance online publication. DOI: 10.1371/journal.pone.0276248 PMID: 36753513

Webster, M., Cairncross, G., Gertler, S., Perry, J., Wainman, N., & Eisenhauer, E. (2005). Phase II trial of SarCNU in malignant glioma: Unexpected pulmonary toxicity with a novel nitrosourea A phase II trial of the national cancer institute of canada clinical trials group *.

Wei, K.C., Hsu, P.W., Tsai, H.C., Lin, Y.J., Chen, K.T., Toh, C.H. (2021). Safety and tolerability of asunercept plus standard radiotherapy/temozolomide in Asian patients with newly-diagnosed glioblastoma: a phase I study. *Scientific Reports*, 15;11(1):24067.

Wei, D., Zhang, N., Qu, S., Wang, H., & Li, J. (2023). Advances in nanotechnology for the treatment of GBM. *Frontiers in Neuroscience*, *17*, 1180943. Advance online publication. DOI: 10.3389/fnins.2023.1180943 PMID: 37214394

Wei, J., Zhu, K., Yang, Z., Zhou, Y., Xia, Z., Ren, J., & Chen, X. (2023). Hypoxia-induced autophagy is involved in radioresistance via HIF1A-associated beclin-1 in glioblastoma multiforme. *Cell Death Discovery*, *9*(1), 1. Advance online publication. DOI: 10.1038/s41420-023-01315-8 PMID: 36588105

Weiser, J. R., & Saltzman, W. M. (2014). Controlled release for local delivery of drugs: Barriers and models. *Journal of Controlled Release*, *190*, 664–673. DOI: 10.1016/j.jconrel.2014.04.048 PMID: 24801251

Wen, J., Ding, Y., Zheng, S., Li, X., & Xiao, Y. (2024). Sevoflurane suppresses glioma cell proliferation, migration, and invasion both in vitro and in vivo partially via regulating KCNQ1OT1/miR-146b-5p/STC1 axis. *Cancer Biology & Therapy*, *25*(2), 105–116. DOI: 10.1080/15384047.2024.2304216 PMID: 32996777

West, C. M., & Barnett, G. C. (2011). Genetics and genomics of radiotherapy toxicity: Towards prediction. *Genome Medicine*, *3*(8), 52. Advance online publication. DOI: 10.1186/gm268 PMID: 21861849

Westphal, M., Hilt, D. C., Bortey, E., Delavault, P., Olivares, R., Warnke, P. C., Whittle, I. R., Jääskeläinen, J., & Ram, Z. (2003). A phase 3 trial of local chemotherapy with biodegradable carmustine (BCNU) wafers (Gliadel wafers) in patients with primary malignant glioma. *Neuro-Oncology*, *5*(2), 79–88. DOI: 10.1093/neuonc/5.2.79 PMID: 12672279

Weth, F. R., Hoggarth, G. B., Weth, A. F., Paterson, E., White, M. P., Tan, S. T., Peng, L., & Gray, C. (2024). Unlocking hidden potential: Advancements, approaches, and obstacles in repurposing drugs for cancer therapy. *British Journal of Cancer*, *130*(5), 703–715. DOI: 10.1038/s41416-023-02502-9 PMID: 38012383

Whitaker, A. M., Schaich, M. A., Smith, M. S., Flynn, T. S., & Freudenthal, B. D. (2017). Base excision repair of oxidative DNA damage: From mechanism to disease. *Frontiers in Bioscience (Landmark Edition)*, *22*(9), 1493–1522. DOI: 10.2741/4555 PMID: 28199214

Wick, W., Puduvalli, V. K., Chamberlain, M. C., van den Bent, M. J., Carpentier, A. F., Cher, L. M., Mason, W., Weller, M., Hong, S., Musib, L., & Hedley, D. W. (2010). Phase III study of enzastaurin compared with lomustine in the treatment of recurrent intracranial glioblastoma. *Journal of Clinical Oncology*, *28*(7), 1168–1174. DOI: 10.1200/JCO.2009.23.2595 PMID: 20124186

Wick, W., Weller, M., Van Den Bent, M., Sanson, M., Weiler, M., Von Deimling, A., Plass, C., Hegi, M., Platten, M., & Reifenberger, G. (2014). MGMT testing—The challenges for biomarker-based glioma treatment. *Nature Reviews. Neurology*, *10*(7), 372–385. DOI: 10.1038/nrneurol.2014.100 PMID: 24912512

Wilke, C., Grosshans, D., Duman, J., Brown, P., & Li, J. (2018). Radiation-induced cognitive toxicity: Pathophysiology and interventions to reduce toxicity in adults. *Neuro-Oncology*, *20*(5), 597–607. DOI: 10.1093/neuonc/nox195 PMID: 29045710

Woo, P. Y. M., Li, Y., Chan, A. H. Y., Ng, S. C. P., Loong, H. H. F., Chan, D. T. M., Wong, G. K. C., & Poon, W. S. (2019). A multifaceted review of temozolomide resistance mechanisms in glioblastoma beyond O-6-methylguanine-DNA methyltransferase. *Glioma (Mumbai, India)*, *2*(2), 68–82. DOI: 10.4103/glioma.glioma_3_19

Wrensch, M., Minn, Y., Chew, T., Bondy, M., & Berger, M. S. (2002, October 1). Epidemiology of primary brain tumors: Current concepts and review of the literature. *Neuro-Oncology*, *4*(4), 278–299. DOI: 10.1093/neuonc/4.4.278 PMID: 12356358

Wright, J., Chugh, J., Wright, C. H., Alonso, F., Hdeib, A., Gittleman, H., Barnholtz-Sloan, J. S., & Sloan, A. E. (2016). Laser interstitial thermal therapy followed by minimal-access transsulcal resection for the treatment of large and difficult to access brain tumors. *Neurosurgical Focus, 41*(4), E14. Advance online publication. DOI: 10.3171/2016.8.FOCUS16233 PMID: 27690658

Wu, H., Yang, L., Liu, H., Zhou, D., Chen, D., Zheng, X., & Liu, Y. (2021). Exploring the efficacy of tumor electric field therapy against glioblastoma: An in vivo and in vitro study. *Cancer Management and Research, 13*, 1587–1604. DOI: 10.2147/CMAR.S289206 PMID: 34710276

Wu, J., Chu, Y., Jiang, Z., & Yu, Q. (2020). Losartan protects against intermittent hypoxia-induced peritubular capillary loss by modulating the renal renin–angiotensin system and angiogenesis factors. *Acta Biochimica et Biophysica Sinica, 52*(1), 38–48. DOI: 10.1093/abbs/gmz136 PMID: 31836883

Wu, W. E., Chang, E., Jin, L., Liu, S., Huang, C.-H., Kamal, R., Zhang, J., & Yang, X. (2023). Multimodal in vivo tracking of chimeric antigen receptor T cells in preclinical glioblastoma models. *Scientific Reports, 13*(6), 388–395. DOI: 10.1038/s41598-023-27741-8 PMID: 36729074

Wu, Z., Ho, W. S., & Lu, R. (2022). Targeting mitochondrial oxidative phosphorylation in glioblastoma therapy. *Neuromolecular Medicine, 24*(1), 18–22. DOI: 10.1007/s12017-021-08678-8 PMID: 34487301

Xiang, Z., Xie, Q., & Yu, Z. (2023). Exosomal DNA: Role in reflecting tumor genetic heterogeneity, diagnosis, and disease monitoring. *Cancers (Basel), 16*(1), 57. DOI: 10.3390/cancers16010057 PMID: 38201485

Xiao, L., Li, X., Fang, C., Yu, J., & Chen, T. (2023). Neurotransmitters: Promising immune modulators in the tumor microenvironment. *Frontiers in Immunology, 14*, 1118637. DOI: 10.3389/fimmu.2023.1118637 PMID: 37215113

Xia, Y., Sun, M., Huang, H., & Jin, W.-L. (2024). Drug repurposing for cancer therapy. *Signal Transduction and Targeted Therapy, 9*(1), 92. DOI: 10.1038/s41392-024-01808-1 PMID: 38637540

Xie, J.. (2021). Nanomaterial-Based Platforms for CRISPR/Cas9 Delivery: From Bench to Bedside. *Frontiers in Bioengineering and Biotechnology, 9*, 765080. DOI: 10.3389/fbioe.2021.765080

Xie, X., Zhang, Y., Wang, Z., Wang, S., Jiang, X., Cui, H., & Guo, Q. (2021). ATM at the crossroads of reactive oxygen species and autophagy. *International Journal of Biological Sciences, 17*(12), 3080–3090. DOI: 10.7150/ijbs.63963 PMID: 34421351

Xie, Z., Chen, M., Lian, J., Wang, H., & Ma, J. (2023). Glioblastoma-on-a-chip construction and therapeutic applications. *Frontiers in Oncology*, *13*, 1183059. Advance online publication. DOI: 10.3389/fonc.2023.1183059 PMID: 37503321

Xin, H., Jiang, X., Gu, J., Sha, X., Chen, L., Law, K., Chen, Y., Wang, X., Jiang, Y., & Fang, X. (2011). Angiopep-conjugated poly(ethylene glycol)-co-poly(ε-caprolactone) nanoparticles as dual-targeting drug delivery system for brain glioma. *Biomaterials*, *32*(18), 4293–4305. DOI: 10.1016/j.biomaterials.2011.02.044 PMID: 21427009

Xu, C., Hou, P., Li, X., Xiao, M., Zhang, Z., Li, Z., & Liu, Y. (2024). Comprehensive understanding of glioblastoma molecular phenotypes: Classification, characteristics, and transition. *Cancer Biology & Medicine*, 1–19. Advance online publication. DOI: 10.20892/j.issn.2095-3941.2023.0510 PMID: 38712813

Xu, C., Yuan, X., Hou, P., Li, Z., Wang, C., Fang, C., & Liu, Y. (2023). Development of glioblastoma organoids and their applications in personalized therapy. *Theranostics*, *13*(5), 353–368. DOI: 10.7150/thno.80078 PMID: 37283493

Xu, J., Wang, J., Zhao, M., Li, C., Hong, S., Zhang, J., & Chen, N. (2023). LncRNA LINC01018/miR-942-5p/KNG1 axis regulates the malignant development of glioma in vitro and in vivo. *CNS Neuroscience & Therapeutics*, *29*(2), 691–711. DOI: 10.1111/cns.14053 PMID: 36550594

Xu, L.. (2020). Challenges in active targeting for glioblastoma therapy. *Cancer Treatment Reviews*, *86*, 102031. DOI: 10.1016/j.ctrv.2020.102031

Xu, X., Tan, M., Corcoran, B., Wu, J., Boes, A., Nguyen, T. G., Chu, S. T., Little, B. E., Hicks, D. G., Morandotti, R., Mitchell, A., & Moss, D. J. (2021). 11 TOPS photonic convolutional accelerator for optical neural networks. *Nature*, *589*(7840), 44–51. DOI: 10.1038/s41586-020-03063-0 PMID: 33408378

Xu, X., Wang, L., Xu, H., Yang, X., & Li, Y. (2019). Smart nanotheranostic systems for precise cancer therapy based on stimuli-responsive nanocarriers. *Signal Transduction and Targeted Therapy*, *4*(1), 1–18. DOI: 10.1038/s41392-019-0082-3

Xu, Z.. (2022). Targeted Nanoparticle Delivery Systems in Gene Therapy. *Biomaterials Science*, *10*(4), 877–890. DOI: 10.1039/d0bm01851f PMID: 35024701

Yadav, K., Vijayalakshmi, R., Sahu, K. K., Sure, P., Chahal, K., Yadav, R., Dubey, A., Jha, M., & Pradhan, M. (2024). Exosome-based macromolecular neurotherapeutic drug delivery approaches in overcoming the blood-brain barrier for treating brain disorders. *European Journal of Pharmaceutics and Biopharmaceutics*, *199*, 114298. DOI: 10.1016/j.ejpb.2024.114298 PMID: 38642716

Yalamarty, S. S. K., Filipczak, N., Li, X., Subhan, M. A., Parveen, F., Ataide, J. A., & Torchilin, V. P. (2023). Mechanisms of resistance and current treatment options for glioblastoma multiforme (GBM). *Cancers (Basel), 15*(7), 2116. Advance online publication. DOI: 10.3390/cancers15072116 PMID: 37046777

Yamaura, K., Nelson, A., Nishimura, H., Rutledge, J., Ravuri, S., Bahney, C., Philippon, M., & Huard, J. (2023). The effects of losartan or angiotensin II receptor antagonists on cartilage: A systematic review. *Osteoarthritis and Cartilage, 31*(4), 435–446. DOI: 10.1016/j.joca.2022.11.014 PMID: 36586717

Yan, C., Wang, J., Yang, Y., Ma, W., & Chen, X. (2019). Molecular biomarker-guided anti-angiogenic targeted therapy for malignant glioma. *Journal of Cellular and Molecular Medicine, 23*(8), 4876–4882. DOI: 10.1111/jcmm.14417 PMID: 31210419

Yang, C. Y., Liu, H. W., Tsai, Y. C., Tseng, J. Y., Liang, S. C., Chen, C. Y., Lian, W. N., Wei, M. C., Lu, M., Lu, R. H., Lin, C. H., & Jiang, J. K. (2015). Interleukin-4 receptor-targeted liposomal doxorubicin as a model for enhancing cellular uptake and antitumor efficacy in murine colorectal cancer. *Cancer Biology & Therapy, 16*(11), 1641–1650. DOI: 10.1080/15384047.2015.1095397 PMID: 26436767

Yang, M., Oh, I. Y., Mahanty, A., Jin, W. L., & Yoo, J. S. (2020). Immunotherapy for glioblastoma: Current state, challenges, and future perspectives. *Cancers (Basel), 12*(9), 2334. Advance online publication. DOI: 10.3390/cancers12092334 PMID: 32824974

Yang, Q., Zhou, Y., Chen, J., Huang, N., Wang, Z., & Cheng, Y. (2021). Gene therapy for drug-resistant glioblastoma via lipid-polymer hybrid nanoparticles combined with focused ultrasound. *International Journal of Nanomedicine, 16*, 185–199. DOI: 10.2147/IJN.S286221 PMID: 33447034

Yang, S., Wallach, M., Krishna, A., Kurmasheva, R., & Sridhar, S. (2021). Recent developments in nanomedicine for pediatric cancer. *Journal of Clinical Medicine, 10*(7), 1–22. DOI: 10.3390/jcm10071437 PMID: 33916177

Yang, T., Martin, P., Fogarty, B., Brown, A., Schurman, K., Phipps, R., Yin, Y., Spence, A., & Bellamkonda, R. V. (2015). Exosome delivered anticancer drugs across the blood-brain barrier for brain cancer therapy in Danio rerio. *Pharmaceutical Research, 32*(6), 2003–2014. DOI: 10.1007/s11095-014-1593-y PMID: 25609010

Yang, Y., Cheng, N., Luo, Q., Shao, N., Ma, X., Chen, J., Luo, L., & Xiao, Z. (2023). How Nanotherapeutic Platforms Play a Key Role in Glioma? A Comprehensive Review of Literature. *International Journal of Nanomedicine, 18*(June), 3663–3694. DOI: 10.2147/IJN.S414736 PMID: 37427368

Yang, Z., Wei, D., Dai, X., Stevens, M. F., Bradshaw, T. D., Luo, Y., & Zhang, J. (2019). C8-substituted imidazotetrazine analogs overcome temozolomide resistance by inducing DNA adducts and DNA damage. *Frontiers in Oncology*, *9*, 485. DOI: 10.3389/fonc.2019.00485 PMID: 31263673

Yan, H., Parsons, D. W., Jin, G., McLendon, R., Rasheed, B. A., Yuan, W., Kos, I., Batinic-Haberle, I., Jones, S., Riggins, G. J., Friedman, H., Friedman, A., Reardon, D., Herndon, J., Kinzler, K. W., Velculescu, V. E., Vogelstein, B., & Bigner, D. D. (2009). IDH1 and IDH2 mutations in gliomas. *The New England Journal of Medicine*, *360*(8), 765–773. DOI: 10.1056/NEJMoa0808710 PMID: 19228619

Yan, K. (2024). The role of cancer stem cells in glioblastoma treatment: New strategies for targeted therapy. *Translational Materials Research in Biotechnology and Life Sciences*, *7*, 248–253. DOI: 10.62051/7tjwpt29

Yan, Y., Zhou, S., Chen, X., Yi, Q., Feng, S., Zhao, Z., Liu, Y., Liang, Q., Xu, Z., Li, Z., & Sun, L. (2024). Suppression of ITPKB degradation by Trim25 confers TMZ resistance in glioblastoma through ROS homeostasis. *Signal Transduction and Targeted Therapy*, *9*(1), 58. Advance online publication. DOI: 10.1038/s41392-024-01763-x PMID: 38438346

Ye, J., Fan, Y., Kang, Y., Ding, M., Niu, G., Yang, J., Liu, Y., & Li, X. (2025). Biomimetic dual-driven heterojunction nanomotors for targeted catalytic immunotherapy of glioblastoma. *Advanced Materials*, *37*(9), 2416265. Advance online publication. DOI: 10.1002/adma.202416265

Yekula, A., Minciacchi, V. R., Morello, M., Shao, H., Park, Y., Zhang, X., & Carter, B. S. (2020). Large and small extracellular vesicles released by glioma cells in vitro and in vivo. *Journal of Extracellular Vesicles*, *9*(1), 1689784. Advance online publication. DOI: 10.1080/20013078.2019.1689784 PMID: 31839905

Yekula, A., Taylor, A., Beecroft, A., Kang, K. M., Small, J. L., Muralidharan, K., & Carter, B. S. (2021). The role of extracellular vesicles in acquisition of resistance to therapy in glioblastomas. *Cancer Drug Resistance (Alhambra, Calif.)*, *4*(1), 1–16. DOI: 10.20517/cdr.2020.94 PMID: 35582008

Ye, L., Lv, W., He, W., Li, S., Min, Z., Gong, L., Chen, X., & Zhang, J. (2023). Reduced malignant glioblastoma recurrence post-resection through the anti-CD47 antibody and temozolomide co-embedded in-situ hydrogel system. *Journal of Controlled Release*, *359*, 224–233. DOI: 10.1016/j.jconrel.2023.05.046 PMID: 37290721

Yin, L., Yao, Z., Wang, Y., & Mazuranic, M. (2022). Investigational cyclin-dependent kinase 4/6 inhibitor GLR2007 demonstrates activity against isocitrate dehydrogenase wild-type glioblastoma and other solid tumors in mice xenograft models. *Frontiers in Oncology*, *12*, 915862. DOI: 10.3389/fonc.2022.915862 PMID: 36033522

Yin, Y., & Alivisatos, A. P. (2005). Colloidal nanocrystal synthesis and the organic–inorganic interface. *Nature*, *437*(7059), 664–670. DOI: 10.1038/nature04165 PMID: 16193041

Yoon, S.. (2022). Smart Nanoparticles for CRISPR/Cas9-Based Gene Therapy: A Comprehensive Review. *Nanomedicine; Nanotechnology, Biology, and Medicine*, *29*, 102253. DOI: 10.1016/j.nano.2021.102253

Young, R. M., Jamshidi, A., Davis, G., & Sherman, J. H. (2015). Current trends in the surgical management and treatment of adult glioblastoma. *Annals of Translational Medicine*, *3*(9), 121. Advance online publication. DOI: 10.3978/j.issn.2305-5839.2015.05.10 PMID: 26207249

Yuan, S., Yu, B., & Liu, H. M. (2020). New drug approvals for 2019: Synthesis and clinical applications. In *European Journal of Medicinal Chemistry* (Vol. 205). Elsevier Masson s.r.l. DOI: 10.1016/j.ejmech.2020.112667

Yuan, B., Wang, G., Tang, X., Tong, A., & Zhou, L. (2022). Immunotherapy of glioblastoma: Recent advances and future prospects. *Human Vaccines & Immunotherapeutics*, *18*(5), 2055417. Advance online publication. DOI: 10.1080/21645515.2022.2055417 PMID: 35344682

Yuan, Z., Guo, M., Zhang, Y., Deng, Y., Sun, B., Hou, Y., Wang, Y., Jin, X., Liu, Y., Shi, B., & Yin, J. (2025). MAGL targeted PROTAC degrader simultaneously enhances P53 for synergistic treatment of glioblastoma stem cell. *Cell Death Discovery*, *11*(1), 109. Advance online publication. DOI: 10.1038/s41420-025-02392-1 PMID: 40113745

Yusuf, A., Almotairy, A. R. Z., Henidi, H., Alshehri, O. Y., & Aldughaim, M. S. (2023). Nanoparticles as drug delivery systems: A review of the implication of nanoparticles' physicochemical properties on responses in biological systems. *Polymers*, *15*(7), 1596. Advance online publication. DOI: 10.3390/polym15071596 PMID: 37050210

Yu, W., & Wu, Z. (2019). Use of AAV vectors for CRISPR-mediated in vivo genome editing in the retina. In Castle, M. J. (Ed.), *Adeno-associated virus vectors* (pp. 123–139). Springer., DOI: 10.1007/978-1-4939-9139-6_7

Zaffino, P., Moccia, S., De Momi, E., & Spadea, M. F. (2020). A review on advances in intra-operative imaging for surgery and therapy: Imagining the operating room of the future. *Annals of Biomedical Engineering*, *48*(8), 2171–2191. DOI: 10.1007/s10439-020-02553-6 PMID: 32601951

Zaghmi, A., Drouin-Ouellet, J., Brambilla, D., & Gauthier, M. (2021). Treating brain diseases using systemic parenterally administered protein therapeutics: Dysfunction of the brain barriers and potential strategies. *Biomaterials*, *269*, 120461. DOI: 10.1016/j.biomaterials.2020.120461 PMID: 33218788

Zanders, E. D., Svensson, F., & Bailey, D. S. (2019). Therapy for glioblastoma: Is it working? *Drug Discovery Today*, *24*(5), 1193–1201. DOI: 10.1016/j.drudis.2019.03.008 PMID: 30878561

Zanotto-Filho, A., Braganhol, E., Edelweiss, M. I., Behr, G. A., Zanin, R., Schröder, R., & Moreira, J. C. F. (2012). The curry spice curcumin selectively inhibits cancer cells growth in vitro and in preclinical model of glioblastoma. *The Journal of Nutritional Biochemistry*, *23*(6), 591–601. DOI: 10.1016/j.jnutbio.2011.02.015 PMID: 21775121

Zhai, K., Siddiqui, M., Abdellatif, B., Liskova, A., Kubatka, P., & Büsselberg, D. (2021). Natural compounds in glioblastoma therapy: Preclinical insights, mechanistic pathways, and outlook. *Cancers (Basel)*, *13*(10), 2317. DOI: 10.3390/cancers13102317 PMID: 34065960

Zhan, C., Wei, X., Qian, J., Feng, L., Zhu, J., & Lu, W. (2012). Co-delivery of TRAIL gene enhances the anti-glioblastoma effect of paclitaxel in vitro and in vivo. *Journal of Controlled Release*, *160*(3), 630–636. DOI: 10.1016/j.jconrel.2012.02.022 PMID: 22410115

Zhang, B. (2021). CRISPR/Cas gene therapy. *Journal of Cellular Physiology*, *236*(4), 2459–2481. DOI: 10.1002/jcp.30064 PMID: 32959897

Zhang, H., Li, Z., Gao, C., Fan, X., Pang, Y., Li, T., & Zhang, Z. (2021). Dual-responsive biohybrid neutrobots for active target delivery. *Science Robotics*, *6*(52), eaaz9519. Advance online publication. DOI: 10.1126/scirobotics.aaz9519 PMID: 34043546

Zhang, J., Sun, X., Li, H., Ma, H., Duan, F., Wu, Z., Liu, Y., & Wang, Y. (2023). In vivo characterization and analysis of glioblastoma at different stages using multiscale photoacoustic molecular imaging. *Photoacoustics*, *30*, 100462. Advance online publication. DOI: 10.1016/j.pacs.2023.100462 PMID: 36865670

Zhang, L. P., Kang, L., Li, X., Liu, S., Liu, T., & Zhao, Y. (2021). Pyrazino[2,3-g] quinoxaline-based nanoparticles as near-infrared phototheranostic agents for efficient photoacoustic-im imaging-guided photothermal therapy. *ACS Applied Nano Materials*, *4*(2), 2019–2029. DOI: 10.1021/acsanm.0c03346

Zhang, M.. (2021). CRISPR-Cas9 and Nanoparticles in Gene Therapy: Prospects and Challenges. *Nanomedicine; Nanotechnology, Biology, and Medicine*, *30*(4), 529–540. DOI: 10.1016/j.nano.2020.102317

Zhang, P., Xia, Q., Liu, L., Li, S., & Dong, L. (2020). Current opinion on molecular characterization for GBM classification in guiding clinical diagnosis, prognosis, and therapy. *Frontiers in Molecular Biosciences*, *7*, 562798. Advance online publication. DOI: 10.3389/fmolb.2020.562798 PMID: 33102518

Zhang, Q., Yuan, L.-C., Wu, C.-J., Wu, S.-Y., Ren, S.-Z., Zhao, M.-D., Hu, Y.-Z., & Liu, Z.-X. (2023). Real-time diagnosis of glioblastoma by sensing peroxynitrite with a highly selective and rapid-responding fluorescent probe. *Analytica Chimica Acta*, *1275*, 134502. Advance online publication. DOI: 10.1016/j.aca.2023.341552

Zhang, X. Q., Chen, X., Cheng, X. B., Li, B. Q., Shen, X., Yan, C., Huang, J. Q., & Zhang, Q. (2018). Highly stable lithium metal batteries enabled by regulating the solvation of lithium ions in nonaqueous electrolytes. *Angewandte Chemie International Edition*, *57*(19), 5301–5305. DOI: 10.1002/anie.201801513 PMID: 29465827

Zhang, X., Zhao, L., Zhang, H., Zhang, Y., Ju, H., Wang, X., Ren, X., & Li, W. (2022). The immunosuppressive microenvironment and immunotherapy in human glioblastoma. *Frontiers in Immunology*, *13*, 1003651. Advance online publication. DOI: 10.3389/fimmu.2022.1003651 PMID: 36466873

Zhang, Y.. (2023). Multifunctional Nanoparticles for Cancer Therapy and Imaging: Recent Advances. *Nature Reviews. Materials*, *8*(3), 153–174. DOI: 10.1038/s41578-023-00531-9

Zhang, Y., & Wang, W. (2025). Advances in tumor subcolony formation and mechanisms of growth and invasion. *Journal of Translational Medicine*, *23*(1), 461. DOI: 10.1186/s12967-025-06486-3 PMID: 40259385

Zhang, Z. X., Ren, P., Cao, Y. Y., Wang, T. T., Huang, G. H., Li, Y., Liang, Y., & Liu, Z. (2023). HOXD-AS2-STAT3 feedback loop attenuates sensitivity to temozolomide in glioblastoma. *CNS Neuroscience & Therapeutics*, *29*(11), 3430–3445. DOI: 10.1111/cns.14277 PMID: 37308741

Zhao, Y., Bai, L., Zhang, Z., Wu, Y., Islam, M., & Ren, H. (2024). Transferring knowledge from high-quality to low-quality MRI for adult glioma diagnosis. arXiv. Retrieved May 17, 2025, from https://arxiv.org/abs/2410.18698

Zhao, J., Ma, X., Gao, P., Han, X., Zhao, P., Xie, F., & Liu, Z. (2024). Advancing glioblastoma treatment by targeting metabolism. *Neoplasia : an International Journal for Oncology Research*, *51*, 100985. Advance online publication. DOI: 10.1016/j.neo.2024.100985 PMID: 38479191

Zhao, L., Li, Y., Zhu, J., Sun, N., Song, N., Xing, Y., Huang, H., Zhao, J., & Sun, J. (2019). Chlorotoxin peptide-functionalized polyethylenimine-entrapped gold nanoparticles for glioma SPECT/CT imaging and radionuclide therapy. *Journal of Nanobiotechnology*, *17*(1), 30. Advance online publication. DOI: 10.1186/s12951-019-0462-6 PMID: 30782154

Zhao, M., van Straten, D., Broekman, M. L. D., Préat, V., & Schiffelers, R. M. (2020). Nanocarrier-based drug combination therapy for glioblastoma. *Theranostics*, *10*(3), 1355–1372. DOI: 10.7150/thno.38147 PMID: 31938069

Zhao, T., Li, C., Ge, H., Lin, Y., & Kang, D. (2022). Glioblastoma vaccine tumor therapy research progress. *Chinese Neurosurgical Journal*, *8*(1), 2. Advance online publication. DOI: 10.1186/s41016-021-00269-7 PMID: 35045874

Zhao, W. Y., Zhang, C. X., Liu, L., Mu, L. M., Zeng, F., Ju, R. J., Xie, H.-J., Yan, Y., Zhao, Y., & Lu, W.-L. (2016). Construction of functional targeting daunorubicin liposomes used for eliminating brain glioma and glioma stem cells. *Journal of Biomedical Nanotechnology*, *12*(7), 1404–1420. DOI: 10.1166/jbn.2016.2266 PMID: 29336535

Zhao, W., Zhou, L., Zhao, W., Yang, H., Lu, Z., Zhang, L., & Liu, Y. (2024). The combination of temozolomide and perifosine synergistically inhibit glioblastoma by impeding DNA repair and inducing apoptosis. *Cell Death Discovery*, *10*(1), 1–11. DOI: 10.1038/s41420-024-02085-1 PMID: 38977680

Zhao, Y., Li, D., Zhao, J., Song, J., & Zhao, Y. (2016). The role of the low-density lipoprotein receptor-related protein 1 (LRP-1) in regulating blood-brain barrier integrity. *Reviews in the Neurosciences*, *27*(6), 623–634. DOI: 10.1515/revneuro-2015-0069 PMID: 27206317

Zheng, X., Wang, L., Pei, Q., He, S., Liu, S., & Xie, Z. (2017). Metal–organic framework@porous organic polymer nanocomposite for photodynamic therapy. *Chemistry of Materials*, *29*(5), 2374–2381. DOI: 10.1021/acs.chemmater.7b00228

Zhou, G. (2024). Exploring Ester Prodrugs: A Comprehensive Review of Approaches, Applications, and Methods. *Pharmacology & Pharmacy, 15*(8), 269–284. DOI: 10.4236/pp.2024.158016

Zhou, Q., Zhang, L., & Guo, C.. (2020). Onfekafusp alfa in glioblastoma: Clinical trials and efficacy. *Journal of Clinical Oncology, 38*(23), 2581–2589.

Zhou, W., & Wahl, D. R. (2019). Metabolic abnormalities in glioblastoma and metabolic strategies to overcome treatment resistance. *Cancers (Basel), 11*(9), 1231. DOI: 10.3390/cancers11091231 PMID: 31450721

Zhu, Z., Zhang, H., Chen, B., Liu, X., Zhang, S., Zong, Z., & Gao, M. (2020). PD-L1-mediated immunosuppression in glioblastoma is associated with the infiltration and M2-polarization of tumor-associated macrophages. *Frontiers in Immunology, 11*, 588552. Advance online publication. DOI: 10.3389/fimmu.2020.588552 PMID: 33329573

About the Contributors

Athanasios Alexiou has a BSc in Applied Mathematics from the National and Kapodistrian University of Athens, a Ph.D. in Bioinformatics Algorithms and Mathematical Modeling in Biology, and a two-year Postdoc Research Fellowship in Neuroinformatics Applications from the Ionian University. He is the Head of Research & Education at Funogen Research Company in Greece and AFNP Med Company in Austria, an Adjunct Professor at the University Centre for Research & Development at Chandigarh University in India, and the Department of Science and Engineering at the Novel Global Community Education Foundation (an educational platform registered in Australia). He also collaborates with international research teams (including Yerevan State University, King Abdulaziz University, the University of Sharjah and Damanhour University). Dr. Alexiou's area of research is Cross-Field, with a special focus on Computational Biomedicine. Also, it focuses on developing novel mathematical models and algorithms in neurodegenerative diseases, prognostic Bayesian tools for Alzheimer's disease and Neurodegenerative disorders, sustainable agriculture, nanotoxicity in human health, AI and ML methods, identifying molecular mechanisms of infectious diseases, cancer biomarkers, and the ethical implications of scientific research. He serves as an Associate Editor in highly reputed journals like the Frontiers in Genetics and Pharmacology in the Section of ELSI, the Frontiers in Neuroscience and Psychology Journals, as a Section Editor in the Current Alzheimer Research Bentham Science journal, etc.; he is the author of more than 250 peer-reviewed articles/chapters/books in high impact publications and 5 filled patents; he is the editor of several books in known publishing houses; he has delivered many talks and presentations in international conferences and workshops; he participates in several international funded programs; he serves as a Scientific and Program Committee Member in several conferences and as a Reviewer/Member of the Editorial Board of international journals; he is supervising from diploma to Ph.D. theses and internships' programs; he has over 20 years of mentoring and educational experience. The 33rd Marquis Who's Who International Edition, 2016, includes Athanasios' biography. Dr. Alexiou is a Fellow of the International Institute of Biomedical Science and is highly ranked in the Computational Biomedicine field.

Md. Habibur Rahman, RPh, is a registered pharmacist in Bangladesh and a member of the Novel Global Community Education Foundation (Australia). He earned his Ph.D. in Medical Science from Yonsei University, South Korea, and has worked with several leading pharmaceutical organizations. His research primarily focuses on neuroscience, exploring the molecular mechanisms of clinical dementia with emphasis on biomarker discovery and targeted diagnostics. Recognized among the world's top 2% of scientists (Stanford University ranking), he is also an expert in molecular biology, oxidative stress, and neuroinflammation. Dr. Rahman is adept in advanced molecular and cell biology, animal models, and data analysis, and has mentored international students. He currently serves as Faculty at the Novel Global Community Educational Foundation and Director of the IM Group of Researchers. His achievements include the Hae Rang Best Young Scientist Award and the International Excellence Researcher Award.

Muhasina K.M. is a distinguished researcher in pharmaceutical sciences, specializing in cancer biology, herbal formulations, and multidrug-resistant cancers. She earned her PhD from JSS College of Pharmacy, Ooty as an AICTE Doctoral fellow, focusing on analytical and biological markers for anticancer herbal formulations. Her research explores phytochemicals' molecular mechanisms in targeting triple-negative breast cancer and the role of gut microbiota in disease progression. With expertise in advanced analytical techniques, she has authored numerous high-impact publications and secured multiple patents on herbal drug formulations and AI-based pharmaceutical technologies. Recognized with prestigious awards, she continues to advance cancer therapeutics by developing novel plant-based interventions. Beyond her publications, Dr. Muhasina has secured multiple patents on herbal drug formulations and AI-based pharmaceutical technologies. She has been recognized with prestigious awards, including the Best Research Scholar Award and Late SH. Bhola Nath Nikhra Memorial Young Researcher Award. Her research contributions have been widely acknowledged at national and international conferences, where she has delivered award-winning oral presentations. Dr. Muhasina's career aspiration is to advance cancer therapeutics by identifying novel phytochemicals and herbal formulations to counteract multidrug resistance and metastasis. She aims to bridge pharmaceutical sciences with translational medicine, contributing to developing effective, plant-based therapeutic interventions for cancer and neurological disorders.

Chenmala Karthika is a postdoctoral fellow at the National Institute of Health, USA. She completed her PhD from JSS College of Pharmacy, Ooty. She worked as an ICMR-senior research fellow during her PhD tenure and had published around 35 national and International paper. For the past 5 years, she has been researching cancer and its therapeutic approaches and had some interest in COVID-19 and neurodegenerative disorders.

Priti Tagde, M. Pharm, PhD, is an accomplished academician, researcher, and administrator in the field of pharmaceutical sciences. She is currently serving as Project Coordinator at the Madhya Pradesh State Price Monitoring Unit, Office of Food & Drugs Administration, M.P. With over a decade of teaching and research experience, she has held positions as Professor, Associate Professor, and Assistant Professor at reputed institutes. Her research primarily focuses on nanomedicine and innovative drug delivery systems, including lipid-based nanocarriers for breast cancer treatment. Dr. Tagde has authored books, published numerous research papers in international journals, and holds an Australian patent. She has been invited as a keynote speaker, resource person, and chief guest at national and international forums. Recognized globally, she has received honors such as the Pharma Ratan Young Achiever Award and inclusion among the 100 Most Impactful Healthcare Leaders. She also leads PRISAL, an international NGO fostering pharmaceutical education and research.

***

Rizwan Ahamad received his Master's degree in Pharmacology form Jamia Hamdard, New Delhi, India in 2022. Currently, he is a Doctoral Fellow at Department of Pharmacology, School of Pharmaceutical Education and Research (SPER), Jamia Hamdard, New Delhi, India. His current research interest is in Natural products, computational study, development of nanoformulations and evaluate their pharmacological as well as immunomodulatory activity in animal models. Mr. Rizwan has contributed to the scientific community by publishing numerous research and review papers in esteemed journals during his academic pursuits.

Mohd Akhtar is a Professor in the Department of Pharmacology, SPER, Jamia Hamdard, New Delhi, India, joined Jamia Hamdard in 2002. He also worked as clinical Pharmacist in Saudi Arabia for two and a half years. He did his Ph. D (2006 Neuropharmacology) from Jamia Hamdard. He was a recipient of Senior Research Fellowship (SRF) from ICMR New Delhi for completing his Ph.D. He has more than 24 years of teaching experience and is actively involved in teaching and research. His areas of research include Depression, Alzheimer's disease and cerebral ischemia.

He has more than 4400 citations, h-index: 38 and i10-index: 100. He is life member of IPS, APTI, IPGA, IHPA SOPVI, ISA and NESA. He is also giving his services as a reviewer for various National and International journals.

Rabnoor Alam obtained his master's degree in pharmaceuticals from Dr A.P.J. Abdul Kalam Technical University, located in Lucknow, Uttar Pradesh, India, in 2021. He is presently engaged in his Ph.D. studies as a doctoral fellow in the Department of Pharmaceutics at the School of Pharmaceutical Education and Research (SPER), Jamia Hamdard, New Delhi, India. His research centres on developing chitosan-modified polymeric nanoparticles for the nose-to-brain delivery of sumatriptan, incorporating herbal components along with thorough in vitro and in vivo evaluations. Throughout his academic career, Mr. Alam has made noteworthy contributions to the scientific community by publishing various research articles, review papers, and patents in respected journals.

Mohd. Aqil completed his PhD in Pharmaceutics from Jamia Hamdard, New Delhi, India in 2002. He has supervised 12 PhD scholars and 50 M. Pharm. dissertations. He has published more than 280 papers in national and international journals. Recently he received certificates of recognitions from Jamia Hamdard for his papers published in Journals with high impact factors. Prof. Aqil has authored 13 books and has been granted 7 Indian patents. He has presented his work at more than 130 conferences. He is the editor of the Journal of Pharmacy and Bio-allied Sciences. Prof. Aqil has received the Scientist of the year award from the National Environmental Science Academy for the year 2006. He was a visiting scientist to the School of Pharmacy, London under Exchange of Scientists Program of Indian National Science Academy and the Royal Society, UK in 2006 and was also a recipient of BOYSCAST fellowship of DST, Govt. of India for a Postdoc research tenure at University of Queensland, Brisbane, Australia in 2008.

Arshi Aquil obtained her Master's degree in Pharmaceutics from Jamia Hamdard, New Delhi, India, in 2024. Her research was focused on the development of microformulation for the management of topical disease. During her postgraduate studies, she gained expertise in formulation development, quality assurance, and pharmaceutical research methodologies. Miss Aquil has actively contributed to the scientific community through the publication of several research and review articles in reputed peer-reviewed journals. In addition to her academic accomplishments, she has experience in scientific writing, e-learning content development, and the creation of animated educational materials. She remains committed to advancing pharmaceutical research and aims to contribute to innovations in drug delivery systems and wound care management.

Mimoza Basholli-Salihu is an Associate Professor at the University of Prishtina, Faculty of Medicine. She holds a PhD in Pharmaceutical Technology and has focused her academic and research career on the development of advanced drug delivery systems, including polymer- and lipid-based nanoformulations. Her work aims to improve the bioavailability and therapeutic efficacy of drugs, with applications in cancer treatment, antimicrobial therapy, and pediatric medicine. She leads the Department of Drug Analysis and Pharmaceutical Technology and is actively involved in international research initiatives such as EPTRI and NanoAlb. Through her collaborations with European universities and contributions to scientific publications and conferences, she plays a significant role in advancing pharmaceutical sciences in Kosovo and the wider region.

Amritha Chakkittukandiyil is a passionate pharmacologist, currently working as an Assistant Professor at the National College of Pharmacy, Kozhikode, Kerala. She secured her Ph.D. in pharmaceutical sciences from JSS College of Pharmacy, Ooty, Tamil Nadu, as an ICMR-Senior Research Fellow. Her research was focused on neuroprotective agents for the treatment of Parkinson's disease. She has authored several research articles and review articles in peer-reviewed high-impact journals. Her research contributions were appreciated at various national and international seminars and have secured the best oral and poster presentation awards. She aims to pursue advanced research by actively involving herself in elucidating molecular mechanisms underlying disorders and identifying potential therapeutic candidates through translational research approaches.

Nunzio Denora is a full Professor of Pharmaceutical Technology and Regulatory Sciences at the University of Bari "Aldo Moro" (Italy). He earned his degree in Chemistry and Pharmaceutical Technology from the University of Bari in 2001 and completed his PhD in Pharmaceutical Technology at the University of Palermo in 2004. His research focuses on advanced drug-delivery systems (including microfluidics, 3D printing and nanomedicine) and regulatory aspects of pharmaceuticals. He has published over 190 peer-reviewed articles and holds multiple patents in formulation and diagnostics. Denora serves on the editorial board of key pharmaceutics journals (e.g., International Journal of Pharmaceutics) and participates in European initiatives in pharmaceutical technology and paediatric translational research.

Amit Kumar Dutta is currently working as an Assistant Professor in the Department of Chemistry, Bangabasi Morning College (Affiliated to University of Calcutta). He has Completed M.Sc. from University of Calcutta in 2007 with Inorganic Chemistry specialization and obtained Ph.D. degree in the area of Nanocatalysis from Bengal Engineering and Science University, Shibpur (presently, IIEST, Shibpur) in 2012 under the supervision of Prof. Bibhutosh Adhikary. His area of research interest is the use of semiconducting nano-materials in photo-catalysis and bio-sensing applications. He has published 36 research papers in different peer-reviewed journals and 6 book chapters. He has completed one UGC project (INDIA) and currently one research scholar is working with him.

Dafina Fondaj is a doctoral researcher in pharmaceutical sciences at University of Bari "Aldo Moro" (Italy), with a research focus on microfluidic production of hybrid biomimetic nanoparticles for pharmaceutical applications. Her academic background includes earlier studies at University of Prishtina (Kosovo) before moving into advanced pharmaceutical technology work in Bari.

Toskë Kryeziu is a pharmacist and academic affiliated with the Faculty of Medicine at the University of Prishtina, where he serves as a teaching assistant in the Department of Pharmacy and as Academic Development Coordinator. He earned his PhD in Pharmaceutical Sciences in December 2023 with a dissertation focused on the development and evaluation of cytotoxic nanosystems delivering essential oils in cancer cell lines. His doctoral research was conducted through a multidisciplinary collaboration involving the University of Prishtina, the University of Graz, and Trakya University. In 2024, he completed a postdoctoral research fellowship at King's College London, Institute of Pharmaceutical Science, supported by the NanoKos initiative. In 2025, he participated in a CEEPUS-supported teacher mobility program at the University of Graz, where he contributed to research supervision and academic exchange in the field of pharmaceutical sciences. His research interests lie in pharmaceutical nanotechnology, particularly in liposomal and nanoemulsion-based delivery of plant-derived compounds with anticancer activity. Dr. Kryeziu has co-authored multiple peer-reviewed publications and actively participates in international academic exchange programs. His work contributes to advancing nanomedicine strategies for cancer therapy, with a growing reputation in the Balkan and European scientific communities.

Mohd Mujeeb is working as Professor and Ex-Head at Department of Pharmacognosy and Phytochemistry, School of Pharmaceutical Education and Research, Jamia Hamdard, New Delhi, India. He has supervised 15 PhD candidates and 45 M. Pharm students. With over 7912 citations and h-index of 45, Prof. Mujeeb published more than 200 research and reviews articles in many reputed and high-impact journals. His research interest are development of plant based formulation, optimization of extraction methods of bioactive compounds.

G M Masud Parvez, is a researcher working on analytical method development. He is expert on PK/PD studies of different drugs and biomolecules. His expertise is on HPLC, LCMS, GCMS, FTIR, TGA, DSC and many other analytical instruments. He also works on Biomedical regulatory affairs and his expertise is reviewing IND application procedures, regulatory inspections and patient safety studies.

S. Venkatesh, M. Pharm., Ph. D., He is currently working as an Professor and Head in the Department of Pharmacology, National College of Pharmacy, Kozhikode, Kerala, India. He has over 16+ years of Academic experience. He has authored 25 Peer reviewed International/National Journal Publications and 15 Paper/Poster presented in International/National Conferences. He has Completed Ph. D in Vellore Institute of Technology (Deemed to be University), Vellore, Tamilnadu, India. His research work focused on various Animal screening models and guided 18 Post graduates research projects past 16+ years.

Prerna Saxena has received her Master's degree from JSS College of Pharmacy, Mysuru, India in 2022 in Department of Pharmacognosy. Currently, she is pursuing PhD at Department of Pharmacognosy, School of Pharmaceutical Education and Research (SPER), Jamia Hamdard, New Delhi, India. Her research focuses on specializing in the study of Medicinal Plants, Natural Product Chemistry, Pharmacological Screening of Bio active Compound and Development & Characterization of nano formulations. Ms. Prerna actively contributes to the advancement of pharmacognostic research through academic engagement.

Aida Loshaj Shala is a Professor Assistant in the Department of Pharmacy, Faculty of Medicine, University of Prishtina. She obtained her Magister of Pharmacy degree and subsequently completed her PhD in Pharmaceutical Sciences at the Faculty of Pharmacy, Ss. Cyril and Methodius University in North Macedonia. Her academic career began in 2007 as a Research Assistant, followed by progressive advancement to her current professorial role. Her research portfolio comprises numerous peer-reviewed publications spanning pharmaceutically active essential oils, nanoemulsions, neurodegenerative processes, therapeutic formulations, and proteomics, reflecting an interdisciplinary focus at the interface of pharmacology, biotechnology, and innovative drug-delivery systems. Beyond academic research, she has played a pivotal role in strengthening national pharmaceutical quality infrastructure, most notably through the establishment and leadership of the Laboratory for Quality Control of Medicines at the Kosovo Agency for Medicines and Medical Devices. She also holds specialized professional qualifications in medicines quality control and has undertaken training in regulatory harmonization with European regulatory bodies. In addition to her scientific and regulatory contributions, she is engaged in international research governance. She serves on the Board of Directors of TEDDY, the European Network of Excellence for Paediatric Research, and co-leads a thematic research platform focused on paediatric medicine formulations.

Nazreen Tabassum, a Ph.D. Research Scholar at Department of Pharmaceutics, SPER, Jamia Hamdard, New Delhi, India currently. She obtained her Master's degree in Pharmaceutics from Jamia Hamdard, New Delhi, India, in 2024. Her research primarily focuses on the development of advanced nanoformulations which targeted treatment of brain diseases. Miss Tabassum has actively contributed to the scientific community through the publication of several research, review articles and book chapters in reputed peer-reviewed journals.

Deepak Vasudev Sajini is a highly motivated and passionate researcher with extensive experience in in vitro and in vivo experimental models. He is currently working as an Assistant Professor and Research Coordinator at National College of Pharmacy, Kozhikode, Kerala. He pursued his Ph.D. in Pharmaceutical Sciences from JSS College of Pharmacy, Ooty, Tamil Nadu. During his Ph.D., he acquired Rs. 16 lakhs of research fund from ICMR and Rs. 1.2 lakhs from JSS AHER for the project. He has published several research and review articles in peer-reviewed high-impact journals. His research contributions were widely acknowledged at various national and international seminars and have secured the best oral presentation award at Kazakhstan.

Index

H

I

M

N

www.ingramcontent.com/pod-product-compliance
Lightning Source LLC
LaVergne TN
LVHW080910300926
849162LV00003B/630